Health and Wellness

Health and Wellness

Seventh Edition

Gordon Edlin

John A. Burns School of Medicine
University of Hawaii

Eric Golanty

Las Positas College

Kelli McCormack Brown

Department of Community and Family Health
University of South Florida

Jones and Bartlett Publishers

Sudbury, Massachusetts
Boston   Toronto   London   Singapore

World Headquarters
Jones and Bartlett Publishers
40 Tall Pine Drive
Sudbury, MA 01776
978-443-5000
info@jbpub.com
www.jbpub.com

Jones and Bartlett Publishers Canada
2406 Nikanna Road
Mississauga, Ontario L5C 2W6
CANADA

Jones and Bartlett Publishers International
Barb House, Barb Mews
London W6 7PA
UK

All resource addresses, telephone numbers and Web addresses found in *Health and Wellness*, Seventh Edition have been checked and are correct at time of printing. Jones and Bartlett Publishers is not responsible for changes in resource addresses, telephone numbers or Web addresses.

Library of Congress Cataloging-in-Publication Data
Edlin, Gordon, 1932–
    Health and wellness / Gordon Edlin, Eric Golanty, Kelli McCormack
Brown. — 7th ed.
        p.   cm.
    Includes bibliographical references and index.
    ISBN 0–7637–2055–0
    1. Health.   2. Holistic medicine.   I. Golanty, Eric.   II. Brown,
Kelli McCormack.   III. Title.
    RA776 .E24   2002
    613—dc21

                                              2001050560
                                              CIP

Student Edition ISBN 0-7637-2055-0

Chief Executive Officer: Clayton Jones
Chief Operating Officer: Don W. Jones, Jr.
Executive Vice President and Publisher: Robert Holland
V.P., Design and Production: Anne Spencer
V.P., Manufacturing and Inventory Control: Therese Bräuer
Editor-in-Chief, College: J. Michael Stranz
Acquisitions Editor: Laurie A. Klausner
Production Editor: Julie C. Bolduc

Editorial Assistant: Corinne G. Hudson
Text Design: Merce Wilzek
Marketing Manager: Nathan Schultz
Composition: GTS Companies
Cover Design: Anne Spencer
Printing and Binding: Courier
Cover Printing: Courier

Unless otherwise acknowledged, all photographs are the property of Jones and Bartlett Publishers
Cover Photo Credits
(woman weightlifting) © 1996 PhotoDisc, Inc. All rights reserved. Images provided by © 1996 PhotoDisc, Inc./Keith Brofsky; (pregnant woman) © 1996 PhotoDisc, Inc. All rights reserved. Images provided by © 1996 Jack Hollingsworth Photography; (young family) © 1999 PhotoDisc, Inc. All rights reserved. Images provided by © 1999 Ryan McVay; (grandfather and grandson) © 1999 PhotoDisc, Inc. All rights reserved. Images provided by © 1999 Steve Mason; (peas and sunflower) © 1998 PhotoDisc, Inc. All rights reserved. Images provided by © 1998 Siede Preis; (apple) © 1999 PhotoDisc, Inc. All rights reserved. Images provided by © 1999 C Squared Studios.

Text photo credits follow the index, which constitutes a continuation of the copyright page.

Printed in the United States of America
05 04 03 02 01   10 9 8 7 6 5 4 3 2 1

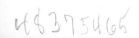

Brief Contents

Contents

Part 2   Eating and Exercising Toward a Healthy Lifestyle   79

Part 3   Building Healthy Relationships   153

Part 4 Understanding and Preventing Disease   243

12 Reducing Infections and Building Immunity: Knowledge Encourages Prevention   245

13 Cancer: Understanding Risks and Means of Prevention   277

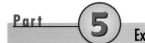

Part 5   Explaining Drug Use and Abuse   341

Part 6   Making Healthy Choices   399

Feature Contents

Global Wellness

Dollars and Health Sense

Preface for the Student

Our goal in writing this textbook is to provide you with the information you need to understand and implement the basic principles of physical, mental, and spiritual wellness. We have provided the most up-to-date tools, information, exercises, and humor to motivate you toward making healthy changes in your life and developing a lifestyle that will promote lifelong wellness. We believe that the key to health is self-responsibility for one's behaviors (both positive and negative)—for overeating or undereating, for drinking alcohol or smoking, for taking drugs or engaging in stressful activities, and for living in harmony with the environment. We also believe that health involves our entire being and is not a matter of repairing broken parts.

What does it mean to be healthy and well? Often, we equate health with being a certain ideal weight, exercising regularly, not smoking, or never catching a cold. But a holistic view of health encompasses many more of our behaviors. Answer the following questions and see if your opinion about your health changes:

- If you drink, do you drink responsibly (e.g., you do not get drunk or drink and then drive)?

- Do you get enough sleep (at least 8 hours a night)?

- Are you able to cope with stressful situations without getting angry, anxious, or depressed?

- Are your interpersonal relationships satisfying?

- If you are sexually active, do you use fertility control and practice safer sex?

- Does your diet consist of fast food, pizza, and ice cream?

- Do you exercise regularly?

- Do you take time to enjoy nature?

- Are you involved in your community?

Remember, we all engage in unhealthy behaviors from time to time, but you should know that these behaviors are things that you can change. Wellness is a process, not a place. We hope that, in your use of this textbook, you will become aware of your unhealthy behaviors, and we hope that we can motivate you to change and give you some strategies for making that change. We want you to achieve lifelong wellness through self-responsibility.

We have developed a number of features to help you in your study of the material.

Each chapter begins with a list of **Learning Objectives** to help you focus on the most important concepts in that chapter.

Learning Objectives

1. Describe what it means to be healthy.
2. Describe the medical, environmental, and holistic, or wellness, models of health.
3. Explain the wellness continuum and its impact on personal health.
4. Identify and describe the six dimensions of wellness.
5. Describe the personal qualities that are associated with the six dimensions of wellness.
6. Explain the philosophy of holistic health.
7. List the three most common actual causes of death and explain how lifestyles and behaviors contribute to disease.
8. Explain how modern lifestyles contribute to nearsightedness (myopia).
9. Understand how spirituality enhances health.
10. Explain the importance of the national health objectives for the year 2010.

Key Terms are defined on the page on which they are introduced as well as in the glossary at the end of the book. For review, terms are available in a print format in the **Built-in Workbook** and in a flash card format on the text's Web site (www.jbpub.com/hwonline).

Epigrams enliven each chapter with both serious and humorous quotations about health.

Certain key topics in each chapter are highlighted with a **Web Icon**, 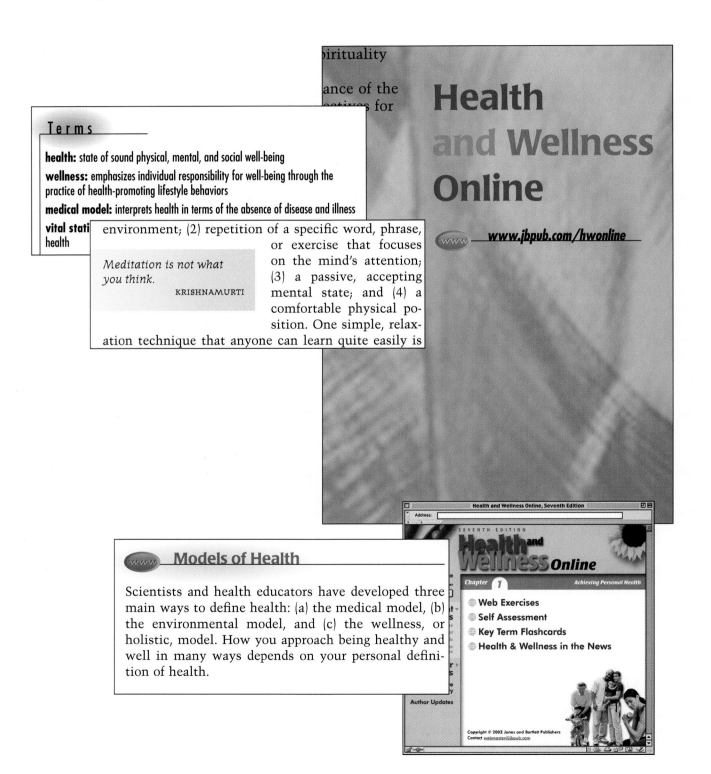 indicating that additional or up-to-date information is available on the Web site. **Health and Wellness Online** (www.jbpub.com/hwonline) is a valuable resource for you to use for research, to prepare for tests, or just to find out more about a topic.

Health and Wellness Online

www.jbpub.com/hwonline

Terms

health: state of sound physical, mental, and social well-being

wellness: emphasizes individual responsibility for well-being through the practice of health-promoting lifestyle behaviors

medical model: interprets health in terms of the absence of disease and illness

vital stati[s...] health

environment; (2) repetition of a specific word, phrase, or exercise that focuses on the mind's attention; (3) a passive, accepting mental state; and (4) a comfortable physical position. One simple, relaxation technique that anyone can learn quite easily is

Meditation is not what you think.
KRISHNAMURTI

Models of Health

Scientists and health educators have developed three main ways to define health: (a) the medical model, (b) the environmental model, and (c) the wellness, or holistic, model. How you approach being healthy and well in many ways depends on your personal definition of health.

Health and Wellness Online, Seventh Edition

Address:

SEVENTH EDITION
Health and Wellness Online

Chapter 1   *Achieving Personal Health*

- Web Exercises
- Self Assessment
- Key Term Flashcards
- Health & Wellness in the News

Author Updates

Copyright © 2002 Jones and Bartlett Publishers
Contact webmaster@jbpub.com

Current and interesting topics are highlighted in boxes to give a complete perspective in your study of health and wellness. **Managing Stress** boxes give you practical strategies for coping with stress; **Wellness Guides** offer tips, techniques, and steps toward a healthy lifestyle and self-responsibility; and **Global Wellness** boxes explore health and wellness topics as they affect different cultures. **Dollars and Health Sense** boxes, new to this edition, focus on ways companies promote products that are detrimental to health—worthless nutritional supplements; dangerous, ineffective, or unnecessary prescription drugs; environmentally destructive substances; and other money-making schemes that harm health.

Global Wellness

Iodine Deficiency Is the Most Common Cause of Mental Deficits Worldwide

Iodine is an essential trace element in the human diet. Supplementing table salt with iodine in most countries of the world has eliminated the terrible effects of iodine deficiency in most populations. However, in many areas of Africa, Asia, Latin America, and parts of Eastern Europe, people's diets are deficient in iodine. The most severe consequence of iodine deficiency is severe mental retardation called *cretinism*.

Conclusive proof of the importance of iodine in the diet comes from an experiment carried out in Papua, New Guinea. Over a four-year period, some families received an injection of iodine and other families received placebo injections. Only one case of cretinism occurred among 412 newborns of mothers who had received iodine injections. Among women who had not received iodine injections, 21 of 406 babies were born with cretinism.

The primary sign of iodine deficiency is the the World Health Organization estimated that 200 million people had goiter and another 20 million had mental deficits resulting from iodine deficiency. In most areas of the world, the soil does not contain iodine and plants grown in these regions are also deficient. Efforts are under way to supply everyone in the world with iodized salt or oil to prevent

Wellness Guide

Health Issues for College Students

What health issues face North America's 15 million college students? Here's what college and university health educators and medical professionals think the answers are (Grace, 1997).

Sexual health. More than any others, sexual issues have the potential to affect the health of college students. These include sexually

Substance abuse. The abuse of alcohol, drugs, tobacco, and food is related to trying to gain peer acceptance, unhealthy role modeling in families and in society at large, and trying to cope with psychological distress. Students whose parents abuse substances often have a tendency for substance abuse. Alcohol abuse is related to the

lead to stress-related physical illnesses. Competitive academic environments can create feelings of inferiority, insecurity, and emotional distress.

Food and weight. Many students are highly concerned about their body size and shape and may become malnourished to meet their perceptions of social ideality. Eating disorders, such as bulimia and anorexia nervosa, affect a large number of students.

Health care. A large proportion of college students in the United States have limited access to health care because their colleges do not have comprehensive services for students or they do not have private health insurance.

Accidents and injuries. Many students are susceptible to automobile accidents (often alcohol-related) and sports injuries.

Managing Stress

The Rainbow of Human Energy

In truth, we know that we cannot separate the mind from the body, nor can we separate the mind from emotions, or the body from the soul. All aspects are integrated. Through the recent insights of quantum physics, we know that everything, including our thoughts and feelings, consists of energy. This is what the wisdom keepers and shamans have known for millennia. Renowned physicist David Bohm addressed the spiritual nature of health in terms of quantum physics. He used the term *coherence* to describe the harmony among the energies of body, mind, and spirit, which gives a sense of wholeness that can only be described as "inner peace." As we continue to explore the issues of health and illness, some interesting facts come to light which support the holistic concept that the whole is greater than the sum of the parts. Spontaneous remissions and

healing through prayer are two of many phenomena that cannot be explained by the mechanistic model. In fact, the new paradigm suggests that we are not a mind in a body, but a *body in a mind*.

Try the following ex concept of coherence in moment to reflect on yo you are, not just your b thinking about your phys organs, bones, tissue, a organs, tissues, and flui with each other (coherer in your body, like the ne headed north. Next, im surrounds and permeate energy is aqua. This rep your emotional body. Im

energy around your body like warm Caribbean water. Imagine what it would feel like to sense harmony between your emotions and physical body. Next, imagine that superimposed over this aqua-blue

Dollars and Health Sense

Drugs for Worries and Bad Habits

In the past 25 years worries and "bad habits" of various kinds have become reclassified as mental disorders that need to be medically treated, usually by drug therapy. By redefining worries and bad habits as diseases, physicians, hospitals, and drug companies now earn vast amounts of money treating these problems.

Now a significant proportion of the population is being treated with an antidepressant, antianxiety, or antiphobic pill, or with drugs to control unhealthy habits such as smoking cigarettes, drinking alcohol, or overeating. We live in a time when it is widely accepted that "bad molecules" produced in our brains or bodies cause us to drink and eat too much,

to worry excessively, or to be overly shy. If a bad molecule can be identified, then a "good drug" can be developed that will counteract the effects of the bad molecule. As more and more unhealthy behaviors and anxieties become molecularized and medicalized, the medical/pharmaceutical industry continues to grow and prosper.

There are still some bad habits left waiting to be medicalized and treated. For example, gambling is widely regarded as a bad habit, especially compulsive gambling. Researchers are looking for an inherited gene carried by compulsive gamblers that is responsible for their obsession. Moving from an identified gene to a drug to combat its effects is

only a matter of time, money, and effort on the part of a dedicated drug company. And considering the number of people who like to gamble, the rewards could be enormous.

Compulsive shopping (strongly encouraged by advertisements and sales clerks) is another bad habit, especially if you don't have the money to pay for your charged purchases. Drug companies are currently testing drugs in order to identify ones that put a damper on the uncontrollable urge to buy. Consumers will soon have the choice of running out to buy some new clothes or spending the money on a prescription that will suppress the urge.

Chapters conclude with **Critical Thinking About Health**—a set of questions that present thought-provoking or controversial situations and ask you to examine your opinions and explore your biases.

End-of-chapter material includes **Health in Review**, a brief review of the chapter, **Health and Wellness Online,** a glimpse at the resources available on the Web; **References;** and **Annotated Suggested Readings.**

The text also includes appendixes on **relaxation exercises** and **stress management techniques** (including guides to yoga and t'ai chi).

Finally, a **Built-in Workbook** includes chapter reviews to test your knowledge of the material and self-assessments and activities to explore your own health.

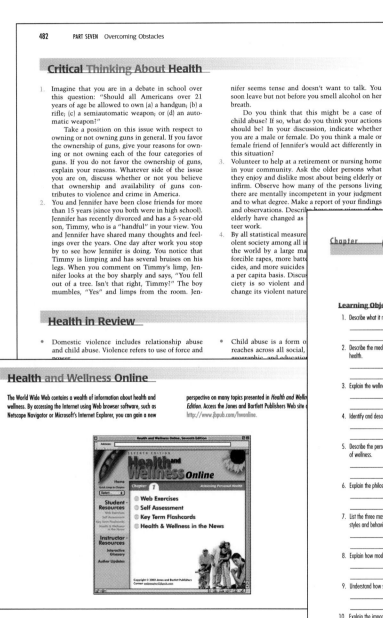

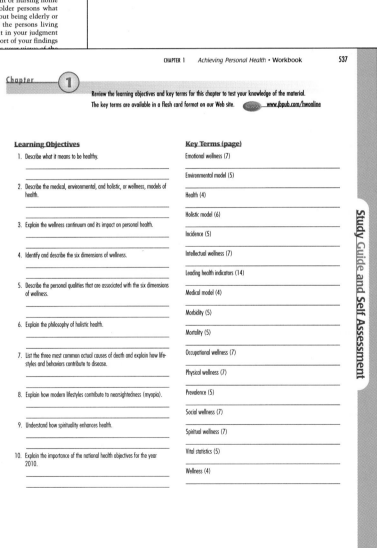

A Note of Thanks

Throughout all of the editions of *Health and Wellness,* many people have contributed support and guidance. This book has benefited greatly from their comments, opinions, thoughtful critiques, expert knowledge, and constructive suggestions. We are most appreciative for their participation in this project.

Reviewers

Pat Alsader, Planned Parenthood of West Central Illinois

David Anspaugh, Memphis State University

Judy B. Baker, East Carolina University

N. K. Bhagavan, University of Hawaii Medical School

Nancy J. Binkin, Centers for Disease Control and Prevention, Atlanta

David Birch, Indiana University

Donald Calitri, Eastern Kentucky University

Barbara Coombs, San Francisco City College

Linda Chaput, W. H. Freeman, New York

Dorothy Coltrin, De Anza College

Geoffrey Cooper, Harvard Medical School

Judy Drolet, Southern Illinois University at Carbondale

Philip Duryea, University of New Mexico

Seymour Eiseman, California State University – Northridge

Carol Ellison, Berkeley, California

Marianne Frauenknecht, Western Michigan University

Nicole Gegel, Illinois State University

Mal Goldsmith, Southern Illinois University at Edwardsville

Allan C. Henderson, California State University – Long Beach

Sherry Hineman, University of California – San Diego

Leo Hollister, Stanford Medical Center

Stanley Inkelis, Harbor General Hospital

William Kane, University of New Mexico

Mark Kittleson, Southern Illinois University at Carbondale

Tim Knickelbein, Normandale Community College

Dawn Larsen, Mankato State University

Will Lotter, University of California, Davis

Beverly Saxton Mahoney, The Pennsylvania State University

Mary Martin, University of California – San Francisco

Marion Micke, Illinois State University

Anne Nadakavukaren, Illinois State University

Marion Nestle, University of California – San Francisco

Roberta Ogletree, Southern Illinois University at Carbondale

Larry Olsen, The Pennsylvania State University

David Phelps, Oregon State University

Richard Plant, South Middlesex Community College

Bruce Ragon, Indiana University

Kerry J. Redican, Virginia Technical University

Dwayne Reed, Buck Center for Research in Aging

Janet Reis, University of Illinois at Urbana–Champaign

Brian Luke Seaward, University of Colorado – Boulder

Sam Singer, University of California – Santa Cruz

Susan Spreecher, Illinois State University

David Stronk, California State University – Hayward

John Struthers, Planned Parenthood of Sacramento County

Bryan Williams, University of Arkansas

Carol Wilson, University of Nevada at Las Vegas

Richard Wilson, Western Kentucky University

Acknowledgements

This book could not have been published without the efforts of the staff at Jones and Bartlett Publishers and the *Health and Wellness* team: Laurie Klausner, Acquisitions Editor; Julie Bolduc, Production Editor; Nathan Schultz, Marketing Manager; Nicole Healey, IT Manager; Corinne Hudson, Editorial Assistant; and GTS Companies. We would also like to thank Brian Luke Seaward, Ph.D., University of Colorado, Boulder; James Walsh; Esther M. Weekes; Martin Schulz; Shae Bearden; Rocky Young; Bharti Temkin; Laura Jones-Swann, M.ED., LCDC, Texas Tech University; and Scott O. Roberts, Ph.D., FAACVPR, Texas Tech University. To all we express our appreciation.

Gordon Edlin
John A. Burns School of Medicine
University of Hawaii
Honolulu, Hawaii 96822

Eric Golanty
Las Positas College
Livermore, California 94550

Kelli McCormack Brown
Department of Community and Family Health
University of South Florida
Tampa, Florida 33612-3805

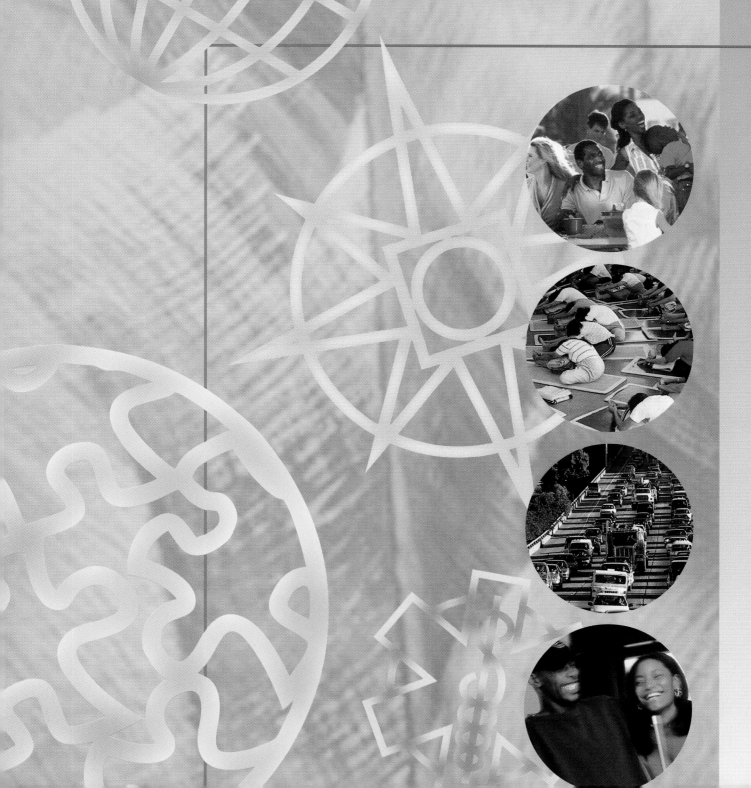

Part 1

Achieving Wellness

Learning Objectives

1. Describe what it means to be healthy.
2. Describe the medical, environmental, and holistic, or wellness, models of health.
3. Explain the wellness continuum and its impact on personal health.
4. Identify and describe the six dimensions of wellness.
5. Describe the personal qualities that are associated with the six dimensions of wellness.
6. Explain the philosophy of holistic health.
7. List the three most common actual causes of death and explain how lifestyles and behaviors contribute to disease.
8. Explain how modern lifestyles contribute to nearsightedness (myopia).
9. Understand how spirituality enhances health.
10. Explain the importance of the national health objectives for the year 2010.

Study Guide
and
Self Assessment

How Well Are You?

Health
and Wellness
Online

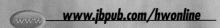 **www.jbpub.com/hwonline**

Achieving Personal Health

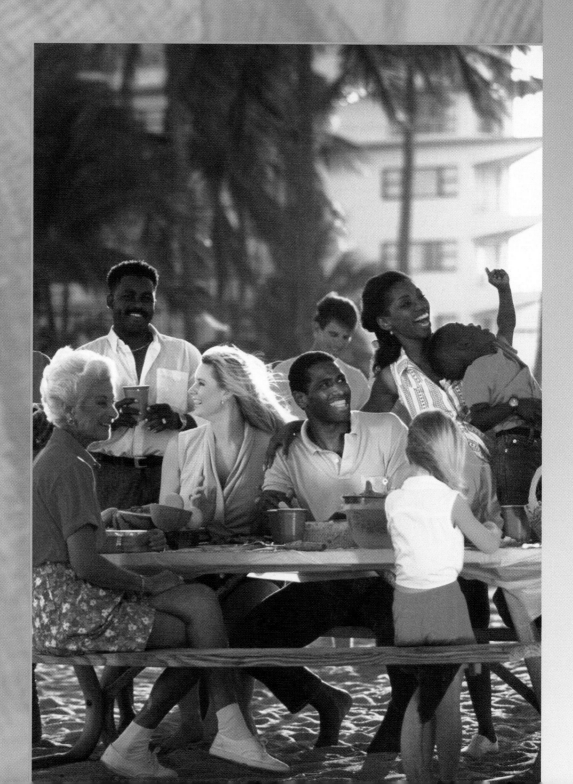

Ask people what they mean by "being healthy" or "feeling well" and you probably will get a variety of answers. Most people usually think of health as the absence of disease. But what about someone who has a relatively harmless genetic disorder, such as an extra toe? Is this individual less healthy than a person with the usual number of toes? Different perhaps, but not necessarily less healthy. Are you less well when you are struggling with a personal problem than when you are out having fun? Finding an acceptable, generally useful definition of health or wellness is not a simple task.

> *The only way to keep your health*
> *is to eat what you don't want . . .*
> *Drink what you don't like . . .*
> *And do what you'd rather not.*
> MARK TWAIN

It is true that not feeling sick is one important aspect of health. Just as important, however, is the idea that health is a sense of optimum well-being—a state of physical, mental, emotional, social, and spiritual wellness. Contained in this view is the idea that health can be obtained by living in harmony with yourself, with other people, and with the environment. Health is gained and maintained by exerting self-responsibility for reducing exposure to health risks and for maximizing good nutrition and exercise.

Throughout this book, we show you ways to maximize your health by understanding how your mind and body function, how to avoid harmful chemicals, how to make informed decisions about health and health care, and how to be responsible for your actions and behaviors. Learning to be responsible for the degree of health and energy you want while you are young helps to ensure lifelong wellness and the capacity to cope with sickness when it does occur.

Defining Health and Wellness

Health, like love or happiness, is a quality of life that is difficult to define and virtually impossible to measure. **Health** is defined differently among experts, but all definitions have a common theme: self-responsibility and adopting a healthy lifestyle.

> Health is a state of complete physical, mental, and social well-being and not merely the absence of disease or infirmity.
> —*World Health Organization, 1947*

> [Health is] an integrated method of functioning which is oriented toward maximizing the potential of which the individual is capable. It requires that the individual maintain a continuum of balance and purposeful direction with the environment where he/she is functioning.
> —*Dunn, 1967*

Wellness has been defined as

> an approach to personal health that emphasizes individual responsibility for well-being through the practice of health-promoting lifestyle behaviors.
> —*Hurley and Schlaadt, 1992*

Wellness is many times referred to in a broader context than health, which sometimes means only physical health. For the purposes of this book, we consider health multidimensional, involving the whole person's relation to the total environment. We refer to wellness as a process of moving toward optimal health.

Models of Health

Scientists and health educators have developed three main ways to define health: (a) the medical model, (b) the environmental model, and (c) the wellness, or holistic, model. How you approach being healthy and well in many ways depends on your personal definition of health.

The Medical Model

The **medical model's** main tenet is that health is the absence of one or more of the "five Ds"—death, disease, discomfort, disability, and dissatisfaction. In other words, if you are not sick or dying, you are considered to be in the best attainable state of health. Followers of the medical model rely almost exclusively on biological explanations of disease and illness and tend to interpret disease and illness in terms of malfunction of individual organs, cells, and other biological systems, e.g., liver disease, heart disease, or sickle cell anemia.

Terms

health: state of sound physical, mental, and social well-being

wellness: emphasizes individual responsibility for well-being through the practice of health-promoting lifestyle behaviors

medical model: interprets health in terms of the absence of disease and illness

vital statistics: numerical data relating to birth, death, disease, marriage, and health

morbidity: ratio of persons who are diseased to those who are well in a given community

mortality: death rate: number of deaths per unit of population (e.g., per 100; 10,000; or 1,000,000) in a specific region, age range, or other group

prevalence: predominance of a particular disease

incidence: frequency of occurrence of a particular disease

environmental model: modern analyses of ecosystems and environmental risks to health, such as socioeconomic status, education, and various environmental factors

Within the medical model, the health of a population is measured in terms of **vital statistics,** which are data on the degree of illness **(morbidity)** and the numbers of deaths **(mortality)** in a given population. Vital statistics include **prevalence** (the predominance of a disease in a population) and **incidence** (the frequency at which certain diseases occur). These statistical measurements allow comparisons between populations and also within the same population over time.

The medical model tends not to deal with social problems that affect health and only with difficulty integrates mental and behavioral issues that do not derive from diseased organs. In the medical model, health is restored by curing a disease or by restoring function to a damaged body part. Because of its exclusive focus on biological processes, the medical model is of limited value. It does not help us understand psychological and social factors that affect health and contribute to disease.

The reliance on biological interpretations of illness has contributed greatly to the success of the medical model. Anyone who has been cured of a serious infection by taking antibiotics or undergone a lifesaving surgical procedure can attest to that. On the other hand, that same reliance on biological thinking has not furthered understanding of health and illness in terms of psychological and social factors, nor has it been very successful in fostering health by preventing disease caused by unhealthy lifestyles and destructive behaviors.

The Environmental Model

The **environmental model** of health emerged with modern analyses of ecosystems and environmental risks to human health. In this model, health is defined in terms of the quality of a person's adaptation to the environment as conditions change.

> *Happiness is good health and a bad memory.*
> INGRID BERGMAN

This model (Figure 1.1) includes the effects on personal health of socioeconomic status, education, and multiple environmental factors.

Unlike the medical model, which focuses on diseased organs and biological abnormalities, the environmental model focuses on conditions outside the individual that affect his or her health. These conditions include the quality of air and water, living conditions, exposure to harmful substances, socioeconomic conditions, social relationships, and the health-care system.

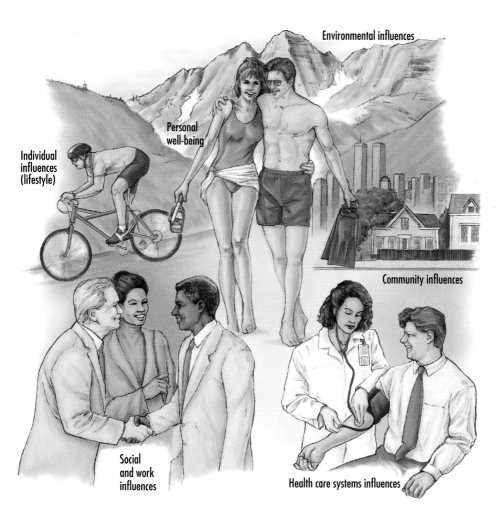

Environmental influences

Personal well-being

Individual influences (lifestyle)

Community influences

Social and work influences

Health care systems influences

FIGURE 1.1   Environmental Health Model   This model takes into account all factors that interact with one another to affect one's health.

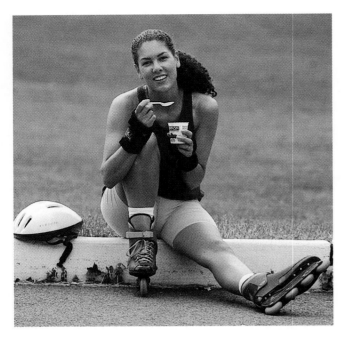

A healthy lifestyle depends on exercise and good nutrition.

In many respects the environmental model of health is similar to ancient Asian and Native American philosophies that associate health with harmonious interactions with fellow creatures and the environment. In particular, as the environment changes, one's interaction with it must change to remain in harmony. Illness is interpreted as disharmony of human and environmental interactions.

The Holistic Model

The holistic, or wellness, model defines health in terms of the whole person, not in terms of diseased parts of the body. The **holistic model** encompasses the physiological, mental, emotional, social, spiritual, and environmental aspects of individuals and communities. It focuses on optimal health, prevention of disease, and positive mental and emotional states.

The holistic model incorporates the idea of spiritual health, which is not considered in the medical model. Unlike the medical model, which assumes that a person who is not sick or not suffering from a disease is as healthy as possible, the holistic model proposes that health is a state of optimum or positive wellness.

Wellness is much more than physical health; it addresses mental, emotional, and spiritual aspects of a person, as well as the relationships among these dimensions. The wellness continuum helps delineate between the medical concept of health and the wellness concept (Figure 1.2). Most people find themselves in the neutral area of the continuum. Most of us, however, can remember moving toward disability and also moving toward optimal health or high-level wellness.

One may move from a state of illness or disease back to the neutral point many times with the help of medical care. The wellness continuum also includes prevention, which means taking positive actions to prevent acute and chronic illnesses.

Wellness is not static; it is a dynamic process that takes into account all the decisions we make daily, such as which foods we eat, the amount of exercise we get, whether we drink alcohol before driving, wear safety belts, or smoke cigarettes. Every choice we make potentially affects health and wellness.

In this book we discuss aspects of all of the different models of health wherever appropriate. The models themselves are abstractions of ideas, but in real life one needs to use whatever is practical to optimize health and well-being. Health depends very much on each person's perception. People with a disease may live joyful, positive, healthy lives; people without a disease may be despondent, unhappy, and feel sick. People need attainable goals to promote wellness and to live harmoniously with family, friends, and the environment.

Truth does not change over time. Jesse Williams (1937), one of the founders of modern health education, described health as

> that condition of the individual that makes possible the highest enjoyment of life, the greatest constructive work, and that shows itself in the best service to the world. . . . Health as freedom from disease is a standard of mediocrity; health as a quality of life is a standard of inspiration and increasing achievement.

This is a goal we believe in, and the content of this book reflects this view.

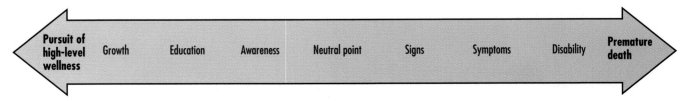

Pursuit of high-level wellness	Growth	Education	Awareness	Neutral point	Signs	Symptoms	Disability	Premature death

FIGURE 1.2 **The Wellness Continuum** The wellness continuum allows you to visualize the difference between wellness and the medical approaches to health.

Managing Stress

Harmony and Peace

Many Native American cultures and tribes incorporate the idea of harmonious interactions with nature, animals, and other people in their religions.

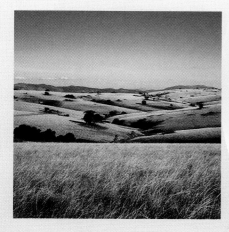

The first peace,
which is the most important,
is that which comes from
within the souls of men when they
realize their relationship,
their oneness, with the universe
and all its powers,
and when they realize that
at the center of the universe dwells
Wakan-Tanka, and that
this center is really everywhere,
it is within each of us.
This is the real peace, and the others are
but reflections of this.
The second peace is that which is
made between two individuals,
and the third is that
which is made between two nations.
But above all you should
understand that there can never be peace
between nations until there is
first known that true peace which . . .
is within the souls of men.

Black Elk
The Sacred Pipe

Source: From *The Sacred Pipe: Black Elk's Account of the Seven Rites of the Oglala Sioux,* by Joseph Epes Brown. Copyright © 1953, 1989 by the University of Oklahoma Press.

Dimensions of Health and Wellness

Because wellness is dynamic and continuous, no dimension of wellness functions in isolation. When you have a high level of wellness or optimal health, all dimensions are integrated and functioning together. The person's environment (including work, school, family, community), and his or her physical, emotional, intellectual, occupational, spiritual, and social dimensions of wellness are in tune with one another to produce harmony. Health educators commonly refer to six dimensions of health and wellness: emotional, intellectual, spiritual, occupational, social, and physical:

- **Emotional wellness** requires understanding emotions and coping with problems that arise in everyday life.
- **Intellectual wellness** involves having a mind open to new ideas and concepts. If you are intellectually healthy, you seek new experiences and challenges.
- **Spiritual wellness** is the state of harmony with yourself and others. It is the ability to balance inner needs with the demands of the rest of the world.
- **Occupational wellness** is being able to enjoy what you are doing to earn a living and contribute to society, whether it be going to college, working as a secretary, doctor, construction manager, or accountant. In a job, it means having skills such as critical thinking, problem solving, and communicating well.
- **Social wellness** refers to the ability to perform social roles effectively, comfortably, and without harming others.
- **Physical wellness** is a healthy body maintained by eating right, exercising regularly, avoiding harmful habits, making informed and responsible decisions about health, seeking medical care when needed, and participating in activities that help prevent illness.

Terms

holistic model: encompasses the physiological, mental, emotional, social, spiritual, and environmental aspects of health

emotional wellness: understanding emotions and knowing how to cope with problems that arise in everyday life, and how to manage stress

intellectual wellness: having a mind open to new ideas and concepts

spiritual wellness: state of balance and harmony with yourself and others

occupational wellness: enjoyment of what you are doing to earn a living and contribute to society

social wellness: ability to perform the expectations of social roles effectively, comfortably, and without harming others

physical wellness: maintenance of your body in good condition by eating right, exercising regularly, avoiding harmful habits, and making informed, responsible decisions about your health

Managing Stress

The Rainbow of Human Energy

In truth, we know that we cannot separate the mind from the body, nor can we separate the mind from emotions, or the body from the soul. All aspects are integrated. Through the recent insights of quantum physics, we know that everything, including our thoughts and feelings, consists of energy. This is what the wisdom keepers and shamans have known for millennia. Renowned physicist David Bohm addressed the spiritual nature of health in terms of quantum physics. He used the term *coherence* to describe the harmony among the energies of body, mind, and spirit, which gives a sense of wholeness that can only be described as "inner peace." As we continue to explore the issues of health and illness, some interesting facts come to light which support the holistic concept that the whole is greater than the sum of the parts. Spontaneous remissions and

healing through prayer are two of many phenomena that cannot be explained by the mechanistic model. In fact, the new paradigm suggests that we are not a mind in a body, but a body in a mind.

Try the following exercise: Keeping in mind the concept of coherence in this new paradigm, take a moment to reflect on your whole being—all that you are, not just your body. You can begin by thinking about your physical body—your senses, organs, bones, tissue, and fluids. Visualize all the organs, tissues, and fluids working in cooperation with each other (coherence). Imagine that every cell in your body, like the needle of a compass, is headed north. Next, imagine that a layer of energy surrounds and permeates your body. This layer of energy is aqua. This represents what is known as your emotional body. Imagine this layer of blue

energy around your body like warm Caribbean water. Imagine what it would feel like to sense harmony between your emotions and physical body. Next, imagine that superimposed over this aqua-blue layer is a layer of energy deeper in color—indigo blue. This color represents your intellect and the powers of the mind. When all thoughts are focused in the same direction, you have coherence at this level of energy as well. Finally, visualize that superimposed on the layer of indigo blue is a layer of violet, a color that often represents the spiritual nature of humanity. As you envision these colors, think and sense coherence—the integration, balance, and harmony of your mind, body, spirit, and emotions. Know that there is no separation of body, mind, and spirit and the whole is truly greater than the sum of the parts.

Health as Positive Wellness

If freedom from sickness isn't all there is to health, then what else is involved? The World Health Organization (WHO) defines health as "a state of complete physical, mental, and social well-being and not merely the absence of disease and infirmity." This definition is so broad and covers so much that some people find it meaningless. Its universality, however, is exactly right. People's lives, and therefore their health, are affected by every aspect of life: environmental influences such as climate; the availability of nutritious food, comfortable shelter, clean air to breathe, and pure water to drink; and other people, including family, lovers, employers, coworkers, friends, and associates of various kinds.

The WHO definition of health takes into account not only the condition of your body but also the state of your mind. Your mental processes are perhaps the most important influences on your health, because they determine how you deal with your physical and social surroundings, what attitudes about life you have, and how you interact with others.

Health as the totality of a person's existence is the holistic view, which recognizes the interrelatedness of the physical, psychological, emotional, social, spiritual, and environmental factors that con-

tribute to the overall quality of a person's life. No part of the mind, body, or environment is separate and independent.

The philosophy of holistic health is not incompatible with the practice of conventional medicine. Rather, it emphasizes a view that has gained wide acceptance among members of the medical community—that each person has the capacity and the responsibility for optimizing his or her sense of well-being, for self-healing, and for the creation of conditions and feelings that help prevent disease. Holistic health is hardly a revolutionary idea; the Old English root of our word *health* (*hal*, meaning sound or whole) implies that there is more to health than freedom from sickness.

Positive wellness involves (a) being free from symptoms of disease and pain as much as possible; (b) being active, able to do what you want and what you must at the appropriate time; and (c) being in good spirits and feeling emotionally healthy most of the time. These characteristics indicate that health is not something suddenly achieved at a specific time, like getting a college degree. Rather, health is a *process*—indeed, a way of life—through which you develop and encourage every aspect of your body, mind, and feelings to interrelate harmoniously as much of the time as possible.

The Philosophy of Holistic Health

The philosophy of holistic health emphasizes the unity of the mind, spirit, and body. Therefore, symptoms of illness and disease may be viewed as an imbalance in a person's total state of being and not simply as the malfunction of a particular part of the body. Consider, for example, a common minor illness: the headache. About 80% to 90% of American adults experience at least one headache each year. Although a headache can be the result of brain injury or the symptom of another illness, more often it is caused by emotional stress that produces a tightening of the muscles in the head and neck. These contracting muscles increase the blood pressure in the head, thereby causing the pain of headache.

Most people try to relieve a headache by taking aspirin or some other analgesic drug that can alter the physiological mechanisms that produce the pain. In contrast, someone using the holistic approach would first try to determine the *source* of the tensions—worry, anger, or frustration—and then work to reduce or eliminate the tensions. Similarly, an upset stomach cannot be regarded as simply the result of excessive secretion of stomach acid, requiring an antacid to bring relief. In many cases, the upset results from unexpressed hostility or fear. You are probably aware that such common events as taking an examination or having a dispute with someone can cause uncomfortable feelings in the stomach.

The holistic approach emphasizes self-healing, the maintenance of health, and the prevention of illness,

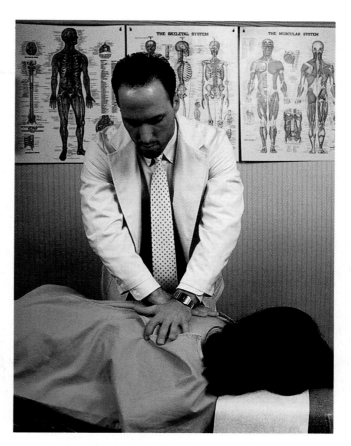

Many alternative medical practices, such as chiropractic, massage, and acupuncture, are now considered legitimate medical treatments and are often covered by insurance.

Wellness Guide

Whole-Person Wellness

A person with emotional wellness is able to:

- Maintain a sense of humor.
- Recognize feelings and appropriately express them.
- Strive to meet emotional needs.
- Take responsibility for his or her behavior.

A person with intellectual wellness is able to:

- Communicate effectively in speaking and in writing.
- See more than one side of an issue.
- Keep abreast of global issues.
- Exhibit good time-management skills.

A person with spiritual wellness is able to:

- Examine personal values and beliefs.
- Search for meanings that help explain the purpose of life.
- Have a clear understanding of right and wrong.
- Appreciate natural forces in the universe.

A person with occupational wellness is able to:

- Feel a sense of accomplishment in his or her work.
- Balance work and other aspects of life.
- Find satisfaction in being creative and innovative.
- Seek challenges at work.

A person with social wellness is able to:

- Develop positive relationships with loved ones.
- Develop relationships with friends.
- Enjoy being with others.
- Effectively communicate with others who may be different.

A person with physical wellness is able to:

- Exercise regularly and select a well-balanced diet.
- Participate in safe, responsible sexual behavior.
- Make informed choices about medicinal use and medical care.
- Maintain a positive, health-promoting lifestyle.

rather than the treatment of symptoms and disease. A holistic approach integrates medical technology into a broader treatment that looks not only at a person's symptoms, but also at the sources of disharmony. From the holistic point of view, illness is the result of some imbalance in the harmonious interaction of the body, mind, and environment. Thus, to the extent that we can follow a program of positive wellness and create a healthy environment, we can be free of disease.

Some of the great advances in medicine have resulted from considering illness solely in terms of the affected bodily organ. Indeed, devoting medical attention to one specific ailing part of the body is sometimes the most efficient way to treat a medical problem, which is why we have specialists who are experts in treating diseases of different body parts, such as heart specialists, gastrointestinal specialists, podiatrists, gynecologists, and so on.

Some health professionals have criticized those who advocate holistic health practices and holistic medicine, arguing that the concepts and methods are antiscientific and hence harmful. Holistic medicine is not antiscientific. By encouraging individuals to take personal command of their health, including how they use medical services, holistic health practices are likely to be less harmful than some modern medical practices, such as unnecessary surgery (see chapter 19).

 ## Taking Responsibility for Your Health

Not so many years ago, people were subject to a variety of diseases over which they had little or no

TABLE 1.1   Ten Leading Causes of Death for All Ages, All Races, and Both Sexes, 1900, 1987, and 1998

1900	1987	1998
1. Tuberculosis	Heart disease	Heart disease
2. Pneumonia	Cancer	Cancer
3. Diarrhea and enteritis	Stroke	Stroke
4. Heart disease	Injuries	Chronic obstructive pulmonary disease (COPD)
5. Liver disease	Bronchitis and emphysema	Accidents, including motor vehicle accidents
6. Injuries	Pneumonia and influenza	Pneumonia and influenza
7. Stroke	Diabetes	Diabetes
8. Cancer	Suicide	Suicide
9. Bronchitis	Chronic liver disease	Kidney disease
10. Diphtheria	Arteriosclerosis	Chronic liver disease and cirrhosis

Source: National Center for Health Statistics, July 2000.

control. In the early part of the twentieth century, infectious diseases caused by organisms were the leading causes of death in the United States (Table 1.1). Modern public health methods and modern drugs, such as antibiotics, were not available. In 1918, millions of people around the world died from influenza, the cause of which was unknown at that time.

Today, the leading causes of illness and death are not due to infections, but to "lifestyle diseases." These diseases, such as heart disease and cancer, result from people's behaviors, and the ways in which

Wellness Guide

Oh My Aching Head!

Headaches are one of the most common causes of human discomfort. Although headaches can be a symptom of a brain disease or injury, the vast majority of headaches are caused by anxiety, tension, and emotional distress.

Tension headache is the most common type of headache. It is caused by persistent contractions of the muscles in the neck and scalp, brought on by anxiety, stress, or allergic reactions to drugs and foods. Tension headaches may last for hours, may occur frequently, and may be a problem over the course of several years. The pain of a tension headache often can be relieved by experiencing a

few minutes of deep mental relaxation or by massaging the tense muscles in the neck and scalp.

Migraine headache, or vascular headache, is characterized by throbbing pain that can last for hours and even days. Migraine headaches are accompanied by altered blood flow to the brain's blood vessels. Massaging the neck and scalp can help relieve the pain, as can mental relaxation and visualizing normal blood flow to the head. Autosuggestion and visualizing the hands becoming warmer may also help relieve pain, because some blood flow is diverted from the brain to the hands, thereby reducing blood pressure in the brain.

Identifying and eliminating the sources of tension and anxiety in your life is the surest way to prevent headaches. Some people have learned to use "having a headache" as a means of avoiding unpleasant situations, such as school or work obligations. As children they may have observed their parents coping with tension and stress by "getting a headache," and so they too learned that "having a headache" can be used to avoid anxiety-provoking experiences. Have you developed such an avoidance mechanism?

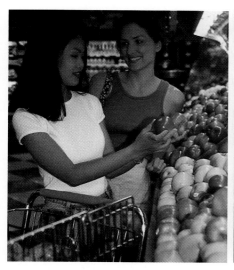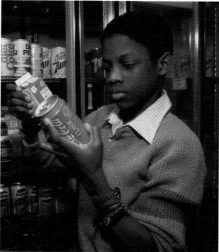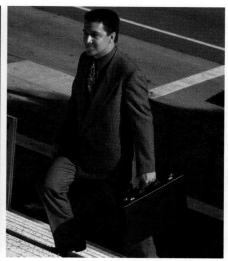

Simple behaviors in our everyday lives can positively affect health: eat 5 servings of fruits and vegetables every day, read food labels to make wise choices; and walk to work whenever possible.

they choose to live. The idea that lifestyle is a major cause of disease and death in modern societies is not new. A generation ago, Lewis Thomas (1978), an eminent physician and author, observed that our lifestyles were killing us.

> The new theory is that most of today's human illnesses, the infectious ones aside, are multifactoral in nature, caused by two great arrays of causative mechanisms: the influence of things in the environment; and one's personal lifestyle. For medicine to become effective in dealing with such disease, it has become common belief that the environment will have to be changed, and personal ways of living also have to be transformed, and radically.

There is no bacterium that causes heart disease. Heart disease results from today's lifestyles, which include overeating (see chapter 6), cigarette smoking (see chapter 17), lack of exercise (see chapter 7), high levels of stress (see chapter 3), and high blood pressure and high levels of blood cholesterol (see chapter 14). Cancer is associated with both nutritional (see Chapter 5) and human-activity environmental factors (see Chapter 13). Improper nutrition, smoking cigarettes, and exposure to hazardous substances in the environment initiate biological changes that can result in cancer. An unhealthy lifestyle is also at the root of suicide and homicide (alcohol, drugs, and stress), accidents (alcohol use and stress), and cirrhosis of the liver (alcohol abuse).

Lifestyle and Health

When a person dies, the cause of death is generally identified in terms of the organ system that failed and resulted in the person's death, e.g., heart disease, cirrhosis of the liver, cancer of the lung. This may not, however, identify the root causes of that death. For example, saying someone died of lung cancer does not tell us that the *actual* cause of death was smoking. When deaths are examined for their actual causes and not simply what is reported on death certificates, the results show that approximately *half* of the 2.1 million deaths in the United States each year are due to lifestyle factors (Table 1.2), and by extension, that many, many deaths could be prevented if people lived more healthfully (McGuinnis and Foege, 1993).

Leading the list of life-shortening behaviors is tobacco use, which is responsible for more than 400,000 American deaths per year. Smoking cigarettes and cigars, chewing tobacco, and being exposed to second-hand smoke contribute substantially to deaths caused by cancer of all kinds, heart disease, high blood pressure, stroke, bronchitis, chronic obstructive pulmonary disease (COPD), pneumonia, low birth weight, and burns from fires. The enormous toll on life and health exacted by tobacco use is the reason that health agencies, doctors, and governments overwhelmingly recommend limiting tobacco use (see chapter 17).

Next to tobacco use, unhealthy diet and activity patterns contribute the most to death in the U.S. Consumption of high levels of cholesterol and saturated fat in foods is associated with heart disease, several types of cancer, and stroke. High-calorie consumption coupled with low levels of physical activity predisposes people to overweight, diabetes, and high blood pressure. A sedentary lifestyle is responsible for 23% of deaths from the leading chronic diseases (heart disease, high blood pressure, stroke, and diabetes).

Drug use and abuse are responsible for 120,000

TABLE 1.2   Number of Preventable Deaths in the United States in 1990

Estimates are from data including actual numbers (firearm deaths) and calculated risks (tobacco deaths). More than 1 million deaths are caused by lifestyles and behaviors—all preventable deaths.

	Deaths	
Cause	Estimated No.	Percentage of Total Deaths
Tobacco	400 000	19
Diet/activity patterns	300 000	14
Alcohol	100 000	5
Microbial agents	90 000	4
Toxic agents	60 000	3
Firearms	35 000	2
Sexual behavior	30 000	1
Motor vehicles	25 000	1
Illicit use of drugs	20 000	<1
Total	1 060 000	50

Source: McGuinnis and Foege (1993). Actual causes of death in the United States. *Journal of the American Medical Association, 270,* 2207–2212.

American deaths each year. Misuse of alcohol accounts for nearly 100,000 deaths each year directly from alcohol toxicity and medical complications therefrom (e.g., liver and pancreatic disease), motor vehicle and other types of accidents, and homicides. Another 20,000 deaths annually are attributable to the use of both legal and illegal drugs other than alcohol. These include deaths from deliberate overdose, accidental overdose, and fatal accidents caused by intoxication.

The transmission of infectious agents accounts for over 120,000 deaths. Unsafe sex and injection drug use contribute to thousands of new cases of AIDS each year. Transmission of hepatitis B virus by unsafe sex and injection drug use and of other strains of hepatitis virus via fecal contamination of food results in thousands of cases of fatal liver failure. Overuse of antibiotics has produced bacterial strains that are resistant to antibiotics, resulting in infections that are difficult (and occasionally impossible) to treat.

Social factors cause fatalities, also. For example, exposure to toxic agents in the workplace and elsewhere account for 60,000 deaths per year. Firearms used in homicides, suicides, and accidental shootings are responsible for 35,000 deaths. Motor vehicle

Dollars and Health Sense

Large Corporations Profit from Products That Make People Sick

Heart disease, stroke, lung cancer, colon cancer, type 2 diabetes, and chronic obstructive pulmonary disease account for nearly half of all deaths in the United States. These diseases are caused in large part by unhealthy lifestyle choices: eating poorly, smoking cigarettes, being overweight, and not exercising. Unfortunately, many large corporations profit from individuals' unhealthy lifestyles— indeed, some encourage unhealthy behavior as the basis of their business.

The tobacco industry is the prime example of companies profiting financially from harming others. No other industry makes a product that, when used as directed, causes disease and death. In the late 1990s, the major tobacco companies were sued by the federal government, state governments, and individuals for lying to the public for nearly 50 years about the addictive properties of their products and

the harm that tobacco use causes. Knowing that long-term smokers (i.e., their best customers) tend to begin smoking as teens, the tobacco industry uses sophisticated marketing methods to lure young people to smoke and to get them hooked. The tobacco industry is a friend to no one.

Whereas it is not as obvious as with tobacco, some food companies—particularly fast-food companies—also profit from harming their customers. A typical serving of fast food (e.g., burger, fries, and a soft drink or shake) contains around 1000 calories. Approximately one-third to one-half of those calories are from fat, a prime contributor to heart and blood vessel disease. Fast food also contains large amounts of cholesterol and salt, which also contribute to heart and blood vessel disease. Studies show that the blood vessels of young people who consume typical fast foods show the beginning

stages of disease, with the degree of damage proportional to the amount of fast food consumed. Moreover, the calories in a typical serving of fast food provide about half or more of most individuals' energy requirement for one day. This is why a steady diet of fast food can lead to weight problems and associated illnesses like type 2 diabetes.

Although fast food companies have yet to be legally challenged for causing disease, one day they may be. After all, 20 years ago, it seemed that the tobacco industry was invulnerable to legal attack, but that changed over time.

You need not wait for legal challenges to be a healthy person, however. You can become aware that in some instances the quest for corporate profits is based on encouraging people to adopt unhealthy living habits, and you can choose a healthier way to live.

Wellness Guide

Health Issues for College Students

What health issues face North America's 15 million college students? Here's what college and university health educators and medical professionals think the answers are (Grace, 1997).

Sexual health. More than any others, sexual issues have the potential to affect the health of college students. These include sexually transmitted diseases (7% to 10% of college students carry an undiagnosed STD), unintended pregnancy, and sexual assault, especially acquaintance or date rape.

Sexuality is also related to issues of self-esteem, peer acceptance, loneliness, and relieving academic stress with superficial sexual relationships, all of which have the potential to produce psychological harm and establish negative attitudes and behavior that may impair future sexual and intimate relationships.

Substance abuse. The abuse of alcohol, drugs, tobacco, and food is related to trying to gain peer acceptance, unhealthy role modeling in families and in society at large, and trying to cope with psychological distress. Students whose parents abuse substances often have a tendency for substance abuse. Alcohol abuse is related to the majority of sexual assaults, unintended pregnancies (from not using contraceptives properly or at all), and the transmission of STDs (from not practicing safe sex).

Mental health. Failure to achieve, academic stress, lack of social support, difficulty adjusting to young adulthood, and pressures to fit in socially all contribute to emotional problems (especially anxiety and depression) that may impair a student's academic performance and sense of well-being. They can also

lead to stress-related physical illnesses. Competitive academic environments can create feelings of inferiority, insecurity, and emotional distress.

Food and weight. Many students are highly concerned about their body size and shape and may become malnourished to meet their perceptions of social ideality. Eating disorders, such as bulimia and anorexia nervosa, affect a large number of students.

Health care. A large proportion of college students in the United States have limited access to health care because their colleges do not have comprehensive services for students or they do not have private health insurance.

Accidents and injuries. Many students are susceptible to automobile accidents (often alcohol-related) and sports injuries.

accidents cause another 47,000 deaths. Lack of access to medical care—a condition that affects the one third of American families who have no health insurance—contributes to thousands of deaths each year as well.

Type 2 Diabetes as a Lifestyle Disease

Diabetes is a disease in which the level of sugar in the blood cannot be regulated, which causes a variety of symptoms including degeneration of some organs in the body and even death. There are two forms of diabetes: type 1, or insulin-dependent diabetes, requires injections of insulin to control symptoms of the disease; type 2, or non–insulin-dependent diabetes, generally can be controlled by diet, exercise, or drugs other than insulin. Type 1 diabetes was formerly called "juvenile-onset" diabetes because it tends to start in childhood and adolescence. Type 2 diabetes was formerly called "maturity-onset" diabetes because it tends to start in adulthood.

Evidence that type 2 diabetes is a disease of lifestyle comes from studies of populations that have dramatically altered their lifestyle over a brief time span. For example, Yemenite Jews who emigrated to Israel in 1949 had one of the lowest rates of type 2 diabetes in the world—less than 1 case per 1,000 individuals.

Thirty years later, the same population, now adapted to a Western lifestyle in Israel, had a rate of almost 12 cases of type 2 diabetes per 1,000 individuals.

Another example is the prevalence of diabetes among the Pima Indians of the southwestern United States. In the last century, these Native Americans lived mostly on maize, beans, wild game, and vegetables. They were active, lean, and strong. Today many Pima Indians are sedentary, corpulent, and have the highest rate of diabetes in the world—341 cases per 1,000 individuals (Eaton, 1990). As a result of their changed lifestyle, more than one in three Pima Indians suffers from diabetes.

Type 2 diabetes is an increasingly prevalent lifestyle disease. It is associated with being overweight: for every 20% increase in overweight, the chance of diabetes doubles. Improving nutrition and maintaining normal body weight can help prevent diabetes.

Nearsightedness

Another dramatic example of how modern lifestyles affect health concerns vision. Many children and a majority of adults in modern societies wear glasses or contact lenses to correct for nearsightedness (myopia). When our ancestors had to forage and hunt for food, acute vision was probably essential to survival and, of course, corrective lenses were unknown. During early development, a child's eye adapts to the visual information the eyes receive from the environment. Looking at distant objects tends to produce normal vision or eyes that are slightly farsighted. Today, almost all children watch TV and computer screens for many hours a day and also read books, magazines, and newspapers—all of which require close-up vision. These activities tend to cause myopia in many children.

The influence of modern lifestyles on vision was documented by measuring the vision of young people in rural China compared with the vision of Chinese students in Hong Kong (Wallman, 1994). Most of the young people in the rural environment had normal vision or were slightly farsighted (Figure 1.3). In contrast, most of the Chinese students in Hong Kong were nearsighted, many to a considerable degree. Thus, if one considers 20/20 vision desirable, our modern lifestyle, which involves computers, TV, and reading, is likely to affect eye development and may produce myopia. Until we understand more about the environmental and genetic cues that affect visual development, children should be encouraged to spend time outdoors, where their eyes are more likely to focus on distant objects.

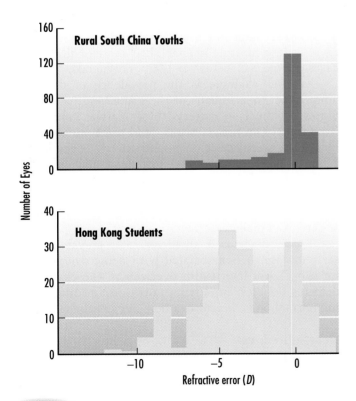

FIGURE 1.3   Comparison of visual acuity of 18- to 28-year-old students in Hong Kong with youths in rural areas of China. Most of the rural youths have normal vision, while most of the Hong Kong students are myopic.

Source: Reprinted with permission from *Nature, 371,* 201–202. Copyright 1994 Macmillan Magazines Limited. Courtesy of Josh Wallman and Carly Lam.

National Health Objectives

In 1979 the first *Surgeon General's Report on Health Promotion and Disease Prevention* was released. Its purpose was to emphasize prevention of disease by focusing on personal responsibility for one's own health and reducing unhealthy behaviors. The report indicated that, for people to be healthy, social changes must also take place to deal with poverty, lack of education, inadequate housing, hunger, drug use, and so on.

Since the initial Surgeon General's report in 1979, the U.S. government has periodically issued health objectives for the country. The most recent of these is called Healthy People 2010, which is designed to help individuals of all ages increase life expectancy and improve their quality of life, as well as to eliminate health disparities among different segments of the population (Office of Disease Prevention and Health Promotion, 2000). Healthy People 2010 consists of 467 specific health objectives grouped into 28 focus areas (Figure 1.4). Specific goals include reducing the number of new cancer cases, lessening the illness and death caused by cancer, promoting the health of people with disabilities, and improving food safety, and reducing food-borne illnesses.

Several of the specific goals of Healthy People 2010 have been grouped into 10 categories, called the **Leading Health Indicators,** which reflect the major public health concerns in the United States (Figure 1.5). The Leading Health Indicators illuminate individual behaviors, physical and social environmental factors, and important health system issues that greatly affect the health of individuals and communities. The Leading Health Indicators are intended to

1. Access to Quality Health Services
2. Arthritis, Osteoporosis and Chronic Back Conditions
3. Cancer
4. Chronic Kidney Disease
5. Diabetes
6. Disability and Secondary Conditions
7. Educational and Community-Based Programs
8. Environmental Health
9. Family Planning and Sexual Health
10. Food Safety
11. Health Communication
12. Heart Disease and Stroke
13. HIV
14. Immunizations and Infectious Diseases
15. Injury and Violence Prevention
16. Maternal, Infant, and Child Health
17. Medical Product Safety
18. Mental Health and Mental Disorders
19. Nutrition
20. Occupational Safety and Health
21. Oral Health
22. Physical Activity and Fitness
23. Public Health Infrastructure
24. Respiratory Diseases
25. Sexually Transmitted Diseases
26. Substance Abuse
27. Tobacco Use
28. Vision and Hearing

FIGURE 1.4   Focus Areas for Healthy People 2010

1. **Healthy Weight.** Percentage of the population with a body mass index that is no more than 20% lower and no more than 20% higher than that recommended for age and gender.
2. **Physical Activity.** Percentage of the population regularly participating in exercise that offers significant cardiovascular benefits.
3. **Immunization.** Percentage of the adult, teenage, and childhood population that is up-to-date for the currently recommended immunization schedule.
4. **Teen Smoking.** Prevalence of any use of tobacco products among youth up to age 17.
5. **Substance Abuse.** Percentage of youth aged 12–17 that used alcohol or illicit drugs during the previous 12 months.
6. **Mental Health.** Percentage of the population with diagnosed clinical depression or severe depressive symptoms.
7. **Preventable Injury Deaths.** Percentage of preventable deaths attributed to injuries.
8. **Clean Air and Water.** Percentage of the population living in areas where air and water quality meet or exceed federal standards.
9. **Access to Health Care.** Percentage of the population with health insurance and/or a regular source of medical care.
10. **Social Environment.** Percentage of the population with household incomes less than 100% of the federal poverty limit, or percentage of the population aged 18–24 that has completed high school.

FIGURE 1.5 Healthy People 2010 Leading Health Indicators

help everyone more easily understand the importance of health promotion and disease prevention and to encourage wide participation in improving health.

Spirituality and Health

Much of our culture's traditional thinking about health tends to view states of wellness and illness as being affected only by physical processes that are amenable to objective, scientific study. Many people believe, however, that spiritual feelings and experiences—those that are not necessarily achieved by the application of logic and critical thought but that are more intuitive and subjective—can affect a person's health. Indeed, nearly all physicians endorse the idea that a spiritual dimension to life can aid healing (Harvard Health Letter, 1998), and research shows that people with higher levels of intrinsic spirituality tend to be healthier (McBride et al., 1998).

Terms

Leading Health Indicators: ten categories of health goals that represent the major public health concerns in the United States.

Spiritual experiences tend to engender feelings of compassion and empathy; peace of mind; relatedness and communion with a force, power, or set of values larger than oneself; and harmony with the environment (Dyson et al., 1997). These feelings are believed to be a cornerstone of health because they represent a balance between the inner and outer aspects of human experience. For some, the spiritual dimension of life is embodied in the practice of a specific religion. For others, the spiritual dimension is nonreligious and simply part of a personal philosophy. Many practices can help people experience the spiritual realms of existence— prayer, meditation, yoga, musical and artistic endeavors, and helping others are but a few common ones.

> We do not see things as they are . . .
> We see things as we are.
> TALMUD

Becoming more spiritually aware, regardless of the chosen path, can lead to a healthier life. Being in touch with your spiritual feelings helps you handle life's ups and downs with understanding and compassion for yourself and others. You become open to love in the highest sense of its meaning, which is acceptance and tolerance. You begin to love yourself despite your problems and hang-ups. You love your family and friends when relations are strained. You see beauty and harmony in more and more aspects of living. And occasionally—however fleetingly—you may experience the truly wondrous feeling of being completely and joyfully alive.

Making Healthy Changes

A major assumption of health education is that nearly everyone has a basic desire to be healthy and well, but that many people acquire habits of thought and behavior that may make them less well rather than more. One goal of health education, therefore, is to encourage people to give up less-healthy attitudes and behaviors and adopt ones that lead to greater health, wellness, and satisfaction in life.

> One day while out walking, the Buddha and some of his students encountered a line of ants in their path. One of the students said, "Master, why are the ants crossing the road?" The Buddha replied, "Because they want to be happy."

It is said that knowledge is power, but with regard to living healthfully, that isn't always the case. Almost everyone knows that smoking cigarettes, driving after drinking alcohol, and eating junk food are unhealthy, but many people do those things anyway. Simply knowing what to do is no guarantee that a person will do it. One reason for this is that an unhealthy attitude or behavior is rewarding in some way, even if it is harmful in some other way (for example, smoking cigarettes to relieve stress). Also, a variety of biological, social, and psychological forces help maintain an attitude or behavior. A smoker may want to stop, but if many of his or her friends smoke, stopping may jeopardize the smoker's friendships. For a change to occur, the person has to believe that the benefits of change outweigh the costs. Rituals such as New Year's resolutions and slogans such as "just do it" offer unrealistic models of how habits are changed. Desire and will power alone are insufficient; research, planning, and enlisting social support are required as well.

Health behavior change models are classified as individual change models, interpersonal change models, and community models or interventions. We will look at two individual change models and how they apply to an ability to make positive, healthy changes or maintain a healthy lifestyle.

The Health Belief Model

The Health Belief Model (HBM) was originally developed as a systematic method to explain and predict preventive health behavior, but it has been revised to include general health motivation for the purpose of distinguishing illness and sick-role behavior from health behavior. Key aspects of the model are described as:

- **Perceived susceptibility.** Each individual has his or her own perception of the likelihood of experiencing a condition that would adversely affect his or her health. Individuals vary widely in their perception of susceptibility to a disease or condition. Those at the low end of the extreme deny the possibility of contracting an adverse condition. Individuals in a moderate category admit to a statistical possibility of disease susceptibility. Individuals at the high extreme of susceptibility feel there is real danger that they will experience an adverse condition or contract a given disease.

- **Perceived seriousness.** Perceived seriousness refers to the beliefs a person holds concerning the effects of a given disease or condition on his or her state of affairs. These effects can be considered from the point of view of the differences that a disease would create—for instance, pain and discomfort, loss of work time, financial burdens, difficulties with family, problems with relationships, and susceptibility to future conditions. It is important to include these emotional and financial burdens when considering the seriousness of a disease or condition.

- **Perceived benefits of taking action.** Taking action toward the prevention of disease or toward dealing with an illness is the next step after an individual has accepted the susceptibility of a disease and recognized its seriousness. The direction of action that a person chooses will be influenced by his or her beliefs regarding the action.

- **Barriers to taking action.** Action may not take place even though an individual may believe that the benefits to taking action are significant. This may be because of barriers, which can include inconvenience, cost, unpleasantness, pain, or upset. These characteristics may lead a person away from taking the desired action.

- **Cues to action.** An individual's perception of the levels of susceptibility and seriousness provide the force to act. Benefits, minus barriers, provide the path of action. However, "cues to action" may be required for the desired behavior to occur. These cues to action may be internal or external.

The Transtheoretical Model

One of the most influential models of health behavior change is the Transtheoretical Model, or Process of Change Model (Prochaska, DiClemente, & Norcross, 1992). This model recognizes that change occurs through the following stages:

- **Precontemplation.** The person is not considering changing a particular behavior any time in the foreseeable future. Many individuals in this stage are unaware or underaware of their problems. Information is important during this stage.

- **Contemplation.** The person becomes aware that change is desirable but has not committed to act. The person often focuses on why it would be difficult to change. Information on options on how to change the behavior can be helpful during this stage.

- **Preparation.** The person desires change and commits to making that change in the near future, usually within the next 30 days. Instead of thinking why he or she can't take action, the focus is on what can be done to begin. The person creates a realistic plan for making a change, including overcoming obstacles. This stage may include announcing the change to friends and family, researching how to make the change, making a calendar, or setting up a diary or journal to record progress and obstacles to progress.

- **Action.** The person implements the plan. The old behavior and the environmental situations that reinforced that behavior are stopped and new behaviors and environmental supports are adopted. Obstacles are expected and noted, and strategies for overcoming them are implemented. Progress through this stage may take six months or more.

- **Maintenance.** The person strengthens the change, recognizing that lapses and even temptations to give up will occur. "Ebb and flow" are to be expected and not to be seen as failures. The person can remind himself or herself of the many benefits of and gains from the behavior change to help combat relapse.
- **Termination.** The person is not tempted to return to the previous behavior.

It's Up to You

If you want to be healthy and well, it's up to you. The medical care system—doctors and other medical providers, pharmaceutical companies, hospitals, clinics, insurance companies, and to some degree the government—can help you when you are sick, but only you can make life goals to be healthy and well; to take responsibility for the ways that your thoughts, feelings, and behaviors affect your life; to care for rather than harm yourself; and to choose to learn and adopt health-promoting behaviors.

Scientists at the University of California at Berkeley undertook a multi-year study to determine, among other things, behaviors that contribute to health and longevity (Breslow and Enstrom, 1980). Their findings include:

- no smoking
- getting seven to eight hours sleep per night
- maintaining body weight not less than 10 percent and not more than 30 percent of recommended for height and body frame
- regular exercise
- little or no alcohol consumption
- eating breakfast regularly
- little between-meal snacking

It is clear from many kinds of health research that each one of us needs to do more to maintain and improve our individual health. This conclusion was also clearly expressed by an eminent authority on health policy:

> Americans think of illness and disability as a condition that can be fixed by an expert, in this case a physician. Accordingly, they want more medicine, more research, and more physicians—all with lower cost and equitable distribution. This was the case in 1930 and it is still the case today. . . . However, the fact that each individual is ultimately responsible for the maintenance of his or her own health is a lesson that most Americans still need to learn.
>
> (Ginzberg, 1999)

Critical Thinking About Health

1. As pointed out in this chapter, the major health issues of college students are sexual health, mental health, substance abuse, weight, accidents and injuries, and health care. Discuss which of these issues is of most concern to you personally. Explain your reasons and worries. How can you deal with your concerns in a way that will improve your health?

2. Describe one lifestyle or behavior that you routinely engage in that you regard as destructive to your health (smoking, for example). Discuss your reasons for continuing to engage in this unhealthy behavior. Consider what you might do to change this behavior and list the steps you would take to accomplish the healthy change. Do you believe that you can make the healthy change?

3. Suppose that someone you know is suffering from frequent, severe headaches (several times a week) and does not know what to do about the problem other than to take acetaminophen or aspirin. Based on your own health experiences, explain the advice that you would give such a friend. Consider all the alternatives discussed in this chapter and any others that you think might be helpful. Develop an approach to ending this person's headaches that you think is both appropriate and likely to solve the problem. Give reasons for the approach that you recommend.

4. Imagine that you are the Surgeon General of the United States, who formulates national health policy. (A former Surgeon General, C. Everett Koop, formulated the crusade against tobacco smoking a generation ago.) Describe what you believe is the primary health problem in the U.S. today. Justify your choice with as many facts as you can find. Describe the steps you believe should be taken by government, private companies, organizations, and individuals to eradicate this health problem.

Health in Review

- Health is not only the absence of disease but also is living in harmony with oneself, friends and relatives, and the environment.
- Health means being responsible for preventing personal illness and injuries as well as knowing when to seek medical help.
- The three models used to describe health are medical, environmental, and holistic, or wellness.
- The wellness continuum ranges from high-level wellness to premature death.
- A holistic approach to health emphasizes prevention of disease and injury and self-responsibility for nutrition, exercise, and other aspects of lifestyle that promote wellness.
- The dimensions of wellness are emotional, intellectual, spiritual, occupational, social, and physical.
- Many chronic diseases (e.g., diabetes, heart disease, cancer) are primarily attributable to unhealthy living habits. Taking responsibility for your health while you are young is the best way to reduce the risk of chronic disease later in life.
- Unhealthy lifestyles and behaviors are responsible for half of all deaths in the United States each year.
- Spiritual awareness is an essential part of maintaining wellness and preventing illness.
- *Healthy People 2010* is a set of national health objectives characterized by enhancing the quality of life, reducing the incidence of preventable diseases and premature deaths, and reducing disparity in health status among different demographic groups.
- Changing health behaviors requires knowledge, planning and social support. The Health Belief Model and the Transtheoretical Model describe the process of health behavior change.

Health and Wellness Online

The World Wide Web contains a wealth of information about health and wellness. By accessing the Internet using Web browser software, such as Netscape Navigator or Microsoft's Internet Explorer, you can gain a new perspective on many topics presented in *Health and Wellness, Seventh Edition*. Access the Jones and Bartlett Publishers Web site at http://www.jbpub.com/hwonline.

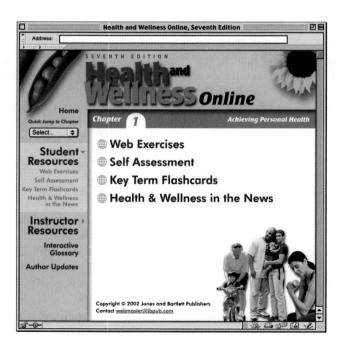

References

Breslow, L., and Enstrom, J. E. (1980). Persistence of health habits and their relationship to mortality. *Preventive Medicine, 9*, 469–483.

Camacho, T. C., and Wiley, J. A. (1983). Health practices, social networks, and change in physical health. In: Berkman, L., and Breslow, L., *Health and Ways of Living: The Alameda County Study*, New York: Oxford University Press.

Dyson, J., Cobb, M., and Forman, D. (1997). The meaning of spirituality: A literature review. *Journal of Advances in Nursing, 26*, 1183–1188.

Ginzberg, E. (1999). Ten encounters with the U.S. health sector, 1930–1999. *Journal of the American Medical Association, 282*, 1665–1668.

Grace, T. W. (1997). Health problems of college students. *Journal of American College Health, 45*, 243–250.

Making a place for spirituality. (1998). *Harvard Health Letter 23(4)*, 1–3.

McBride, J. L., Borrks, A. G., and Pilkington, L. (1998). The relationship between a patient's spirituality and health experiences. *Family Medicine, 30*, 122–126.

McGuinnis, J. M., and Foege, W. H. (1993). Actual causes of death in the United States. *Journal of the American Medical Association, 270*, 2207–2212.

Office of Disease Prevention and Health Promotion, U.S. Department of Health and Human Services (2000). Healthy People 2010. (http://www.health.gov/healthypeople/Default.htm)

Robinson, S., and Johnston, D. G. (1995). Advantages of diabetes. *Nature, 375*, 640.

Wallman, J. (1994). Nature and nurture of myopia. *Nature, 371*, 201–202.

Suggested Readings

Anders, G. (1996). *Health against wealth.* New York: Houghton Mifflin. A journalist's examination of the health care industry and the need for people to take responsibility for their own health.

Breslow, L. (1999). From disease prevention to health promotion. *Journal of the American Medical Association, 281*, 1030–1033. Discusses why health promotion is more important than disease prevention.

Ginzberg, E. (1999). Ten encounters with the U.S. health sector, 1930–1999. *Journal of the American Medical Association, 282*, 1665–1668. An eminent authority on health policy discusses what he has learned in a career spanning 70 years.

Hurley, J. S., and Schlaadt, R. G. (1992). *The Wellness lifestyle.* Guilford, CT: Dushkin Publishing Group. A book that helps you think critically about your lifestyle and offers suggestions for change.

Miller, E. (1997). *Deep healing: The essence of mind/body medicine.* New York: Hay House. Stories, reflections, and case studies that illustrate how mental imagery, positive thinking, and other basics of mind-body medicine contribute to health and longevity.

Ornish, D. (1998). *Love and survival: The scientific basis for the healing power of intimacy.* New York: HarperCollins. Discusses how personal intimacy and other aspects of emotional well-being contribute to better health, including stronger immune systems, better cardiovascular functioning, and longer life expectancies.

Study Guide and Self Assessment

Visualization Eliminates the Pain

Health and Wellness Online

 www.jbpub.com/hwonline

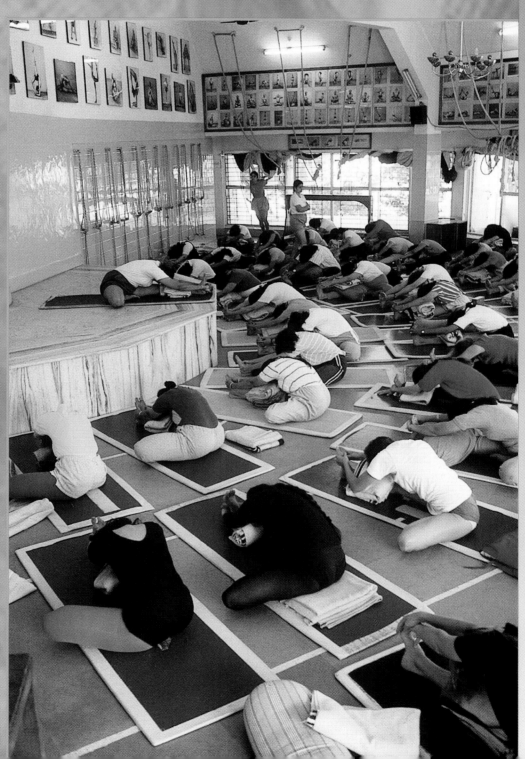

Chapter 2

Mind-Body Communications Maintain Wellness

No human body exists without a mind; no mind exists without a body. Our minds and bodies communicate with each other by means of chemical messengers (e.g., hormones, neurotransmitters) and electrical signals from the nervous system—this has great significance for our health. What goes on in our minds affects the physiological functions of our bodies—digestion, blood pressure, respiration rate, muscle tension, sexual arousal, and many other processes—and, in turn, physiological functions of the body affect how we think and feel.

> *You can observe a lot just by watching.*
> YOGI BERRA

Disturbances in thought and feeling centers in the brain can disrupt the normal activities of the nervous, endocrine (hormone), and immune systems. When this occurs, processes that lead to disease and sickness may be activated. People affect their health by what they think and feel as well as by what they eat and where they live. Becoming aware of how your organs respond to thoughts and feelings can help you to maintain health and promote healing when you become sick.

No medicine or treatment has more healing power than the human mind. This may sound like an exaggeration, but countless cases of people curing themselves of serious diseases by changing their thoughts and feelings have been described, and spiritual cures have been carefully documented over the centuries.

Many easily learned mind-body techniques, such as hypnosis, meditation, biofeedback, guided imagery, autogenic training, breath therapy, progressive relaxation, prayer therapy, and yoga, can be of value in maintaining health and in restoring wellness if you should become sick. Everyone should be familiar with mind-body relaxation techniques, so that they can be used in times of illness and stress or simply to maintain wellness.

In Western culture we are accustomed to thinking about curing sickness in terms of drugs, surgery, or other medical treatments. In other cultures, past and present, healing has been accomplished by magic, ritual, faith, and spiritual practices. Nontraditional ap-

Global Wellness

Yin and Yang—Finding Balance

Taoist philosophy and traditional Chinese medicine embody ideas of balanced energy and internal harmony that are, in many respects, analogous to the Western concept of homeostasis. Harmony is expressed by a balance between the forces of yin and yang (Figure 2.1). Yin and yang represent the opposing and complementary aspects of the universal *chi* that is present in everything, including our bodies. Yang forces are characterized as light, positive, creative, full of movement, and having the nature of heaven. Yin forces are characterized as dark, negative, quiet, receptive, and having the nature of earth.

Chinese medicine classifies the organs of the body as predominantly yin or yang. Hollow organs, such as the stomach, intestines, and bladder, are yang; solid organs, such as the heart, spleen, liver, and lungs, are yin. Food and herbs are also classified as having mostly yin or yang properties. When yin and yang forces are in balance in an individual, a state of harmony exists, and the person experiences health and wellness. However, if either yin or yang forces come to predominate in a person, a state of disharmony is produced and disease may result.

In Asian philosophies and medicine, body and mind are regarded as inseparable. Yin and yang apply to both mental and physical processes. Treatment involves the whole person and is designed to reestablish harmony of the mind and body. The balance of yin and yang forces must be restored so that health returns.

Tai chi chuan and *qigong* (pronounced jē-kung) are two Chinese mind-body exercise techniques that are being practiced by more and more people to help maintain health and to ward off disease. These exercises are especially useful for older persons whose bodies can no longer tolerate vigorous exercise. People who practice qigong experience lower blood pressure, improved circulation, and enhanced immune system functions.

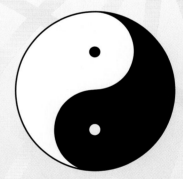

FIGURE 2.1   The Yin-Yang Symbol
This symbol represents the harmonious balance of forces in nature and in people. The white and dark dots show that there is always some yin in a person's yang component and vice versa. The goal in life and nature, according to the Chinese view, is to maintain a harmonious balance between yin and yang forces.

proaches to healing do work and do cure people of many illnesses. Even in our culture we recognize that a patient's attitude plays an important role in the success of a treatment and in recovery. Mental and spiritual healing practices are effective because thoughts, beliefs, faith, and convictions *do* change body chemistry and physiology. Each one of us can learn to use positive thoughts, healthy feelings, and faith to prevent disease and to promote healing in time of sickness.

Homeostasis and Health

Many of the vital functions in the body, such as breathing, heartbeat, blood circulation, digestion, and elimination, require no conscious effort. Rarely do you think about how often to breathe, or whether your heart needs to beat faster or slower to accomplish a task. Your body has mechanisms for controlling and integrating its functions without conscious control, so that it maintains a relatively constant internal physiological environment. The tendency for body systems to interact and to maintain a constant physiological state is called **homeostasis.**

Homeostatic mechanisms maintain blood pressure in most people within the normal limits of 70 to 130 millimeters of mercury, a temperature of 98.6°F, a heart rate between 50 and 90 beats per minute, and blood glucose (sugar) levels around 80 milligrams per 100 milliliters of blood. Although these processes are regulated automatically, they can be deregulated by stress, anger, emotional upset, and thoughts.

Homeostatic mechanisms also prompt many of our behaviors by indicating needs such as hunger, thirst, or sleep. Centers in the brain monitor the amount of nutrients in the blood and the amount of water in the body's tissues. When nutrients are low or the body is in need of water, these centers become activated, and you feel hungry or thirsty. When the body is cold, the brain tells it to shiver in order to generate heat; if the body is overheated, the brain tells it to perspire in order to reduce its temperature.

When you are well and healthy, your body systems function harmoniously. It is similar to the members of a team playing together in a coordinated way to accomplish the goals of the game. If one of your organs is not functioning properly, however, the other organs may not be able to function correctly either, and you may become ill. Thus, in Western medicine disease may be regarded as the disruption of homeostasis, or internal disharmony. Chinese and other Asian cultures define physiological balance as an energy called **chi,** which must be distributed harmoniously throughout the mind and body to maintain health.

Terms

homeostasis: the tendency for body systems to interact in ways that maintain a constant physiological state

chi: a Chinese term referring to the balance of energy in the body

Wellness Guide

Using Your Mind to Heal Your Body

Everyone has accidentally cut or burned his or her hands at one time or another. Perhaps you were chopping vegetables and the knife slipped, or perhaps you reached for a pan on the stove, forgetting that the handle was hot. The usual response to such accidents is anger at being careless or forgetful and anger at the sudden pain. We jump around, curse, and generally act in ways that exacerbate the injury and delay healing. A much better response to minor accidental injuries that do not require immediate medical attention is the following.

In case of a cut, place a clean cloth over the wound and press gently to help stop the bleeding. Then sit or lie down. Close your eyes and allow yourself to become mentally and physically quiet. Visualize the injured part with your mind and see it as it was just *before* the accident. See the skin coming back together. Feel the pain recede. Notice that there is no bleeding. Continue doing this for 5 minutes or longer until you feel calm. If the accident caused a burn, place an ice bag or cool, wet cloth over the wound. Then lie down and visualize the

skin becoming cooler and looking like the normal skin around the burn.

By immediately calming the mind after an injury, inflammation and other harmful physiological reactions in the area are reduced. Healing processes begin immediately when you send positive, calming thoughts and images to the injured area. Continue to visualize healing in the injured area.

The Autonomic Nervous System

The brain influences health and healing through a special group of nerves that control virtually all of the body's organs and functions. This group of nerves is the **autonomic nervous system** (ANS) and regulates many physiological processes (Figure 2.2). The ANS is divided into the *sympathetic* and the *parasympathetic* divisions which tend to work in opposition to one another. For example, sympathetic nerve activity increases heart rate; parasympathetic nerve activity reduces it. Sympathetic nerves decrease digestive activity; parasympathetic nerves increase it.

The autonomic nervous system derives its name from the fact that its activities normally operate without conscious control. For example, a person in a deep coma caused by damage to the outer layers of the brain could maintain a heartbeat, continue to breathe, digest food, and carry out other body functions controlled by the ANS. Centers in the brain, well below the conscious level, send signals to the body that maintain functions vital to life.

Although the ANS functions without conscious control, the signals it sends to the body can be changed by thoughts and feelings. Emotional upset can bring on an upset stomach, panic has an immediate effect on breathing and heart rate, and stress can constrict blood vessels, causing headaches or high blood pressure.

The ability to use the mind to alter physiological processes under the control of the ANS is not restricted to a few exceptional people. With **biofeedback training,** almost anyone can learn to change the temperature in one hand compared with the other or to alter the electrical pattern of the brain's activity. In biofeedback training, the person observes his or her physiological response on a monitor and tries to adjust thought processes in any way that changes the response in the desired direction.

Incorporating mind-body techniques into mainstream medicine has accelerated in the past few years (Taylor et al., 1997). Physicians' awareness of the value of mind-body techniques in healing is largely the result of our increased understanding of the mechanisms that govern mind-body interactions. In recent years researchers have identified dozens of small molecules called **neuropeptides** that transmit changes in moods and emotions in the brain to organs in many parts of the body, particularly the digestive system (Figure 2.3). Cells in the feeling center of the brain *(limbic system)* have receptors for neuropeptides that are identical to cell receptors in the esophagus, stomach, and intestines. That is why a strong emotion in the brain can be felt as a choking in the throat, a pain

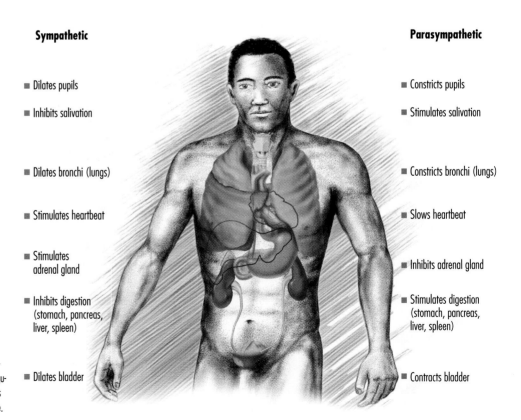

Sympathetic

- Dilates pupils

- Inhibits salivation

- Dilates bronchi (lungs)

- Stimulates heartbeat

- Stimulates adrenal gland

- Inhibits digestion (stomach, pancreas, liver, spleen)

- Dilates bladder

Parasympathetic

- Constricts pupils

- Stimulates salivation

- Constricts bronchi (lungs)

- Slows heartbeat

- Inhibits adrenal gland

- Stimulates digestion (stomach, pancreas, liver, spleen)

- Contracts bladder

FIGURE 2.2 **Functions Controlled by the Autonomic Nervous System** The sympathetic nerves and the parasympathetic nerves regulate functions that normally are not under conscious control, such as breathing, digestion, and heart rate.

in the stomach, or faulty digestion in the intestines. The expression "I can feel it in my gut" is, in fact, a scientifically accurate description.

Rapid advances are being made in identifying the molecular mechanisms that are used in mind-body communications. New studies confirm the ancient idea that the mind is the most powerful healing force we possess. We all need to learn how to use the power of our minds in positive ways. On the negative side, the mind can cause illness if we are depressed, angry, or sad for extended periods of time.

Hormones

Hormones are chemicals produced in the body that affect a wide range of body functions, such as growth, development of sexual organs, the menstrual cycle, di-

gestion in the stomach, and the level of sugar in the blood, to mention just a few (Table 2.1). Hormones are synthesized and released from special glands located throughout the body (Figure 2.4). The synthesis of

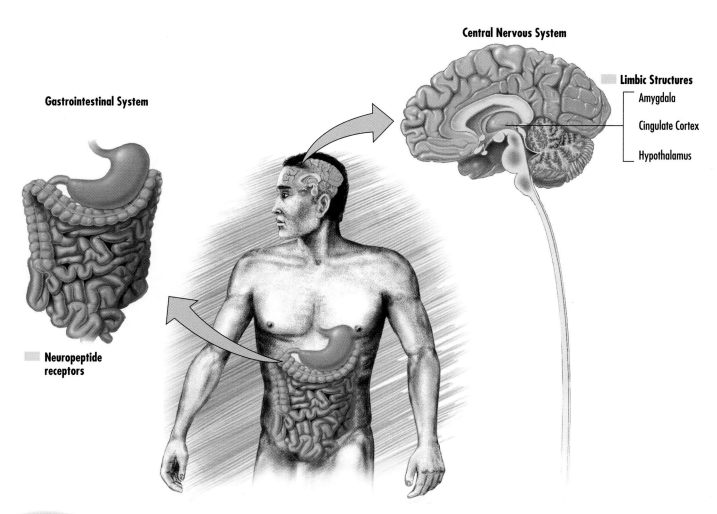

FIGURE 2.3   The Limbic System   The emotional centers of the brain located in the limbic structures communicate with the gastrointestinal system and other organs by means of small chemicals called neuropeptides. These chemicals are carried throughout the body in blood and other body fluids. Neuropeptides bind to receptors on different cells and adjust their pattern of chemical reactions. Chemical messages sent from the brain to the body and from the body to the brain ultimately play an important role in our physiology and health.

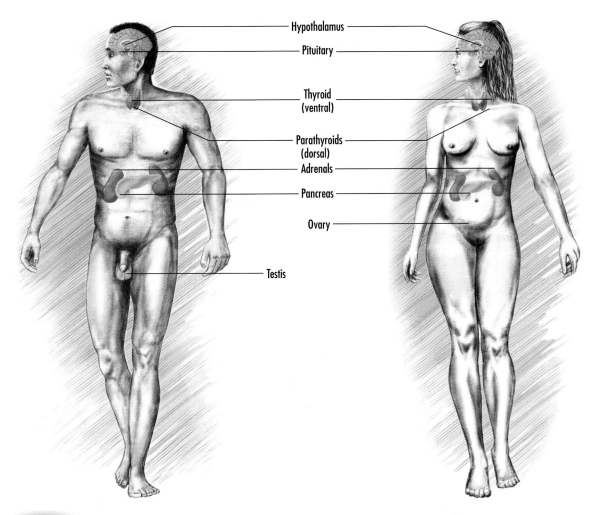

Hypothalamus

Pituitary

Thyroid
(ventral)

Parathyroids
(dorsal)

Adrenals

Pancreas

Ovary

Testis

FIGURE 2.4   Where Hormones Are Released   Hormones are released from different glands throughout the body. The synthesis and release of these hormones are regulated by the mind and autonomic nervous system. Hormones carry chemical messages that tell organs in the body how to respond to stimuli.

hormones and their release in the body is regulated by the mind and nervous system.

Your five senses (sight, hearing, touch, taste, and smell) constantly record whether the environment is safe or hostile, familiar or unfamiliar, pleasurable or painful. In order to be able to respond appropriately to environmental stimuli, the mind must interpret the experiences moment by moment and send chemical signals to the organs of the body. Hormones carry the chemical messages that tell the body how to respond.

For example, when the mind interprets a situation as threatening or frightening, regardless of whether the danger is real or imagined, hormones are released that make the body alert and ready for action. Fear produces an increased heart rate and blood pressure, sweaty palms, changes in breathing, tension in muscles, and so forth. That is why fear, especially if it is prolonged or ongoing, can damage health and increase the risk of sickness.

When people commonly mention stress, they are usually referring to experiences that the mind has difficulty resolving. As a result, the "stress" is converted to hormonal and other chemical changes that affect how the body functions; homeostasis is disturbed. Feelings such as anger, anxiety, frustration, hostility, and guilt may cause adverse hormonal changes. For example, anxiety or guilt can block the release of hormones that are necessary for a sexual response. Because the mind governs the overall chemistry of the body, it is the most important determinant of wellness or illness.

The Mind Can Create Illness or Wellness

The power of the mind to affect the health of the body is illustrated by **psychosomatic illnesses.** When a person is subjected to stress or emotional upset, changes in the body may manifest as diseases (Figure 2.5). The

TABLE 2.1   The Functions of Various Glands and Organs That Produce Hormones

Gland and hormones	Function
Hypothalamus and pituitary glands	
Growth hormone	Stimulates growth of bones and other structures
Adrenocorticotropic hormone (ACTH)	Stimulates release of hormones from the adrenal glands
Thyroid-stimulating hormone	Stimulates growth of the thyroid gland and release of thyroxin
Luteinizing hormone	Stimulates ovaries and the release of ovarian hormones in women; stimulates testes to produce hormones in men
Follicle-stimulating hormone	Stimulates ovum production in women; stimulates sperm production in men
Prolactin	Stimulates milk production in breasts
Testes	
Testosterone	Controls maleness
Ovaries	
Estrogen	Controls aspects of female sexuality and reproduction
Progesterone	Controls aspects of female sexuality and reproduction
Pancreas	
Insulin	Regulates blood sugar levels
Thyroid gland	
Thyroxin	Regulates metabolism
Parathyroid glands	
Calcitonin	Regulates calcium and phosphorus levels
Adrenal glands	
Aldosterone	Regulates water balance in the body
Cortisol	Increases blood glucose
Adrenalin (Epinephrine)	Increases heart rate; activates muscles

terms *psycho* (mind) and *soma* (body) emphasize the connection between the mind and the body with respect to health.

Many people believe that if a person has a psychosomatic illness, he or she is imagining it, that it is "all in the mind." This is not true. The symptoms of a headache brought on by stress can be just as severe as one brought on by being hit over the head with a bat. In one case, stress has caused a change in the flow of blood through the head, and in the other case, blood vessels may have been damaged by the injury. Psychosomatic illnesses are as real as a cold brought on by a virus.

Western medicine is not well equipped to deal with psychosomatic illnesses. Although physicians can treat the symptoms, they are not well trained to help with the underlying mental states that cause the illness. On the other hand, Buddhist and Chinese medicine take the position that all sickness, to some degree, is brought on by a person's state of mind. In Western medicine, if a physician cannot find an organic cause for symptoms, the patient may be advised to see a psychologist or given a drug to mask symptoms.

This view should not be interpreted to mean that sickness is brought on *just* by a person's state of mind, but that our psychological state, at any time, may invite illness. In order for an emotional or mental state to change physiology, a process called **somatization** must occur. Somatization refers to the occurrence of physical symptoms in a person without the presence of disease or injury that can be detected medically.

Psychological and social problems may contribute to pain, fatigue, nausea, diarrhea, sexual dysfunction, and other symptoms that are classified as **somatization disorders** (McCahill, 1995). It is estimated that 25% to 75% of all patients who visit primary care physicians suffer from somatization disorders. These are difficult to treat, time-consuming for physicians to diagnose, and expensive for the health care system. The diagnostic criteria for a somatization disorder are shown in Table 2.2; the chief complaint is pain of long duration in several parts of the body that cannot be explained by any medical condition or injury.

The lives that many people choose to live or are forced to live by financial or family circumstances can cause mind-body disruption that eventually produces pain and sickness. People suffering from somatization disorders are not feigning sickness; they have lost mind-body harmony to a serious degree.

Exam Anxiety

One breakdown in mind-body harmony that everyone has experienced is exam anxiety. People in American society equate educational success, academic degrees, and professional licenses with the attainment of important life goals, particularly financial ones. As a consequence, competition among students at all levels is intense. Students believe that grades and exam scores will determine how successful their lives will be in terms of jobs, careers, and money.

Terms

psychosomatic illnesses: physical illnesses brought on by negative mental states such as stress or emotional upset

somatization: occurrence of physical symptoms without any bodily disease or injury being present

somatization disorder: prolonged pain and other symptoms that are not due to disease or injury

FIGURE 2.5   Psychosomatic Illnesses
Many diseases and disorders of the body are partly caused by thoughts and feelings in the mind that produce psychosomatic illnesses.

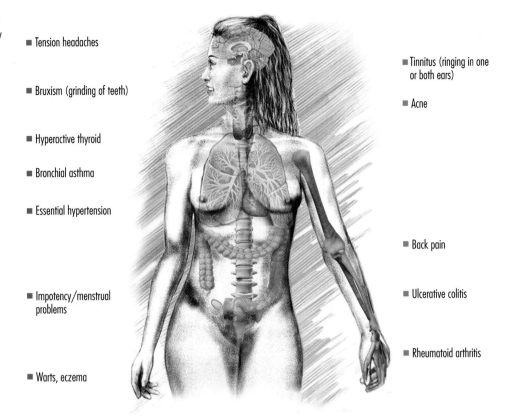

- Tension headaches
- Bruxism (grinding of teeth)
- Hyperactive thyroid
- Bronchial asthma
- Essential hypertension
- Impotency/menstrual problems
- Warts, eczema

- Tinnitus (ringing in one or both ears)
- Acne
- Back pain
- Ulcerative colitis
- Rheumatoid arthritis

Because of academic pressures and anxiety about exams, many students experience health problems. They may suffer from frequent headaches, stomach and bowel problems, eating disorders, recurrent infections, and other symptoms of stress (see chapter 3). Students whose exam anxiety affects their health need to make personal adjustments to reduce the anxiety while they pursue their goals.

The first thing to realize is that exam anxiety is learned behavior and probably began very early in school. Perhaps parents or teachers scolded you or warned you about the consequences of poor performance. Like any undesirable learned behavior, exam anxiety can be unlearned or the stressful response to taking an exam can be changed. The anxiety a student feels about an exam is often related to the importance he or she attaches to the exam or grade *(If I get a B in this course, my life is ruined!)*. The first step to reduce exam anxiety is to realize that life does not hinge on the results of one exam or one course, or even several. Another powerful technique to reduce this type of anxiety is to practice a visualization exercise before taking an exam.

The Placebo Effect

The healing that results from a person's belief in a harmless substance or a treatment that has no medical

TABLE 2.2   Diagnostic Criteria for Somatization Disorder

A. History of physical complaints begins before age 30, lasts for several years, and results in the request for treatment or in significantly impaired social, occupational, or other types of functioning.

B. Each of these four criteria must be met, with individual symptoms occurring at any time:
  1. History of pain related to at least four sites or functions
  2. History of at least two gastrointestinal symptoms other than pain
  3. History of at least one sexual or reproductive symptom other than pain
  4. History of at least one symptom or deficit suggesting a neurologic condition not limited to pain (a conversion symptom, a dissociative symptom, or loss of consciousness other than fainting)

C. One of these two criteria must be met:
  1. Symptoms in B cannot be explained by a medical condition or the effects of a substance.
  2. When there is a related medical condition, the physical complaint or the resulting social or occupational impairment is in excess of what would be expected from the history, physical examination, or laboratory findings.

D. Symptoms are not intentionally produced or feigned.

Source: American Psychiatric Association. (1994). *Diagnostic and statistical manual of mental disorders* (4th ed.). Washington, DC: American Psychiatric Association. Copyright 1994, American Psychiatric Association. Reprinted with permission.

value is called a **placebo effect.** The term *placebo* first appeared in the 116th Psalm in the Old Testament. The English translation of the biblical word is "I shall please." In 1785, *placebo* appeared in a medical dictionary, where it was defined as "a commonplace medicine or treatment." Later the term came to mean a make-believe medicine or a sugar pill. Today anything that a person takes or believes in that has a healing effect can be called a placebo. Prayer, meditation, suggestion, hypnosis, good luck charms, laughter, elixirs, and sugar pills all act as placebos to heal and cure.

How powerful is the placebo effect? What kinds of illness and disease respond to placebos? Although the curative power of placebos has been demonstrated scientifically in many experiments, few people really appreciate what placebos can accomplish in curing diseases. Remember that in any placebo effect, it is really the mind that is changing physiology and causing the cure.

Drugs or Placebos: Which Are More Effective?

Depression is often present in patients who seek medical attention for other symptoms; it is especially common among patients who have a somatization disorder. Whether the depression contributes to the physical symptoms or results from them is usually impossible to determine. In either event, the depression should be treated. A variety of drugs are now available for treating depression, including Prozac, one of the most widely publicized antidepressants.

Before being approved by the Food and Drug Administration (FDA), all drugs (including those used to treat depression) must be tested in a double-blind, placebo-controlled study. Figure 2.6 shows the results of such a study comparing the efficacy of two antide-

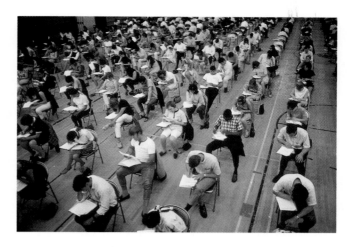

Academic pressures and test taking can produce anxiety and stress.

pressant drugs with placebo pills given as a control; notice that for 3 months depressed patients got almost as much relief from the placebo as from the antidepressant drugs. Why the effect wears off after several months is anyone's guess; perhaps the control group sensed that they were receiving placebos.

Terms

placebo effect: healing that results from a person's belief in a treatment that has no medicinal value

---

Managing Stress

Visualization Reduces Exam Anxiety

The following exercise can reduce the stress and anxiety of taking exams. It can result in improved scores and a reduction in symptoms produced by stress.

1. Find a comfortable place in your house or room and a time when you will not be disturbed by other people. Sit in a comfortable chair or lie down on a couch or floor. The main thing is to get physically comfortable. If music helps you relax, play some of your favorite music softly.

2. Close your eyes and ask your mind to recall a place and time where you felt contented. It might be a vacation time, being with someone, or being alone in a beautiful environment. Use

your imagination and memory to reconstruct the scene where you felt happy and healthy. Notice that you had no concerns there at that time. Let yourself become involved with the scene. The process is similar to having a daydream or a fantasy. While your mind is focused on pleasurable memories, your body automatically relaxes.

3. When you feel quite relaxed, refocus your mind on the upcoming exam. See yourself taking the exam while feeling relaxed and confident. Because your mind and body are relaxed and comfortable, your mind automatically associates the same feelings with the image of taking the exam. Visualize the exam room, the other

students, yourself answering the questions; let your mind focus on as many details as possible.

4. Now project your mind into the future to the actual day and place of the exam. Notice how relaxed you feel as you take the exam; the anxiety you used to experience seems to have vanished. Continue with the visualization until you see yourself turning in the exam and feeling confident and pleased with your performance.

5. Do this exercise for several days prior to any exam that causes anxiety. You will be surprised at the absence of nervousness and stress on exam day. You will be even more pleased at the improvement in your grades.

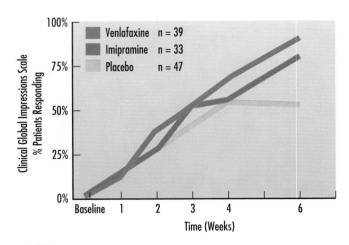

FIGURE 2.6 **Placebo Study** A double-blind, placebo-controlled study comparing two antidepressant drugs, venlafaxine and imipramine, with placebo in reducing the symptoms of clinical depression. (*n* is the number of patients in each group.) For at least 1 month, just as many patients received relief of their symptoms with a placebo as with either antidepressant drug.

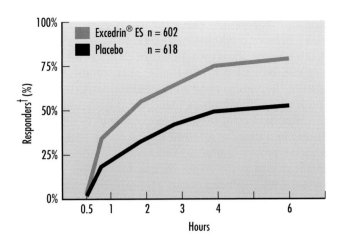

FIGURE 2.7 Double-blind, placebo-controlled study comparing Excedrin® and placebo in relieving the pain of migraine headache†. A responder is a patient with moderate or severe pain whose pain was reduced to mild or none following treatment. Note that more than half of over 600 patients with migraine headache had mild or no pain after taking a placebo pill.

The effectiveness of placebos in treating depression was supported when development of a new antidepressant drug was canceled by Merck after clinical trials showed that their new drug, MK-869, was actually *less* effective than the placebo pill in treating patients with depression (Enserink, 1999). In addition, an analysis of 19 antidepressant drugs showed that the placebo effect accounted for, on average, 75 percent of the relief of any of the drugs currently being prescribed to treat depression. This indicates that depression is caused by mental states that most patients are capable of reversing on their own, simply by believing that they are receiving an effective therapy.

One might argue that placebos are only effective in reversing diseases of the mind but not the body. This does not seem to be true, however. Pain is a symptom that responds exceptionally well to the placebo effect, which often provides as much relief as analgesic or even opioid drugs (see Figure 2.7). In relieving pain, placebos, like drugs, affect physiology rather than merely change the mind's perception of the pain. The effect of the placebo in pain relief can be blocked by administering a drug called naloxone, which blocks the action of pain-relieving drugs (Christensen, 2001).

Another remarkable placebo effect was reported in which a protein (vascular endothelial growth factor, or VEGF) was being tested on patients with angina (i.e., chest pain due to restricted supply of blood to the heart). The drug was supposed to stimulate the growth of new blood vessels in the heart and relieve angina. After 10 months of treatment with VEGF, patients were evaluated for chest pain during a treadmill test. Patients who received the placebo had less pain and performed longer on the treadmill test than patients who had received VEGF.

Other biological processes or illnesses that respond to a placebo include ulcers, postoperative pain, seasickness, headaches, coughs, rheumatoid arthritis, blood cell counts, hay fever, hypertension, and warts. The number of people responding to placebos for any kind of symptom range from about 30 to 70 percent; most studies report about a 50 percent response. What does this mean? For almost any disease or symptom, a person has a 50 percent chance of being cured simply by believing in the power of a placebo pill, prayer, a suggestion from a physician, an herbal tea, or magic.

Because the placebo effect is so powerful in healing, we discuss it in other chapters to emphasize the power of the mind in overcoming many diseases and conditions. For example, placebos have reversed tumor progression in some cancer patients (chapter 13). And placebos are about half as effective as drugs in blocking nicotine addiction (chapter 17).

The Dark Side of Placebos

Why, if placebos are so effective in healing, are they not used more by physicians in treating patients? One reason is an ethical dilemma for physicians: a placebo might work for one patient but not for another. While the same could be true for a prescribed drug, the physician is protected legally by prescribing a drug that has been clinically tested and approved by the FDA. However, no legal protection exists for a physician prescribing a placebo if the patient decides to sue, claiming that the treatment did not meet accepted medical standards.

Yet another reason that placebos are not part of medical practice is that placebos can be dangerous, just as drugs can be dangerous. Patients can become addicted to placebo pills used for pain relief and suffer withdrawal symptoms when they stop using them.

Also, like prescription drugs, placebo pills can cause side effects, which further complicates their use. For example, in one experiment, 40 volunteer asthmatic patients were asked to inhale a placebo spray, which they were told contained an allergen. Twelve of the volunteers had full-blown asthma attacks and seven had lesser symptoms (Brown, 1998). The asthma attacks were reversed by inhalation of another placebo spray, which they were told would relieve the symptoms.

Words can produce a placebo effect in the same way as a pill. Because of this fact, you should always seek out health practitioners whom you trust and who use positive, constructive healing suggestions and who encourage you to become involved in self-healing practices. Avoid health practitioners who voice negative and pessimistic recommendations. No one needs to hear negative suggestions such as "You'll probably have to take these pills for the rest of your life," or "I doubt that you'll be able to move around much after an accident like that." In the presence of a physician many patients become very open to suggestions, both positive and negative, because their minds are intently focused on what the doctor is saying. Such a focused state of mind is similar to that obtained in meditation or hypnosis. It is more helpful to practice being alert and critical when discussing your health concerns or diagnostic test results with a health professional. Of course, this is not always easy to do, especially when the information being conveyed causes distress or fear.

A tragic, but dramatic, example of mind-body communication and the power of a negative placebo effect involved a patient who died apparently from reading a single word (Hewlett, 1994). This person had a history of chronic lymphatic leukemia, a form of blood cancer that usually is easily controlled with drugs. The patient had been well for more than 3 years with only intermittent need for medication. However, he had never actually been informed of the original diagnosis of his condition.

One day he was in his physician's office on a routine visit and happened to read the physician's notes, which were lying on the desk. He saw the word *leukemia* in his file. He missed his next scheduled office visit and shortly thereafter showed up in the hospital's emergency room. Within 3 weeks he died in the hospital. No cause of death could be discovered at autopsy, and his leukemia was still in remission. The patient apparently *believed* that he had terminal cancer just from seeing the word *leukemia* in his medical records. The mind *does* heal; the mind *does* kill.

Faith and Healing

Thousands of years ago the priest-healers of ancient civilizations and the shamans of primitive tribes used the beliefs of their people to heal by incantation, to exorcise evil spirits, and to vanquish demons who were thought to cause disease. The existence of shamans, faith healers, and medicine men in cultures throughout human history suggests that their healing methods must have been generally successful. Egyptian papyri show that although the priest-physicians of ancient Egypt prescribed herbs and performed surgeries, their treatments relied on the belief of the people in the healing power of the gods. Priests would put patients into a trance in a temple and tell them that when they awakened, they would be healed. And often they were.

> *Faith. You can do little with it and nothing without it.*
> SAMUEL BUTLER

The Greeks and Romans also had gods, oracles, and temples of healing. Their priests also used trance and sleeplike mental states to impart healing suggestions to receptive minds. Sometimes "miraculous cures" resulted. Greek and Roman emperors and priests also healed by the "laying on of hands"; people were healed because they believed that their rulers had divine powers. King Pyrrhus of Epirus is reputed to have cured sick patients solely by the touch of his big toe.

All religions teach that divine persons have the power to heal. The New Testament recounts many examples of the healing power of Jesus.

> That evening they brought him many who were possessed with demons, and he cast out the spirits with a word, and healed all who were sick.
> —*Matthew 8:14*

> And he said to her, "Daughter, your faith has made you well; go in peace and be healed of your diseases."
> —*Mark 5:34*

Over the centuries, faith and prayer have healed many people. Some ascribe healing to the power of God; others explain it by the power of belief in producing a placebo effect.

Today's patients have faith in the knowledge of their physicians and the drugs they prescribe just as people of ancient civilizations believed in their priests and herbs. The improvement in any patient's condition is a combination of faith in the healer and the efficacy of the treatment.

Religion and Health

Associations between religious practices and health have been studied for more than a century. Recent studies have shown that Seventh Day Adventists and Mormons are healthier and have lower mortality rates than people in the general population. These religions prohibit tobacco and alcohol use and promote largely vegetarian diets. These factors contribute to the overall health of people generally.

Studies also have found evidence suggesting that the more dedicated people are in attending church services, the healthier they are irrespective of other factors. One large study that followed attendance at religious services over a period of 28 years concluded that church-goers do indeed have lower mortality rates than non-churchgoers (Strawbridge et al., 1997). This might be due to increased social contacts, better health practices, more stable marriages, or a combination of factors.

Nearly 30 U.S. medical schools offer courses on religion, spirituality, and health, but not all physicians are convinced that physicians should advocate church attendance. Part of the concern stems from the overall weakness of scientific studies that find a positive effect of church attendance on health. As some critics point out:

> Attempts to use religion instrumentally, as one uses antibiotics or surgical procedures to treat diseases, may be deeply offensive to some people. . . . Most important, we are concerned that attempts to obtain scientific evidence of health benefits of religious activity and to use such activity instrumentally in achieving beneficial health outcomes not only are superficial but also suggest that the value of religion derives from its effects on health. Religion . . . is a spiritual way of being in the world (Sloan et al., 2000).

However the scientific arguments about religion and health are interpreted, polls show that more than half of all Americans believe that their faith has helped them recover from a particular illness or injury.

Hypnosis and Healing

The modern use of hypnosis as a medical technique began with the Viennese physician, Franz Anton Mesmer, who practiced in the late eighteenth and early nineteenth centuries. History has preserved the term *mesmerism* for the trancelike state that Mesmer produced in his patients. Many years later, a Scottish physician, James Braid, introduced the term *hypnosis* (from the Greek *hypnos,* meaning sleep) and began to practice **hypnotherapy,** the use of hypnosis to cure sickness.

Mesmer called his technique for healing "animal magnetism" because he had his patients hold onto metal rods that supposedly transmitted healing energy while they were in trance. Mesmer was so successful that other physicians in Vienna forced the authorities to order him to stop using his unorthodox methods. In 1778 Mesmer moved to Paris where he again was successful in attracting patients. Eventually, the French authorities appointed a scientific panel, which included Benjamin Franklin (U.S. ambassador to France at the time), to investigate Mesmer and his methods. The panel concluded that there was no scientific basis to animal magnetism and that Mesmer was a fraud. This conclusion was reached even though the panel did not dispute Mesmer's success in curing many patients. Discredited by physicians and scientists, Mesmer died in obscurity in 1815.

Despite being officially discredited, mesmerism (now called hypnotism) flourished throughout England, Europe, and the United States in the nineteenth century. In 1847, J. W. Robbins, a Massachusetts physician, reported using hypnotherapy to treat eating disorders and to help people stop smoking. Dr. Robbins used aversive suggestions while patients were in trance and also gave them posthypnotic suggestions. Many of the same procedures are used today in treating these and other behavioral disorders.

In the late nineteenth century, two French physicians showed that healing could be accomplished solely by suggestion and that cures resulted from the patient's expectation of being cured. Hippolyte-Marie Bernheim, who used hypnotherapy successfully with

Wellness Guide

Healing Prayers

Most people pray when they or loved ones become seriously ill or injured. Prayer certainly helps to relieve a sense of helplessness and despair that inevitably arises during a period of life-threatening illness. But can prayer actually help the healing process? A recent study examined the effectiveness of intercessory prayer on the outcomes of seriously ill patients admitted to the coronary care unit of a hospital (Harris et al., 1999). Patients were randomized to receive remote, intercessory prayer or not to receive such prayer (the placebo group). The first names of patients in the prayer group were given to outside intercessors who prayed for them daily for four weeks. Patients did not know they were being prayed for, nor did the intercessors know or meet the patients.

The results of the study showed that patients who were prayed for had fewer complications and a shorter hospital stay than patients not receiving intercessory prayer. So, the next time you want to pray for someone who is seriously ill, you can do so with the expectation that it might just help.

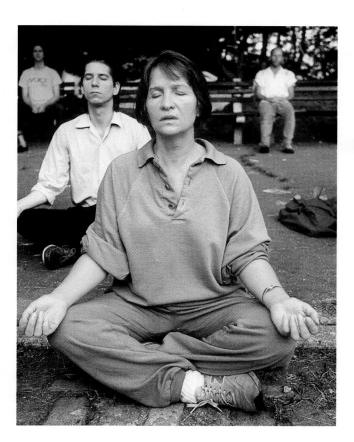

Meditation can be done anywhere, anytime.

pend on the degree of mental relaxation involved. For reasons that are not entirely clear, a mind engaged in the conscious thoughts of daily living is not as open to suggestion as one that is internally relaxed by hypnosis, meditation, or other mental relaxation techniques.

The Relaxation Response

In 1975 Herbert Benson and his colleagues at Harvard Medical School (Benson et al., 1975) studied the effects of various relaxation techniques on human physiology. They discovered that hypnosis; **meditation,** in which the person focuses on breathing, a sound, or an image; and **yoga,** a combination of physical movements and mental focusing, all produce similar physiological responses. They found that persons practicing these techniques had lower blood pressure and heart rate, reduced oxygen consumption, more relaxed muscles, and reduced perspiration.

Benson called the sum of these physiological effects the **relaxation response.** He found that, regardless

thousands of patients, argued that almost all healing resulted from suggestions he gave receptive patients while they were in trance.

Effective use of suggestion in healing seems to de-

Terms

hypnotherapy: the use of hypnosis to treat sickness

meditation: relaxed state of mind produced by focusing the mind on internal images, sounds, or passing thoughts

yoga: a combination of physical movements and mental exercises that relax the mind and the body

relaxation response: the physiological changes in the body that result from mental relaxation techniques

Managing Stress

Progressive Muscle Relaxation

In the technique called progressive relaxation, you lie on your back in quiet, comfortable surroundings with your feet slightly apart and palms facing upward. Before beginning the exercise allow the thoughts of the day and any worries to leave your mind. Then you are ready to begin.

1. Close your eyes; squeeze your lids shut as tightly as you can. Hold them shut for a count of five; then slowly release the tension. Notice how your eyes feel as they relax. Keep your eyelids lightly closed; breathe slowly and deeply.

2. Turn your palms down. Bend your left hand back

at the wrist, keeping your forearm on the floor. Bend your hand as far as it will go until you feel tension in your forearm muscles. Hold for a count of five; then release the tension. Notice the warm, relaxed sensation that enters your wrist. Repeat with your right hand.

3. With palms up, make a tight fist in your left hand by tightening the muscles of the arm and fingers. Hold for a count of five; release the tension. Notice the tingling, relaxed sensation in your hand and arm. Repeat with your right hand.

4. Focus your attention on your left leg; slowly bring the top of your foot as far forward as you can while keeping your heel on the floor. Notice the tension in the muscles of your lower leg. Hold for a count of five; release the tension. Repeat with your right leg.

5. Point the toes in your left foot away from you as far as you can. Notice the tension in your calf muscles. Release the tension slowly. Repeat with your right foot.

Similar exercises can be performed to tense and relax other muscles.

of the relaxation technique used, the relaxation response embraced four common elements: (1) a quiet environment; (2) repetition of a specific word, phrase, or exercise that focuses on the mind's attention; (3) a passive, accepting mental state; and (4) a comfortable physical position. One simple, relaxation technique that anyone can learn quite easily is **progressive muscle relaxation.**

> *Meditation is not what you think.*
> KRISHNAMURTI

Meditation

Meditation has been associated with both Eastern and Western religions for centuries. Meditation is simply focused awareness. If you examine what is going on in your mind at any given moment, odds are you will find it flitting from one thought to another: "Did I remember to turn off the stove before I left the house?" "My feet are killing me; I shouldn't have worn these shoes." "I wonder what mood she's going to be in tonight?" "Did the kids say something about going to a sleepover this weekend?" Our minds are generally constantly active and often involved in worrying or thinking about emotional upsets, financial concerns, or the pressures of daily activities.

Quieting the mind is healthy and meditation is a way to accomplish that. Focused awareness can be achieved in a number of ways, and there are many different kinds of meditation. *Zen meditation* (zazen) involves sitting still with legs crossed while trying to empty the mind of its chatter. *Transcendental meditation* teaches practitioners to focus on a particular phrase (called a **mantra**) that is repeated internally; focusing the mind's attention on a single phrase excludes other random thoughts. *Insight meditation* (Vipassana) teaches meditators simply to observe the flow of thoughts that pass through the mind with detachment. Buddhists, especially Tibetan Buddhists, often meditate by focusing their attention on a religious image (called a **mandala**). Prayer is a form of meditation in that it focuses awareness on God. Thus, meditation is something that everyone has experienced even if they have not called it meditation.

Meditation does not have to be done in a religious setting, nor is it complicated. To begin meditating, follow these simple suggestions:

- Choose a quiet place in your home or outside.
- Find a comfortable sitting position with your back straight. (Lying down is not recommended since it is strongly associated with sleep.)
- Be sure that you have at least 10 to 30 minutes during which you will not be disturbed.

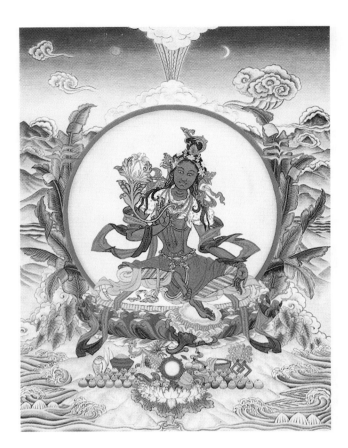

A mandala is a complex visual image used to focus attention and facilitate meditation. ("Green Tara," an original painting by Maile Yawata)

- A good way to begin meditation is to focus your attention on breathing. Begin by becoming aware of the way you are breathing. Is it slow and deep? Is it quick and shallow? Is it through one nostril or both?

Gradually try to breathe by using your stomach muscles to move your diaphragm. Some people recommend the 4/7/8 pattern of breathing—inhale through the nose for a count of 4, hold for a count of 7, and exhale for a count of 8 through pursed lips. If this sequence is not comfortable, make up your own and focus on taking each breath the same way.

Practice this meditation twice a day, particularly if you are upset, tired, or in pain. Once you are comfortable with a breathing meditation, you may want to explore other forms of meditation. Meditation has many documented health benefits—lowered blood pressure, decreased heart rates, less stress, increased blood flow, reduced pain, and relief of many chronic conditions such as asthma, arthritis, and irritable bowel syndrome.

The faster the world becomes, the more we need to slow down.

Wellness Guide

Using Your Mind to Improve Health

- Become more aware of the power your mind has to improve health, hasten healing, and help you perform better in school and in other activities. Belief in yourself, in prayer, or in a particular treatment can facilitate healing and help prevent sickness.

- Use mental images that feel right to you to reduce exam anxiety and to improve performance in sports or other activities. Avoid negative mental images and thoughts such as "I feel lousy," or "I'm too tired to run," or "I just know I can't do that." Use your mind to create positive images and thoughts. You can reverse what seems to be a "bad" day by suggesting to yourself that things are going to change and improve.

- Practice a daily mental relaxation technique in a place that is comfortable and quiet. Use the time to "talk" to your body to promote healing or to change behaviors. Visualize scenes from the past or the future that you know are healthy and constructive. As you become more adept at using your mind, you will find new ways to use mental relaxation in all aspects of your life. (*Notice how we inserted a positive suggestion.*)

The Power of Suggestion

Anytime the mind becomes focused and relaxed, it also becomes more open to suggestion. This can be very beneficial or it can create problems, depending on the kind of suggestions being received by the mind. Suggestions given as warnings, especially to children who are particularly vulnerable to suggestion, can affect behaviors and cause health problems throughout life. For example, here are some common admonitions given to children that can cause health problems, because young children *believe* what they are told.

- Put on your boots when you go out in the snow or you will catch cold.
- If you keep eating cookies, you'll get fat.
- If you don't try harder, you'll be a failure in life.
- If you climb those trees, you'll fall and get hurt.
- If you go out at night, the ghosts will get you.

Each of these suggestions predicts a negative outcome. To a child's mind, which is usually in a trance-like, suggestible state, these negative suggestions become fixed in the unconscious mind and may have a harmful effect even many years later.

The mind can be made more open to suggestion by many things we are exposed to in daily life. For example, movies and television focus attention with both images and sound. As a consequence, they can induce a trancelike state and cause us to cry, laugh, and become angry or upset; they can actually manipulate our emotions through light and sound. No one dies on a movie screen, but we often react as if they did. The violence and horror people watch at movies and on TV often do affect both physical and emotional states. As a result of watching some frightening scene, people may actually become sick days, weeks, or years later when something reminds the subconscious mind of the scene and brings back the fear.

Advertisers know how to take advantage of viewers' suggestible, hypnotic states of mind. Television programs usually are interrupted at an emotional peak in the story by advertising a product while viewers are still in a suggestible state of mind. Many people believe they are not influenced by advertising, but marketing studies indicate otherwise. Most advertisers try to persuade people to buy products they usually do not need. It is important to become more aware of how suggestible you are and to protect yourself from both obvious and subtle suggestions that can damage your health and peace of mind.

Image Visualization

One of the most effective ways to promote wellness and change undesirable behaviors is through the use of **image visualization.** Many mind-body healing techniques employ some form of image visualization. For example, frightening scenes from the past, especially from early childhood, can be reexperienced while a person is in a state of mental relaxation brought on by hypnosis or some other technique. As the scenes and

Terms

progressive muscle relaxation: a specific technique that produces relaxation by tensing and relaxing muscles

mantra: a sound or phrase that is repeated in the mind to help produce a meditative state

mandala: an artistic, religious design used as an object of meditation

image visualization: use of mental images to promote healing and change behaviors

emotional upsets are visualized in the mind, they can be reinterpreted and reprogrammed to change their negative effects on health and behaviors. Mental imagery can also be used to reduce pain; hasten healing; improve performance in sports; change smoking, drinking, or eating behaviors; and help control compulsive urges to gamble. At one time or another in our lives, we all daydream or run an "internal movie," fantasizing our hopes and fears. During such fantasies we visualize experiences and create feelings. Image visualization can change body temperature, blood flow, heartbeat, breathing rate, production of hormones, and other body processes regulated by the brain.

Most psychologists who work with athletes to improve physical performance use image visualization. The so-called inner games of tennis, golf, skiing, and skating are based on image visualization. Baseball players in a batting slump use relaxation and visualization to "see" themselves getting hits. Basketball players use the technique to "see" their free throws going cleanly through the hoop.

Image visualization is also the secret to improved sexual responses and enjoyment. Sexual arousal begins in the mind and negative thoughts or fears can stifle the sexual responses. The sex organs are particularly sensitive to images generated in the mind. Most sex therapists use relaxation techniques and image visualization to help clients improve their sexual experiences. Tension related to sexual performance is usually the main reason for not experiencing the desired sexual sensations. In all areas of your life, begin to use your mental powers more to enhance health and improve performance in daily tasks.

> *We are what we pretend to be, so we better be careful what we pretend to be . . .*
> KURT VONNEGUT
> *MOTHER NIGHT*

Critical Thinking About Health

1. Identify one time in your life when you have been seriously ill (not counting colds or minor injuries). Describe the nature of the illness and the time it took to become well again. Discuss all of the factors that you think may have contributed to your becoming sick, including stress, emotional problems, poor nutrition, and so forth. Then discuss all of the factors that you believe contributed to your becoming well again, including medical care, prayer, alternative medicines, and other factors. What were the most important factors that led to your becoming sick; what were the most important ones in the healing process?

2. Find a selection of medical journals in the library and look at the drug company advertisements. Try to locate ones that show a comparison of the drug's effectiveness with a placebo. Determine how effective the placebo was from the data given (usually shown in a graph). Then compare the effectiveness of the drug with the placebo. If the placebo was effective, explain why you think it was so effective in this instance. Give your views on whether doctors should prescribe a placebo pill for some conditions before prescribing an active drug.

3. Do you experience test anxiety to such a degree that you become physically or emotionally upset before or after taking an exam? If so, describe your symptoms and feelings. If you have an exam that makes you anxious coming up in the next few weeks, try the exercise described in the "Managing Stress" box, *Visualization Reduces Exam Anxiety*, for at least a week before taking the exam. After the exam describe your experience in detail and indicate whether you performed better than you expected on the exam.

4. Describe any experiences you have had with meditation, hypnosis, yoga, qigong, image visualization, or any other form of mental focusing and relaxation. Describe how you became involved with this activity and for what purpose you used it. Did it help you solve a particular health or emotional problem? Would you recommend this technique to others?

Health in Review

- The human mind can cause changes in body chemistry through thoughts and feelings, which may have a positive or negative effect on your health.
- Optimal health is achieved when the mind and body communicate harmoniously.
- The unconscious regulation of all vital processes in the body is called homeostasis.
- Disease can be regarded as disruption of homeostasis or disruption of the harmonious interaction of mind and body.
- The mind and organs of the body communicate continuously via the autonomic nervous system, which maintains vital body functions such as heart rate, level of blood sugar, and temperature.
- Psychosomatic illnesses are physical symptoms caused by stress, anxiety, and emotional upsets.

- Somatization disorders are caused by psychosocial problems.
- The placebo effect often is almost as powerful as drugs in treating symptoms of illness.
- Religious activity is often associated with a healthier lifestyle.
- Hypnosis and meditation can play a positive role in healing psychosomatic illnesses.
- Belief, faith, and suggestion all have the power to heal because the mind can change disturbed body functions and reestablish homeostasis.
- A key to maintaining or improving health and wellness is to learn and practice a mental relaxation technique.
- Image visualization can be used to reduce anxiety and stress, modify behaviors, and enhance performance.

Health and Wellness Online

The World Wide Web contains a wealth of information about health and wellness. By accessing the Internet using Web browser software, such as Netscape Navigator or Microsoft's Internet Explorer, you can gain a new perspective on many topics presented in *Health and Wellness, Seventh Edition.* Access the Jones and Bartlett Publishers Web site at http://www.jbpub.com/hwonline.

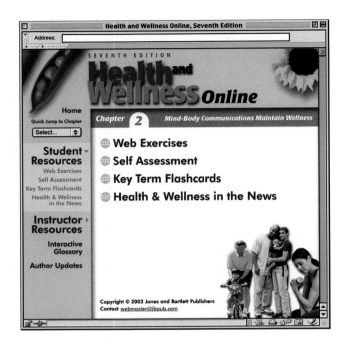

References

Benson, H., Greenwood, M., and Klemchuk, H. (1975). The relaxation response: Psychophysiologic aspects and clinical applications. *International Journal of Psychiatric Medicine, 6,* 87–98.

Brown, W. A. (1998, July 15). Harnessing the placebo effect. *Hospital Practice,* 107–116.

Christensen, D. (2001). Medicinal mimicry. *Science News, 159,* 74–76.

Enserink, M. (1999). Can the placebo be the cure? *Science, 284,* 238–240.

Harris, W. S., et al. (1999). A randomized, controlled trial of the effects of remote, intercessory prayer on outcomes in patients admitted to the coronary care unit. *Archives of Internal Medicine, 159,* 2273–2278.

Hewlett, C. (1994). Killed by a word. *Lancet, 344,* 695.

Sloan, R. P., et al. (2000). Should physicians prescribe religious activities? *New England Journal of Medicine, 342,* 1913–1916.

Strawbridge, W. J., Cohen, R. D., Shema, S. J., and Kaplan, G. A. (1997). *American Journal of Public Health, 87,* 957–961.

Taylor, E., Lee, C. T., and Young, J. D. E. (1997, May 15). Bringing mind-body medicine into the mainstream. *Hospital Practice,* 183–196.

Suggested Readings

Brown, W. A. (1998, January). The placebo effect. *Scientific American*, 90–95. A short article documenting the power of the placebo effect in relieving pain and curing a remarkable range of illnesses. Read this one to convince yourself of the power of your mind.

Christensen, D. (2001). Medicinal Mimicry—Sometimes placebos work—but how? *Science News*, *159*, 74. A brief discussion of the placebo effect and experiments that try to uncover the mechanisms by which it alters physiology.

Cohen, K. S. (1997). *The way of Qigong*. New York: Ballantine. The definitive guide to qigong—what it is, how it works, and what it can do for you.

Hendricks, G. (1995). *Conscious Breathing*. New York: Bantam Books. Explains the benefits of breathing meditations and describes many advanced techniques for practicing conscious breathing.

LeShan, L. (1999). *How to Meditate*. Boston: Back Bay Books. A good introduction to the practice of meditation and its benefits.

Miller, E. E. Source Cassette Learning Systems (www.DrMiller.com). A good source for cassettes that facilitate meditation, image visualization, self-hypnosis, stress reduction, and healing.

Learning Objectives

1. Define the terms stress, stressor, eustress, distress, and stress-related illness.
2. Describe the changes in behavior, autonomic nervous system, and immune system that are caused by stress.
3. Name several stress-related illnesses.
4. Identify and explain the three components of stress.
5. Explain how frustration, inner conflict, and social pressures cause stress.
6. Discuss three common reactions to stress.
7. Discuss several factors that influence the degree of stress a person experiences.
8. Explain the fight-or-flight response.
9. Describe the three phases of the general adaptation syndrome.
10. Describe how stress affects the immune system.
11. Explain how stress can be managed.

Study Guide and Self Assessment

What Are Your Stress Reactions?
How Susceptible Are You to Stress?
Do You Have Hurry Sickness?

Health and Wellness Online

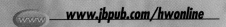 **www.jbpub.com/hwonline**

Chapter 3

Managing Stress: Restoring Mind-Body Harmony

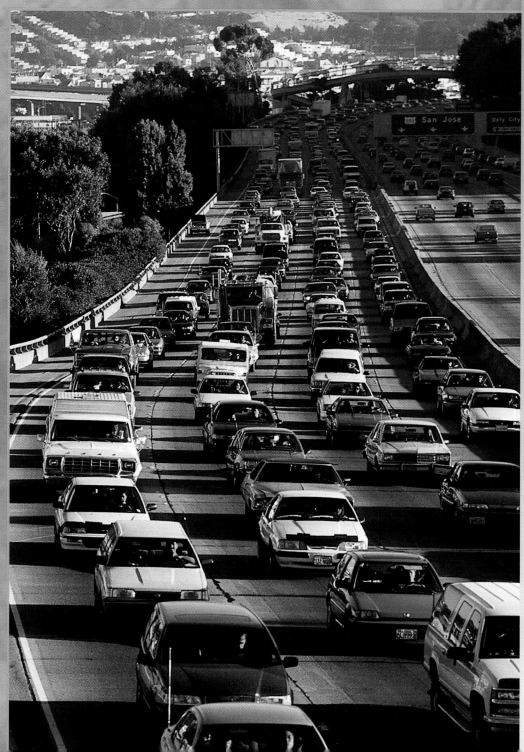

Life is filled with a never-ending array of challenges. Some of them are obstacles to accomplishing necessary daily tasks or cherished life goals. Others are opportunities for growth and positive changes in our lives. When confronted with a particular challenge—whether it be earning good grades in school, obtaining a well-paying job, becoming a parent, becoming involved in a social relationship, or living with an uncompromising roommate—we may feel excited, anxious, sad, depressed, angry, or afraid. Such feelings may cause symptoms like sleeplessness, gastrointestinal upset, headache, and muscular tension, all of which signal a disruption of psychobiological balance. Usually this disruption is brief, because we find ways to meet the challenge and to restore our well-being. Confronting and resolving a challenge often becomes a positive growth experience. Other times, however, disruption in mind-body harmony is prolonged or severe, and we are said to be "under stress" or "stressed out." Prolonged, unresolved stress can contribute to the development of several kinds of disorders.

In this chapter we discuss the various definitions of *stress* and how the manifestation of stress may lead to illness. We also suggest ways to reduce stress and to prevent stress-related illness.

> *Heavy thoughts bring on physical maladies; when the soul is oppressed, so is the body.*
>
> MARTIN LUTHER

The Definition of Stress

Although most people have at some time considered themselves "under stress" or "stressed out," it is important to take note of the difference in how the word *stress* is used. When someone is "under stress," stress refers to the *cause* of the disruption of mind-body harmony; for example, "She was under stress from having to take five exams in two days." On the other hand, "stressed out" refers to the *experience* of the disruption in mind-body harmony; for example, "During final exams she was so stressed out that she suffered from stomach cramps, diarrhea, and insomnia."

Because it is confusing to use the word *stress* to represent both causes and results of challenging or disruptive life experiences, we use the term **stressor** in this chapter to refer to circumstances and events that produce disruptions in mind-body harmony. We use the term **stress** to refer to the symptoms resulting from stressors.

Defining stress in terms of a person's response focuses attention on an individual's experience rather than on external factors (the stressors). By doing this, the avoidance or prevention of stress is largely under the control of the individual, and it is suggested that stress-related illnesses can be prevented. In many instances, people can minimize their interaction with or even avoid a stressor. They can change how they perceive a challenging situation and thereby lessen their degree of distress. And they can use physical, mental, and social resources to help them meet the challenge without incurring a stress-related illness.

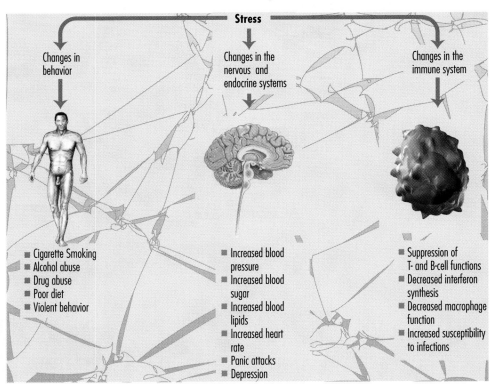

FIGURE 3.1   Stress Causes Physiological Changes Relationships between stress and changes in the nervous, endocrine, and immune systems.

Stress

Changes in behavior
- Cigarette Smoking
- Alcohol abuse
- Drug abuse
- Poor diet
- Violent behavior

Changes in the nervous and endocrine systems
- Increased blood pressure
- Increased blood sugar
- Increased blood lipids
- Increased heart rate
- Panic attacks
- Depression

Changes in the immune system
- Suppression of T- and B-cell functions
- Decreased interferon synthesis
- Decreased macrophage function
- Increased susceptibility to infections

How Stress Contributes to Illness

Stress-related illnesses, such as high blood pressure (hypertension), asthma, gastrointestinal upset, and skin problems are considered psychophysiological or psychosomatic disorders. These illnesses are not phantoms, as the term *psychosomatic* is sometimes thought to mean, but are real physical conditions.

When we experience a challenging situation, the nervous, endocrine (hormone), and immune systems respond to meet the challenge. These responses are aspects of normal physiology that are meant to deal with short-term stressful situations. Illness arises when the body's stress-response mechanisms are continually activated. Then, organs wear down and become diseased, and lowered immunity leads to increased susceptibility to infections and other diseases (Figure 3.1).

Stress also contributes to illness by fostering unhealthy behaviors. To manage stressful feelings, for example, some people smoke cigarettes, drink alcohol (or take other drugs), overeat, undereat, or overwork. Furthermore, people with high levels of stress may not engage in health-promoting activities, such as exercising regularly, eating properly, and getting enough sleep.

Stress has three components (Figure 3.2):

1. *Activators:* occurrences, situations, and events that are potential stressors
2. *Reactions:* interpretations of activators as taxing or exceeding one's mental, physical, and social resources to cope with them successfully. For example, taking six courses in a school term becomes an activator when the student interprets that course load as potentially overwhelming and becomes anxious about completing the work successfully. This work load would not be an activator of stress to someone who did not interpret it as overwhelming.

3. *Consequences:* the psychobiological effects of a reaction to stress. These can include attempting to change the stressful situation; quelling stressful feelings with alcohol, drugs, cigarettes, tranquilizers, overwork, or other unhealthy behaviors; or, if the person is unable or unwilling to alter interaction with the activator or reaction, facing the possibility of a stress-related illness.

Stress Activators

Activators are situations that have the potential to disrupt a person's emotional or mental state. Activators or stressors can be major external events (war, flood, famine), unpleasant interactions with people (divorce, job loss), or they may result from changes in the body resulting from accidents, disease, or aging. An unmet emotional need or happy events such as marriage or winning a lottery can also activate stress.

Life Changes as Activators

Stress researchers have developed a variety of methods to identify and measure the potential for life

Terms

stressor: any physical or psychological event or condition that produces stress

stress: the sum of physical and emotional reactions to any stimulus that disturbs the organism's homeostasis

activators: potential stressors; occurrences, situations, or events perceived as stressful

reactions: interpretations of activators as taxing or overwhelming

consequences: the effects of one's action; the effects of stress response

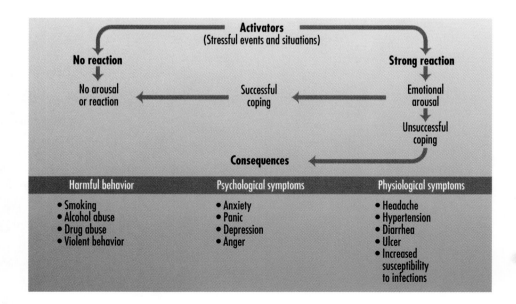

FIGURE 3.2   The Stress-Illness Relationship   It is through one's reaction that a given situation is experienced as stressful.

experiences to be stress activators. One of the most common of these is the Social Readjustment Rating Scale (SRRS), which lists 43 common life events and, for each event, a corresponding number of life change units (LCUs) (Holmes and Rahe, 1967). LCUs represent the relative amount of psychological and physiological adjustment required to meet the challenge produced by the particular life event. For example, in the SRRS, the death of a spouse requires the most adjustment, with an arbitrary numerical LCU value of 100. Marriage carries a value of 50 LCUs, and a vacation has a value of 13 LCUs. Notice that both positive (marriage, vacation) and negative (death of spouse) events are on the scale.

Research has shown that accumulating more than 150 LCUs on the SRRS within 6 months correlates with a high probability that a person will experience a negative health change. The nature of the health change cannot be predicted, only that one is likely to occur. Negative health changes include heart attacks, accidents, infectious diseases, worsening of a previous illness, injuries, and metabolic disease.

The Recent Life Changes Questionnaire (RLCQ) (Table 3.1) is an updated version of the SRRS (Miller and Rahe, 1997). (Most published studies still refer to the SRRS.) The RLCQ contains 74 life events that are representative of the stressors of people living in American society today. Accumulation of more than 300 LCUs within 6 months or 500 LCUs within 1 year is indicative of a high degree of recent life stress.

Recognizing that people's reactions to various life situations differ in intensity, Irwin Sarason and his colleagues (1985) developed the Life Experience

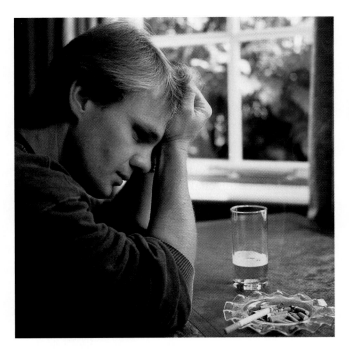

Stress can cause unhealthy behaviors, such as drinking and smoking.

Survey (LES) for students. The LES lists life events that are potential activators of stress, many of which also appear on the SRRS. The LES does not assign a value to events; rather, each respondent is asked to rate the degree of distress experienced with each event. Results of research with the LES are similar to the results obtained with the SRRS (Table 3.2).

Wellness Guide

Disorders That Can Be Caused or Aggravated by Stress

Gastrointestinal disorders	*Skin disorders*	*Metabolic disorders*
Constipation	Eczema	Hyperthyroidism
Diarrhea	Pruritus	Hypothyroidism
Duodenal ulcer	Urticaria	Diabetes
Anorexia nervosa	Psoriasis	
Obesity		*Cardiovascular disorders*
Ulcerative colitis	*Musculoskeletal disorders*	Coronary artery disease
	Rheumatoid arthritis	Essential hypertension
Respiratory disorders	Low back pain	Congestive heart failure
Asthma	Migraine headache	
Hay fever	Muscle tension	*Menstrual irregularities*
Tuberculosis		
		Cancer
		Accident proneness

TABLE 3.1   The Recent Life Changes Questionnaire

Life event	Life change units Men	Women	Life event	Life change units Men	Women
Death of son or daughter	135	103	Moderate illness	47	39
Death of spouse	122	113	Loss or damage of personal property	47	35
Death of brother or sister	111	87	Sexual difficulties	44	44
Death of parent	105	90	Getting demoted at work	44	39
Divorce	102	85	Major change in living conditions	44	37
Death of family member	96	78	Increase in income	43	30
Fired from work	85	69	Relationship problems	42	34
Separation from spouse due to marital problems	79	70	Trouble with in-laws	41	33
Major injury or illness	79	64	Beginning or ending school or college	40	35
Being held in jail	78	71	Making a major purchase	40	33
Pregnancy	74	55	New, close personal relationship	39	34
Miscarriage or abortion	74	51	Outstanding personal achievement	38	33
Death of a close friend	73	64	Troubles with co-workers at work	37	32
Laid off from work	73	59	Change in school or college	37	31
Birth of a child	71	56	Change in your work hours or conditions	36	32
Adopting a child	71	54	Troubles with workers whom you supervise	35	34
Major business adjustment	67	47	Getting a transfer at work	33	31
Decrease in income	66	49	Getting a promotion at work	33	29
Parents' divorce	63	52	Change in religious beliefs	31	27
A relative moving in with you	62	53	Christmas	30	25
Foreclosure on a mortgage or a loan	62	51	Having more responsibilities at work	29	29
Investment and/or credit difficulties	62	46	Troubles with your boss at work	29	29
Marital reconciliation	61	48	Major change in usual type or amount of recreation	29	28
Major change in health or behavior of family member	58	50	General work troubles	29	27
Change in arguments with spouse	55	41	Change in social activities	29	24
Retirement	54	48	Major change in eating habits	29	23
Major decision regarding your immediate future	54	46	Major change in sleeping habits	28	23
Separation from spouse due to work	53	54	Change in family get-togethers	28	20
An accident	53	38	Change in personal habits	27	24
Parental remarriage	52	45	Major dental work	27	23
Change residence to a different town, city, or state	52	39	Change of residence in same town or city	27	21
Change to a new type of work	51	50	Change in political beliefs	26	21
"Falling out" of a close, personal relationship	50	41	Vacation	26	20
Marriage	50	50	Having fewer responsibilities at work	22	21
Spouse changes work	50	38	Making a moderate purchase	22	18
Child leaving home	48	38	Change in church activities	21	20
Birth of grandchild	48	34	Minor violation of the law	20	19
Engagement to marry	47	42	Correspondence course to help you in your work	19	16

Source: Adapted with permission from M. A. Miller and R. H. Rahe (1997). "Life changes scaling for the 1990s." *Journal of Psychosomatic Research, 43,* 279–292, with permission from Elsevier Science.

TABLE 3.2   Stress Associated with Common Life Changes Experienced by Students

Event	LES score[a]
Death of close family member	100
Death of a close friend	73
Divorce between parents	65
Jail term	63
Major personal injury or illness	63
Marriage	58
Fired from job	50
Failed important course	47
Change in health of family member	45
Pregnancy	45
Sex problems	44
Serious argument with close friend	40
Change in financial status	39
Trouble with parents	39
Change of major	39
New girlfriend or boyfriend	38
Increased workload at school	37
Outstanding personal achievement	36
First quarter or semester in college	35
Change in living conditions	31
Serious argument with instructor	30
Lower grades than expected	29
Change in sleeping habits	29
Change in social activities	29
Change in eating habits	28
Chronic car trouble	26
Change in number of family get-togethers	26
Too many missed classes	25
Change of college or work	24
Dropped more than one class	23
Minor traffic violations	20

Source: I. G. Sarason, B. R. Sarason, and J. H. Johnson, "Stressful Life Events: Measurement, Moderators, and Adaptation," in Susan R. Burchfield, ed., *Stress* (Washington, D.C.: Hemisphere, 1985).

[a]LES Life Experience Survey.

Surveys such as the SRRS and LES are culture-bound; that is, their effectiveness in predicting health problems associated with activators depends on the similarity of the people in the survey group. The potential for health changes depends on the meaning and importance people place on certain events. Because individuals from different social strata or ethnic groups have different values, beliefs, and attitudes, they often respond differently to the same activator.

Daily Events as Activators

Stress results from the cumulative effects of daily hassles, which irritate us, cause us to worry, and create psychic and bodily tension. Hassles include frustrations, inner conflicts, and social pressures and demands.

Frustration is the feeling resulting from being blocked from attaining a personal goal, like getting stuck in a traffic jam when you're trying to get somewhere. Besides being uncomfortable, frustration produces potentially illness-causing physiological changes (increased heart rate, changes in hormone levels, and lowered immune function). Frustration can lead to feelings of aggression (the motivation to overcome an obstacle). Acting on feelings of frustration and aggression, a stuck motorist might honk the horn, yell at other stopped motorists, be angry with himself or herself for choosing this particular route, or pound on the steering wheel. None of these actions are likely to get traffic moving again; instead, they are likely only to increase frustration. It would be healthier to reduce frustration by changing the importance of the goal ("The world won't end because I'm late for work") or changing the goal to something that can be accomplished ("I'm stuck so I'm going to listen to this relaxation audiotape or enjoy a few minutes of meditation.") Releasing frustration healthfully is better than "bottling it up inside," which tends to make people sick.

Inner conflict is represented by having to choose between two incompatible goals. The choice can be between two desired goals (approach-approach conflict), two undesirable goals (avoidance-avoidance conflict), or a goal that has both desired and undesired outcomes (approach-avoidance conflict). Having to choose between two desired goals, like deciding which film to see or what toppings to put on a pizza, causes little stress. Having to choose between two undesirable goals—"being between a rock and a hard place"—is very stressful.

Approach-avoidance situations often produce vacillation, inaction, or procrastination. For example, someone wanting to ask someone out may vacillate because of fear of rejection. To get unstuck from approach-avoidance conflict, psychologists generally advise lessening focus on the negative ("Rejection might hurt but I'm still a nice person") and increasing focus on the positive ("It'll be great if she or he says yes"). Procrastinators can stop judging themselves as inferior and instead focus on lessening the reason they avoid pursuit of their goal.

Pressure is the expectation or demand that we behave in a certain way. Pressure can be external (social or peer pressure) or internal (the perfectionist inside you). Pressure is stressful because it increases anxiety. Failure to conform risks rejection from the group, and failure to perform risks loss of self-esteem.

Antidotes to the negative effects of the frustration and inner conflict associated with daily stressors are daily uplifts from the things in life that give you pleasure: spending time with someone you like, having fun, enjoying a good movie, taking a walk, or reading a good book.

Reactions to Activators

Reactions depend largely on the individual's personality and emotional makeup and not on the nature of the activator. Everyone interprets the world and events differently. Each of us is born with a capacity for certain behaviors, which are greatly modified and shaped by what we learn and experience. Each of us reacts to a particular situation according to individual values, beliefs, and attitudes.

Because of these differences, a situation that may be stressful and upsetting to one person may not even bother another. Experiencing stress requires that an individual interpret a given situation as significant ("This situation is important to me") and that he or she decide what to do with the situation ("What can I do about it?"). For most people, situations that are interpreted as stressful include (a) harm and loss, (b) threat, and (c) challenge.

Harm-and-loss situations include the death of a loved one, theft or damage to one's home, physical injury or loss of an organ, physical assault, or loss of

Terms

harm-and-loss situations: stressful events that include death, loss of property, injury, and illness

Wellness Guide

Time Management

A major cause of college student stress is the sense that there's too much to do and not enough time to do it. Since you can't make more time, the way to ease this pressure is to make the best use of the time you've got. Here are some tips for time management:

- *Perform a time audit.* For at least 3 representative days in your week (a whole week is better), write down everything you do during each of the 24 hours. Make a chart. Identify "windows" of time that could be put to better use and alter your activities accordingly.

- *Be energy efficient.* Schedule important activities for the times of the day when you are most alert and attentive. For example, if you're a morning person, take morning classes and study in between them. Schedule exercise and socializing for the afternoon. Night people might do the opposite.

- *Keep a to-do list.* At the beginning of each day, or the night before, write down all the things you have to do.

- *Prioritize tasks: first things first.* Classify tasks according to their *urgency* and *importance,* and do them in this order: (a) urgent and important;

(b) not urgent but important; (c) urgent but not important; and (d) not urgent or important. Distinguishing the urgent and important tasks from the urgent but not important tasks is often difficult because urgency is a state of mind that makes everything seem important. Before prioritizing the items on your to-do list, take a few minutes to become mentally and physically quiet. This will allow you to place truly urgent and important items at the top of your to-do list.

- *Don't sweat the small stuff.* Eliminate unimportant tasks from your list. Don't do, worry about, or think about anything that doesn't match your most important values or long-term life goals.

- *Control interruptions.* Discourage drop-in visiting; don't answer the pager or the phone (if it's important, the person will call back); stay away from TV, computer games, and the Internet.

- *Schedule time for you.* Even if it's only a few moments a day, take time for activities that you find meaningful, e.g., reading, prayer, meditation, journal writing, letter writing, musical or artistic pursuits. This will keep you from burning out.

- *Schedule time for fun.* Don't forget to play and socialize.

- *Sleep.* Not sleeping enough is like overdrawing money from a bank account: eventually you have to pay it back. Furthermore, when "overdrawn" at the sleep bank, you function at 50% to 70% efficiency, which makes school work take longer and adds to the sense that there isn't enough time.

- *Tame any tendencies toward perfectionism.* Don't try to make everything perfect. Every task has a point of diminishing returns—when the time and energy you put in is out of proportion to what you can reasonably hope to get back.

- *Understand any tendencies to procrastinate.* Procrastination often grows out of the fear of failure or exposure (people seeing you or your work and judging it harshly). When you hear your litany of excuses for not working at a task, ask yourself what you fear. Be your own best friend and encourage yourself to move ahead. Break the task into smaller parts and take them on one by one. Reward yourself when each one is finished.

DILBERT   By Scott Adams   © 1998 United Features Syndicate, Inc.

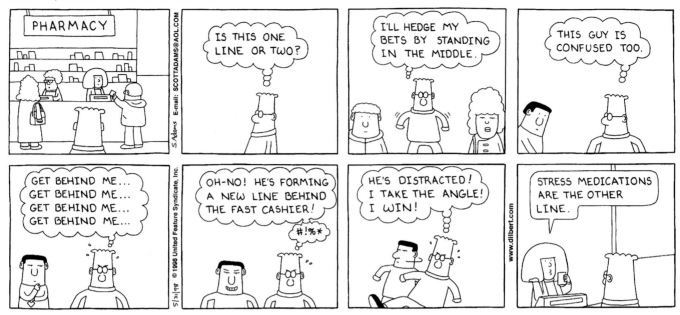

self-esteem. Harm-and-loss situations create stress because an important physical or psychological need is not satisfied. Emotions that signal harm or loss include sadness, depression, and anger. Eight of the first ten items on the RLCQ involve harm and loss.

Threat situations are perceived and interpreted as likely to produce harm or loss whether any harm or loss actually occurs. The experience is one of continually warding off demands that tax one's abilities to cope with life. Emotions associated with threat include anger, hostility, anxiety, frustration, and depression.

Challenge situations are perceived and interpreted as opportunities for growth, mastery, and gain. Very often such situations involve major life transitions such as leaving one's family to start life on one's own, graduating from college, or getting married. Even though they are interpreted as good, life transitions can be stressful because they require considerable psychological and physical adjustment. Often a life transition involves both sadness and excitement: sadness for the loss of what is familiar and excitement in anticipation of the new. Psychologists refer to the stress that comes from positive challenges as **eustress** and the stress associated with negative life challenges or the anticipation of them as **distress.**

Interpreting a situation as threatening or challenging often leads to asking oneself, "what can I do about it?" The degree of stress may depend on your answer. Believing we can manage a stressful situation is more likely to lessen stress than believing that the situation is overwhelming. In laboratory experiments, for example, animals given the opportunity to avoid or delay a mild electric shock develop only slightly more ulcers than do animals who receive no shock at all. People who work in jobs that involve a lot of pressure to perform but allow little opportunity for deciding how the tasks of the job are to be accomplished experience greater stress than do workers who have more control over decision-making (Karasek and Theorell, 1989). Efforts to manage a situation are called **coping.**

Several factors influence the degree of distress a person experiences. Among them are predictability, control, belief in the outcome, and social support.

Predictability   Research shows that knowing when a stressful situation will occur produces less stress than not knowing. Individuals may be just as stressed when the event occurs, but knowing when it will occur allows them to relax afterward. Knowing that something stressful may occur but not knowing when (like a "pop" quiz in a class) puts the individual on constant alert. For example, during World War II, London was bombed every night, but the London suburbs were not. Londoners had fewer ulcers than suburbanites, presumably because they knew bombings would occur.

Control   Individuals who believe they can influence the course of their lives (internal locus of control) are likely to suffer less stress than individuals who believe their destiny is influenced largely by factors outside of themselves (external locus of control). The crucial factor is not whether the locus of control is internal or external, but the belief that one can influence one's destiny.

Belief in the Outcome People who believe that things are improving (optimistic) experience less stress than do people who believe that things are getting worse (pessimistic).

Social Support Having someone to talk to and believing that that person can be supportive with physical, emotional, and intellectual resources lessens stress. For example, patients who talk with their surgeons about their fears before surgery require less anesthetic during the operation and have a smaller stress response than patients who go through such procedures feeling uninformed and unsupported.

The Consequences of Our Reactions

Although the human mind interprets a given situation as harmful, threatening, or challenging, the nervous and endocrine systems, which link the brain and the rest of the body, bring about the changes in physiology that lead to harmful behaviors or to disease. The feelings associated with stressful experiences (fear, anger, sadness, etc.) activate the nervous and endocrine systems, which in turn produce changes in the immune system and in physiology. Illnesses arise when the nervous and endocrine systems are continually activated or overstimulated. Anxiety, sadness, frustration,

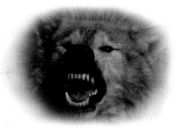

Heart
Increases in heart rate and force of contractions

Blood
Constriction in abdominal viscera and dilation in skeletal muscles

Eye
Contraction of radial muscle of iris and relaxation of ciliary muscle

Intestines
Decreased motility and relaxation of sphincters

Skin
Contraction of pilomotor muscles and contraction of sweat glands

Spleen
Contraction

Brain
Activation of reticular formation

FIGURE 3.3 **The Fight-or-Flight Response** All humans display this response when confronted with challenges they interpret as frightening or threatening.

and other emotions alter the functions of the heart, blood vessels, immune system, and other organs. If prolonged, such alterations can produce heart disease, high blood pressure, and an increased susceptibility to infectious disease and, possibly, cancer (see chapters 12, 13, and 14).

The Fight-or-Flight Response

The challenge-response systems activate the **fight-or-flight response.** All mammals, including humans, are capable of displaying this particular response when confronted with challenges they interpret as frightening or a threat to survival. The response is characterized by a coordinated discharge of the **sympathetic nervous system** and portions of the **parasympathetic nervous system** and by the secretion of a number of hormones, especially **epinephrine** and **cortisol.** When a person (or other animal) experiences a threatening situation, the associated emotions (usually fear or rage) that arise in the limbic system portion of the brain are translated automatically into the appropriate physiological responses through nervous and hormonal pathways mediated by the **hypothalamus.**

As Figure 3.3 shows, some prominent aspects of the fight-or-flight response are an elevation of the

Terms

threat situations: events that cause stress because of a perception that harm or loss may occur

challenge situations: positive events that may involve major life transitions and may cause stress

eustress: stress resulting from pleasant stressors

distress: stress resulting from unpleasant stressors

coping: attempts to manage a stressful situation

fight-or-flight response: a defensive reaction that prepares the organism for conflict or escape by triggering hormonal, cardiovascular, metabolic, and other changes

sympathetic nervous system: a division of the autonomic nervous system that reacts to danger or challenges by almost instantly putting body processes into high gear

parasympathetic nervous system: a division of the autonomic nervous system that tones down the excitatory effects of the sympathetic nervous system; slows metabolism and restores energy reserves

epinephrine: a hormone secreted by the medulla (inner core) of the adrenal gland; also called adrenaline

cortisol: a steroid hormone secreted by the cortex (outer layer) of the adrenal gland

hypothalamus: a part of the brain that activates, controls, and integrates the autonomic nervous system, the endocrine system, and other bodily functions

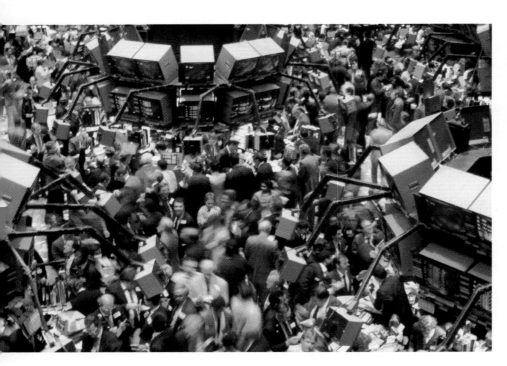

Several heart attacks occur every year on the floor of the New York Stock Exchange, making it one of the highest-density heart attack zones in the U.S. The Exchange has installed a defibrillator near the bank of phones used to place orders for stock trading, and it has trained workers to use the defibrillator and perform CPR when a heart attack occurs.

heart rate and blood pressure (to provide more blood to muscles), constriction of the blood vessels of the skin (to limit bleeding if wounded), dilation of the pupil of the eye (to let in more light, thereby improving vision), increased activity in the reticular formation of the brain (to increase the alert, aroused state), and liberation of glucose and free fatty acids from storage depots (to make more stored energy available to the muscles, brain, and other tissues and organs).

Everyone is capable of the fight-or-flight response; it is part of the human biological makeup. Individuals display this reaction to some extent when they narrowly escape from a dangerous mishap or when they get angry or frustrated and lose their tempers. The heart rate quickens, the person becomes more alert and tense, and he or she experiences a rush of excitement from increased secretion of epinephrine into the blood. In short, the person becomes ready to take action to deal with the situation.

In our modern civilized society, however, literally fleeing from a threatening situation or engaging in physical combat is often an inappropriate—and sometimes impossible—response. Social norms dictate that people handle many difficult situations "civilly." Moreover, many threats are symbolic. The fear of losing a job, social status, or a lover is not the same as being confronted by a ferocious animal or thug, but the anxiety can produce similar stress-related physiological responses. Thus, one of the consequences of having a highly evolved brain with the ability for symbolic thought and the intellectual capacity to produce a "civilized" society is the existence of social norms

that make people unwilling or unable to take direct action when confronted with threatening situations.

The General Adaptation Syndrome

Hans Selye, a pioneer in stress research, found that continued physiological responding to stressors led to a characteristic response called the General Adaptation Syndrome (GAS). The GAS is a three-phase response to a stressor (Figure 3.4). The three phases are stage of alarm, stage of resistance, and stage of exhaustion.

1. *Stage of alarm:* A person's ability to withstand or resist any type of stressor is lowered by the need to deal with the stressor, whether it is a burn, a broken arm, the loss of a loved one, the fear of failing a class, or losing a job.
2. *Stage of resistance:* The body adapts to the continued presence of the stressor by producing more epinephrine, raising blood pressure, increasing alertness, suppressing the immune system, and tensing muscles. If interaction with the stressor is prolonged, the ability to resist becomes depleted.
3. *Stage of exhaustion:* When the ability to resist is depleted, the person becomes ill. Because many months or even years of wear and tear may be required before the body's resistance is exhausted, illness may not appear until long after the initial interaction with the stressor.

Experiments with laboratory animals have demonstrated that profound changes in vital body organs—principally the adrenal glands, the thymus gland, the

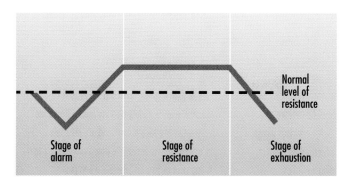

FIGURE 3.4   The Three Phases of the General Adaptation Syndrome   In the stage of alarm, the body's normal resistance to stress is lowered from the first interactions with the stressor. In the stage of resistance, the body adapts to the continued presence of the stressor and resistance increases. In the stage of exhaustion, the body loses its ability to resist the stressor any longer and becomes exhausted.

lymph nodes, and the lining of the stomach—can be caused by activation of the GAS. For example, stomach ulcers often result in humans or other animals from a prolonged interaction with a stressor. In a study of more than one hundred air traffic controllers, more than half were found to have gastrointestinal illnesses. Among those who were ill, more than half had peptic ulcers. The constant stress from worrying about airplane crashes and collisions caused ulcers in many of the persons who were susceptible to the effects of the stress.

Posttraumatic Stress

Some forms of stress are so severe that they produce a serious, long-lasting psychological condition called **posttraumatic stress disorder (PTSD).** This condition can result from the stress produced by combat in war, living through a natural disaster, such as a devastating hurricane or tornado, as well as rape, physical assault, or life-threatening illness. About 4% of the U.S. population are estimated to have PTSD as a result of traumatic and terrifying experiences. Some of the diagnostic criteria for PTSD include: (1) flashbacks to the traumatizing event(s) or recurrent thoughts and dreams of the experience; (2) difficulty sleeping, outbursts of anger, and being hyperalert and easily startled; and (3) little interest in daily activities, feeling cut off from others, and a sense of having a limited future.

PTSD came into prominence among combat veterans of the Vietnam war, and even 20 years later many of the veterans diagnosed with PTSD have an

excessively high rate of circulatory, digestive, respiratory, and musculoskeletal disorders, as well as susceptibility to infectious diseases (Boscarino, 1997). How the severe stress of wartime combat, natural disasters, and physical and sexual abuse produces these illnesses is not understood. But PTSD does show that severe or prolonged stress can initiate biological changes that result in serious diseases.

Not everyone who is exposed to life-threatening or traumatic events will develop PTSD; some persons are able to cope better or are genetically or psychologically less susceptible to PTSD. Although there are several theories as to what causes PTSD, none really explains the array of psychological and biological symptoms in PTSD patients. However, any of several forms of psychological counseling can help individuals who have PTSD to cope with their traumatic experiences. What seems to matter most is not the form of psychological therapy but the rapport between the patient and the counselor. Antidepressant and sedative drugs also may be prescribed to alleviate symptoms while the person is learning to cope with the traumatic experiences.

Stress and the Immune System

A variety of studies have shown that stress can impair the functions of the immune system. For example, students who experience considerable stress prior to taking exams show reduced blood levels of immune system cells (e.g., natural killer cells, T-cells) (see chapter 12), thus making exam stress a risk factor for colds and flu. Stress also slows the body's ability to mount an immune response to a vaccine. Also, men whose wives have recently died have been shown to have lower-than-normal levels of immune cells. This finding may explain the observation that among older adults a surviving spouse has a higher-than-expected risk of death during the period of bereavement. In addition to bereaved spouses, unhappily married, never married, and recently divorced people have reduced immune functioning, as do individuals experiencing job loss.

Stress-related impairment of the immune system is mediated by hormonal and neurological responses to stress. A variety of hormones secreted by the hypothalamus in the brain, the pituitary gland, and the adrenal glands bind to cells of the immune system and alter their functions. Activation of the sympathetic nervous system fibers that connect the brain to tissues and organs that produce immune-system cells and

> *The man who fears suffering is already suffering from what he fears.*
>
> MONTAIGNE

Terms

posttraumatic stress disorder (PTSD): physical and mental illnesses resulting from severe trauma

Wellness Guide

Twenty Tips for Managing Stress

Once you have recognized the fact that you are under too much stress, you are well on your way to coping with it. Although there are no pat answers, no instant solutions, no one-day stress-off programs, there are a number of ways you can manage stress.

1. *Work off stress.* If you're angry or ready to blow up, physical activities are a terrific outlet. This is a time to vent that energy. Whether you go out and chop wood, take a run, wash the floor, or tackle a time- and energy-consuming project you've put off, chances are that you'll feel better and also will have accomplished something useful.

2. *Talk to someone you truly trust.* Confiding in another person and talking out your problem, even if there is no immediate solution, usually makes you feel better. If there is no one you trust, not even a relative or clergyperson, call one of the reputable hotlines that operate around the country twenty-four hours a day. They are staffed with counselors who can listen and discuss any problem with a great deal of understanding and compassion. Look them up in a telephone directory under such listings as Alcoholics Anonymous, Gamblers Anonymous, Help.

3. *Learn to accept what you cannot change.* Sometimes problems cannot be avoided or solved right now. Whether it's a serious illness in the family, a divorce, an economic setback, or a death, simply accepting what has happened will lessen the stress.

4. *Avoid self-medication.* Many easily available substances, from aspirin to alcohol, are often abused in an effort to avoid the stress by blotting out pain. They are not a solution to a problem, and if taken in excess, become a problem in themselves. Think about what you are doing if you have an urge to "drown your sorrows."

5. *Get enough sleep and rest.* Sometimes we are so busy we tend to cut down on things we need most. Sleep is a wonderful cure-all, a time to recharge your body's batteries, and usually one of the first things sacrificed to stress. Keep in mind that lack of sleep makes you cranky and irritable. If you find that you can't sleep, after a week or ten days, consult your family physician.

6. *Take time to play.* All work won't make you dull; it's more likely to make you a nervous wreck. Working extra hours tends to be counterproductive past a certain point. Make

the time to relax, even if it's only to take a short nap. Schedule a sanity break. If you are too busy to take a weekend off, schedule minivacations during the day. Treat yourself to an hour or two off whether it's to play racquetball, shop for something personal, or take a walk around the block.

7. *Do something for others.* It may sound foolishly optimistic, but doing some good things for others makes you feel good and helps you put your life into perspective.

8. *Take one thing at a time.* Sometimes we are so overwhelmed that we try to do everything at once—and nothing gets accomplished. Take a few minutes to make a list of what has to be done, establish priorities, and tackle one project at a time, the most essential thing first. Completing the most important, pressing project will give you a sense of accomplishment, relieve some stress, and give you the strength to dive back into your workload.

9. *Agree with someone.* Sometimes we get so irritable that we wind up fighting with everyone. If life has turned into a battleground—from the bedroom to the boardroom—stop and agree with someone. Let someone have his or her way, even if you

---

molecules also can alter immune functions. The immune system responds negatively to stress; it responds positively to relaxation.

Managing Stress

The best way to manage stress is to replace stressful ways of living with beliefs, attitudes, and behaviors that promote peace, joy, and mind-body harmony. That does not mean you must become reclusive or try to eliminate all sources of conflict and tension from your life.

> *Hope does not lie in a way out but in a way through.*
> ROBERT FROST

People need tension to be creative and grow psychologically and spiritually. It may mean, however, changing some self-harming ways of thinking and behaving. Seeking help from a teacher, counselor, psychotherapist, clergyman, or coach can help you recognize sources of stress and ways to deal with them.

One way to manage stress is to alter or eliminate interaction with the stressor, for example, by changing jobs, changing a college major, accepting that a career that makes you happy is more important than one that promises a large income. Because stress is mediated by beliefs and attitudes, another way to manage it is to alter your perception of the situation. Ask yourself, "Am I seeing this potentially stressful situation realistically? And even if I am, is it really that threatening?"

really don't agree. He or she may turn around and agree with you on something else and the sense of working together, of cooperation, will change the emotional environment from one of hostility and stress to one of teamwork. Feeling like you are besieged by an army of enemies and idiots hurts you more than it hurts anyone else.

10. *Manage your time better.* The overwhelming feeling that there simply aren't enough hours in the day can defeat you before you begin. Perhaps it means take-out food instead of cooking; maybe it means asking your spouse to work out a new system of sharing; maybe you've really taken on too much. You need to develop a system that works *for* not against you.

11. *Plan ahead.* If you see a period of increased stress coming—a big project, holidays, vacation, moving, even a promotion—plan now to rest and be ready. Or postpone what can be delayed.

12. *If you become sick, don't carry on as if you're not.* No matter how pressing your work, don't be a martyr. Stay home. Get enough rest until you can resume your duties. If you go back prematurely, you risk a relapse. If you don't take time off, you risk a breakdown. If your work is so vital that nothing can function without you, have work sent to your home.

13. *Develop a hobby.* Even if you are either totally happy and work is a thrill or you are too busy to have a hobby, you aren't indulging yourself but doing yourself a favor by changing the focus of your interest. It lessens stress to have a hobby. Quite simply, it's good therapy.

14. *Believe the answer lies within you.* No one can give you a stress-free life, although they can offer advice. It is up to you to take that advice and incorporate it into your lifestyle. Just as no one can tell you what happiness or peace is or describe chocolate to you, so you have to search out your own inner desires and needs and make them work for you.

15. *Eat well and exercise.* You can't simply relax and hope stress will go away. A liveable stress level is only attainable if you integrate stress management with proper nutrition (see chapter 5) and exercise (see chapter 7).

16. *Don't put off relaxing.* Some people promise themselves that "tomorrow" or "next week" I'll take care of myself and take a break. That simply won't work. You have to relax every single day, even if it's for a few minutes between appointments or some deep breathing on your way home from work.

17. *Don't be afraid to say no.* If you are asked to do someone a favor, or complete an extra project, and it really is too much, say so. Taking on too much can in itself be the stress that breaks you down.

18. *Know when you are tired.* Being able to stop work when you are fatigued rather than pushing yourself beyond your limits will reduce unnecessary stress.

19. *Learn to delegate responsibility.* Sometimes you can't do everything yourself and yet the work must get done. Don't be afraid to ask for help.

20. *Be realistic about perfection.* When there is a tremendous amount of work to be done, don't dwell on doing and redoing it until it is perfect. This isn't to advocate being slipshod, but to accept that a fourth or fifth draft of a report that was due yesterday is putting an unnecessary amount of stress on yourself.

Source: What You Should Know About Stress, Diet and Exercise, Now!: The RIA Guide to Feeling Good (New York: The Research Institute of America, Inc., 1984). Reprinted with permission by the Research Institute of America, 90 Fifth Avenue, New York, NY 10011.

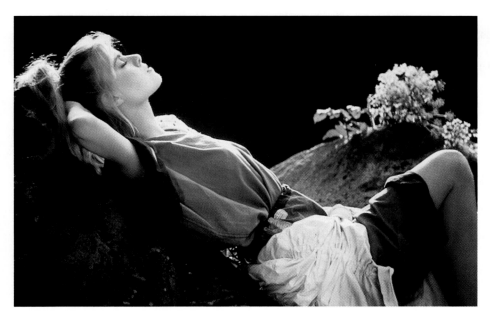

Taking time to just "lie back" and "let go" helps eliminate stress.

Managing Stress

Do It the "Write" Way

When we're stressed and troubled, quite often we get so caught up in our emotions that we lose perspective on what's going on. We only know that we're distressed. This is where writing down thoughts and feelings can help.

Research has shown that writing about one's traumatic experiences can lessen stress, improve immune functioning, and foster health and well-being (Pennebaker, 1997). Apparently, writing about psychologically painful experiences releases the stress and anxiety associated with trying to keep painful, unpleasant feelings out of conscious awareness. Writing about trauma helps one sort, understand, and eventually put the experience into the past.

You don't have to experience a trauma to benefit from writing out your thoughts and feelings. Doing so can help you clarify why you feel a certain way and how your thoughts, perceptions, and reactions to situations are affecting your life. Writing forces you to look at your life honestly. Also, writing lets you express yourself privately without concern about a listener's reaction.

"Write for health" by making regular entries in a *journal,* which is similar to a diary except you express thoughts and feelings instead of recording daily events.

- Use a special notebook for your journal.
- Write in a quiet place.
- Keep your journal private so you can be honest with yourself.
- Write continuously. Don't worry about grammar or spelling.
- Be expressive. Don't worry about making sense.

By perceiving a situation as less difficult (turning a mountain into several molehills), you lessen the chance of feeling overwhelmed.

Another way to lessen stress is to change beliefs and goals. Winning may be an athlete's highest goal, but worrying about losing may bring about an illness. The solution is not to give up sports but to change priorities, perhaps by emphasizing the joy of participation and not the outcome of competition.

You can also change beliefs about yourself. Give yourself credit for things you have done that have lessened stress in your life rather than thinking it was blind luck. This will increase your sense of **self-efficacy,** the belief and confidence that you can master many situations that you encounter. Some stressful situations cannot be overcome, but be aware of tendencies toward needlessly feeling helpless in the face of a challenge.

Stress can be reduced by seeking support from people you trust. Talk to friends, teachers, counselors—whomever you believe can understand, lend a sympathetic ear, and offer sound feedback and advice if you request it.

Still another way to manage stress is to alter the mental and physical experience of stress. Many people do this by consuming alcohol, smoking cigarettes, taking tranquilizers and sleeping pills, and over- or undereating. Because these behaviors do not focus on the problem that is causing stress, at best they offer only short-term relief of symptoms and can lead to drug addiction or an eating disorder. Replace destructive behaviors with a stress-reduction technique that produces a psychophysiological condition, called the relaxation response, opposite of the fight-or-flight response (see chapter 2).

People use a variety of strategies to manage stress. In general, practical problems and situations perceived as high threats call forth active strategies and social support. Situations perceived as involving loss tend to call forth strategies using religion, faith, and passive acceptance.

Frequently individuals use more than one strategy (versatile coping) and occasionally they use none (passive coping). Versatile coping tends to be effective in situations involving practical events (taking an exam, losing a job, legal problems). Passive coping tends to be effective when action is unlikely to change the situation, such as dealing with the ravages of a flood or earthquake. In such instances, passivity is adaptive inasmuch as one accepts one's fate and "cruises" with the situation until an opportunity for change presents itself. Avoidance and thinking a lot about a stressful situation without actively doing anything about it tend to be ineffective means of coping.

Terms

self-efficacy: your belief that you are capable of handling the situation; self-esteem

Managing Stress

<u>Two Monks and the River</u>

Two monks set out on their last day's journey to their monastery. At mid-morning they came upon a shallow river, and on the bank there stood a beautiful young maiden.

"May I help you cross?" asked the first monk.

"Why, yes, that would be most kind of you," replied the maiden.

So the first monk hoisted the maiden on his back and carried her across the river. They bowed and went their separate ways.

After an hour or two of walking, the second monk said to the first monk, "I can't believe you did that! I just can't believe it! We take vows of chastity, and you touched a woman. You even asked her! What are we going to tell the abbot when we get home? He's going to ask how our journey was, and we can't lie. What are we going to say?"

Another couple of hours passed and the second monk erupted again. "How could you do that? She didn't even ask. You offered! The abbot's going to be incredibly angry."

By late afternoon the two were nearing their home, and the second monk, now filled with anxiety, said, "I can't believe you did that! You touched a woman. You even carried her on your back. What are we going to tell the abbot?"

The first monk stopped, looked at the second monk and said, "Listen, it's true that I carried that maiden across the river. But I left her at the river bank hours ago. You've been carrying her all day."

Critical Thinking About Health

1. Three groups of people were vaccinated against a test substance (one that could not make anyone sick). Group 1 consisted of students during final exams; group 2, people complaining of loneliness; group 3, people whose spouse had cancer. Each group was further subdivided into two subgroups. One subgroup in each major group was given 6 weeks of weekly support group meetings plus education about reducing the stress of their circumstance. The other subgroup in each major group was given no support or education. Below are the results of the strength of the immune response to the test vaccine.

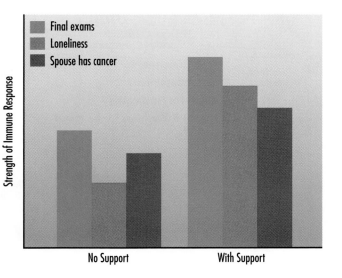

a. Explain the results of the experiment.
b. Suggest a hypothesis to explain the results of the experiment.
c. What do the results suggest about how you can better deal with stress in your life?

2. Johann Wolfgang von Goethe (1749–1832), the German author of *Faust* and other literary works, once wrote: "Things which matter most must never be at the mercy of things which matter least."
a. What is your interpretation of Goethe's idea?
b. How does letting things which matter most be at the mercy of things which matter least contribute to stress?
c. How susceptible are you to stress from letting things which matter most be at the mercy of things which matter least? What could you change to reduce that stress?

3. Offer an explanation for the following: In the 1980s, researchers studied the health of adults living in two communities that were separated by a river. North River was a prosperous farming region, and South River was an industrial region in which the major employer, an auto plant, had permanently closed. The results of the research showed that children living in South River had many more doctor visits for infections and allergies than did children in North River. Also, adults in South River had more motor vehicle accidents and colds and flu during winter months than adults in the North River did. (Hint: Refer to Figure 3.2.)

4. On the Recent Life Changes Questionnaire, the death of a child, spouse, sibling, or parent carries the highest LCU values.
   a. Offer an hypothesis to explain that result. In your hypothesis, take into account the nature of those kinds of relationships and what is lost when someone dies.
   b. Given that the loss of a loved one is associated with the highest LCU values, how should someone who experiences that kind of loss navigate life so as to reduce their stress and the risk of becoming ill?
   c. What is the best way to cope with the loss of a loved one?

Health in Review

- Life presents situations that can disrupt mind-body harmony. Such situations and events are called stressors.
- Prolonged stress can impair functioning of the body's organs and immune system and may result in illness.
- Activators are situations and events that have the potential to become stressors depending on how a person interprets them.
- Reactions are an individual's interpretation of activators. The nature and degree of a person's reactions depends on how threatening or challenging she or he perceives a situation to be.
- Consequences are the psychological and physiological effects of a reaction. An appraisal of how difficult it is to deal with a situation determines how well a person is able to cope.
- The onset of stress-related illness is the result of interpreting a situation as personally disruptive, threatening, or challenging and believing that personal resources to meet the challenge are insufficient.
- Stress results from the cumulative effects of daily problems, including frustrations, inner conflicts, and social pressures and demands.
- The fight-or-flight response is the body's way of dealing with the challenges it encounters.
- The general adaptation syndrome has three phases: (a) alarm, (b) resistance, and (c) exhaustion.
- Stress can be reduced by disengaging from stressors, and/or by altering perceptions and goals, and thereby reducing the potential for stress-related illness.
- Stress can be reduced by techniques that produce a peaceful state of being, such as image visualization, meditation, exercise, yoga, and just taking it easy.

Health and Wellness Online

The World Wide Web contains a wealth of information about health and wellness. By accessing the Internet using Web browser software, such as Netscape Navigator or Microsoft's Internet Explorer, you can gain a new perspective on many topics presented in *Health and Wellness, Seventh Edition*. Access the Jones and Bartlett Publishers Web site at http://www.jbpub.com/hwonline.

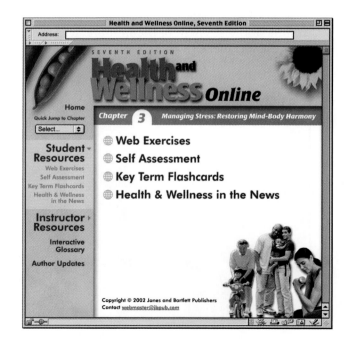

References

Boscarino, J. S. (1997). Diseases among men 20 years after exposure to severe stress: Implications for clinical research and medical care. *Psychosomatic Medicine, 59,* 605–614.

Holmes, T. H., and Rahe, R. H. (1967). The social readjustment rating scale. *Journal of Psychosomatic Research, 11,* 213–218.

Miller, M. A., and Rahe, R. H. (1997). Life changes scaling for the 1990s. *Journal of Psychosomatic Research, 43,* 279–292.

Pennebaker, J. C. (1997). *Opening up: The healing power of expressing emotions.* New York: Guilford Press.

Sarason, I. G., Sarason, B. R., and Johnson, J. H. (1985). Stressful life events: Measurement, moderators, and adaptation. In S. R. Burchfield (Ed.), *Stress* (pp. 279–299). Washington, DC: Hemisphere.

Suggested Readings

Davis, M. (2000). *The Relaxation & Stress Reduction Workbook.* Oakland, CA: New Harbinger. Offers many self-assessment tools and calming techniques to help overcome anxiety and promote physical and emotional well-being.

Hubbard, J. R., and Edward, A. (Eds.). (1998). *Handbook of stress medicine: An organ system approach.* New York: CRC Press. An explanation of how stress causes illness and how improved care and prevention can hold down medical costs.

McEwen, B. S. (1998). Protective and damaging effects of stress mediators. *New England Journal of Medicine, 338,* 171–179. A review of the long-term physiological response to stress.

Rabin, B. S. (1999). *Stress, Immune Function, and Health: The Connection.* New York: Wiley-Liss. A discussion of the long-term effects of stress on the immune system and human health.

Sapolsky, R. M. (1998). *Why Zebras Don't Get Ulcers: An Updated Guide to Stress.* New York: W. H. Freeman & Co. A primer about stress, stress-related disease, and the mechanisms for coping with stress by a Stanford University neuroscientist.

Schedlowski, M., and Tewes, U. (eds.). (1999). *Psychoneuroimmunology: An Interdisciplinary Introduction.* New York: Plenum. A textbook with contributions from international leaders in the field that examines the complex functional relationships between the nervous system, the neuroendocrine system, and the immune system.

Study Guide and Self Assessment

Identify Your Fears or Phobias
Keep a Sleep and Dream Record
Saying No

Health and Wellness Online

www.jbpub.com/hwonline

Chapter 4

Maintaining Emotional Wellness

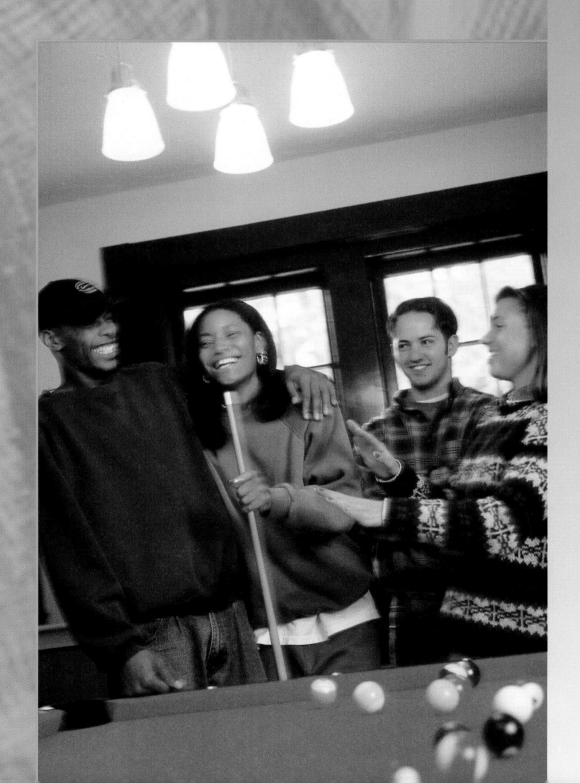

Much of human behavior is motivated by basic human needs. When individuals succeed in meeting their basic needs, they experience pleasant emotions, such as joy, pleasure, satisfaction, and contentment. When they do not, however, they experience unpleasant emotions, such as frustration, anger, sadness, grief, and shame.

Although basic needs are intrinsic to humans, the ways in which people satisfy them are not. Everyone may need to eat, but not everyone obtains food in the same way. Neither does everyone choose to eat the same kind of food. Similarly, people engage in a variety of activities, occupations, relationships, and recreational pursuits to meet their needs.

> *You never feel better than when you start feeling good after you've been feeling bad.*
> WILLIAM LEAST-HEAT MOON
> *BLUE HIGHWAYS*

Infants have a limited need-fulfilling repertoire. A child can cry when wanting to be fed or comforted and can smile or coo to invite touch and play. Beginning in childhood, individuals learn to understand the nature of their needs and develop strategies for interacting with the environment to meet them.

There are two types of basic human needs: **maintenance needs** involve physical safety and survival; **growth needs** involve social belonging, self-esteem and mental, psychological, and spiritual stimulation. Mental and emotional health are functions of how successfully a person meets her or his basic needs and deals with circumstances in which these needs are not met. Thoughts, beliefs, and attitudes that help us appropriately interpret and respond to internal needs, as well as environmental challenges, are involved. We should have emotional experiences that accurately help us interpret the environment and our interactions with it, as well as a biologically healthy brain and nervous system, not one that is undernourished, diseased, or disequilibrated with drugs or alcohol.

According to psychologists, there is a **hierarchy of needs** that describes a process through which people navigate life. These include physiological needs, safety, love, self-esteem, and self-actualization (Figure 4.1). When the needs for food, clothing, and shelter have been met, less urgent needs become a priority. As people meet their needs, they move up the hierarchy. A person attains **self-actualization** (the highest level), by living to the fullest. People who are self-actualized have met their basic needs and reached their full human potential (Maslow, 1970).

To be emotionally healthy, we do not necessarily have to be like everyone else. Being true to ourselves leads to greater satisfaction in life than social conformity. Also, being mentally healthy does not mean that

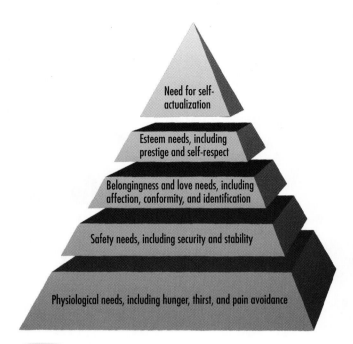

FIGURE 4.1   **Maslow's Hierarchy of Human Needs**

we never feel angry, anxious, lonely, depressed, confused, or overwhelmed. These are normal human emotions. Furthermore, being mentally healthy does not mean that we never need support, advice, or other kinds of help. In fact, inner strength is being able to recognize our limits and to seek and accept help so we can restore harmony when our mental and emotional resources are taxed.

Understanding Thoughts and Emotions

One foundation of mental health is seeing the world realistically. This perspective helps people devise strategies to meet their needs.

How we see the world is determined by the mental process called **cognition,** (from the Latin *cogito,* meaning "I know"). Cognition includes the following mental processes:

- *Perception:* interpreting data gathered by the sensory receptors (sight, smell, hearing, taste, touch, movement)
- *Learning:* integrating new perceptions with previous ones and storing them in memory as values, beliefs, and attitudes
- *Reasoning and problem solving:* formulating plans of action

Some thoughts, beliefs, and attitudes are **conscious,** which means that an individual can be aware of them.

Wellness Guide

Hints for Emotional Wellness

People who have a positive self-image

. . . are not incapacitated by their emotions of fear, anger, love, jealousy, or guilt.

. . . can take life's disappointments in stride.

. . . have a tolerant attitude toward themselves and others; they can laugh at their shortcomings and mistakes.

. . . respect themselves and have self-confidence.

. . . are able to deal with most situations that come along.

. . . get satisfaction from simple, everyday pleasures.

People who feel positive about other people

. . . are able to give love and accept others the way they are.

. . . have personal relationships that are satisfying.

. . . expect to like and trust others and take it for granted that others will like and trust them.

. . . respect the many differences they see in people.

. . . do not need to control or push other people around.

. . . feel a sense of responsibility to friends and society.

People who are able to meet life's demands

. . . do something about their problems as they arise.

. . . accept their responsibilities.

. . . shape their environment whenever possible; otherwise they adjust to it.

. . . plan ahead but do not fear the future.

. . . welcome new ideas and experiences.

. . . use their natural capacities and talents.

. . . set attainable and realistic goals for themselves.

. . . get satisfaction from what they accomplish.

Others are **unconscious,** which means that they are not in our everyday awareness. Unconscious thoughts can be accessed through hypnosis, dreams, fantasies, and various forms of creative experience.

Cognition is usually associated with emotions. Emotions are patterns of energy in the brain that can arise spontaneously or in response to cognitive evaluations of what we experience, have experienced, or believe we may experience. Emotions provide a sense of what is pleasant or unpleasant, which helps us evaluate an experience. This sets the stage for appropriate behavior. Emotions also provide the energy or motivation for behavior, and they play a part in evaluating the outcome of behavior.

Here is an example of how cognition and emotions affect behavior. An exam is scheduled in an economics course. If a student believes that success on the exam is beneficial (i.e., doing well meets a need), she is likely to feel challenged and anxious. These emotions motivate her to study. If she does well on the exam, she is likely to feel happy. If she attributes her success to the fact that she studied, she is likely to study for the next exam and feel good about herself and her ability to master schoolwork.

Another student in the same economics class believes that performance on the exam will determine all future success in school and in life. This erroneous belief is likely to produce anxiety to the point of panic, which may be so intense that he is unable to concentrate; he may even be sick or psychologically incapacitated on the day of the test (see chapter 2). This experience may be so unpleasant that he may drop economics or even drop out of school. He might have helped himself by changing his belief about the significance of the test, which would have altered his emotional experience. This could have produced a different set of behavioral choices. With a different perspective, he might have done quite well on the exam.

 ## Developing Coping Strategies

There are times in life when everything seems to be going well, and it is possible to experience reasonably long periods of great joy. Change is a fact of life, however, and satisfaction is rarely permanent. Even if all your physical needs are met, you live in harmonious relationships, and your work is meaningful and

Terms

maintenance needs: human needs that include physical safety and survival requirements, such as food and water

growth needs: a human need that includes social belonging, self-esteem, and spiritual growth

hierarchy of needs: a progression of human requirements, including physiological needs, safety, love, self-esteem, and self-actualization

self-actualization: a state in which a person has achieved the highest level of growth in Maslow's hierarchy of needs

cognition: the act or process of knowing in the broadest sense

conscious: knowing or perceiving something within oneself

unconscious: whatever is in the mind but out of conscious awareness

Managing Stress

Humor Therapy

It's true that laughter is the best medicine. On average, the typical person laughs about 15 times per day. This number can shrink dramatically, however, when people are influenced by emotions such as anger, fear, or grief. Just as unresolved emotions can ultimately have a negative effect on the body, positive emotions can also influence our state of health. The importance of humor on health was recognized as far back as ancient Greece. Plato was a strong advocate of humor as a means to lighten the burdens of the soul and to improve one's state of health. From medieval court jesters to circus clowns, humor has long been a factor influencing mind-body healing wisdom. Only now is medical science learning what people have known intuitively for centuries—laughter is good medicine.

Thanks to the pioneer work of Norman Cousins and others who have followed in his footsteps to develop the field of psychoneuroimmunology, we know that our emotions can trigger physiological responses, including the release of special neuropeptides, which seem to have a healing effect all their own. The result of several bouts of laughter can actually bring about a sense of homeostasis to help calm the body and, in effect, bring a sense of inner peace.

The real message of humor therapy is that we must learn to establish a sense of emotional balance, to feel the range of feelings—anger, fear, joy, love, and so on. Shortly before he died, Norman Cousins said that it wasn't humor that healed him; it was love. Humor, he said, was a way in which compassion could do its healing work.

Here are some ways to tickle your funny bone and get your quota of 15 laughs per day.

1. Create a tickler notebook of cartoons, stories, photographs, and other items that bring a smile to your face. Refer to it often, especially when you're down in the dumps.

2. Walk into a greeting card shop and buy five of the funniest cards you find.

3. Tell a close friend the most embarrassing event that has ever happened to you.

4. Buy 10 red roses and go to the nearest hospital or nursing home and distribute them to the first 10 people you see.

5. Over the weekend, go to a video store and pick up some comedy videos. Have a humorfest at home.

6. Read a funny novel.

7. Listen to a comedy audiotape or CD.

8. Hang out at a children's playground and watch little kids play for a half hour.

9. Fill your tub with hot water, bubble bath, and a rubber duck. And play!

10. Call some old friends you haven't talked to in a while, catch up on their lives; tell them a funny joke; then tell them you love them.

---

fulfilling, you still probably experience some degree of frustration and conflict because you initiate changes in your life in the pursuit of new and enriching experiences to satisfy your growth needs.

Coping strategies are ways of dealing with the emotional distress that comes from not having your needs met. In general, there are three categories of coping strategies; you can alter (a) the interaction with the cause of the distress, (b) thoughts and beliefs regarding the significance of the need that is not being met, or (c) the distressing feeling, without changing the situation or how you think about it.

To reduce emotional distress by changing your interaction with the situation, you could:

- Attack the situation head-on ("I'm anxious about asking her out, but I'll go ahead and do it").
- Avoid the situation ("I'm too nervous about possible rejection. I'll do it some other time").
- Adapt to the situation ("I get nervous every time I ask someone out, but that's normal. So what?").

To change your thoughts and beliefs about the significance of the unmet need, you could:

- Judge your situation to be less distressing than someone else's ("At least I'm meeting people. Poor John works so much he doesn't get to meet anyone").
- See your distress as necessary or temporary ("This is the way it is," or "Eventually I'll find somebody and I won't have to go through this anymore").
- Focus on positive aspects of a situation and minimize the negative ("If she says yes, I'm sure we'll have a great time").
- Devalue the goal and believe you will do fine no matter the outcome ("If he says no, it won't be the end of the world").

Reducing emotional distress by changing or reducing the intensity of the feeling itself could in-

Terms

coping strategies: ways people devise to prevent, avoid, or control the emotional distress of unfulfilled needs

defense mechanisms: mental strategies for avoiding unpleasant emotions

volve releasing emotional energy through an alternative activity:

- Exercise helps with frustration and anger.
- Meditation helps with sadness and anger.
- Talking to a receptive and empathic person can help with grief, shame, and anxiety.

Defense Mechanisms

Defense mechanisms are strategies people use to distort the perception and awareness of reality to avoid unpleasant thoughts, memories, emotions, and situations. A common defense mechanism is denial, which is not believing a truth. An example of denial is a smoker not believing she is at risk for lung cancer even though she knows that smoking causes cancer. This person denies reality to prevent awareness of the truth, possibly to avoid the fear of death.

Defense mechanisms protect us from thoughts and beliefs that we find threatening. The distorted reality feels safe because of the distortion. Strategies for meeting needs that are based on a faulty foundation result in needs not met. This may lead to disappointment, depression, self-blame, and withdrawal or avoidance of involvement in similar situations.

Distorting reality is not always bad. Sometimes it is necessary because of trauma or abuse. In such instances, denial helps a person cope with what would otherwise be a highly stressful psychological situation. Other times, denial can be a way to take a mental vacation. From the perspective of mental health,

however, the key is knowing when you are "on a fantasy trip" and when you are not and not letting certain defensive ways of thought become habitual. You can do this by learning to observe how your mind works. Such self-knowledge is a goal of meditation, yoga, modern psychotherapies, and other practices that help to focus on awareness and engage one's consciousness.

Facilitating Coping

Even when emotions make us aware that something in our lives is not going well, we do not always know what the problem is, or what is the best way to deal with it, or how to overcome fear of change or long-standing inertia. People should not suffer in silence or believe themselves to be flawed or "crazy." Support and advice are available from trusted family members, friends, teachers, clergy, and mental health professionals, such as counselors, psychotherapists, and physicians. Reaching out to such people helps those in distress gain a new perspective on their problems and to see a workable solution.

Psychotherapists are professionals who have undergone considerable training to help people deal with their emotional distress. Whether a person has feelings of inferiority, is troubled by painful dependency in a love relationship, or is immobilized by fear, a therapist can facilitate change that can make a person's life better. The change comes about not only by talking, but also by helping the distressed person adopt new behaviors and attitudes. It is one thing to know intellectually the source of a personal problem

Wellness Guide

Common Defense Mechanisms

Recognizing the following defense mechanisms will help you in maintaining emotional wellness.

Repression: keeping distressing thoughts and feelings unconscious

Example: A rape victim who has no memory of the assault

Projection: attributing one's own thoughts and feelings to someone else

Example: A student who dislikes her roommate but feels the roommate dislikes her

Displacement: diverting an emotion from the original target or source to another

Example: You are angry with your parents but yell at your best friends.

Reaction formation: believing and experiencing the opposite of how you really feel

Example: You are friendly to someone you dislike.

Rationalization: creating a plausible but false reason for your behavior

Example: Failing the course was due to the teacher's poor teaching methods.

Identification: imagining that someone's or some group's attributes are your own

Example: People who identify with a winning football team by wearing the team's colors, singing the team's song, and talking about the plays "we" made

Isolation and dissociation: compartmentalizing thoughts and emotions in different parts of awareness

Example: A man who gives successful and lucrative seminars to teach negotiation skills to business people, but frequently feuds with his neighbors

Denial: absolute rejection of a truth or of objective reality

Example: A college student who drinks a six-pack of beer every day but believes he has no problem with alcohol

and even what to do about it, but it may be quite another to face these unpleasant emotions and adopt new behaviors ("the map is not the road").

The value of psychotherapy, regardless of the method, is that the distressed person has faith in the professional's ability to facilitate change. This faith produces a situation of trust that enables the distressed person to be honest about himself or herself and to disclose painful and unflattering thoughts, memories, and emotions that would not likely be shared with a friend or relative.

Fears, Phobias, and Anxiety

Everybody experiences fear at some time or another. Fear is a powerful emotion that arises in situations that are interpreted as dangerous. The purpose of fear is to alert you to take protective action—usually to fight, flee, or seek assistance. For example, if you were hiking in the woods and encountered a snake, you would naturally interpret this situation as dangerous, which would produce the emotion of fear, which, in turn, would motivate some self-preserving behavior—probably an attempt to escape. If, however, you recognize that the snake is harmless, your interpretation of the situation as dangerous and the ensuing emotion of fear would have been erroneous. Notice how important the cognitive act of interpretation is in experiencing fear.

> Skate to where the puck is going to be, not where it has been.
>
> WAYNE GRETSKY

If fear is the response to a situation interpreted as threatening, **anxiety** is the response to an *imaginary situation*—usually something in the future that has not yet happened—that is interpreted as threatening. The purpose of anxiety is to warn you of *potentially* threatening situations and can take many forms (Figure 4.2). For example, anxiety about encountering a snake while on a hike, while heightening your awareness of this potential danger, could make the hike very unpleasant or prevent the hike from taking place at all, even if there were no snakes to encounter.

The word phobia comes from the Greek *phobos*, meaning "to take flight." Thus, a phobia causes us to avoid the object or situation that we fear—to flee from it both metaphorically and actually. A **phobia** involves an intense, irrational fear that something can threaten a person's life. The phobia can be a fear of anything: spiders, worms, snakes, bees, roses, a color, flying, boats, darkness—the list of phobias is very long. Some common phobias are *acrophobia* (fear of heights), *mysophobia* (fear of dirt and germs), *ophediophobia* (fear of snakes), and *zoophobia* (fear of animals). A particularly disabling phobia is *agoraphobia*, which is a

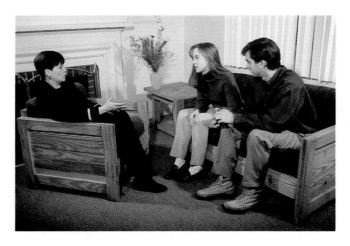

Talking with a counselor can help solve emotional problems.

fear of open spaces. People with agoraphobia are often so fear-stricken that they are unable to leave their homes to even run an errand or go shopping.

A person with a phobia invariably knows that the fear is irrational and illogical, yet is unable to control the feelings of anxiety even when thinking about the feared object or situation. Phobias often are triggered in childhood by a frightening event that may or may not be consciously remembered. For example, being stung by a bee while sniffing a rose in the garden at age four may result years later in fear produced by the smell of roses or a phobia to bees.

Specific phobias, including agoraphobia, can be treated by a variety of image visualization techniques, with hypnotherapy to uncover the unconscious sensitizing event or events, and by systematic desensitization therapy. Because a phobia only exists in the mind, the mind is where the healing must take place. Imagination is a powerful tool. By imagining the thing that is feared while safe and relaxed at home or in the therapist's office, the mind gradually learns to be comfortable with the object or situation that evokes fear. For example, a person with agoraphobia might begin at home by lying down and visualizing opening the door and looking out. After several days of open-door visualization, he or she might further imagine walking down the stairs, and so on, until he or she can visualize going to the corner store while feeling safe and comfortable. After imagining the trip outside, the next step is to actually open the door and step outside. The key to systematic desensitization is to monitor the anxiety and only take the step that feels safe. A trusted counselor or friend is essential in this process.

Social phobia (also known as social anxiety disorder) is characterized by an ongoing, pervasive fear of being observed and evaluated by others in all social situations most of the time. Individuals diagnosed with social phobia are constantly apprehensive that they will do or say something embarrassing or humiliating to themselves or to others. They compensate for these feelings by avoiding most social situations or interactions with others or, if unavoidable, enduring them with great anxiety and stress. Affected persons typically have few friends, drop out of school, have difficulty in work environments or in holding jobs, drink alcohol or use drugs to dull the anxiety, and often develop other psychological problems.

Social phobia is now regarded as a common, serious mental health problem, ranking third behind major depression and alcoholism; it is estimated that as much as 5 percent of Americans suffer from shyness severe enough to be designated social phobia. It should be emphasized that a diagnosis of social phobia entails more than just being shy or nervous in personal interactions at work or in social settings. It usually involves isolating oneself from even simple kinds of interactions: being unable to talk to authority figures such as a teacher or boss, avoiding informal interactions with coworkers, not accepting social invitations, and inability to talk even in small groups. However, advertisements from the drug company that makes Paxil (paroxetine hydrochloride), the leader among drugs used to treat social phobia, would have you believe that almost any form of shyness means you suffer from social phobia and need to take their drug (Stein et al., 1998). It might be wise to shy away from such advertisements.

Panic disorder should not be confused with phobia (fear of specific things like flying or snakes) or common anxiety disorders. Panic disorders frequently affect healthy young adults who suddenly experience intense sensations of a pounding heart, shortness of breath, sweating, and a fear of dying or losing control (Feldman, 2000). Because of these symptoms, panic disorder was formerly known as *irritable heart* or *hyperventilation syndrome.*

Panic disorder affects as many as 3 percent of healthy adult Americans and seriously disrupts their quality of life. Persons with panic disorder often wind

Terms

anxiety: the fear of an imaginary threat
phobia: a powerful and irrational fear of something
social phobia: fear of being observed and evaluated by others in social situations
panic disorder: severe anxiety accompanied by physical symptoms

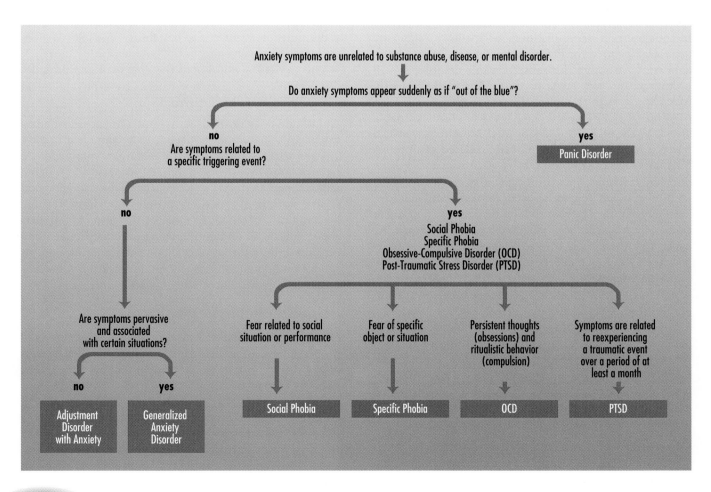

FIGURE 4.2   **The Variety of Anxiety Disorders**   *Source:* Adapted from American Psychiatric Association *DSM-IV-PC,* 1994.

Dollars and Health Sense

Drugs for Worries and Bad Habits

In the past 25 years worries and "bad habits" of various kinds have become reclassified as mental disorders that need to be medically treated, usually by drug therapy. By redefining worries and bad habits as diseases, physicians, hospitals, and drug companies now earn vast amounts of money treating these problems.

Now a significant proportion of the population is being treated with an antidepressant, antianxiety, or antiphobic pill, or with drugs to control unhealthy habits such as smoking cigarettes, drinking alcohol, or overeating. We live in a time when it is widely accepted that "bad molecules" produced in our brains or bodies cause us to drink and eat too much,

to worry excessively, or to be overly shy. If a bad molecule can be identified, then a "good drug" can be developed that will counteract the effects of the bad molecule. As more and more unhealthy behaviors and anxieties become molecularized and medicalized, the medical/pharmaceutical industry continues to grow and prosper.

There are still some bad habits left waiting to be medicalized and treated. For example, gambling is widely regarded as a bad habit, especially compulsive gambling. Researchers are looking for an inherited gene carried by compulsive gamblers that is responsible for their obsession. Moving from an identified gene to a drug to combat its effects is

only a matter of time, money, and effort on the part of a dedicated drug company. And considering the number of people who like to gamble, the rewards could be enormous.

Compulsive shopping (strongly encouraged by advertisements and sales clerks) is another bad habit, especially if you don't have the money to pay for your charged purchases. Drug companies are currently testing drugs in order to identify ones that put a damper on the uncontrollable urge to buy. Consumers will soon have the choice of running out to buy some new clothes or spending the money on a prescription that will suppress the urge.

up in hospital emergency rooms suffering from dizziness, bowel distress, and symptoms of a heart attack. In the case of a panic disorder, all medical diagnostic tests are negative for disease, but the symptoms often continue. Although the cause of panic disorder is still unknown, research suggests that a disturbance of neurotransmitters in the brain are responsible.

One of the most effective ways to control a panic attack is through deep, abdominal breathing that can prevent hyperventilation and other related symptoms. Yoga breathing techniques are a good way to begin or one can consult a breathing specialist who can teach techniques that help an affected person avoid shallow, rapid breathing. The fact that panic disorder appears at certain periods of life, that no biological or genetic cause is known, and that it is effectively relieved by psychotherapy or placebo should encourage people to focus on lifestyle changes that will free them of the serious and debilitating consequences of panic disorder (Barlow et al., 2000).

Generalized anxiety disorder is characterized by persistent and excessive worry and feelings of anxiety. Only in the last 20 years has the diagnosis of generalized anxiety disorder been recognized as a mental disorder distinct from phobia, panic disorder, or social phobia (see Figure 4.2). However, generalized anxiety disorder now has its own set of diagnostic criteria:

- Excessive worry and anxiety over work or school performance that has continued for at least six months.
- The patient is unable to control or cope with the anxiety and feels that it interferes with performance at work or in other aspects of daily life.

- The anxiety must be accompanied by at least three of the following: restlessness or being "on edge," fatigue, difficulty concentrating, irritability, muscle tension, and problems sleeping.
- The anxiety is not due to the effects of any drug (legal or illegal) and is not caused by a physiological condition (e.g., hyperthyroidism).

Where does normal worry end and excessive anxiety begin? There does not seem to be any clear or easy answer to this question. For example, many people have ongoing worries (generalized anxiety) about being able to pay their bills, keep their jobs, or get good grades in school. Anxious people may have trouble sleeping or be "on edge" most of the time. Is one person mentally ill and another mentally well depending on how anxious they are about their money, job, or school problems? This is the dilemma for psychotherapists who treat people with ongoing worries.

Obsessive-Compulsive Disorder

Obsessive-compulsive disorder (OCD) is characterized by persistent, unwelcome thoughts or images (*obsessions*) which often are accompanied by the urgent need to engage in certain rituals that cannot be controlled (*compulsions*). Rituals such as handwashing, counting, checking, or cleaning are often performed in hope of preventing obsessive thoughts or making them go away. Performing these rituals, however, provides only temporary relief, and not performing them markedly increases anxiety. OCD affects about 2 percent of the U.S. population. The condition typically begins during adolescence or early childhood. It is

Global Wellness

Depression Is Worldwide

Missing my dear mother, as a son,
my liver and intestines are painfully broken!
Crying for my old mother, as a son,
my tears pour into my chest!
Thinking about my old mother, as a son,
to swallow food and tea is difficult!
Searching for my old mother, as a son,
I cannot sleep day and night!

Si-Lang, *Searching for Mother*
Tenth Century Beijing Opera

Melancholy and depression know no geographic boundaries, as this thousand-year-old Chinese aria describing the physical aspects of depression shows.

Depression has been documented in virtually all cultures, although its prevalence varies (Young, 1997). Depression in Asia, for example, is less prevalent than in North America and Europe. Rates of depression in the U.S. even vary by cultural group: The lifetime prevalence of depression among people of African and Hispanic ancestry is about 12%; among people of European ancestry, it's 17%.

Besides prevalence rates, depression manifests differently among cultures. Several Native American cultures tend to experience depression as social loneliness. A typical Caucasian North American or European is likely to experience depression in terms of psychological symptoms, such as melancholy, moodiness, and lack of interest in pleasure. However, in Asian cultures, depression tends to be experienced as physical complaints (as in the Chinese aria above), such as fatigue, loss of appetite, and sleep problems.

Help-seeking behavior for depression also varies among cultures. Latin American men and mainland Chinese tend not to seek help for depression, fearing that doing so will stigmatize them as weak. In Japan and Hong Kong, where depression tends to be experienced as a physical ailment, people tend to consult with a doctor for relief of physical symptoms. Latin American women and European-Americans are more likely to consult mental health practitioners.

---

sometimes accompanied by depression, eating disorders, substance abuse, attention deficit hyperactivity disorder, or other anxiety disorders. Symptoms of OCD can also coexist and may even be part of a spectrum of neurological disorders, such as Tourette's syndrome. OCD likely has a neurobiological basis and is not caused by family problems or by attitudes learned in childhood, such as an inordinate emphasis on cleanliness or a belief that certain thoughts are dangerous or unacceptable. Treatments for OCD involve medications and behavioral therapy.

Depression

According to the National Institute of Mental Health, each day approximately one person in seven experiences **depression,** characterized by feelings of dejection, guilt, hopelessness, self-recrimination, loss of appetite, insomnia, loss of interest in sex, reduced interest in previously enjoyable activities, withdrawal from social contacts, inability to concentrate and make decisions, lowered self-esteem, and a focus on negative thoughts and the bad things in life. If asked how they feel, depressed people usually say something like, "Life's a drag" or "What's the use of doing anything?"

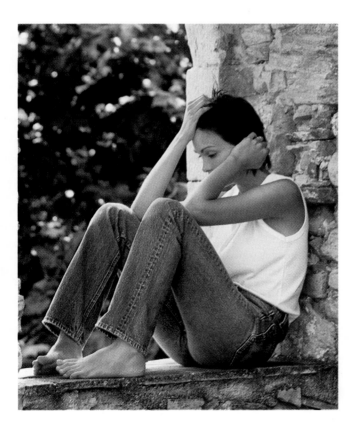

Many things may make us feel depressed temporarily.

Terms

generalized anxiety disorder: persistent and often nonspecific worry and anxiety

obsessive-compulsive disorder: persistent, unwelcome thoughts or images and the urgent need to engage in certain rituals that cannot be controlled

depression: a mental disorder characterized by sadness, feelings of inadequacy, and low self-esteem

Depression can occur as a normal response to the loss of something that a person values or is attached to, such as a loved one, a job, good health, or self-esteem (e.g., when a person does not succeed at a task she or he deems important). When individuals experience a loss, it is "normal" for them to feel sad and depressed, and to grieve the loss. Sadness and grief are the human spirit's way to heal the hurt of loss and open the way for new attachments. When depression is associated with a loss, the depressed individual may be simultaneously aware that the experience is transitory and, along with grief, feel that there is hope for the future. This kind of depression tends to lift after the grieving ends.

In contrast to the "normal" depression that may accompany loss, some people experience a long-lasting depressive state, or periodic episodes of deep depression, that are not self-limiting and may hinder and even jeopardize a person's life. These depressions may be a response to stress, severe psychological trauma, injury, disease, biological malfunctions of some part of the brain, or a combination of factors. In some persons, major episodes of depression are accompanied by periods of excited euphoria ("mania"), resulting in a condition referred to as **bipolar disorder.**

Some individuals are susceptible to depression during the winter months because a lack of sunlight disturbs the production of neurotransmitters in the brain that affect mood. This "seasonal affective disorder" (SAD) is sometimes remedied by increased exposure to stronger-than-normal indoor lighting that mimics sunlight or relocation to southern latitudes where there is more light.

Depression can also accompany the experience of being very sick or injured. In such cases, depression results from a combination of factors, such as grieving the loss of health; coping with the stress of being sick; lack of exercise and normal routine; disruption of regular social activities; or alterations in physiology that may change brain chemistry. Medications may also make one susceptible to depression. Some people experience a mild form of depression called **dysthymia.** Like major depression, dysthymia is associated with disturbances in sleep, appetite, and the ability to concentrate.

> *Your health is bound to be affected if day after day you say the opposite of what you feel.*
>
> BORIS PASTERNAK,
> DOCTOR ZHIVAGO

One of the characteristics of severe depression is a considerable degree of negative thinking, characterized by severe self-criticism; negative views about the self, the world, and the future; and a variety of logic errors in assessing the self and the world (Burns, 1992). Some of these logic errors include:

- *All or none thinking:* seeing things as polar extremes (e.g., all good and all bad)
- *Overgeneralizing:* interpreting one setback as evidence that *every* similar situation will *forever* turn out badly
- *Negative filtering:* focusing only on the negative while filtering out the positive
- *Disqualifying the positive:* transforming positive occurrences into negative experiences

Becoming aware of negative thoughts (often called *negative self-talk*) opens the way to adopting positive self-images and more realistic appraisals of the world. These, in turn, help to lessen the depressive state. Cognitive behavioral therapy is a very successful method for helping depressed people change their negative thought patterns.

Another characteristic of depression is that it can intensify itself, thus creating a depressive cycle. The depressed person's negative thoughts, social withdrawal, and loss of interest in pleasurable experiences serve to reinforce feelings of worthlessness, helplessness, gloom, and doom. Recovery from depression requires both interrupting the depressive cycle and correcting the life situation that brought on the depression.

One way to deal with depression is to get life moving again. This is accomplished by establishing and achieving simple, attainable goals that can be done in a brief period of time. The goals should involve movement that restores fundamental breathing and other mind-body rhythms, which may alter the chemistry of the brain to facilitate pleasant (instead of unpleasant) moods. Many a depressed person has found relief in taking up a regular exercise program.

Also, depressed individuals should interact with people who offer support. Remaining in seclusion only reinforces feelings of loss and worthlessness. It is also helpful not to engage in long conversations with friends and family about how lousy life is. Recreational activity can divert attention from negative thinking and weaken the depressive cycle.

Several types of medication are extremely effective in helping people recover from depression. These medications include: tricyclic antidepressants, selective serotonin reuptake inhibitors, and monamine oxidase inhibitors. Pharmacotherapy for depression often involves an initial phase of medication to interrupt the depressive cycle and restore a sense of balance and control over life, followed by psychological counseling (usually cognitive behavioral therapy)

Terms

bipolar disorder: major episodes of depression accompanied by periods of excitement

dysthymia: a long-lasting, mild form of depression

Wellness Guide

If a Friend Is Considering Suicide

If you suspect that a friend is considering suicide, how can you help? You can take any of several possible courses of action. All involve you making a concrete intervention. Intervention is tough. It is much easier to tell yourself that things will get better, or tomorrow is another day. Rationalization and procrastination are not useful behaviors in a situation that involves depression or potential suicide. Let's look at some options available to you.

- Talk to your friend. Tell him or her that you are concerned. Describe the behavior that is causing you to worry. Ask if you can help (but don't give up if your friend says no).
- Ask your friend directly if he or she is thinking about suicide. You may be shocked if your friend answers yes, but, remember, even someone who sees suicide as a potential solution always has a wish to live. If your friend admits thinking of suicide, ask if he or she has thought of a plan.
- Negotiate a "no-suicide" agreement before leaving your friend. Ask your friend to agree not to commit suicide at any time. If your friend will not agree to this contract or tries to change it to a certain time, then he or she is at increased risk. Report this situation to a professional counselor at once. Stay with your friend or arrange for someone else to stay with him or her until professional help arrives.
- If your friend agrees to a "no-suicide" pact, go to your college health service or residence hall advisor, speak with a counselor or physician, and describe your friend's behavior. The professional will know the best way to handle the situation. And remember, even if you feel you are interfering or breaking a confidence, you may be saving a life. An intervention made now can prevent suicide.
- Talk to other friends, a residence hall advisor, or even a teacher—anyone who will assist you to verbalize your concerns and decide how to help. The most important action is to do something after you become aware of the potentially dangerous outcome.

to find nonmedical ways to sustain well-being (Whooley and Simon, 2000).

Because depression involves inactivity, withdrawal, hopelessness, and self-defeating thoughts and behaviors, it is often difficult for individuals to activate themselves on a program of self-healing. At such times, the encouragement of a caring friend or family member and the guidance of a therapist, counselor, or other helper can be invaluable. Others can help a depressed person confront the causes of the depression and become aware of and try to minimize negative self-talk—negative views about the self, the world, and the future; self-critical inner dialogue, and logic errors in the assessment of self and events.

Suicide

One of the most worrisome aspects of depression is the risk of suicide. In the United States, suicide ranks among the 10 most frequent causes of death, accounting for approximately 30,000 deaths per year. The number of reported suicides is thought to represent only 10% to 15% of suicide attempts. People over 65 make up the largest age group of suicides. Among young people (15 to 24 years old), suicide ranks third behind accidents and murder as a cause of death.

Suicide is not a disease, nor is it a disorder that can be inherited. Suicides are not caused by the weather or a full moon. Generally people consider suicide because they feel overwhelmed and painfully distressed by life and they believe suicide to be their only option. Sometimes people attempt suicide not because they really want to die but because they want to express anger at others or signal others for help. In such instances, suicide attempts are characterized by limited self-destructive acts, such as taking less than a lethal dose of sleeping pills or arranging that the attempt be discovered in time for the person to be saved.

Occasionally a person expresses thoughts of suicide to a friend or relative. This can be extremely distressing to the listener, who may react with disbelief, panic, or avoidance. In attempting to deal with his or her own uncomfortable feelings, a listener might say things like, "Cheer up, you've got a lot to live for," or "You're better off than I am," or "You can't be serious!" These and similar statements have the effect of denying the distressed person's feelings. Psychologists recommend instead that listeners speak directly to suicidal thoughts ("Tell me more about why you want to kill yourself"), offer the distressed person nonjudgmental sympathy and concern, and firmly but patiently direct the distressed person to professional help immediately.

Often suicidal individuals offer excuses for not seeing a professional and may even try to blackmail a friend into silence with threats ("I'll kill myself if you tell anyone"). The friend must hold firm and, if necessary, make an appointment with a counselor or psychiatrist at the student health center or hospital emergency room and deliver the distressed person there, or telephone a suicide prevention hotline.

Wellness Guide

Some Tips for Dealing with Anger

Here are some suggestions for expressing anger constructively.

- *Recognize your anger.* Pay attention to anger in yourself when you become aware of it. Then take some time to determine which of your thoughts are causing it. Are you hurt, frustrated, frightened? What happened that made you angry?

- *Own your anger.* Try not to blame someone else for your angry feeling by means of thoughts or statements like, "It's all your fault!" or "If it weren't for you," or "If only you'd have . . ." Don't put it onto someone else unless you're sure it belongs there.

- *Find anger's origins.* Even if you are very angry, try not to act immediately on those feelings. Instead, set aside a time to think about them and how best to express them.

- *Resolve the anger.* Try not to let anger build up over time. If you do, you may become resentful, which may cause you to distance emotionally or physically or to displace the anger onto someone else, like a child or a co-worker.

- *Don't ambush.* Attacking with anger when it's least expected is unfair and invites resentment or a counterattack, not reconciliation.

- *Be specific.* When you're talking about emotional conflicts, name exactly what's causing the anger and stick to that issue. Don't bring up past hurts. Don't discuss second and third topics until the first one is settled. If other issues arise, write them down so you can discuss them later. Make it a habit to keep pencil and paper handy when issues are discussed. Don't give in to the temptation to bring up secondary issues in order to retaliate for hurt feelings or as a way to avoid resolving the issue at hand.

- *Don't hit below the belt.* Don't attack your partner with something you know will hurt because you think you're losing an argument.

- *Attack the problem, not each other.* Don't engage in character assassination with put-downs and accusations. Use "I" statements to communicate resentments. If someone attacks with a put-down, rather than retaliate, the recipient can say "Ouch, that hurt." This can be a cue to redress the attack and go on with the issue under discussion. If this doesn't happen, the discussion will probably be sidetracked from the main point to the put-down, and a fight about hurt feelings may ensue.

- *Be respectful and respectable.* When working to resolve an issue, try to maintain an attitude of respect. Try to understand the other's point of view. Ask the other person to respect you and your feelings, even though you disagree.

- *Take some time.* Sometimes you can sense that an anger-causing issue isn't getting resolved in the discussion. It's all right to acknowledge that and to take a few hours or days to reconsider things, then discuss the issue again. Sometimes emotions are too intense and it's not possible to think clearly. Sometimes you just need time to reflect and figure things out.

- *Physical affection is okay.* Sex or any other affectionate behavior before an issue is resolved is acceptable, as long as it's not taken as a sign that the issue is resolved. Both of you must understand this. Affectionate behavior shows that arguing about something can be accommodated within a caring relationship.

- *Both sides win.* After an issue has been discussed and the partners seem agreed on the outcome, if one or both feels a grudge, then the argument has produced a winner and a loser, and the relationship has been harmed. Holding a grudge is a sign that the issue is not resolved. Try again.

At the time a person contemplates suicide, life seems absolutely hopeless. But few life problems are beyond solution. Life crises improve and distressing emotions pass. Time does heal many hurts. And the experience gained by working through a distressing time of life can bring confidence, insight, and understanding. Acquiring experience and understanding, a person is better able to cope with life's problems and is better able to help others deal with their challenges.

Anger

Anger occurs when we've been attacked, blamed, hurt, or have experienced a loss; when we *imagine* we've been attacked, blamed, hurt, or have experienced a loss; when we imagine we *may* be attacked, blamed, hurt, or experience a loss; or when the pursuit of an important goal is blocked. Anger is an excitatory emotion, providing the motivational energy to protect ourselves or things we care about or to overcome obstacles to our goals. We use anger to stop physical or psychological abuse and to protect ourselves from the hurt of loss. Sometimes we get angry because we perceive something as threatening that really isn't. In this case, we make ourselves angry by what we think.

Many people have difficulty dealing with anger in themselves or in others. They fear the intensity of the emotion. They fear the possibility of violence that may accompany its expression. They fear retaliation or rejection.

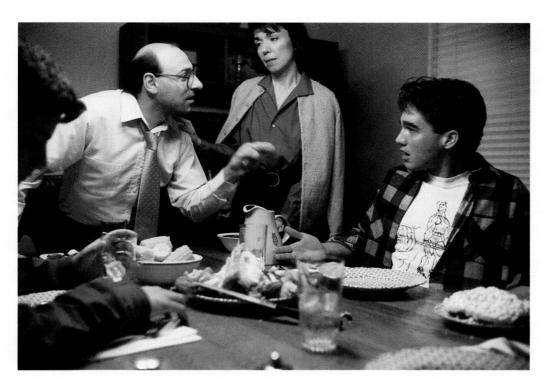

Family arguments disrupt the emotional well-being of parents and children.

One constructive way to work with anger is to understand the source of the emotion. For example, to deal with frustration you can reassess the merits of the goal you cannot attain or reconsider the strategy you've employed for attaining it. It may feel right to blame someone else for your troubles, but a reevaluation of how you contribute to the situation may be more productive.

The next time you feel angry, take a "time out" for a few seconds, minutes, or days if necessary. Ask yourself what you've experienced that's led you to be angry. Are you really being harmed or threatened or are you making yourself angry because you've interpreted a situation as such? If you feel frustrated about not being able to accomplish a goal, is your goal realistically attainable? Have you expected too much of yourself? Have you expected too much of someone else? Is your strategy for attaining your goal workable? Is something else better? Did you communicate your goals, needs, plans, and desires to people whose help you wanted or expected?

Sleep and Dreams

All living things exhibit cycles of rest and activity, which in humans are represented by the daily sleep-wake cycle. Everyone has a sleep-wake cycle that corresponds to their optimal degree of physical, mental, and spiritual well-being. Studies show that adequate sleep enhances attentiveness, concentration, mood, and motivation. Sleep deprivation, on the other hand, impairs a person's ability to be productive, good-humored, satisfied with life, and even to laugh at a joke! Lack of sleep can gravely impair judgment; sleeplessness is second only to drunkenness as a cause of automobile accidents. Long-term sleep deprivation can be fatal.

Sleep researchers believe that a majority of Americans are sleeping 60 to 90 minutes a night less than the seven, eight, or nine hours that would leave them refreshed and energetic during the day. Individuals "cheat on their sleep" to create time for other things in the busy schedules that characterize modern life. Sleep is considered expendable, and *not* sleeping is considered a sign of ambition and drive. Furthermore, around-the-clock TV and radio entertainment can distract people from sleeping. Before the advent of the electric light bulb about 100 years ago, people tended to sleep about nine hours a night. When it got dark, people slept. Because sleep is so strongly linked to one's total state of well-being, focusing on healthy sleep habits can produce greater mind-body harmony.

Sleep Problems

Because of life's never-ending array of challenges, just about everyone has trouble sleeping once in a while. Experiences that commonly disrupt sleeping patterns include being sick, jet-lagged, nervous about an upcoming exam, or excited about something new; having consumed too much food, alcohol, or caffeine; or losing a loved one. Fortunately, most people tend to adjust to these situations, and their sleep rhythms return to normal (for them) in a few days. A large percentage of Americans, however, have problems with sleeping that last several weeks to years. The most common sleep problems are not sleeping enough (insomnia), sleeping during the day (excessive daytime sleepiness), and unusual activities associated with sleep (parasomnias).

Insomnia

The majority of people with long-term sleep problems have **insomnia.** They have trouble falling asleep or staying asleep, or they awaken after a few hours of sleep and cannot go back to sleep. The daytime results of insomnia are fatigue, the desire to nap, impaired ability to concentrate, impaired judgment, and a lack of zest for life. Although insomnia may be related to disease or injury in the brain's sleep centers, most often it is the result of a physical illness, chronic pain, stress, depression, anxiety, obsessive-compulsive ruminations, panic attacks, post-traumatic stress disorder, and drug or alcohol abuse.

Sometimes, as a result of insomnia, individuals have a difficult time staying awake during the day. They may feel sleepy most of the time, may "nod off"

easily during a routine activity, or may nap at the slightest opportunity. Because they get insufficient sleep at night, about 20% of college students can fall asleep almost instantaneously if permitted to lie down in a darkened room. Extreme tendency to fall asleep during the day is called **narcolepsy.**

Parasomnias

Parasomnias occur in many forms and have the potential to interrupt restful sleep. Nightmares are dreams that arouse feelings of fear, terror, panic, or anxiety. Sleepwalking, or **somnambulism,** is a condition occurring primarily in children and often associated with anxiety, fatigue, or stress. The person performs motor activity, usually leaving bed and walking around, while sleeping and has no memory of it on awakening. Other vigorous behaviors, such as punching, kicking, and night terrors (episodes that begin with a loud cry followed by rapid heart rate, sweating, and feelings of panic), will also interrupt sleep. Another abnormality is **sleep apnea,** in which individuals stop breathing while sleeping; typically, breathing resumes within 30 seconds.

Since the majority of sleep problems represent some form of disharmony within ourselves or with

---

Wellness Guide

Getting a Good Night's Sleep

Here are some suggestions for getting a good night's sleep.

- *Establish a regular sleep time.* Give your own natural sleep cycle a chance to be in synchrony with the day-night cycle by going to bed at the same time each night (within an hour more or less) and arising *without being awakened by an alarm clock.* This will mean going to bed early enough to give yourself enough time to sleep. Try to maintain your regular sleep times on the weekend. Getting up early during the week and sleeping late on weekends may upset the rhythm of your sleep cycle.

- *Create a proper (for you) sleep environment.* Sleep occurs best when the sleeping environment is dark, quiet, free of distractions, and not too warm. If you use radio or TV to help you fall asleep, use an autotimer to shut off the noise after falling asleep.

- *Wind down before going to bed.* About 20 to 30 minutes before bedtime, stop any activities that cause mental or physical arousal, such as work or exercise, and take up a "quiet" activity that can create a transition to sleep. Transitional activities could include reading, watching "mindless" TV, taking a warm bath or shower, meditation, or making love.

- *Make the bedroom for sleeping only.* Make the bedroom your place for getting a good night's sleep. Try not to use it for work or for discussing problems with your partner.

- *Don't worry while in bed.* If you are unable to sleep after about 30 minutes in bed because of worry about the next day's activities, get up and do some limited activity such as reading a magazine article, doing the dishes, or meditating. Go back to bed when you feel drowsy. If you cannot sleep because of thinking about all that

you have to do, write down what's on your mind and let the paper hold onto the thoughts while you sleep. You can retrieve them in the morning.

- *Avoid alcohol and caffeine.* Some people have a glass of beer or wine before bed in order to relax. Large amounts of alcohol, while sedating, block normal sleep and dreaming patterns. Because caffeine remains in the body for several hours, people sensitive to caffeine should not ingest any after noon.

- *Exercise regularly.* Exercising 20 to 30 minutes three or four times a week enhances the ability to sleep. You should not exercise vigorously within three hours of bedtime, however, because of the possibility of becoming too aroused to sleep.

Source: Adapted from M. L. Reite, K. E. Nagel, and J. R. Ruddy, *The Evaluation and Management of Sleep Disorders* (Washington, DC: American Psychiatric Press, 1990).

our surroundings, restoring harmony is a way to return to our natural rest-activity cycle. This can be accomplished by employing mind-body health practices such as meditation, exercise, and proper nutrition. For extreme sleep disorders, professional help should be sought.

Some people turn to alcohol, sleeping pills, tranquilizers, and other drugs; however, they offer only short-term symptomatic relief for sleep disorders. Without a holistic approach and fundamental changes in one's lifestyle and attitudes, relying on drugs to restore natural sleep rhythms may be harmful and may lead to physical dependency and habituation.

Understanding Our Dreams

We all dream while we sleep. Even animals dream. Although some people deny they dream, this is because they do not recall their dreams when awake. On the other hand, some people have vivid recall of the several dreams they have each night (a skill that can be learned).

Dreams tend to occur in the stage of sleep called **rapid eye movement (REM) sleep** (Figure 4.3). While asleep, people cycle through the four stages several times. Dreams usually occur between Stage 4 (deep sleep) and the return to Stage 1 (light sleep) of the next cycle.

No one knows why we dream. Some researchers have suggested that REM sleep states are necessary for brain growth, daily information processing, and cellular rejuvenation. Others believe that dreams are the brain's way of processing and eliminating information and memories that are no longer useful. Whatever the reasons, dreams are necessary for health. Experimental subjects who were deprived of the chance to dream (they were awakened by experimenters during REM sleep) developed bizarre behaviors and psychotic symptoms. The individuals returned to normal after at least one night of catching up on the missed REM time.

For thousands of years dreams have been used in many cultures to restore mental and physical health. The temples of Asclepius were used by ancient Greeks for more than a thousand years as places where people went to have healing dreams and to have them interpreted by the priests and priestesses.

Indications that dreams can be healthy come from studies of the Senoi, a Malaysian tribe known as the "dream people." The Senoi live in a nonaggressive, noncombative, communal society. The tribe's members have a remarkable degree of mental and emotional health, which is attributed by some to the daily ritual of discussing and interpreting their dreams. Both children and adults gather each morning to recount their dreams to one another, singly and in groups. According to Senoi custom, the events, anxieties, and people in a dream are real and must be acknowledged and dealt with. Such behavior is similar to our custom of looking for meaning in dreams, especially as a component of psychotherapy.

Interpreting Your Dreams

In our culture, numerous theories of dream interpretation have been proposed. Perhaps the best known are those of Sigmund Freud and Carl Jung, who proposed universally applicable rules for uncovering the meaning of symbols and events in dreams. Most modern dream researchers do not believe in universal symbolism, however. Instead, they believe that the symbolism and meaning in a dream are unique. Dreams are private conversations with ourselves, communicated in a private language of images that often are bizarre, dramatic, emotional, and exaggerated.

Terms

insomnia: prolonged inability to obtain adequate sleep

narcolepsy: extreme tendency to fall asleep during the day

parasomnias: activities that interrupt restful sleep

somnambulism: sleepwalking

sleep apnea: state of troubled or interrupted breathing while sleeping

rapid eye movement (REM) sleep: stage of sleep in which dreams occur

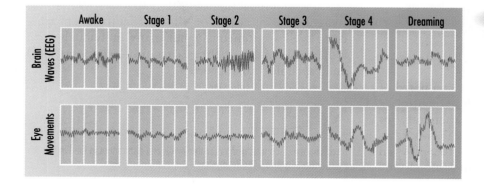

FIGURE 4.3   Tracings of the Electrical Signals Produced During the Stages of Sleep Tiny electrodes are placed on a person's scalp and eyelids. They detect electrical signals within the brain and movements of the eyes. Notice that rapid eye movement (REM) occurs during a dream period.

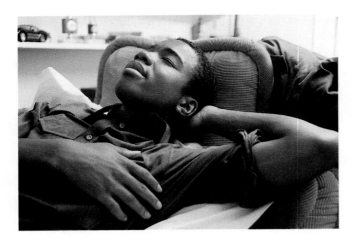

Sufficient sleep and dreams are essential to mental health.

Much dream research suggests that dreams are reflections of recent happenings, thoughts, and feelings that are not dealt with in our daily consciousness. Many people are too busy to attend to everything they experience, think, and feel. Sometimes, they purposely do not deal with reality because it is unpleasant. In a dream, however, you "come clean" with yourself. You bring forth subtle feelings and impressions that were not attended to while awake. You engage your innermost thoughts and feelings about fears, worries, conflicts, and problems that you chose not to deal with when awake. Thus, many problems (and sometimes their solutions!) are presented in dreams.

Dreams may also be a literal representation of reality that went unattended. For example, if you dream of a mouse, perhaps you saw a mouse in your kitchen, or perhaps you noticed some movements out of the corner of your eye and thought of a mouse. In either case, your discomfort at the thought of a mouse in your house caused you to block the thought from consciousness.

Another device for finding the message in a dream is to focus on the emotions in the dream and not on the dream's content. Although you may have dreamed of dancing an incredibly brilliant solo on a stage to an audience's wild applause, the actual emotion in the dream may have been fear. The dream, therefore, is probably about fear, not pride or accomplishment.

Mental Disorders

The brain, like all other body organs, is composed of molecules and cells whose functioning is controlled by biological processes. It is possible, therefore, for brain tissue to be affected by chemical imbalance, injury, infection, toxins, and genetic disorders. When brain injury or disease occurs, thoughts, mood, and

TABLE 4.1   Signs of Schizophrenia

Aspect of life	Typical symptoms
Emotions	Inappropriate responses to stimuli
	Blunted or flat emotions
	Fear of warmth or closeness
	Erratic and negative feelings
Thought	Inability to tell real from unreal
	Delusions and hallucinations
	Disorganized and confused thoughts
	Tangential or circumstantial conversation
	Bizarre ideas and language
Interpersonal relationships	Thoughts only of self, autism
	Unpredictable responses when approached
	Social isolation
	Lack of response
	Withdrawal
	Impaired role functioning
Behavior	Deteriorated level of functioning, immobilization
	Inability to make decisions
	Poor judgment
	Bizarre or peculiar behavior
	Lethargy, loss of initiative
	Poor personal hygiene and grooming

behaviors can be impaired. In most cases, the biological basis for mental disorders is unknown.

Schizophrenia is a debilitating mental disorder characterized by hallucinations, delusions, an inability to maintain logical and coherent thought patterns, diminished emotional and social experience, and a diminished sense of purpose (Table 4.1). Typically schizophrenia manifests in teenage years and progresses into adulthood. The disease occurs at the same rate (0.85%) in virtually all societies in the world; it is responsible for 2.5% of total U.S. health expenditures. The cause of schizophrenia is unknown, although scientists believe that biological (possibly inherited) factors are partially responsible. While medications and psychosocial rehabilitation can help lessen symptoms, there is no cure. About one third of schizophrenics become well spontaneously, but many individuals with a diagnosis of schizophrenia require ongoing medical and psychological support.

Terms

schizophrenia: a mental disorder that involves a disturbance in thinking, in perceiving reality, and in functioning

Critical Thinking About Health

1. Dr. Razmataz's book, "30 Days to Exceptional Mental Health," had been on the best-seller charts for 10 weeks, but after his appearance on TV's "Inside This Week," sales went through the roof. Entertainers, business executives, professional athletes, and political leaders extolled the value of his program to lessen needless worry, improve sleep, and enhance mood, self-esteem, memory, and mental acuity.

    Dr. Razmataz based his program on 10 years of research he conducted as director of the Ersatz Mental Health Clinic. In his book and his media appearances, Dr. Razmataz explained that the type and severity of a particular mental illness was caused by either the over- or underactivity of the genes that controlled the production of the six basic neurotransmitter chemicals in the brain. The key to his method was determining a patient's genetic profile and matching it to one of six specific organic food diets.

    Questions:
    a. What factors are mentioned in the description above that might suggest to someone that Dr. Razmataz's method is credible and efficacious?
    b. Which of these factors do you find influence you when you are making a health decision?
    c. What additional information, if any, would you want before trying Dr. Razmataz's method yourself or recommending it to someone else? How would you find such information?

2. List five characteristics of a mentally healthy person. If you were a parent, how would you ensure that your child(ren) grow(s) up to manifest the five characteristics on your list? Also discuss how individuals can contribute to the mental health of people in their community.

3. John hasn't liked being Margie's supervisor since her first day of work. She just doesn't get it. And since she's the boss's niece, there is little he can do. In the past six months, whenever Margie is on John's shift-team, his finds himself so distressed that he doesn't want to go to work.
    a. The chapter describes several ways to cope with emotional distress including (a) changing the situation that is causing the distress, (b) altering the significance one places on the distressing situation, and (c) lessening the distressing emotions. Discuss how John could employ each of these coping strategies to lessen his emotional distress. Also, describe the consequences for John of implementing each coping strategy.
    b. When you experience emotional distress, which of the three coping strategies do you employ most often? Do you notice situations in which one coping strategy works better than in others?

4. Many people equate mental and emotional well-being with happiness. If they feel happy, they identify themselves as emotionally well. In your opinion, what is the relationship of emotional well-being and happiness? How do unpleasant emotions, such as sadness, grief, shame, guilt, and anger, affect one's sense of emotional well-being? Would you argue that the path to mental and emotional well-being is the pursuit of happiness? If not, in your view, what constitutes the path to mental and emotional well-being?

Health in Review

- Mental and emotional health depend on how well individuals meet their maintenance and growth needs and cope with situations in which their needs are not met.
- People understand their needs by interpreting what they sense from the environment and in their bodies. As they mature, people develop ideas about and learn strategies to meet their emotional needs.
- Emotions tell us whether we are satisfied by, and the level of satisfaction from, our experiences, plans, and outcomes of behavior.
- Emotional distress occurs when needs are not met. People cope with emotional distress by changing their modes of interaction with the environment, changing the importance of their unmet needs, or changing the distressing feelings.
- Counselors, therapists, and others can help clarify the source of emotional distress and find healthy ways to cope with it.
- Fear, anxiety, and depression are common emotional problems.
- Common phobias include acrophobia, agoraphobia, claustrophobia, mysophobia, ophediophobia, and zoophobia.
- Depression is often characterized by feelings of dejection, guilt, hopelessness, self-recrimination,

- loss of appetite, insomnia, loss of interest in sexual activity, withdrawal from friends, inability to concentrate, lowered self-esteem, and a focus on the negative.
- Other mental disorders include panic disorder, social phobia, and obsessive-compulsive disorder.
- Suicide is the third leading cause of death among persons aged 15 to 24 years, of all races and both genders.
- Many of the signs of depression occur in someone suicidal. Many suicidal people talk about suicide when life appears hopeless.

- Sleep and dreams are fundamental to human health. Sleep has four stages. REM sleep, during which dreams occur, happens during the cycle of sleep from deep to lighter stages.
- Many people use their dreams to help them understand and deal with distressing situations and confusing emotions.
- Schizophrenia is a mental disorder characterized by delusions, inability to think logically and coherently, diminished social and emotional experiences, and loss of sense of purpose.

Health and Wellness Online

The World Wide Web contains a wealth of information about health and wellness. By accessing the Internet using Web browser software, such as Netscape Navigator or Microsoft's Internet Explorer, you can gain a new perspective on many topics presented in *Health and Wellness, Seventh Edition.* Access the Jones and Bartlett Publishers Web site at http://www.jbpub.com/hwonline.

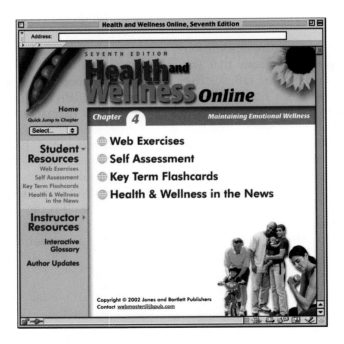

References

Barlow, D. H., et al. (2000). Cognitive-behavioral therapy, imipramine, or their combination for panic disorder: a randomized controlled trial. *Journal of the American Medical Association, 283*, 2529–2536.

Burns, D. (1992). *Feeling good.* New York: Avon.

Feldman, M. D. (2000, July 5). Managing psychiatric disorders in primary care: Anxiety. *Hospital Practice*, 77–84.

Maslow, A. L. (1970). *Motivation and personality.* New York: Harper & Row.

Murray, B., et al. (1998). Paroxetine treatment of generalized social phobia (social anxiety disorder). *Journal of the American Medical Association, 280*, 708–713.

Trungpa, C. (1977). Acknowledging death. In P. Olson and J. L. Fosshage (Eds.), *Healing: Implications for psychotherapy.* New York: Human Science Press.

Whooley, M. A., and Simon, G. E. (2000). Managing depression in medical outpatients. *New England Journal of Medicine, 343*, 1942–1950.

Young, D. M. (1997). Depression. In W. S. Tseng and J. Streltzer (Eds.), *Culture and psychopathology.* New York: Brunner/Mazel.

Suggested Readings

Acocella, J. (2000, May 8). The empty couch—what is lost when psychiatry turns to drugs. *The New Yorker*, 82–118. A thoughtful article addressing the serious problems stemming from excessive use of therapeutic drugs in the treatment of mental disorders.

Bourne, E. J. (2000). *The Anxiety & Phobia Workbook.* Presents step-by-step guidelines, questionnaires, and exercises to help sufferers learn skills and make lifestyle changes to help them get relief from the most distressing symptoms.

Dement, W. C., and Vaughan, C. (2000). *The Promise of Sleep: A Pioneer in Sleep Medicine Explores the Vital Connection Between Health, Happiness, and a Good Night's Sleep.* New York: Dell. One of the most renowned sleep experts offers the latest sleep information so people can "reclaim healthy sleep" in their own lives.

Kupfer, D. J., and Reynolds III, J. D. (1997). Current concepts: Management of insomnia. *New England Journal of Medicine, 336*, 341–345. A thorough review of the causes and management of sleep problems.

Roberts, F. M. (1998). *The therapy sourcebook.* New York: Lowell House. Discusses different kinds of therapy to treat mental illness resulting from cognitive, behavioral, psychological, and biological disorders. Also lists resources.

Schiraldi, G. R. (1999). *The Post-Traumatic Stress Disorder Sourcebook: A Guide to Healing, Recovery, and Growth.* Lincolnwood, IL: Contemporary Books. Information on diagnosis and treatment is at one's fingertips with nuggets of wisdom and clinical insights.

Whybrow, P. C. (1998). *A mind apart.* New York: HarperCollins. A penetrating look at how the mind goes awry and becomes ill. Dr. Whybrow discusses mental illness with insight and compassion.

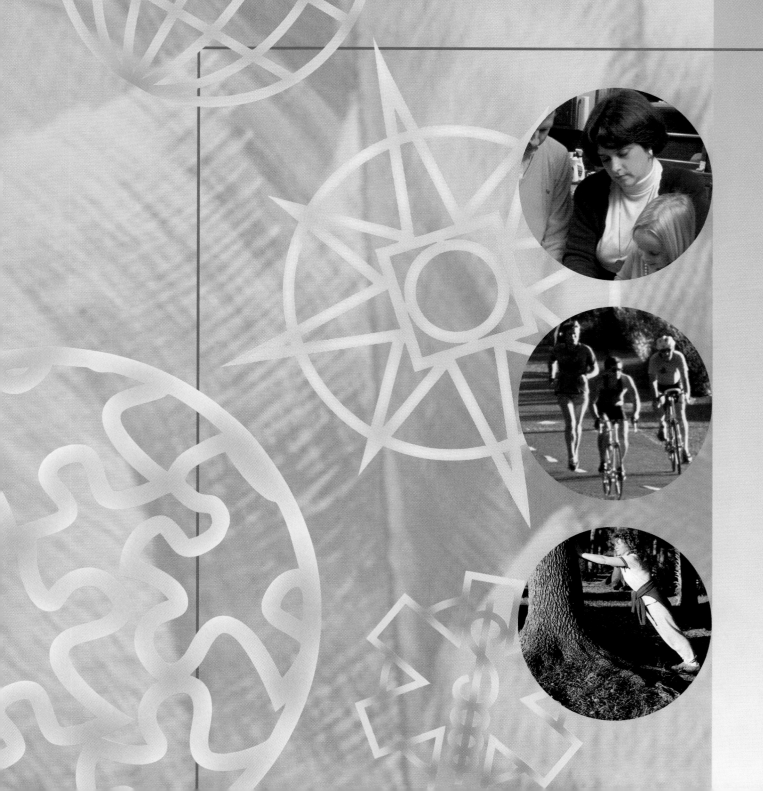

Part 2

Eating and Exercising Toward a Healthy Lifestyle

Learning Objectives

1. List the various factors that influence dietary choices.
2. Describe the dietary guidelines proposed by health organizations.
3. Describe the three kinds of vegetarian diets and several reasons for vegetarianism.
4. Describe which foods are at the bottom of the food guide pyramid and which are at the top and give the reasons for that placement.
5. Describe the ingredients and nutrition facts labels on manufactured foods.
6. Describe the three functions of food.
7. Define calorie.
8. List the seven components of food, and identify common foods that contain each component.
9. Describe the difference between simple and complex carbohydrates.
10. Define and identify sources of antioxidants.

Study Guide and Self Assessment

Health and Wellness Online

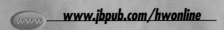 **www.jbpub.com/hwonline**

Chapter 5

Choosing a Nutritious Diet

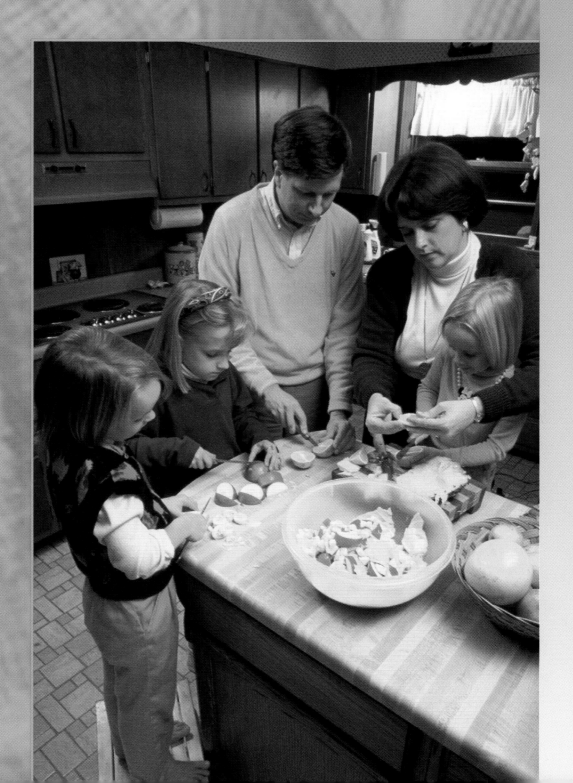

Of the many things you can do to enhance your well-being, none is more important than maintaining proper nutrition. Many people are aware that good nutrition is essential and sincerely want to eat healthfully. But the plethora of claims and counterclaims about nutrition and health and the aggressive marketing of food products tend to confuse rather than enlighten. Indeed, one study found that about 40% of Americans are tired of hearing about what foods they should and shouldn't eat and have become skeptical of official dietary guidelines (Patterson et al., 2000).

Moreover, many factors other than knowledge of nutrition influence a person's dietary choices—family, ethnic, and cultural eating patterns; social factors (eating what friends eat); food fads; and time pressures that limit thoughtful food shopping and meal preparation and make convenience foods attractive. Stress also influences food choices by encouraging consumption of foods high in fat and sugar to soothe jangled nerves and emotions.

> *If breakfast is such an important meal, why don't people dress for it?*
> LILY TOMLIN

Dietary Guidelines for Eating Right

To encourage and promote healthy dietary choices, the U.S. government, the World Health Organization, and organizations such as the American Heart Association and the American Cancer Society (Table 5.1) promote guidelines for good nutrition. These guidelines are based on the latest scientific evidence for good nutrition, obtained by examining the biological effects of specific dietary components and by comparing dietary patterns and disease frequencies in different populations. For example, compared to the standard American diet with its associated high levels of heart disease and cancer, the high-carbohydrate, low-fat diet of rural China is associated with less heart disease and fewer cancers of all kinds (Campbell and Junshi, 1994). Seventh Day Adventists, who consume high-carbohydrate, low-fat diets, also have less heart disease and cancer than other Americans. The same is true of the people of Mediterranean countries (Greece, southern Italy), whose traditional diet is high in fruits, vegetables, and legumes and low in animal fat.

The U.S. Departments of Agriculture and Health and Human Services (2000) produce dietary guidelines (Figure 5.1) designed to help prevent diseases that result from poor nutrition, including:

- Heart disease, cancer of various organs, and obesity from diets high in fat
- Cancer of the colon from consumption of too much meat
- Diseases of the gastrointestinal tract from not consuming sufficient fiber
- High blood pressure from consuming too much salt
- Tooth decay from consuming too much sugar

The Food Guide Pyramid

To help implement the dietary guidelines, the U.S. government created the Food Guide Pyramid, which recommends diets that emphasize grains, fruits, and vegetables, with moderate to little consumption of meat and dairy products, and only the sparest consumption of sweets and fats (Figure 5.2).

The Food Guide Pyramid places the most healthful foods at the bottom and the least healthful foods at the top. This arrangement helps people remember the composition of a healthful diet without having to count calories and grams. All people have to remember is to "eat low on the pyramid" by basing meals on pastas, breads, rice, fresh vegetables, and fruit. The slogan "five-a-day" was coined by nutritionists as a reminder to consume a total of five servings of fruits and vegetables each day. A study involving over 40,000 American

TABLE 5.1   American Heart Association and American Cancer Society Dietary Guidelines

American Heart Association's Dietary Guidelines with your heart in mind	American Cancer Society's Dietary Guidelines for reducing your risk of cancer
• Eat five or more servings of fruits and vegetables per day.	• Eat five or more servings of fruits and vegetables each day.
• Eat six or more servings of grain products per day.	• Eat other foods from plant sources, such as breads, cereals, grain products, rice, pasta, or beans, several times each day.
• Eat fat-free and low-fat milk products, fish, legumes (beans), skinless poultry, and lean meats.	• Choose foods low in fat.
• Balance the number of calories you eat with the number you use each day.	• Limit consumption of meats, especially high-fat meats.
• Limit intake of foods high in calories and low in nutrition.	• Be at least moderately active for 30 minutes or more on most days of the week.
• Eat less than 6 grams of salt (sodium chloride) per day (2,400 milligrams of sodium).	• Stay within your healthy weight range.
• Limit foods high in saturated fat, trans-fat, and cholesterol, such as full-fat dairy products, fatty meats, tropical oils, partially hydrogenated vegetable oils, and egg yolks.	• Limit consumption of alcoholic beverages, if you drink at all.

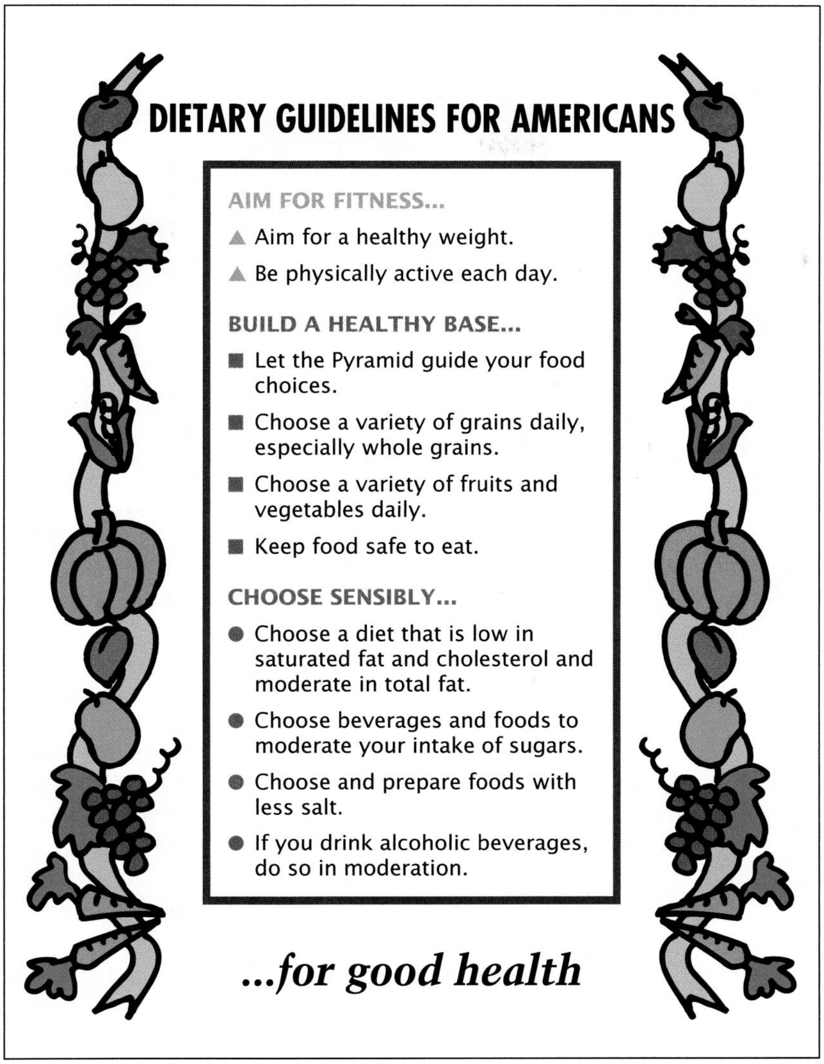

DIETARY GUIDELINES FOR AMERICANS

AIM FOR FITNESS...

▲ Aim for a healthy weight.

▲ Be physically active each day.

BUILD A HEALTHY BASE...

■ Let the Pyramid guide your food choices.

■ Choose a variety of grains daily, especially whole grains.

■ Choose a variety of fruits and vegetables daily.

■ Keep food safe to eat.

CHOOSE SENSIBLY...

● Choose a diet that is low in saturated fat and cholesterol and moderate in total fat.

● Choose beverages and foods to moderate your intake of sugars.

● Choose and prepare foods with less salt.

● If you drink alcoholic beverages, do so in moderation.

...for good health

FIGURE 5.1 **Dietary Guidelines for Americans**

Source: U.S. Department of Agriculture and U.S. Department of Health and Human Services.

women showed that the risk of dying from cancer was lowest among those whose diets emphasized consumption of fruits, vegetables, whole grains, low-fat dairy, and lean meats and poultry (Kant et al., 2000).

Traditional Asian, Mediterranean, and vegetarian diets also emphasize the consumption of foods of plant origin, while limiting (or eliminating) foods of animal origin and sweets. Vegetarians need to modify their consumption of foods according to a modified food pyramid (Figure 5.3).

The typical college student's diet follows an inverted food guide pyramid; sweets, fats, and meats make up a large portion of the diet, while grains, fruits, and vegetables are virtually absent. One popular food that does conform to the food guide pyramid is pizza. The dough (made of wheat flour) is at the base, representing the grain group; the tomato sauce, mushrooms, olives, peppers, garlic, and onion represent the vegetable group; the cheese represents the dairy group; and salami, pepperoni, anchovies, and other meats represent the meat group.

The Food Guide Pyramid has been criticized because it accommodates politically powerful meat and dairy industries and it does not offer sufficient information to guide healthy food choices. For example, meat and dairy products, which can contain high percentages of fat, are lumped together with beans and other legumes, which are high in fiber and contain little or no fat. Some products in the grain group are manufactured with considerable sugar and salt, but these additives are not reflected in the recommendations.

On the other hand, the pyramid's proponents point out that the pictorial display placing the most healthful food at the broad base and the least healthful at the tip is easy to remember. They believe it allows people to stop counting calories and grams and build diets based on foods found at the bottom of the pyramid: these include whole grains, fresh fruits, and fresh vegetables, which provide adequate nutrients and calories for good health.

Making daily food choices can be frustrating and confusing. However, using the food guide pyramid

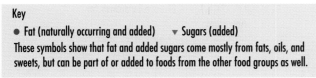

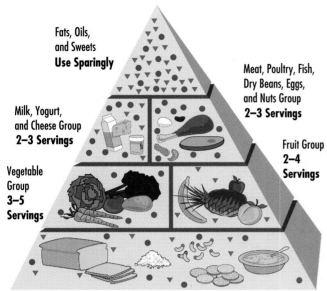

Bread, Cereal, Rice, and Pasta Group 6–11 Servings

FIGURE 5.2   **Food Guide Pyramid: A Guide to Daily Food Choices**   Each of these food groups provides some, but not all, of the nutrients you need. No one food group is more important than another—for good health, you need them all. Go easy on fats, oils, and sweets, the foods at the tip of the pyramid.

Source: U.S. Department of Agriculture and U.S. Department of Health and Human Services.

 Food Labels

The U.S. government requires that all manufactured foods carry two food labels: the **ingredients label** (Figure 5.4) and the **nutrition facts label** (Figure 5.5). The ingredients label lists the chemical composition of the food, i.e., all the substances that the manufacturer uses, including other foods (e.g., grains, eggs), natural and artificial sweeteners, natural and artificial fats, water, natural and artificial thickeners, natural and artificial flavorings, food colorings, and preservatives. The ingredients label lists substances in descending order by weight; the substance in the greatest amount is listed first and that in the least amount is listed last.

The ingredients label does not specify how much—either by weight or percentage—of an ingredient is in a food, only its amount relative to the other ingredients. Also, by listing each individual substance, the ingredients label may not indicate the true relative amount of sugar or fat in the food. For example, a snack food's

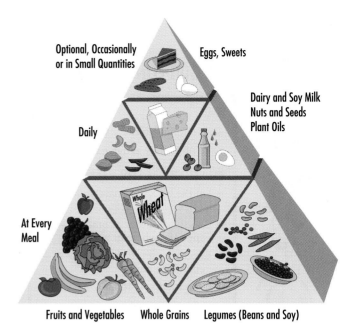

FIGURE 5.3   **The Vegetarian Food Guide Pyramid**   Notice that some foods are eaten at every meal, others daily, and some occasionally or in small quantities. Lactoovovegetarians can follow the regular food guide pyramid by replacing meats with two to three servings of dry beans, nuts, seeds, peanut butter, tofu, or eggs. Soy milk should be fortified with calcium and vitamins B_{12} and D. Vegans (no animal products) should consume 3 to 5 tablespoons of vegetable oil, 1 tablespoon blackstrap molasses, and 1 tablespoon of brewer's yeast daily.

Source: Cornell University, University of Rochester Medical Center, and the Human Connection.

ingredients label could list separately sucrose, fructose, and corn sweetener, all of which are sugars.

Unlike the ingredients label, the nutrition facts label provides *quantitative* information on certain nutrients in the food (ones whose consumption should be monitored for good health) and the calorie content of the food. The amounts indicated for each nutrient and the calorie count are for a "serving," which is all or a portion of the food in the package, as determined by the manufacturer. The manufacturer's definition of a serving is given at the top of the nutrition facts label as the "serving size."

In addition to the actual amounts of nutrients and calories, the nutrition facts label lists the **percent daily value** (PDV) for each nutrient, which is the percentage of the recommended daily amount that is contained in the food. (The percent daily value on the nutrition facts label is for someone who requires 2000 calories of food energy per day; people with higher or

Ingredients: Wheat flour, sugar, rolled oats, corn sweetener, molasses, partially hydrogenated safflower oil, salt, pantothenic acid, reduced iron, yellow No. 6, yellow No. 5, pyridoxine, ascorbic acid (vitamin C), BHT, riboflavin, folic acid.

FIGURE 5.4   **The Ingredients Label**   The government requires that food manufacturers list the substances within their products by weight from greatest to least.

Global Wellness

The Mediterranean Diet

The Mediterranean diet is associated with longer life and reduced risk of heart disease and cancer. It's a diet based on whole grains, fresh fruits and vegetables, minimal animal and trans-fat, and little red meat.

What is a Mediterranean diet?

- meals based on whole grain foods: breads, pasta, couscous, polenta, bulgur
- abundant fresh vegetables and fruits
- generous amounts of beans, nuts, and seeds
- olive oil as the principal source of fat
- use of garlic, onions, and herbs as condiments
- moderate use of fish
- moderate use of dairy
- minimal use of red meat
- low-to-moderate intake of alcohol

What makes the Mediterranean diet healthy?

- low in saturated fat and cholesterol
- energy supplied by unsaturated fat (in olive oil and nuts)

- no trans-fats (artificial fats in packaged pastries and margarine)
- high in fiber
- high in antioxidants
- low in refined sugar and flour
- high in plant-based vitamins and micronutrients

Researchers in France have determined that the Mediterranean diet lowers the risk of heart disease and many types of cancer. Even though a large percentage of calories is derived from fat, mono- and polyunsaturated fats predominate, the kind that raise HDL (so-called "good" cholesterol). Almost absent are animal fats (saturated fats and cholesterol) and manufactured trans-fats, which raise LDL (so-called "bad" cholesterol). The Mediterranean diet's high levels of antioxidants and other micronutrients reduce the risk of cardiovascular disease and cancer.

The typical American dinner, with a slab of meat in the center and one or two "sides," consisting of an overcooked vegetable and a butter-drenched potato, is a far cry from a typical Mediterranean dinner: pasta made of unrefined flour topped with a variety of minimally cooked vegetables (tomatoes, onions, peppers), some beans (peas, fava beans), and a sprinkle of hard cheese (Parmesan or Romano). For dessert, the Mediterranean diet calls for almonds and fresh fruit instead of cake, cookies, or ice cream.

It's too much to ask Americans to replace generations of dietary habits overnight. However, there are ways to incorporate some of the healthier aspects of the Mediterranean diet without radically changing customary eating patterns:

- cut back on fast food, which is generally 50% saturated fat and cholesterol.
- replace cake/ice cream desserts with fruit salad and nuts
- replace meat-centered meals with grain- and bean-centered ones
- replace doughnuts and sugar-laden snacks with fruit and mixed nuts

Bon Appetit!

lower calorie requirements have a larger or smaller PDV.) Near the bottom of the nutrition facts label is the recommended daily amount of nutrients, listed by weight (in grams) for 2000- and 2500-calorie diets.

To help consumers determine health-related claims on food labels, the U.S. government requires manufacturers to adhere to certain definitions (Table 5.2 on page 89).

The Three Functions of Food

Food has three functions:

1. To provide the chemical constituents of the body
2. To provide the energy for life
3. To be pleasurable, including satisfying hunger; the appeal of its smell, taste, sight, and texture; its association of food with enjoyable social activities

Body Structure and Function

Your body is made up of billions of atoms and molecules arranged in particular combinations and proportions. Most of the atoms and molecules that now make up your body were not part of you even a few weeks ago, because living things continually exchange their chemical constituents with the environment. Food provides the "raw materials" for your body's cells to manufacture the specific chemical substances that make you *you*.

Adequate amounts of 40 chemical substances, called the **essential nutrients** (Table 5.3 on page 89), must be supplied continually to the body. Failure to

Terms

ingredient label: label on a manufactured food that lists the ingredients in descending order by weight

nutrition facts label: label on a manufactured food that lists the quantity of certain nutrients in the food and the percent daily value for those nutrients

percent daily value: percentage of the recommended daily amount of a particular nutrient found in a food

essential nutrients: chemical substances obtained from food and needed by the body for growth, maintenance, or repair of tissues; not made by the body; must be obtained from food

do so can result in a nutritional deficiency disease, such as **goiter** from lack of iodine. Some forms of **anemia** result from insufficient dietary iron, and vitamin A deficiency is the most common cause of blindness in children worldwide.

Researchers have determined how much of the essential nutrients are required to prevent deficiency diseases. Many countries and the World Health Organization have produced dietary standards based on that research. In the United States, these requirements are called the **recommended [daily] dietary allowances,** or **RDA,** which lists values for protein, eleven vitamins, and seven minerals (Appendix). The assumption behind the RDA is that if the listed nutrients are consumed in recommended amounts, all other necessary nutrients will be, too. The RDA also lists values for pregnant women, lactating women, and children. The RDA is set for people in reasonably good health, i.e., not suffering from a major disease or under undue stress.

Surveys indicate that many Americans do not consume recommended RDA amounts of calcium, vitamin B_6, magnesium, zinc, copper, and potassium. People can determine if their diets contain the RDA of particular

Terms

goiter: an enlargement of the thyroid gland resulting from lack of iodine, causing a swelling in the front part of the neck

anemia: a deficiency of red blood cells; often caused by insufficient iron

recommended [daily] dietary allowances (RDA): levels of nutrients recommended by the Food and Nutrition Board of the National Academy of Sciences for daily consumption by healthy individuals, scaled according to gender and age

Wellness Guide

How to Use the Food Guide Pyramid

What Counts as One Serving?

Breads, Cereals, Rice, and Pasta

1 slice of bread

1/2 cup of cooked rice or pasta

1/2 cup of cooked cereal

1 ounce of ready-to-eat cereal

Vegetables

1/2 cup of chopped raw or cooked vegetables

1 cup of leafy raw vegetables

Milk, Yogurt, and Cheese

1 cup of milk or yogurt

1-1/2 to 2 ounces of cheese

Fruits

1 piece of fruit or melon wedge

3/4 cup of juice

1/2 cup of canned fruit

1/4 cup of dried fruit

Meat, Poultry, Fish, Dry Beans, Eggs, and Nuts

2-1/2 to 3 ounces of cooked lean meat, poultry, or fish

Count 1/2 cup of cooked beans, or 1 egg, or 2 tablespoons of peanut butter as 1 ounce of lean meat (about 1/3 serving)

Fats, Oils, and Sweets

LIMIT CALORIES FROM THESE, especially if you need to lose weight

The amount you eat may be more than one serving. For example, a dinner portion of spaghetti would count as two or three servings of pasta.

How Many Servings Do You Need Each Day?

	No. of servings		
	Women and some older adults (about 1,600 calories)*	Children, teenage girls, active women, most men (about 2,200 calories)*	Teenage boys and active men (about 2,800 calories)*
Bread group	6	9	11
Vegetable group	3	4	5
Fruit group	2	3	4
Milk group	2–3[†]	2–3[†]	2–3[†]
Meat group	2, for a total of 5 ounces	2, for a total of 6 ounces	3, for a total of 7 ounces

*These are the calorie levels if you choose low-fat, lean foods from the five major food groups and use foods from the fats, oils, and sweets group sparingly.

[†]Women who are pregnant or breastfeeding, teenagers, and young adults to age 24 need three servings.

Source: U.S. Department of Agriculture and U.S. Department of Health and Human Services, 1992.

FIGURE 5.5   **The Nutrition Facts Label**

Nutrition Facts

Serving Size 1/2 cup (114 g)
Servings Per Container 4

Amount per Serving

Calories 90	Calories from Fat 30
	% Daily Value*
Total Fat 3g	5%
Saturated Fat 0g	0%
Cholesterol 0mg	0%
Sodium 300g	13%
Total Carbohydrate 13g	4%
Dietary Fiber 3g	12%
Sugars 3g	
Protein 3g	

Vitamin A	80%	•	Vitamin C	60%
Calcium	4%	•	Iron	4%

* Percent Daily Values are based on a 2,000
calorie diet. Your daily values may be higher or
lower depending on your calorie needs:

	Calories	2,000	2,500
Total Fat	Less than	65g	80g
Sat Fat	Less than	20g	25g
Cholesterol	Less than	300mg	300mg
Sodium	Less than	2,400mg	2,400mg
Total Carbohydrate		300g	375g
Fiber		25g	30g

Calories per gram:
Fat 9   •   Carbohydrate 4   •   Protein 4

More nutrients may be listed on some labels.

Serving Size
Is your serving the same size as the one on the label? If you eat double the serving size listed, you need to double the nutrient and calorie values. If you eat one-half the serving size shown here, cut the nutrient and calorie values in half.

Calories
Are you overweight? Cut back a little on calories! Look here to see how a serving of the food adds to your daily total. A 5'4", 138-lb. active woman needs about 2,200 calories each day. A 5'10", 174-lb. active man needs about 2,900. How about you?

Total Carbohydrate
When you cut down on fat, you can eat more carbohydrates. Carbohydrates are in foods like bread, potatoes, fruits and vegetables. Choose these often! They give you nutrients and energy.

Dietary Fiber
Grandmother called it "roughage," but her advice to eat more is still up-to-date! That goes for both soluble and insoluble kinds of dietary fiber. Fruits, vegetables, whole-grain foods, beans and peas are all good sources and can help reduce the risk of heart disease and cancer.

Protein
Most Americans get more protein than they need. Where there is animal protein, there is also fat and cholesterol. Eat small servings of lean meat, fish and poultry. Use skim or low-fat milk, yogurt, and cheese. Try vegetable proteins like beans, grains and cereals.

Vitamins & Minerals
Your goal here is 100% of each for the day. Don't count on one food to do it all. Let a combination of foods add up to a winning score.

Total Fat
Aim low. Most people need to cut back on fat! Too much fat may contribute to heart disease and cancer. Try to limit your calories from fat. For a healthy heart, choose foods with a big difference between the total number of calories and the number of calories from fat.

Saturated Fat
A new kind of fat? No — saturated fat is part of the total fat in food. It is listed separately because it's the key player in raising blood cholesterol and your risk of heart disease. Eat less!

Cholesterol
Too much cholesterol — a second cousin to fat — can lead to heart disease. Challenge yourself to eat less than 300 mg each day.

Sodium
You call it "salt," the label calls it "sodium." Either way, it may add up to high blood pressure in some people. So, keep your sodium intake low — 2,400 to 3,000 mg or less each day. The AHA recommends no more than 3,000 mg sodium per day for healthy adults.

Daily Value
Feel like you're drowning in numbers? Let the Daily Value be your guide. Daily Values are listed for people who eat 2,000 or 2,500 calories each day. If you eat more, your personal daily value may be higher than what's listed on the label. If you eat less, your personal daily value may be lower.

For the fat, saturated fat, cholesterol and sodium, choose foods with a low % Daily Value. For total carbohydrate, dietary fiber, vitamins and minerals, your daily value goal is to reach 100% of each.

g = grams (About 28 g = 1 ounce)
mg = milligrams (1,000 mg = 1 g)

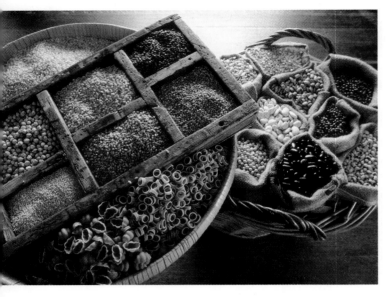

Natural, unprocessed foods provide the best nutrition.

nutrients by consulting tables and websites listing the composition of foods. Packaged food labels also carry information on the nutrient composition of the product.

Energy for Life

Food also provides energy to the body. The ultimate source of energy for complex organisms is sunlight, which is captured by green plants and converted to chemical energy that is stored as plant material. When humans eat plant matter or tissue from plant-eating animals, they obtain this stored chemical energy. Biological energy is used most efficiently when liberated in the presence of oxygen, which is one reason you breathe. In the process, the food material is converted to carbon dioxide, water, and other waste products and eliminated from the body in expired air, urine, feces, and sweat.

Energy transformations in living things are discussed in terms of calories. A **calorie** is the amount of

Wellness Guide

Taking Care of Your Teeth and Gums

Taking care of your teeth and gums means adopting practices for oral health that prevent tooth decay (*dental caries*) and gum disease (*gingivitis* and *periodontitis*). Tooth decay and gum disease are caused by the action of a variety of bacteria that live in the mouth, which produce acids by breaking down the sugars in food. The acids attack the enamel of teeth, causing tooth decay. Other bacteria are involved in the conversion of sugars and some of the material in saliva into a gelatinous substance called *plaque*, which sticks to teeth and gums and fosters more bacterial growth and decay.

Tooth and gum disease could be prevented if (a) the bacteria responsible could be removed from the mouth, (b) the sugars and other substances bacteria use to produce acids and plaque were removed from the mouth, or (c) teeth were protected from the bacterial products.

It is not yet possible to keep all tooth and gum disease—causing bacteria from the mouth or to render them harmless. So, keeping the mouth free of sugar and plaque is the best way to prevent tooth and gum problems. You can accomplish this by:

- Not eating sugar and sugar-containing foods between meals.

- Consuming sweets in liquid rather than solid form when possible.
- Avoiding sticky or slowly dissolving sweets.
- Brushing and flossing teeth after each meal.
- Rinsing the mouth with warm water when unable to brush after a snack or meal.
- Obtaining fluoride (to increase resistance to tooth decay) from toothpastes, mouthwashes, and drinking water.
- Getting periodic dental checkups.

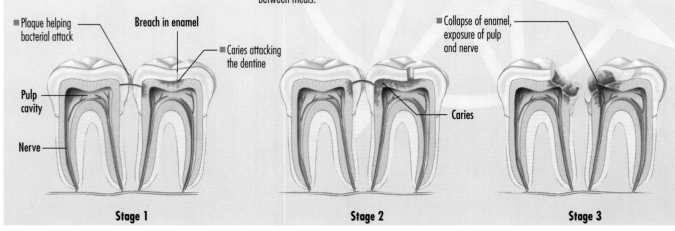

TABLE 5.2 What Words on Product Labels Mean

Calorie-free	Fewer than 5 calories per serving
Light (lite)	1/3 less calories or no more than 1/2 the fat of the higher-calorie, higher-fat version; or no more than 1/2 the sodium of the higher-sodium version
Fat-free	Less than 0.5 g of fat per serving
Low-fat	3 g of fat (or less) per serving
Reduced or less fat	At least 25% less fat per serving than the higher-fat version
Lean	Less than 10 g of fat, 4 g of saturated fat, and 95 mg of cholesterol per serving
Extra-lean	Less than 5 g of fat, 2 g of saturated fat, and 95 mg of cholesterol per serving
Low in saturated fat	1 g saturated fat (or less) per serving and not more than 15% of calories from saturated fatty acids
Cholesterol-free	Less than 2 mg of cholesterol and 2 g (or less) of saturated fat per serving
Low-cholesterol	20 mg of cholesterol (or less) and 2 g of saturated fat (or less) per serving
Reduced cholesterol	At least 25% less cholesterol than the higher-cholesterol version; and 2 g (or less) of saturated fat per serving
Sodium-free (no sodium)	Less than 5 mg of sodium per serving, and no sodium chloride (NaCl) in ingredients
Very low sodium	35 mg of sodium (or less) per serving
Low sodium	140 mg of sodium (or less) per serving
Reduced or less sodium	At least 25% less sodium per serving than the higher-sodium version
Sugar-free	Less than 0.5 g of sugar per serving
High-fiber	5 g of fiber (or more) per serving
Good source of fiber	2.5 to 4.9 g of fiber per serving

TABLE 5.3 The Essential Nutrients*

Amino acids	Fats	Water	Vitamins	Minerals
Isoleucine	Linoleic acid		Ascorbic acid (vitamin C)	Calcium
Leucine	Linolenic acid		Biotin	Chlorine
Lysine			Cobalamin (vitamin B_{12})	Chromium
Methionine			Folic acid	Cobalt
Phenylalanine			Niacin (vitamin B_3)	Copper
Threonine			Pantothenic acid	Iodine
Tryptophan			Pyridoxine (vitamin B_6)	Iron
Valine			Riboflavin (vitamin B_2)	Magnesium
Arginine[†]			Thiamine (vitamin B_1)	Manganese
Histidine[†]			Vitamin A	Molybdenum
			Vitamin D	Phosphorus
			Vitamin E	Potassium
			Vitamin K	Selenium
				Sodium
				Sulfur
				Zinc

*Must be obtained from food.
†Not essential for adults; needed for growth of children.

heat energy required to raise 1 g of water from 14.5 °C to 15.5 °C. A **nutritional calorie,** which is what weight watchers watch, is 1000 calories, or a **kilocalorie.** Books that discuss human nutrition and physical fitness frequently use the word "calorie" when actually referring to a kilocalorie. This book follows the same convention.

Energy from food is derived from the breakdown of carbohydrates, fats, and proteins. Carbohydrates and proteins supply approximately 4 calories per gram, and fats supply approximately 9 calories per gram. Virtually every cell in the body is capable of the series of chemical transformations necessary to extract chemical energy from these nutrient molecules. The process of breaking down molecules to derive energy and to obtain material for the manufacture of cellular molecules is called **metabolism.**

Energy is needed to support three major processes: (1) **basal** (or resting) **metabolism,** which is the energy required to keep the body alive; (2) physical activity (the things you do when you're not completely at rest); and (3) growth. The energy to support basal metabolism keeps cells functioning, maintains the body temperature within its normal limits, and keeps the

heart, lungs, kidneys, and other internal organs functioning. The daily amount of energy required to support basal metabolism is called **basal metabolic rate (BMR)**, or resting metabolic rate (RMR). The BMR for adult women is about 1100 calories per day, and 1300 calories per day for adult men.

In addition to the energy you need for basal metabolism, you use energy in physical activity: walking, running, working, and so on. The amount of energy expended for these activities depends on how strenuous the activity is, how long it is engaged in, the body's size, and the environmental temperature. It takes more energy to be active in hot weather than in

Terms

calorie: the amount of energy required to raise 1 g of water from 14.5 °C to 15.5 °C

nutritional calorie: unit of energy; often used interchangeably with the term kilocalorie

kilocalorie: unit of energy; the amount of heat needed to raise one kilogram of water 1 °C, equivalent to 1000 calories

metabolism: the process of obtaining energy and matter from the chemical breakdown of molecules obtained from food or from the body

basal metabolism: the minimum amount of energy needed to keep the body alive

basal metabolic rate (BMR): the amount of energy needed per day to keep the body functioning while at rest

Wellness Guide

New Rules for Organic Labeling

In 2001, after many years of discussion, the U.S. Department of Agriculture finally set standards for foods labeled "organic." Foods labeled "100% organic" and "organic" cannot be produced using sewage sludge, ionizing radiation, artificial growth hormones, genetically modified crops, and most synthetic fertilizers and pesticides. The labeling requirements apply to both fresh products and processed foods. Foods that are sold, labeled, or represented as organic have to be produced and processed in accordance with the new USDA standards, and they may carry the "USDA Organic" seal.

The labeling requirements are based on the percentage of organic ingredients in a product. Foods and food products labeled "100% organic" must contain (excluding water and salt) only organically produced ingredients. Products labeled "organic" must consist of at least 95% organically produced ingredients. Any remaining ingredients must consist of nonagricultural substances approved on the national list or products that are not commercially available in organic form.

Processed products that contain at least 70% organic ingredients can use the phrase "made with organic ingredients" and list up to three of the organic ingredients or food groups on the product label. For example, soup made with at least 70% organic ingredients and only organic vegetables may be labeled either "soup made with organic peas, potatoes, and carrots" or "soup made with organic vegetables." Processed products that contain less than 70% organic ingredients cannot use the term "organic" anywhere on the principal display panel. However, they may identify the specific ingredients that are organically produced under ingredients on the information panel.

Source: USDA National Organic Program (http://www.ams.usda.gov/nop/).

moderate temperatures, and it takes more energy to maintain body temperature when the weather is cold.

Energy is also needed whenever the body produces more cells than are needed to replace ones that periodically die. Thus, all young people need additional energy for growth and physical activity. Energy is also needed to produce new cells to repair injuries.

Energy requirements for individuals vary depending on a number of factors including: body size and composition; physical activity; growth needs during adolescence and young adulthood; pregnancy or breast feeding; and injury or illness. The RDA for adult American men is 2,800 calories per day; for nonpregnant, nonlactating adult American women, it is 2,200. Nutritionists recommend that carbohydrates from grains, vegetables, and fruits be the principal source of energy, supplying about 60% to 80% of total calories consumed. Fats should make up no more than 30% of total calories consumed. Protein is generally not recommended as a source of energy, but only as a source of building blocks for the body's tissues and organs.

Pleasures of Eating

Everyone has experienced the feeling of hunger and its appeasement by eating something. But hunger is not the only reason for eating in our society. Most of the time we eat because it is "time to eat," because someone has presented us with food, or simply because it feels good to be eating something—especially something fatty or sweet. The ready availability of food is unique to modern societies; a hundred years ago there were no supermarkets, fast-food restaurants, or convenience stores on every block. Also, advertising encourages us to eat more and more often.

 The Seven Components of Food

Food is composed of seven kinds of chemical substances: proteins, carbohydrates, lipids (fats), vitamins, minerals, phytochemicals, and water. Dietary proteins, most types of carbohydrates, and most lipids cannot be used by the body until they are broken down in the digestive system into smaller chemical units (Figure 5.6). In fact, only vitamins, minerals, a few kinds of carbohydrates, and water are absorbed into the body as is.

Proteins

Proteins make up about 20% of body mass. The main function of dietary protein is to provide your body with the amino acids necessary for growth and maintenance of body tissues. Cells, enzymes, hormones, antibodies, muscles and blood require amino acids as building blocks obtained from protein.

Proteins are made up of chemical units called **amino acids,** which come in 20 different forms. Amino acids are classified as **essential** and **nonessential.** Eight essential amino acids are required by adults; those eight and two others are required by infants. Animal sources of protein include milk and milk products, meat, fish, poultry, and eggs. Plant sources include breads and cereal products, legumes,

Global Wellness

Iodine Deficiency Is the Most Common Cause of Mental Deficits Worldwide

Iodine is an essential trace element in the human diet. Supplementing table salt with iodine in most countries of the world has eliminated the terrible effects of iodine deficiency in most populations. However, in many areas of Africa, Asia, Latin America, and parts of Eastern Europe, people's diets are deficient in iodine. The most severe consequence of iodine deficiency is severe mental retardation called *cretinism.*

Conclusive proof of the importance of iodine in the diet comes from an experiment carried out in Papua, New Guinea. Over a four-year period, some families received an injection of iodine and other families received placebo injections. Only one case of cretinism occurred among 412 newborns of mothers who had received iodine injections. Among women who had not received iodine injections, 21 of 406 babies were born with cretinism.

The primary sign of iodine deficiency is the presence of a *goiter,* which is an enlarged thyroid gland that is observable as a large bulge in the neck. Almost all of the iodine in the body is concentrated in the thyroid gland, where it regulates the production of essential thyroid hormones. In 1990 the World Health Organization estimated that 200 million people had goiter and another 20 million had mental deficits resulting from iodine deficiency. In most areas of the world, the soil does not contain iodine and plants grown in these regions are also deficient. Efforts are under way to supply everyone in the world with iodized salt or oil to prevent cretinism and other iodine-deficiency diseases.

Source: Adapted from B. S. Hetzel, "Iodine Deficiency and Fetal Brain Damage," *New England Journal of Medicine, 331,*1770–1771 (December 29, 1994).

---

nuts, and seeds. The primary sources of protein for the majority of the world's population are cereal grains and legumes.

Amino acids are not stored in the body in any appreciable amounts; therefore, proper nutrition requires eating enough protein every day to meet the body's needs for essential amino acids. Adult women should consume about 45 grams per day and adult men about 55 to 60 grams. The average North American adult consumes about twice that amount; the unneeded protein is broken down by the body and excreted in urine or stored as fat.

Because the amino acid composition of most animal protein is similar, people tend to acquire adequate amounts and proportions of the essential amino acids from animal tissue, such as fish, meat, eggs, and dairy products. Most vegetable proteins, however, are deficient in one or more of the essential amino acids, so individuals who eat little or no meat or dairy products must eat foods in which an amino-acid deficiency in one food is compensated for by an amino-acid surplus in another. For example, wheat, rice, and oats contain very little lysine, but have large amounts of methionine and tryptophan. Soybeans and other legumes are relatively high in lysine, but are low in methionine and tryptophan. Meals consisting of both grains and legumes (e.g., rice and beans, corn and beans, wheat and soybeans) can supply adequate amounts of these essential amino acids.

Meat, dairy products, and eggs provide the essential amino acids, but they can be high in fat, and thus contribute to the health problems associated with a high-fat diet (Table 5.4). For this reason, nutritionists recommend consuming nonfat or low-fat dairy products, using butter as a spread and not as an ingredient for cooking, being mindful of the amount of ice cream eaten, and limiting egg consumption to a few eggs per week. Nutritionists also favor trimming fat from meat before cooking, selecting meat with a low-fat content, and eating poultry (with skin removed because it contains fat) and fish, which have proportionately less fat than red meats. They also recommend using meat sparingly by adding it to grain- or bean-based dishes, rather than making it the center of the meal.

Another reason for avoiding a lot of meat is its association with colorectal cancer. Countries with the highest per capita meat consumption—New Zealand, Canada, and the United States—also have the highest rates of colon cancer. The reasons for this association are not clear. One possibility is that commercially grown and distributed meats may contain cancer-causing or cancer-promoting pesticide residues (DDT), industrial chemicals (PCBs), growth hormones (DES), dyes for color enhancement, and preservatives,

Terms

proteins: the foundation of every body cell; biological molecules composed of chains of amino acids

amino acids: compounds containing nitrogen, which are the building blocks of protein

essential amino acids: amino acids that cannot be synthesized by the body and must be provided by food

nonessential amino acids: eleven amino acids required for protein synthesis that are synthesized by humans and are not specifically required in the diet

Wellness Guide

Estimating Your Daily Calorie Needs

Step 1: What is your height?
I am _____ feet _____ inches tall.

Step 2: How many Body Mass Units do you have?
Calculate them this way:
Women: allow 100 Body Mass Units for first 5 feet of height + 5 Body Mass Units for each additional inch
Men: allow 106 Body Mass Units for first 5 feet of

height and 6 Body Mass Units for each additional inch

My total Body Mass Units = _____

Step 3: What is your Activity Factor?
Sedentary = 13
Active =15
Very active = 17

Step 4: What is your estimated daily calorie need?
Multiply your Body Mass Units by your Activity Factor = _____

such as **nitrates** and **nitrites,** often found in hot dogs, ham, sausage, and other cured meats. Another possibility is that bacteria in the colon convert substances necessary for the digestion of fats (bile acids) into cancer-causing agents. A third possibility is that charring meats in cooking converts substances in the meat into cancer-causing heterocyclic amines (HCAs).

> *Vegetables aren't my meat and potatoes.*
> YOGI BERRA

Athletes are often encouraged to increase their intake of protein, sometimes to as much as 30% of total calories—twice the recommended amount for inactive adults. Because body protein (that is, muscle tissue) can become a source of energy during exercise if carbohydrate and fat are not available, some endurance athletes may require more than the recommended amount of protein. A common recommendation for both endurance athletes and those involved in strength training is to consume 0.6 to 0.9 grams of protein per day per pound of body weight. That pro-

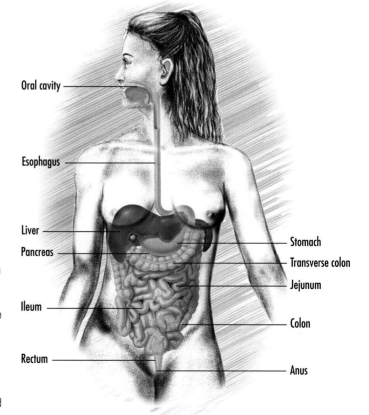

FIGURE 5.6   Human Digestive System
Teeth and glandular secretions in the mouth help break up food, which the esophagus transports to the stomach. The stomach breaks down some of the food molecules and passes the food to the rest of the digestive tube: the duodenum, jejunum, ileum, colon, and rectum. The pancreas secretes enzymes and fluid into the duodenum to help the digestive process. The liver controls release of absorbed nutrients into the body. Undigested material is eliminated from the body at the anus.

Oral cavity

Esophagus

Liver
Pancreas

Ileum

Rectum

Stomach
Transverse colon
Jejunum

Colon

Anus

TABLE 5.4   Fat and Cholesterol Content of Various Meats and Fish

Food (100 g)	Total fat (g)	Polyunsaturated fat (mg)	Cholesterol (mg)
Ground beef, extra lean	16.0	600	82
Ground beef, lean	18.0	700	78
Ground beef, regular	21.0	800	87
Top round	8.8	400	85
T-bone steak	25.0	900	84
Bacon	7.0	800	48
Ham—cured, lean	4.6	400	38
Ham—cured, regular	13.0	1,400	54
Beef liver	4.9	1,100	389
Bologna (slice)	6.6	300	13
Cod	0.6	200	37
Crab	1.0	400	47
Frozen fish sticks (1 stick)	3.4	900	31
Haddock	0.6	200	49
Salmon	2.9	1,200	44
Shrimp	1.5	600	130
Tuna (in water)	0.2	200	0
Tuna (in oil)	7.0	2,500	15
Chicken breast without skin, roasted	3.6	810	85
Chicken breast with skin, fried	8.7	1,900	88

Source: J. A. T. Pennington, *Food Values of Portions Commonly Used*, 16th ed. (Philadelphia: J. B. Lippincott: 1989).

tein can come from lean meat, fish, poultry, vegetables, grains, and beans. It is not necessary to consume so-called "high-protein" liquids. Regular food will do.

Carbohydrates

Carbohydrates are the principal source of the body's energy, and also are used to manufacture some cell components, such as the hereditary material, **deoxyribonucleic acid (DNA).** Because the body can manufacture them from other substances, carbohydrates are not considered essential nutrients. However, not eating enough carbohydrates, recommended by some ill-conceived reducing diets, can force the body to break down muscle tissue to supply energy necessary for life functions.

Most animals have a "sweet tooth," and humans are no exception. That's why food manufacturers often add sugars and other sweeteners to their products. Indeed, many commercial breakfast cereals are 40% sugar by weight. Because added sugar provides calories

Terms

nitrates: preservatives containing any salt or ester of nitric acid. Some individuals are sensitive to nitrates and may suffer from headache, diarrhea, or urticaria after ingesting them

nitrites: preservatives containing any salt or ester of nitrous acid

carbohydrates: the most economical and efficient source of energy; biological molecules consisting of one or more sugar molecules

deoxyribonucleic acid (DNA): a substance occurring in cell nuclei; carrier of the genes; present in all body cells of every species

Dollars and Health Sense

How Sweet the Profits Are!

In 1986, Americans were getting an average of 11% of their daily calories from sugar. Now the average is up to 18%. This sugar is consumed primarily in soft drinks, candies, gum, cookies, and snacks. On average, Americans now drink 53 *gallons* of soda a year, an increase of more than 40% over what was consumed 20 years ago. The gross overconsumption of sugar plays a major role in the increase in obesity and type 2 diabetes.

The profits in sugar-laden products are enormous, and companies spend lavishly to increase consumption of sodas and snacks. Coke and Diet Coke were

supported by $154 million in advertising in 1998; M & M candies by $67 million; Lay's potato chips by $56 million; and Kool-Aid drinks by $19 million (Advertising Age, 1999). Altogether, the soft drink industry spent about $600 million in advertising, and the restaurant industry (mostly fast foods) spent $3 billion. As long as people are willing to fill their diets with a great excess of sugar, their health is going to suffer. It is hard to combat the effects of such advertising and people's desire for sweets, but some solutions have been suggested (Jacobson and Brownell, 2000).

Eighteen states and one major city levy special taxes on the stuff you find in vending machines—sodas, gum, candies, and snacks. While these taxes are too small to affect sales, they generate about $1 billion a year. Perhaps it is time for a substantial national tax on foods of low nutritional value whose primary ingredient is sugar. We already have hefty taxes on cigarettes and alcohol, other substances that cause disease and destroy health. A substantial tax on low nutrition, sugary products might not cut into companies' profits but certainly would save the nation far more in health costs.

Managing Stress

Coping With Stress Through Diet

If academic demands stress you out, you may be able to cope better by altering your diet. The idea is to provide the brain with more tryptophan, which is used by brain cells to manufacture the neurotransmitter serotonin, which helps stabilize mood changes due to stress. Studies indicate that stress may deplete brain serotonin levels (Markus et al., 2000).

Consumption of carbohydrate-rich/protein-poor foods is associated with higher performance on a stressful task than is consumption of carbohydrate-poor/protein-rich foods. Why? Because diets high in protein flood the body with amino acids, and some of these compete with the amino acid tryptophan for entrance into the brain (like too many people trying to move through a revolving door at the same time). The more protein you ingest, the less tryptophan gets into the brain, and the less serotonin you have available to stabilize your mood.

Carbohydrate consumption facilitates the transport of tryptophan into the brain, because it increases the transport of other amino acids into muscle, increasing tryptophan's entry into the brain.

So, try this: A couple of hours before a big exam, have some bread or cookies, but NOT a double cheeseburger.

---

but no essential nutrients, sugar is usually described as contributing "empty calories" to the diet. Excess calories from added sugar are converted to fat, which in some cases may contribute to overweight problems. Populations that consume large amounts of sucrose (refined beet or cane sugar) exhibit high rates of heart disease, obesity, diabetes, and dental caries. Sugar consumption in the United States averages about 156 pounds per person per year.

There are two principal types of carbohydrates: **simple sugars,** found predominantly in fruit, and **complex carbohydrates,** found in grains, fruit, and the stems, leaves, and roots of vegetables. Simple sugars contribute about 20% of total calories in the average American diet. Except for increasing the risk of tooth decay, simple sugars in themselves are not harmful. Problems can arise when simple sugars are consumed in high-fat, low-nutrient snack foods (cakes, candies) and when they replace the more healthful complex carbohydrates in the diet.

Simple Sugars   **Glucose** is the most common simple sugar; it is found in all plants and animals. Glucose circulates in the bloodstream and is commonly referred to as "blood sugar." Another simple sugar is fructose, which is found in fruits and honey. **Fructose** is one of the sweetest sugars, which means you can eat less fructose than other simple sugars and taste an equivalent amount of sweetness. High fructose corn syrup is a common sweetener added to a variety of commercial food products.

Sucrose, which is common table sugar (the "refined" sugar added to many packaged foods), is a combination of glucose and fructose. Sucrose is digested by breaking down the glucose and fructose portions. Because fructose is sweeter than sucrose, you can reduce the amount of sugar in your diet without cutting out sweet tastes by replacing pastries with fresh fruit

and table sugar with honey. Furthermore, you will be gaining other nutrients in the fruit and honey that are not present in refined sucrose.

Lactose, found principally in dairy products, is a sugar consisting of glucose combined with the simple sugar **galactose.** When lactose is digested, the glucose and galactose are separated and the galactose is converted to glucose. Whereas almost all babies have the capacity to digest lactose (it is the major sugar in mother's milk), many older children and adults, particularly of black and Asian heritage, are not able to digest it because they lack a required enzyme, **lactase,** which splits lactose into glucose and galactose. When lactase-deficient people consume dairy products, they experience gastrointestinal upset, diarrhea, and, occasionally, severe illness. These individuals can supplement their diets with products containing lactase (e.g., Lactaid) or by eating yogurt, cheese, and other dairy products in which the lactose has been broken down by the fermentation process. Because dairy products are a major source of calcium in the North American diet, people who avoid dairy products should consume calcium-rich vegetables (e.g., broccoli and peas) and possibly take calcium supplements.

Complex Carbohydrates   These come primarily from grains (wheat, rice, corn, oats, barley); legumes (peas, beans); the leaves, stems, and roots of plants; and some animal tissue. There are two main classes of complex carbohydrates: **starch,** which is digestible, and **fiber,** which is not digestible.

Starch consists of many glucose molecules linked together. It is a way organisms store glucose until it is needed. In plants, starch is usually contained in granules within seeds, pods, or roots. Wheat flour, for example, is made by crushing wheat grain, which separates the outer husk (the bran) from the middle, starch-containing portion (the endosperm), and the inner germ. The white flour commonly used in baking is "70% extraction," which means that 70% of the original grain remains after crushing. In the milling of 70% extraction flour, many nutrients in the wheat grain are lost, so flour manufacturers add back several vitamins and minerals to produce "enriched flour." A "whole-grain flour," on the other hand, is 90% to 95% extraction and does not have to be enriched. In a reasonably varied diet, whatever nutrients not present in flour are obtained in other foods. Those wanting all the nutrients in wheat can choose whole-wheat flour.

Bread made with whole-wheat flour is brown, but not all brown bread is whole-wheat bread. Some manufacturers add molasses or honey to white-flour dough to give it a brown color, and they are allowed to label the product "wheat bread." For this reason, it is important to read the package label before buying.

Starch is also found in potatoes, which have an undeserved reputation for being fattening. Potatoes are no more fattening than any other starchy food unless they are cooked in large amounts of fat or oil, which is used in making french fries and potato chips. One large potato has about 100 calories, less than a medium-sized soft drink. French fries made from a medium potato, however, contain over 300 calories.

Terms

simple sugars: a class of carbohydrates called monosaccharides; all carbohydrates must be reduced to simple sugars to be digested

complex carbohydrates: a class of carbohydrates called polysaccharides; foods composed of starch and cellulose

glucose: the principal source of energy in all cells; also called dextrose

fructose: a simple sugar found in fruits and honey

sucrose: common refined "table" sugar; a molecule of glucose and a molecule of fructose chemically bonded together

lactose: a molecule of glucose and galactose chemically bonded together; found primarily in milk

galactose: a monosaccharide derived from lactose

lactase: enzyme secreted by glands in the small intestine that converts lactose (milk sugar) into simple sugars

starch: complex chain of glucose molecules

fiber: a group of compounds that make up the framework of plants; fiber cannot be digested

glycogen: the form in which carbohydrate is stored in humans and animals

insoluble fiber: cannot be dissolved in water

soluble fiber: can be dissolved in water

cellulose: a carbohydrate forming the skeleton of most plant structures and plant cells; the most abundant polysaccharide in nature and the source of dietary fiber

hemicellulose: substances found in plant cell walls that are composed of various sugars chemically linked together

Animals and humans produce a starch in muscle and liver tissue called **glycogen.** When energy is needed, the glycogen breaks down and its constituent glucose molecules are liberated. Athletes sometimes eat large quantities of carbohydrates the day before competition to build up their supply of glycogen, a practice known as "carbohydrate loading." The practice of carbohydrate loading can be risky, particularly for diabetics.

Fiber is the second main class of complex carbohydrates. There are two kinds of fiber, **insoluble fiber,** which cannot dissolve in water, and **soluble fiber,** which can. Insoluble fiber is made up of **cellulose** and **hemicellulose,** substances that offer rigidity to plant material (wood; stems; the outer coverings of nuts, seeds, grains; the peels and skins of fruits and vegetables). Soluble fiber is composed of pectins, gums, and mucilages. The differences in insoluble and soluble fiber are not significant for health. Nutritionists recommend that individuals consume 20 to 35 grams of fiber daily, regardless of its type (Table 5.5).

Fiber adds bulk to the feces, thereby preventing constipation and related disorders, such as hemorrhoids and hiatal hernia, which can result from prolonged increase in intra-abdominal pressure while defecating. Fiber also facilitates the transport of waste material through the digestive tract, lessening the risk of appendicitis, diverticular disease (out-pocketings in the wall of the lower intestine), and cancer of the colon and rectum. High-fiber diets may also help to lessen the risk of heart disease and some cancers.

TABLE 5.5   Fiber Content of Various Foods

Food	Amount	Fiber (g)
Whole-wheat bread	1 slice	1.6
Rye bread	1 slice	1.0
White bread	1 slice	0.6
Brown rice (cooked)	½ cup	2.4
White rice (cooked)	½ cup	0.1
Spaghetti (cooked)	½ cup	0.8
Kidney beans (cooked)	½ cup	5.8
Lima beans (cooked)	½ cup	4.9
Potato (baked)	medium	3.8
Corn	½ cup	3.9
Spinach	½ cup	2.0
Lettuce	½ cup	0.3
Strawberries	¾ cup	2.0
Banana	medium	2.0
Apple (with skin)	medium	2.6
Orange	small	1.2

Lipids (Fats)

Lipids are a diverse group of substances that have the common property of being relatively insoluble in water. Some of these substances include **cholesterol** and **lecithin,** which are essential constituents of cell membranes; the steroid hormones produced by the reproductive organs and adrenal glands; vitamins A, D, E, and K; and bile acids, which aid the digestion of fats. Despite the current antifat trend, fats are an essential part of the diet. They supply calories, they provide flavor and texture to food, and digesting fat provides feelings of satiety and well-being. One kind of fat, **linoleic acid,** found in vegetable oils such as safflower, sunflower, and corn, is essential, and must be obtained in food. Deficiencies in this substance can produce skin lesions.

Much of the fat consumed in the diet is triglyceride, which is composed of **fatty acids.** These substances are further classified as **saturated, monounsaturated,** or **polyunsaturated,** depending on their chemistry. Saturation refers to the number of hydrogen atoms (and therefore the amount of energy) contained in a fatty acid. A saturated fatty acid carries all the hydrogen atoms it can. A monounsaturated fatty acid (MUFA) carries one less than all the hydrogen atoms it possibly could. A polyunsaturated fatty acid lacks two or more hydrogen atoms. A dietary fat is classified as saturated, monounsaturated, or polyunsaturated, depending on the type of fatty acids it contains in greatest quantity.

Saturated fats are found in whole milk and products made from whole milk; egg yolks; meat; meat fat; coconut and palm oils; chocolate; regular margarine; and hydrogenated vegetable shortenings. Sources of monounsaturated fats include olive oil and some nuts. Polyunsaturated fats are found in safflower, cottonseed, corn, soybean, and sesame seed oils, and fatty fish (Figure 5.7).

Diets high in cholesterol and saturated fat increase the risk of coronary heart disease, some cancers, and obesity. Many nutritionists recommend that adults consume no more than 300 mg of cholesterol per day and limit saturated fat intake to 10% or less of total calories. "Visible" dietary fats include butter, cream, and whole milk. "Hidden" dietary fats include egg yolks, nuts, seeds, olives, avocados, cakes, pies, snack foods, and even lean meat, which can be 4% to 12% fat. Conversely, polyunsaturated fats tend to lower blood cholesterol, which is why nutritionists recommend consuming vegetable oils.

Food manufacturers use a chemical process to transform natural polyunsaturated fatty acids derived from vegetable oils into artificial **trans-fatty acids,** which tend to be solid at room temperature. This is how margarine and vegetable shortenings are made. Because margarine contains no cholesterol or animal fat, many people believe it is a healthier food than butter. In recent years, the fast-food industry switched from beef tallow to vegetable shortening for deep frying, because vegetable shortening was purported to be healthier than animal fat, and is less expensive. The bakery industry uses vegetable shortening for the same reasons to manufacture cookies, donuts, and cakes. There is no evidence, however, that margarine or vegetable shortenings are healthier than animal fats.

Indeed, analysis of dietary patterns of more than 87,000 American nurses showed that those with the highest intake of trans-fatty acids (3.2% of total energy) had the highest risk for heart disease. While you do not need to give up eating margarine, french fries, or donuts to be healthy, you need to practice moderation. Since the amount of trans fatty acids in food products is not listed on the product label, intake of these artificial substances can be limited by using liquid vegetable oils that contain polyunsaturated fatty acids whenever possible. Moreover, vegetables oils are naturally devoid of cholesterol.

Artificial fats are chemicals that are added primarily to packaged pastries and snack foods to provide the taste of fat without contributing calories. Ingesting

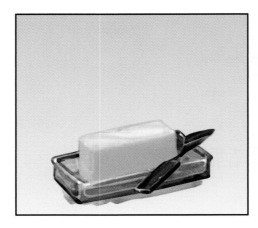 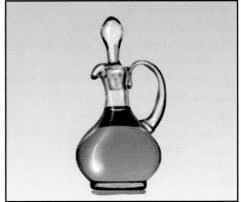

FIGURE 5.7 **Healthy and Unhealthy Fats** Fats that are solid at room temperature are considered less healthy than fats that are liquid because they contain more saturated fat.

these substances is not without risk, however, because they may both inhibit the absorption of fat-soluble vitamins from the gastrointestinal tract and cause diarrhea. The purported benefit of artificial fat—that it contributes to weight management—apparently is overstated, because consumers tend to compensate for the lack of energy derived from fat by ingesting greater amounts of carbohydrates.

Vitamins

Vitamins are substances that facilitate a variety of biological processes. Vitamins do not provide building blocks for the manufacture of the body's tissues nor do they provide calories to fuel the body's functions. This is why the body requires much smaller amounts of vitamins than it does proteins, carbohydrates, and fats. The body cannot manufacture vitamins; they must be obtained from food (Table 5.6). Vitamins are classified as **water-soluble** or **fat-soluble,** depending on their chemistry.

Terms

lipids: fats such as cholesterol and triglycerides

cholesterol: a fatlike compound occurring in bile, blood, brain, nerve tissue, liver, and other parts of the body

lecithin: an essential component of cell membranes

linoleic acid: an essential fat that must be obtained from food

fatty acids: naturally occurring in fats, either saturated or unsaturated (monounsaturated or polyunsaturated)

saturated fat: generally solid at room temperature; comes from animal sources

monounsaturated fatty acid: carries one less than all the hydrogen atoms it possibly could

polyunsaturated fatty acid: carries at least two fewer hydrogen atoms than it would if saturated

trans-fatty acid: an artificial fatty acid manufactured by chemically modifying monounsaturated and polyunsaturated fatty acids

artificial fat: chemicals added to packaged foods to provide the taste and texture of fat but few or no calories

vitamins: essential organic substances needed daily in small amounts to perform specific functions in the body

water-soluble vitamins: soluble in water; there are nine water-soluble vitamins

fat-soluble vitamins: soluble in fat; there are four fat-soluble vitamins

antioxidants: substances that in small amounts inhibit the oxidation of other compounds

homocysteine: a substance derived from the amino acid methionine; high blood levels increase the risk of heart disease; blood levels are reduced with adequate intake of folic acid

minerals: inorganic elements found in the body both in combination with organic compounds and alone

Vitamins A (and its dietary precursor, beta-carotene), C, and E are classed as **antioxidants** because they have the capacity to neutralize the effects of chemicals called free radicals, which can damage biological structures via chemical oxidation. Antioxidant vitamins are found in a variety of fruits and vegetables (not beans) and can be obtained in vitamin supplements. Dietary studies have shown that people who consume foods containing large amounts of antioxidant vitamins have less risk of cancer, heart disease, and cataracts than people who consume small amounts. However, in laboratory studies, antioxidant vitamins C, E, and beta-carotene have not been shown to prevent cancer or cataracts, but vitamin E does block the oxidation of certain molecules that lead to atherosclerosis and heart disease. Possible explanations of these discrepancies include: (1) diets rich in fruits and vegetables contain beneficial substances (e.g., phytochemicals) other than vitamins A, C, and E; (2) many clinical studies are carried out on people who already have cancer or heart disease or carry a high risk for such diseases (e.g., smokers); (3) in order to prevent cancer, antioxidant vitamins may require other plant substances that are not present in pills.

Folic acid (also called folate or folacin), a vitamin found in dark-green, leafy vegetables, beans, and fruits, helps prevent spina bifida and other neural tube defects in newborn babies (see chapter 15). The diets of most American women and elderly persons of both sexes are deficient in folic acid (on average, 200 micrograms per day are consumed; 400 micrograms are recommended), so the federal government requires that manufacturers of cereal-based foods (e.g., breads, breakfast cereals, pastas) fortify their products with it. There is debate whether the amount of folic acid in fortified foods is too low, so pregnant women are advised to ask their prenatal health care providers about taking folic acid supplements.

Folic acid also helps lower the body's manufacture of **homocysteine,** a substance derived from the essential amino acid methionine. High blood levels of homocysteine increase the risk of coronary artery disease and heart attack, so all individuals are advised to obtain adequate amounts of folic acid. The best way to do this is to eat beans and fruits, and possibly take supplements (not to exceed a total of 700 micrograms of folate per day, since too much folate may be toxic).

Minerals

Many body functions require one or more inorganic elements called **minerals** (Table 5.7). Sodium, potassium, and chlorine, for example, are essential for maintaining cell membranes, conducting nerve impulses, and contracting muscle. Magnesium, copper, and cobalt facilitate certain biochemical reactions;

TABLE 5.6 **Water-Soluble and Fat-Soluble Vitamins**

Water-soluble vitamin	Why needed?	Primary sources	Deficiency results in
Ascorbic acid (vitamin C)	Tooth and bone formation; production of connective tissue; promotion of wound healing; may enhance immunity	Citrus fruits, tomatoes, peppers, cabbage, potatoes, melons	Scurvy (degeneration of bones, teeth, and gums)
Biotin	Involved in fat and amino acid synthesis and breakdown	Yeast, liver, milk, most vegetables, bananas, grapefruit	Skin problems; fatigue; muscle pains; nausea
Cobalamin (vitamin B_{12})	Involved in single carbon atom transfers; essential for DNA synthesis	Muscle meats, eggs, milk, and dairy products (not in vegetables)	Pernicious anemia; nervous system malfunctions
Folacin (folic acid)	Essential for synthesis of DNA and other molecules	Green leafy vegetables, organ meats, whole-wheat products	Anemia; diarrhea and other gastrointestinal problems
Niacin	Involved in energy production and synthesis of cell molecules	Grains, meats, legumes	Pellagra (skin, gastrointestinal, and mental disorders)
Pantothenic acid	Involved in energy production and synthesis and breakdown of many biological molecules	Yeast, meats and fish, nearly all vegetables and fruits	Vomiting; abdominal cramps; malaise; insomnia
Pyridoxine (vitamin B_6)	Essential for synthesis and breakdown of amino acids and manufacture of unsaturated fats from saturated fats	Meats, whole grains, most vegetables	Weakness; irritability; trouble sleeping and walking; skin problems
Riboflavin (vitamin B_2)	Involved in energy production; important for health of the eyes	Milk and dairy foods, meats, eggs, vegetables, grains	Eye and skin problems
Thiamine (vitamin B_1)	Essential for breakdown of food molecules and production of energy	Meats, legumes, grains, some vegetables	Beri-beri (nerve damage, weakness, heart failure)
Fat-soluble vitamin	**Why needed?**	**Primary sources**	**Deficiency results in**
Vitamin A (retinol)	Essential for maintenance of eyes and skin; influences bone and tooth formation	Liver, kidney, yellow and green leafy vegetables, apricots	Deficiency: night blindness; eye damage; skin dryness. Excess: loss of appetite; skin problems; swelling of ankles and feet
Vitamin D (calciferol)	Regulates calcium metabolism; important for growth of bones and teeth	Cod-liver oil, dairy products, eggs	Deficiency: rickets (bone deformities) in children; bone destruction in adults. Excess: thirst; nausea; weight loss; kidney damage
Vitamin E (tocopherol)	Prevents damage to cells from oxidation; prevents red blood cell destruction	Wheat germ, vegetable oils, vegetables, egg yolk, nuts	Deficiency: anemia, possibly nerve cell destruction
Vitamin K (phylloquinone)	Helps with blood clotting	Liver, vegetable oils, green leafy vegetables, tomatoes	Deficiency: severe bleeding

iron is essential for the oxygen-carrying function of hemoglobin; iodine is needed to produce thyroid hormone; calcium and phosphorus make up bones and teeth. Selenium may reduce the risk of cancer, perhaps because of its activity as an antioxidant.

Minerals are found in almost all food, especially fresh vegetables. Women and young people are susceptible to iron deficiency, so they must eat iron-rich foods, such as eggs, lean meats, brans, whole grains, and green leafy vegetables. Most women and elderly people ingest too little calcium, which is found in dairy products and some green leafy vegetables such as broccoli and turnip greens (Table 5.8).

Many people consume too much sodium, which may contribute to high blood pressure. The amounts of sodium naturally present in almost every kind of food pose no problem; excess sodium comes from manufactured and restaurant food, to which salt is added to increase flavor, and from the overuse of table salt. Some people consume as many as 20 grams of sodium per day, which is about 10 times the 2 grams

per day the body needs. Athletes are often advised to take salt tablets to replace body salt lost in sweat; this advice is misguided. Except in cases of severe fluid loss, which more often accompanies medical therapies involving diuretics than with sports, salt is readily replaced by eating food.

Phytochemicals

Many vegetables and fruits contain chemical substances, referred to as **phytochemicals,** that are not nutrients *per se* but that positively affect human physiology (Table 5.9). Phytochemicals may help the body destroy and eliminate toxins acquired from the environment or tissue-damaging by-products of metabolism, such as oxygen free radicals. For example,

Terms

phytochemicals: chemicals produced by plants

TABLE 5.7   Essential Minerals

Mineral	Why needed?	Primary sources	Deficiency results in
Calcium	Bone and tooth formation; blood clotting; nerve transmission	Milk, cheese, dark green vegetables, dried legumes	Stunted growth; rickets, osteoporosis; convulsions
Chlorine	Formation of gastric juice; acid-base balance	Common salt	Muscle cramps; mental apathy; reduced appetite
Chromium	Glucose and energy metabolism	Fats, vegetable oils, meats	Impaired ability to metabolize glucose
Cobalt	Constituent of vitamin B_{12}	Organ and muscle meats	Not reported in man
Copper	Constituent of enzymes of iron metabolism	Meats, drinking water	Anemia (rare)
Iodine	Constituent of thyroid hormones	Marine fish and shellfish, dairy products, many vegetables	Goiter (enlarged thyroid)
Iron	Constituent of hemoglobin and enzymes of energy metabolism	Eggs, lean meats, legumes, whole grains, green leafy vegetables	Iron-deficiency anemia (weakness, reduced resistance to infection)
Magnesium	Activates enzymes; involved in protein synthesis	Whole grains, green leafy vegetables	Growth failure; behavioral disturbances; weakness, spasms
Manganese	Constituent of enzymes involved in fat synthesis	Widely distributed in foods	In animals: disturbances of nervous system, reproductive abnormalities
Molybdenum	Constituent of some enzymes	Legumes, cereals, organ meats	Not reported in man
Phosphorus	Bone and tooth formation; acid-base balance	Milk, cheese, meat, poultry, grains	Weakness, demineralization of bone
Potassium	Acid-base balance; body water balance; nerve function	Meats, milk, many fruits	Muscular weakness; paralysis
Selenium	Functions in close association with vitamin E	Seafood, meat, grains	Anemia (rare)
Sodium	Acid-base balance; body water balance; nerve function	Common salt	Muscle cramps; mental apathy; reduced appetite
Sulfur	Constituent of active tissue compounds, cartilage, and tendon	Sulfur amino acids (methionine and cysteine) in dietary proteins	Related to intake and deficiency of sulfur amino acids
Zinc	Constituent of enzymes involved in digestion	Widely distributed in foods	Growth failure

cruciferous vegetables (e.g., broccoli, kale, cauliflower, brussels sprouts, cabbage, mustard greens) are rich in the cancer-preventing phytochemicals *sulforaphane* and *isothiocyanates*. Tomatoes and tomato products (ketchup, tomato sauce), pink grapefruit, papaya, peaches, and watermelon contain a phytochemical called *lycopene*, which protects against oxidative damage and reduces the risk of cancer and heart disease. Green and black tea, onions, apples, and grapes contain a family of phytochemicals called *flavonoids*, which also protect aginst cancer and heart disease.

Water

Water is the principal constituent of blood and is the major component of all cells. Water provides the medium in which all cell chemical activities take place.

Body water is maintained at a relatively constant level by the nervous, endocrine, and urinary systems. If body water volume is low, a person experiences thirst, which motivates drinking. A low volume of body water activates hormonal mechanisms that reduce the production of urine. Excess body water volume activates hormonal mechanisms that increase the output of urine. Increasing output is the function of diuretics, often given to reduce blood pressure, fluid volume after a heart attack, or feelings of bloatedness. The popular maxim that you should drink eight glasses of water a day is partially correct. The average adult loses about that much body water through sweat, moisture in expired air, urine, and feces. This loss is partly offset by drinking water and obtaining water in other fluids and foods.

TABLE 5.8   Calcium in Various Foods
The recommended daily value for adults is 1000 mg.

Food	Serving Size	Milligrams (mg) Calcium
Tofu, calcium processed	1/3 cup	581
Yogurt, plain	8 oz. container	411
Milk, skim and low-fat	1 cup	301
Sesame seeds, whole roasted	1 oz.	297
Cheese, Swiss	1 oz.	288
Cheese, cheddar	1 oz.	216
Cheese, mozzarella	1 oz.	194
Soybeans, cooked	1/2 cup	131
Turnip greens, cooked	1/2 cup	116
Blackeyed peas, cooked	1/2 cup	115
All Bran cereal	1/2 cup	106
Collard greens	1/2 cup	101
Sardines, canned	1 oz.	105
Salmon, canned (with bones)	1 oz.	59

TABLE 5.9   Phytochemicals in Fruits and Vegetables and Their Possible Benefits

Food	Phytochemicals	Possible Benefits
Berries blueberries, strawberries, raspberries, blackberries, currants, etc.	Anthocyanidins, ellagic acid	antioxidants cancer prevention
Chili Peppers	Capsaicin	possible antioxidant topical pain relief
Citrus Fruits oranges, grapefruit, lemon, limes, etc.	Flavanones (tangeretic, nobiletin, hesperitin) Carotenoids	antioxidants
Cruciferous Vegetables broccoli, kale, cauliflower, brussels sprouts, cabbage, mustard greens	indoles isothiocyanates sulphoraphane carotenoids	antioxidants anti-cancer properties
Garlic Family garlic, onions, shallots, leeks, chives, scallions	Allylic sulfides Flavonoids (quercetin)	anti-cancer properties
Soy	daidzein, equol, genestein, enterolactone, and other plant estrogens	reduce risk of breast, prostate cancer reduce risk of heart disease

Body water should be replaced by consuming pure water, milk, or juice, but not sodas. A study found that physically active teenage girls who drank sodas were 4 to 5 times more likely to have had bone fractures than girls who did not drink sodas, possibly because sodas contain phosphoric acid, which affects calcium metabolism and bone mass. Another possibility is that young people may replace milk in their diets with sodas, giving their bodies less calcium with which to strengthen bones. Liquids containing caffeine (coffee, tea, sodas) and alcohol are diuretics, which means that some of the fluid ingested is lost in additional urine output.

Many people drink bottled water believing that it is more healthful than tap water. Not all bottled water comes from "natural" sources as the name of the product may suggest. The source of some bottled water products is a municipal water tap. One should look on the product label to ascertain the source of the water inside.

Dietary Supplements

More than 25,000 products are available in the United States as **dietary supplements**. In the strictest sense, dietary supplements are ingested to provide one or more of the 40 essential nutrients, such as a particular vitamin, mineral, or amino acid (see Table 5.3). For example, someone might take a multivitamin pill every day to ensure that an adequate amount of all vitamins is obtained.

Besides vitamins, however, dietary supplements include a variety of minerals, enzymes, amino acids, herbs, hormones, and nucleic acids (DNA and RNA), the use of which is intended to alter one or more of the body's biological systems to produce a specific physiological or psychological effect. For example, someone might take capsules containing omega-3 fatty acids (fish oil) to try to prevent a heart attack (or *another* heart attack) or stroke by lowering serum lipids. Or, someone may drink herbal tea to feel energized. A dietary supplement intended to prevent or treat an illness or disease is called a **neutraceutical**.

When a dietary supplement is used to augment the nutritional quality of the diet, it is considered a food. When a dietary supplement is used to bring about a particular biological change, it is considered a drug. About 100 million Americans spend a total of $15 to $20 billion each year on dietary supplements.

Dietary Supplements as Food

A varied diet that conforms to the recommendations of the Food Guide Pyramid is likely to provide most people with sufficient essential nutrients for good health. For these people, a nutritional dietary supplement is probably unnecessary, although some may want to take one as a form of "dietary insurance."

People who suspect that their diets are nutritionally inadequate may benefit from taking a daily multivitamin and mineral supplement. For example:

- people who skip meals and eat a lot of processed and fast food
- people who consume an unusual or low-calorie diet for weight loss
- people who consume nutritionally inadequate diets for reasons of economic hardship
- athletes who are concerned about body size
- people who consume large amounts of coffee and/or alcohol

Others who may benefit from dietary supplements include strict vegetarians, who may need vitamin B_{12} because that vitamin comes primarily from animal tissue, people with lactose intolerance (difficulty digesting dairy products), and women of childbearing age who consume insufficient amounts of folic acid. When supplementing the diet with vitamins and minerals,

Terms

dietary supplements: products that provide one or more of the 40 essential nutrients or nonessential vitamins, minerals, enzymes, amino acids, herbs, hormones, and nucleic acids

neutraceutical: a dietary supplement intended to prevent or treat an illness or disease

remember that more is not necessarily better. In high doses, vitamins A, D, K, B_3 (niacin), and B_6 (pyridoxine) may be toxic.

Supplements containing enzymes, other proteins, and nucleic acids are not absorbed intact from the digestive tract; instead, they are broken down into smaller subunits. When a supplement is intended for use in the digestive tract, such as lactase, this is of little concern, as the substance acts prior to being digested. However, an enzyme or nucleic acid will not be absorbed intact into the body, so using them is a waste of money.

Whether a substance is natural or synthetic makes no difference chemically as long as the manufacturer has taken care to be sure that the product is pure. In 1990, thousands of Americans became ill and more than 30 died from consuming a supplement of the amino acid tryptophan because of manufacturing impurities in the product. Moreover, just because a product is labeled "natural" or "comes from plants" does not mean it is safe or effective. A "natural" or "plant" product can have a large number of impurities and may be toxic.

Dietary Supplements as Drugs

Besides being intended to augment the nutritional quality of the diet, many dietary supplements are touted by manufacturers as preventatives or cures for ailments, stress, moods, and recreational drug use. A few supplements that act as drugs have been scientifically tested and found to be safe and effective for certain conditions (Table 5.10).

Unlike prescription and over-the-counter medicines, dietary supplements do not have to be tested before going on the market, so consumers have no assurance of a supplement's contents, that it has no impurities, that it is not harmful, and/or that it actually

does anything beneficial. Some examples of supplement problems are:

Uncertain contents: Independent tests of 10 samples of the supplement DHEA (dihydroepiandrostendione), a male hormone, showed that three contained no DHEA, three had at least 25% less than the amount claimed on the product label, and one contained 50% more than specified on the label. A study of 10 leading brands of St. John's wort, an herb used to treat depression, found that seven contained less than 90% of the amount stated on the product label. Thus, even if a substance in a supplement has been shown scientifically to be beneficial, consumers have no guarantee that the dose is what the product label claims. From a financial point of view, consumers would be spending money for a worthless product. From a health point of view, consumers could be harmed by ingesting too much or too little of a substance.

Harmful impurities: Several products marketed as traditional Chinese medicines were found to contain *aristolochic acid*, a potent carcinogen and kidney toxin. In one instance, more than 100 people in Belgium developed kidney damage as a result of using an herbal product containing aristolochic acids. Either the plant material used in the suspect products was misidentified, or the name of the plant ingredient was confused with that of another plant. In response to this situation, manufacturers were asked by the FDA to review their current manufacturing practices to ensure comprehensive and rigorous testing of ingredients and finished products to prevent the incorporation of potentially harmful impurities.

Harmful supplements: A variety of dietary supplements that were marketed for weight loss (e.g., Triax Metabolic Accelerator, Tricana Metabolic Hormone Analogue, Tria-Cutz, Thyroid Stimulator) contained *tiratricol*, also known as *triiodothyroacetic acid* or TRIAC, a potent thyroid hormone that could cause serious health problems, including thyroid gland malfunction, heart attacks, and strokes. Products containing *gamma butyrolactone*, or GBL (Renewtrient, Revivarant or Revivarant G, Blue Nitro or Blue Nitro Vitality, GH Revitalizer, Gamma G, and Remforce), or *1,4 butanediol*, abbreviated BD (Revitalize Plus, Serenity, Enliven, GHRE, SomatoPro, NRG3, Thunder Nectar, and Weight Belt Cleaner) were found to be harmful because their essential ingredients were converted in the body to *gamma-hydroxybutyrate* (GHB), an illegal substance used to produce intoxication or to enhance body building. GHB use is associated with nausea and vomiting, delusions, depression, vertigo, hallucinations, seizures, difficulty breathing, slowed heart rate, low blood pressure, amnesia, coma, and death. GHB is especially dangerous when

| TABLE 5.10 | Dietary Supplements that Have Been Scientifically Tested and Found to be Effective |

Supplement	Use
Chondroitin Sulfate & Glucosamine	Reduce symptoms of arthritis
Echinacea	Enhance immune functioning
Gingko Biloba	Slow the progression of some forms of dementia
Kava Kava	Calm anxiety
Omega-3 Fatty Acids	Prevent heart disease and stroke
S-Adenosyl Methionine (SAM-e)	Relieve mild to moderate depression
St. John's Wort	Relieve mild to moderate depression
Saw Palmetto	Treat prostate cancer

Dollars and Health Sense

The Marketing of Dietary Supplements

For the last 50 years "effectiveness" meant that there'd be scientific evidence to demonstrate that something worked. Now, effectiveness is measured by how quickly something moves off the shelves.

David Kessler, MD
former FDA Commissioner

In 1906, and again in 1938, the U.S. Congress passed the Pure Food and Drug Act to ensure that foods are safe and medicines are both safe and effective. The federal agency that enforces the law is the Food and Drug Administration (FDA), which requires rigorous testing of drugs before they can be marketed.

In 1994, however, Congress passed a separate law that defines the FDA's regulatory powers over the dietary supplement industry. This law was enacted to prevent the FDA from regulating dietary supplements with the same rigor it does drugs and food additives. However, the agency still can ban a product if it is found to be harmful after being used by the general public. This means that manufacturers and distributors of dietary supplements are able to sell substances that may be worthless or even harmful until they are caught—which usually means a number of people have to get sick first or die.

Proponents of the new law opposed government regulation of substances they believed to be safe (often because they were "from plants," "non-medical," or "natural"). Moreover, they believed that such regulation would limit the variety of products people could take and would drive up the cost of vitamins. Also, people feared that FDA regulation would stop the dietary supplement industry from being a viable alternative to conventional medicine and prescription drugs.

Opponents of the new law argued that without independent scientific testing, consumers cannot be assured that a supplement is safe or effective. They feared people could be harmed by impurities in a product or a product's unknown actions or by outright fraud.

Dr. David Kessler, the former head of the FDA, has stated that the lobbying for passage of the new law was the most intense he had ever seen. The supplement industry told consumers that if the law did not pass, they would have to have a prescription to buy vitamins—if they could get them at all! Millions of frightened people contacted their elected representatives. The lobbying effort was a huge success; the law passed unanimously in Congress.

With more than 25,000 supplements on the market, and with its current budget, the FDA cannot possibly oversee all of the advertising claims made by supplement manufacturers or test even a small fraction of the products. Proponents of an unregulated supplement industry point out that only a handful of people die each year from ingesting supplements, compared to many thousands who die each year from taking prescription medications. Because there is no government oversight, one must be a wise consumer before using a supplement or herbal product. Read a product's label to learn about ingredients and doses. ConsumerLab.com is an independent laboratory that tests many supplements to verify their contents.

---

mixed with alcohol. The U.S. Drug Enforcement Administration documented more than 45 deaths and 5,500 emergency room overdoses associated with GHB.

Because St. John's wort had not undergone rigorous testing before being marketed, it was not known that the herb could stimulate the liver, which inactivates toxic chemicals and drugs. Thus, taking St. John's wort can inadvertently cause the breakdown of medicines taken for other reasons. For example, St. John's wort can lessen body levels of anti-AIDS drugs, immunosuppressant drugs in heart transplant patients, antiseizure medication, breast cancer drugs, and oral contraceptive (birth control) pills. A number of women taking oral contraceptives and St. John's wort have become pregnant, which provided the clue to the undesired effects of the herb.

Food Additives

Manufactured foods contain a variety of additives that alter their texture, flavor, color, and stability. These additives help to increase sales appeal and lengthen shelf life.

Preservatives

About 20% of the world's food supply is lost to spoilage each year. Common preservatives include BHA (butylated hydroxyanisole), BHT (butylated hydroxytoluene), and sodium nitrite. Each of these substances can be toxic and damaging to humans if consumed in excess; however, in amounts commonly present in food, they are presumed safe.

Sulfites in the form of sulfur dioxide, sodium sulfite, sodium or potassium bisulfite, and sodium or potassium metabisulfite are added to many foods to kill bacteria and to slow the food's breakdown. Sulfites are commonly added to wine and to dehydrated soups, vegetables, and fruit (apples, apricots, raisins, pears, and peaches). To keep vegetables looking fresh, they are also used in restaurant salad bars. Some individuals, particularly those with asthma, may be extremely sensitive to sulfite and may experience nausea, diarrhea, respiratory distress, and skin eruptions.

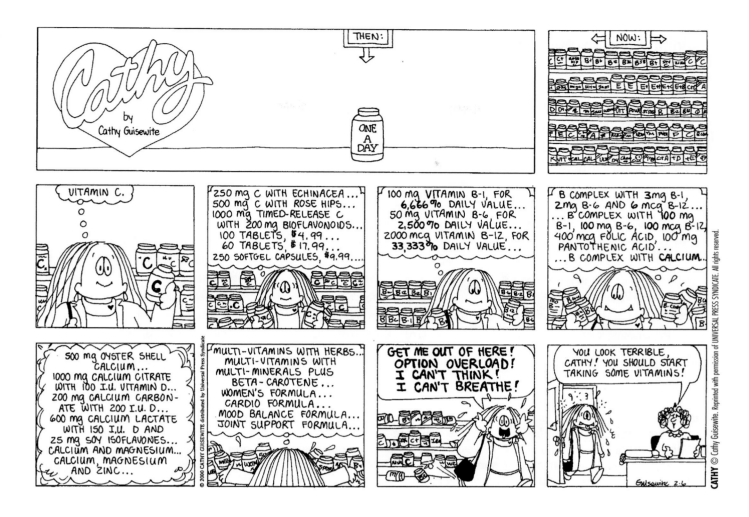

Such problems have led to banning the use of sulfites in restaurants.

Many food additives are nutritionally unnecessary and some may adversely affect health. For example, sugar and salt are added to food to enhance taste and increase sales. Food dyes, some of which have been banned, have been implicated in human cancers and allergies. The FDA estimates that as many as 100,000 Americans are intolerant to **tartrazine,** a yellow dye added to hundreds of manufactured foods, such as frozen breakfast pastries, pill coatings, and some soft drinks.

Consumers concerned about additives should read product labels. Manufacturers must list all the additives in the order of their relative proportions in the food. Do not assume that the words "natural," "organic," or "health food" are free from additives or extra sugar and salt. The only sure way to be certain of the contents of a food is to know how it was produced.

Artificial Sweeteners

Fifty to seventy million Americans use artificial sweeteners. As a presumed ally in the continual battle against being overweight and as a theoretical help to diabetics, artificial sweeteners are in all types of foods. Their widest use, however, is in "diet" soft drinks.

The three major artificial sweeteners—cyclamate, saccharin, and aspartame—have been associated with health risks. In the 1970s, cyclamates and saccharin were linked to cancer. Aspartame (Nutrasweet), made of the amino acids aspartic acid and a modified form of phenylalanine, has been associated with mood changes, insomnia, and seizures. Health-conscious consumers should be aware of the artificial sweeteners used in the products they ingest.

Food Safety

Outbreaks of food poisoning in the U.S. and other countries from bacterial and viral contamination of

Terms

sulfites: used as preservatives for salad, fresh fruits and vegetables, wine, beer, and dried fruit; in susceptible individuals, especially those with asthma, they can cause a severe reaction

tartrazine: a yellow food dye, referred to by the FDA as "FD&C yellow No. 5"

Dollars and Health Sense

How Food Manufacturers Increase Profits

When vitamins, minerals, herbs, or other substances are added to foods to allow the manufacturer to make health claims, the food is called a **functional food**. Americans have been eating functional foods since 1924, when iodine was added to salt to prevent goiter, a disease of the thyroid gland caused by iodine deficiency. For many years after that, some foods (such as enriched flour) were fortified with extra vitamins and minerals but without the manufacturer making health claims. That changed in 1993 when the FDA issued a ruling saying that milk and yogurt, which contain high amounts of calcium, could carry labels claiming that the products helped prevent osteoporosis. Other food manufacturers quickly began adding calcium to other foods—orange juice, waffles, potato chips—so they, too, could make health claims.

Companies were quick to realize that health claims on foods could increase sales. Thus, we now have sodas with kava or ginseng (for relaxation), cereals with psyllium husk (to protect against heart disease or cancer), margarine with plant-derived sterols (to lower cholesterol), ice cream with echinacea (to help the immune system), and soups with St. John's wort (to combat depression). As people strive for better health by taking dietary supplements, food companies try to cash in on the "health-conscious" market (*Consumer Reports*, 1999).

Functional foods may be both dangerous and costly. Herbs added to foods may be dangerous because amounts are not well controlled and, in some instances (e.g., St. John's wort), the herb can interfere with the action of certain medications. Some people may mistakenly believe that more is better and risk overdose with a vitamin, mineral, or plant product by ingesting both dietary supplements and a functional food. Moreover, functional foods often cost more, sometimes a lot more, than equivalent foods without supplements.

---

commercial beef, poultry, and fruit have raised concerns about the safety of the food supply. The bacterium *Escherichia coli* O157:H7 is responsible for thousands of cases of illness and some deaths each year. Each year, nearly 1 million Americans are made ill by *Salmonella* contamination. Symptoms of bacterial food poisoning are headache, nausea, and fever.

The Food and Drug Administration's and the U.S. Department of Agriculture's inspectors oversee nearly 60,000 food manufacturers and processors and billions of tons of imported food—clearly a monumental task. That's why it's imperative for consumers to follow food safety guidelines when they purchase, store, and prepare food.

One method of protecting food involves exposing it to **gamma irradiation** to destroy fungi, bacteria, and other microorganisms. Some opponents of food irradiation argue that the method has not been proven safe. Their concern is that irradiation may produce cancer-causing or toxic by-products or mutant strains of toxic, radiation-resistant microorganisms. Furthermore, vitamins can be destroyed by irradiation. Nonetheless, the government has recommended that all ground meat and poultry be irradiated to destroy harmful bacteria. Irradiation *does not* make food radioactive and therefore consumers are not at risk from radiation. The U.S. government requires a written radiation disclosure statement on the label of irradiated foods; the use of the radura symbol, however, is optional.

Fast Food

Grabbing a fast-food meal is integral to the fast-paced life in America today. Each day approximately 46 million people, or 20% of the U.S. population, eat in a fast-food restaurant. Convenience notwithstanding, fast-food items must be chosen carefully because many contain high quantities of saturated fat, cholesterol, and salt; few complex carbohydrates; and low levels of vitamins A and C (Table 5.11).

The major fast-food companies have responded to consumers' concerns about nutrition by offering salads, baked potatoes, roast beef, and broiled chicken. Roast beef has less fat than hamburger, and broiled chicken breast has less fat than deep fried chicken. Be cautious, though. Fish, a low-fat food, if breaded and fried, may be 50% fat. Salads and baked potatoes can be carriers of high-fat toppings.

www Vegetarian Diets

Vegetarianism has existed as long as humankind and has been advocated by such famous people as

Terms

gamma irradiation: nonchemical method of food preservation

functional food: a food to which additional vitamins, minerals, herbs, or other substances are added to allow the manufacturer to make health claims

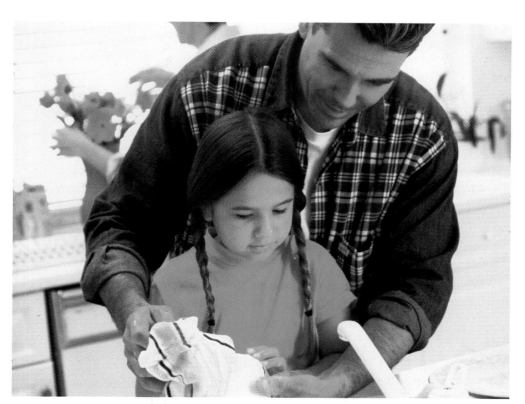

Hand washing is essential to safe food preparation.

Leonardo da Vinci, George Bernard Shaw, Mahatma Gandhi, and Albert Einstein. People choose to be vegetarians for various reasons, including the following:

1. To avoid killing animals—either killing them oneself or killing by others. Some people, who have a strong affection for other animals and feel a certain biological and spiritual kinship with them, object to killing them for food.

2. To contribute to the more efficient utilization of world protein supplies. It takes approximately 10 pounds of livestock feed, usually corn or soybeans, to produce 1 pound of meat. Obviously the 10 pounds of corn or soybeans could feed more people than 1 pound of meat can. With the population of the earth doubling about every 30 years, some people feel a moral obligation to avoid overconsuming food resources in the hope that ways will be found to distribute the world food supply more equitably.

3. To live longer and healthier lives. In many cases, health benefits result from a combination of vegetarianism and nondietary lifestyle factors. Vegetarians, in comparison to nonvegetarians, tend to be leaner, to exercise more, to not smoke cigarettes, and to not abuse alcohol. Vegetarians have a reduced risk for heart and blood vessel disease and for colorectal cancer because of a reduced intake of cholesterol and animal fat. Their increased fiber intake also contributes to the reduced colorectal cancer risk.

TABLE 5.11   Partial Composition of Selected Fast-Food Items

Food	Total Calories	Total fat (grams)	Calories from fat	Cholesterol (milligrams)	Sodium (milligrams)
Big Mac	560	31	280	85	1070
Burrito Supreme	440	18	170	45	1220
French fries (medium/salted)	370	20	180	00	240
Turkey sub sandwich	273	4	34	19	1391
Fried chicken breast	400	24	220	135	1116
Pizza (slice)	300	14	120	25	610
Caesar salad (no dressing)	240	13	120	25	780
Caesar salad (with dressing)	520	43	390	40	1420
Chocolate shake (medium)	320	7	60	20	230

Guidelines for Food Safety

When Purchasing Food

1. Purchase meat and poultry products after all other groceries have been selected and keep packages of raw meat and poultry separate from other foods, particularly foods that will be eaten without further cooking. Consider using plastic bags to enclose individual packages of raw meat and poultry.

2. Make sure meat and poultry products—whether raw, pre-packaged, or cooked from the deli—are refrigerated when purchased.

3. USDA strongly advises against purchasing fresh, pre-stuffed whole birds.

4. Canned goods should be free of dents, cracks, or bulging lids.

5. Take food straight home to the refrigerator. If travel time will exceed 1 hour, pack perishable foods in a cooler with ice and keep groceries and cooler in the passenger area of the car during warm weather.

When Storing Food at Home

1. Verify the temperature of your refrigerator and freezer with an appliance thermometer—refrigerators should run at 40°F or below; freezers at 0°F. Most foodborne bacteria grow slowly at 40°F, which is a safe refrigerator temperature. Freezer temperatures of 0°F or below stop bacterial growth.

2. At home, refrigerate or freeze meat and poultry immediately.

3. To prevent raw juices from dripping on other foods in the refrigerator, use plastic bags or place meat and poultry on a plate.

4. Wash hands with soap and water for 20 seconds before and after handling any raw meat, poultry, or seafood products.

5. Store canned goods in a cool, clean, dry place. Avoid extreme heat or cold, which can be harmful to canned goods.

6. Never store any foods directly under a sink and always keep foods off the floor and separate from cleaning supplies.

When Getting Food Ready to Prepare

1. The importance of hand washing cannot be overemphasized. This simple practice is the most economical, yet often forgotten, way to prevent contamination or cross-contamination.

2. Wash hands (gloved or not) with soap and water for 20 seconds: (a) before beginning preparation; (b) after handling raw meat, poultry, seafood, or eggs; (c) after touching animals; (d) after using the bathroom; (e) after changing diapers; and (f) after blowing the nose.

3. Don't let juices from raw meat, poultry, or seafood come in contact with cooked foods or foods that will be eaten raw, such as fruits or salad ingredients.

4. Wash hands, counters, equipment, utensils, and cutting boards with soap and water immediately after use. Counters, equipment, utensils, and cutting boards can be sanitized with a chlorine solution of 1 teaspoon liquid household bleach per quart of water. Let the solution stand on the board after washing, or follow the instructions on sanitizing products.

5. Thaw meat in the refrigerator, NEVER ON THE COUNTER. It is also safe to thaw in cold water in an airtight plastic wrapper or bag, changing the water every 30 minutes until meat is thawed; Or thaw in the microwave and cook the product immediately.

6. Marinate foods in the refrigerator, NEVER ON THE COUNTER.

7. The USDA recommends that if you choose to stuff whole poultry, you must use a meat thermometer to check the internal temperature of the stuffing. The internal temperature in the center of the stuffing should reach 165°F before removing it from the oven. If you don't have a meat thermometer, cook the stuffing outside the bird. Also, don't put hot stuffing into a frozen bird. By the time it thaws, it will be contaminated inside.

When Cooking

1. Always cook thoroughly. If harmful bacteria are present, only thorough cooking will destroy them; freezing or rinsing the foods in cold water is not sufficient to destroy bacteria.

2. Use a meat thermometer to determine if your meat, poultry, or casserole has reached a safe internal temperature (145°F for roasts and steaks, 180°F for whole poultry, 160°F for ground meat, and 165°F for leftovers). Check the product in several spots to assure that a safe temperature has been reached and that harmful bacteria, such as *Salmonella* and certain strains of *E. coli*, have been destroyed.

3. Avoid interrupted cooking. Never refrigerate partially cooked food to later finish cooking on the grill or in the oven. Meat and poultry products must be cooked thoroughly the first time, and then they may be refrigerated and safely reheated.

4. When microwaving foods, carefully follow the manufacturer's instructions. Use microwave-safe containers, cover, rotate, and allow for the standing time, which contributes to thorough cooking.

When Serving

1. Wash hands with soap and water before serving or eating food.

2. Serve cooked products on clean plates with clean utensils and clean hands. Never put cooked foods on a dish that has held raw products unless the dish is first washed with soap and hot water.

3. Hold hot foods above 140°F and cold foods below 40°F.

4. Never leave foods, raw or cooked, at room temperature longer than 2 hours. On a hot day with temperatures at 90°F or warmer, this time decreases to 1 hour.

When Handling Leftovers

1. Wash hands before and after handling leftovers. Use clean utensils and surfaces.

2. Divide leftovers into small units and store in shallow containers for quick cooling. Refrigerate within 2 hours of cooking.

3. Discard anything left out too long.

4. Never taste a food to determine if it is safe.

5. When reheating leftovers, reheat thoroughly to a temperature of 165°F, or until hot and steamy. Bring soups, sauces, and gravies to a rolling boil.

6. If in doubt, throw it out.

Source: U.S. Department of Agriculture, Food Safety and Inspection Service, November 1996.

There are three kinds of **vegetarian** diets: strict or **veganism,** which excludes all animal products, including milk, cheeses, eggs, and other dairy products; **lacto-vegetarianism,** which excludes meat, poultry, fish, and eggs, but includes dairy products; and **lacto-ovo-vegetarianism,** which excludes meats, poultry, and seafood, but includes eggs and dairy products. Properly planned vegetarian diets can meet the body's nutritional needs, especially by combining sources of protein to assure adequate intake of the essential amino acids. Vegans may need vitamin B_{12} (cobalamin) supplements.

 ## How Nutrition Affects the Brain

The brain requires nutrients in order to function properly. For example, the amount of the neurotransmitter serotonin in the brain is influenced by levels in the blood of the amino acid tryptophan and by the amount of carbohydrate recently eaten. A meal containing tryptophan (derived from dietary protein) and high in carbohydrate increases brain levels of serotonin. Brain levels of the amino acid tyrosine, the precursor of the neurotransmitters dopamine, norepinephrine, and epinephrine, increase after the ingestion of tyrosine-containing protein in a meal. Ingesting choline, a component of lecithin (found in egg yolks, liver, and soybeans), increases the level of the neurotransmitter acetylcholine.

To some degree, moods, feelings of vitality, and sleep patterns may depend on the amount of neurotransmitter molecules ingested and therefore depend indirectly on meals (Fernstrom, 1994). The habit of eating cookies and milk at bedtime may be a way someone increases brain serotonin to help induce a peaceful night's sleep.

> *If your stomach disputes you, lie down amd pacify it with cool thoughts.*
> LEROY "SATCHEL" PAIGE

Some preliminary experiments indicate that tyrosine may help to relieve depression and choline may help to modify certain postural and motor disturbances.

The thoughts, moods, and body sensations of some individuals are highly sensitive to the amount of simple sugars they ingest. Shortly after consuming a couple of donuts or a candy bar, they might experience anxiety, trembling, fatigue, weakness, depression, and inability to concentrate. This response, called **reactive hypoglycemia,** is often the result of a sharp drop in blood sugar when insulin is secreted; this drop, in turn, is produced in response to the large load of sugar in the blood. Something akin to reactive hypoglycemia may be at the root of an eating pattern common to many: consumption of a high-sugar food at breakfast, followed two hours later by a reactive blood sugar low, which motivates a midmorning sugar "hit." The cycle is repeated at noon and midafternoon, and at dinner and late in the evening. To break this cycle, it helps to consume complex carbohydrates with protein and some fat, thereby moderating the rate at which simple sugars enter the body.

Terms

vegetarian: one who consumes no meat, poultry, or fish

vegan: one who excludes all animal products from the diet, including milk, cheese, eggs, and other dairy products

lacto-vegetarian: one who excludes meat, poultry, fish, and eggs, but includes dairy products

lacto-ovo-vegetarian: one who excludes meats, poultry, and fish, but includes eggs and dairy products

reactive hypoglycemia: occurring after the ingestion of carbohydrate, with consequent release of insulin

Critical Thinking About Health

1. Everyone aboard the Zoracian space vehicle XTA-9781 was thrilled when their ship's sensors indicated life forms on a small planet orbiting a medium-sized star in the Milky Way galaxy. To make contact with and explore the planet, a landing party of six underwent molecular rearrangement to take on human form in order both to survive on Earth and communicate and interact with any Earthlings they encountered.

    "When you reach the surface," explained the mission commander, "you will have about eight of their time segments before you must refuel. Energy packets can be obtained in large, stationary pods the locals call supermarkets."

    The crew of the landing party nodded. It seemed similar enough to refueling on their home planet of Zorax not to cause confusion.

    "Except for one thing," the commander cautioned. "There are thousands of kinds of energy packets, from which you will have to choose the appropriate ones."

    "Appropriate ones?" asked the assistant crew-chief.

    "Yes. None of the fuel packets are efficient. You will have to sort and select."

    The crew shifted nervously.

    "Do not worry," said the commander, handing each member of the crew a copy of the Food Guide Pyramid. "Their leaders have prepared refueling guidelines. Take these and use them when the time comes."

    a. How would you explain to the Zoracian landing party why, with the great abundance of food choices in American supermarkets, the U.S. government advises its citizens how to eat properly?
    b. From the Zoracians' point of view, the American food supply, while abundant with many kinds of foods, is inefficient with regard to refueling. Explain why the American food supply is so diverse yet nutritionally inefficient.
    c. What factors influence your food selection?

2. A crusading nutrition journalist points out that the food label on a soup company's best-selling product indicates that the product has 6 grams of fat. Fearing that consumers will stop buying the product, the company responds, and within weeks the label indicates that the product has 3 grams of fat. The company has changed nothing in the product.
    a. Why does the label show that the product contains half the fat?
    b. What limits, if any, would you advocate be placed on what food manufacturers can put on product labels? Where would you draw the line between free enterprise, *caveat emptor* (buyer beware), and the public good?
    c. How much attention do you pay to what is written on food product labels?

3. Explain how an herbicide (weed-killing chemical) could wind up in the breast milk of a woman living hundreds of miles away from the site of herbicide application. Are you concerned about pesticides and additives in the food supply? Why or why not?

Health in Review

- For most of us, good nutrition is a matter of informed choice and is not governed by harsh environmental and economic circumstances.
- The U.S. government commissioned nutritionists and other scientists to create dietary guidelines. These guidelines are aimed at preventing undernutrition and a variety of diseases (e.g., heart disease, many kinds of cancer), which are associated with the high-fat, low–complex carbohydrate diets of Western industrialized nations.
- The U.S. government's required food label is designed to be easy to understand. Reading the food label will help you choose foods that are healthy and that potentially reduce your risk of some diseases.

- In order to be healthy and well, people must obtain 40 essential nutrients from their food in proper amounts and proportions. Food energy, measured in calories, comes principally from sugars, carbohydrates, and fats.
- Dietary supplements can be a form of "dietary insurance" for those who are concerned their diet may be nutritionally inadequate.
- Food is composed of seven kinds of substances: proteins, carbohydrates, fats, minerals, vitamins, phytochemicals, and water. Nutritionists recommend basing our diets on complex carbohydrates and fresh fruits and vegetables to lessen the consumption of saturated fat and to ensure consumption of adequate fiber, vitamins, minerals, and phytochemicals.

- Manufactured foods contain a variety of additives that alter their texture, flavor, color, and stability. Preservatives keep foods from spoiling through the use of sulfites.
- One nonchemical method of food preservation involves exposing food to gamma irradiation to destroy microorganisms.

- Artificial sweeteners are widely used, most commonly in "diet" soft drinks.
- There are several reasons for being a vegetarian, including increased interest in health, ecology, and world issues; economical issues; and the philosophy of not killing animals. A strict vegetarian, or vegan, diet eliminates all animal products, including milk, cheese, eggs, and other dairy products.

Health and Wellness Online

The World Wide Web contains a wealth of information about health and wellness. By accessing the Internet using Web browser software, such as Netscape Navigator or Microsoft's Internet Explorer, you can gain a new perspective on many topics presented in *Health and Wellness, Seventh Edition*. Access the Jones and Bartlett Publishers Web site at http://www.jbpub.com/hwonline

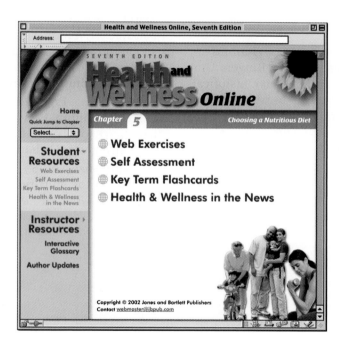

References

Advertising Age (1999, September 27). 100 leading national advertisers. S1–S46.

American Cancer Society: The importance of nutrition in cancer prevention (http://www2.cancer.org/prevention/NutritionandPrevention.cfm)

American Heart Association's eating plan (http://www.deliciousdecisions.org/contents.html)

Campbell, T. C., and Junshi C. (1994). Diet and chronic degenerative diseases: Perspectives from China. *American Journal of Clinical Nutrition, 59(suppl)*, 1153–1161.

Consumer Reports (1999, June). The new foods: functional or dysfunctional? 1–5.

Fernstrom, J. D. (1994). Dietary amino acids and brain function. *Journal of the American Dietetic Association, 94(1)*, 71–78.

Jacobson, M. F., and Brownell, K. D. (2000). Small taxes on soft drinks and snack foods to promote health. *American Journal of Public Health, 90,* 854–857.

Kant, A. K., Schatzkin, A. Graubard, B. I., and Schairer, C. (2000). A prospective study of diet quality and mortality in women. *Journal of the American Medical Association, 283,* 2109–2115.

Markus, C. R., et al. (2000). Carbohydrate intake improves cognitive performance of stress-prone individuals under controllable laboratory stress. *American Journal of Clinical Nutrition, 71,* 1536–1544

Patterson, R. E., et al. (2001). Is there a consumer backlash against the diet and health message? *Journal of the American Dietetic Association, 101,* 37–41.

Schlosser, E. (2001, January). Why McDonald's fries taste so good. *Atlantic Monthly,* 50–56.

U.S. Department of Agriculture, Dietary Guidelines for Americans (2000), 5th Edition. http://www.usda.gov/cnpp/Pubs/DG2000/Index.htm

Suggested Readings

Anderson, J., and Deskins, B. (1997). *The nutrition bible: The comprehensive, no-nonsense, guide to foods, nutrients, additives, preservatives, pollutants, and everything else we eat and drink.* New York: Quill. The title says it all.

Apple, R. D. (1996). *Vitamania: Vitamins in American culture.* New Brunswick, NJ: Rutgers University Press. Explores the scientific, social, historical, and commercial aspects of vitamin use in America. Shows how nutritional information often has been and still is twisted for commercial gain.

Lewis, C. (2001, January/February). A new kind of fish story—the coming of biotech animals. FDA Consumer, 15–20.

Ornish, Dean (2000). *Eat More, Weigh Less: Dr. Dean Ornish's Advantage Ten Program for Losing Weight Safely While Eating Abundantly.* NY: Quill.

You can eat more and weigh less if you know what to eat.

Pollan, M. (2001, May 13). How organic became a marketing niche and a multibillion-dollar industry—Naturally. *New York Times Magazine,* 30–65. Describes how "organic" foods have been turned into TV dinners and other processed foods and still conform to the legal definition of organic.

Schlosser, Eric (2001). *Fast Food Nation.* NY: Houghton Mifflin. Everything you ever wanted to know (and not know) about fast food: Its history, role in the economy, and contribution to the epidemic of obesity.

Scrimshaw, N. S., and SanGiovanni, J. P. (1997). Synergism of nutrition, infection, and immunity. *American Journal of Clinical Nutrition, 66(2),* 464S–477S. How infections affect nutritional status and how nutritional status affects immunity.

Web sites

American Dietetic Association. Provides information and daily tips. (http://www.eatright.org/)

Fast Food Facts. Enables analysis of the nutrient content of common fast foods. (http://www.olen.com/food/)

Nutrition Analysis Tool (NAT). Allows analysis of foods for various nutrients. (http://www.ag.uiuc.edu/~food-lab/nat/)

Nutrition.gov. Provides easy access to all online federal government information on nutrition including nutrition, healthy eating, physical activity, and food safety. (http://www.nutrition.gov)

Quackwatch. Offers information on safety and health issues of dietary supplements. (http://www.quackwatch.com/01QuackeryRelatedTopics/DSH/suppsherbs.html)

U.S. Department of Agriculture food composition data. Estimates of the nutrient composition of 3,200

foods. (http://63.73.158.76/Foodcomposition.htm)

U.S. Department of Agriculture National Organic Program. Provides information on organic food. (http://www.ams.usda.gov/nop/)

U.S. Department of Agriculture Food Safety and Inspection Service. Includes consumer advice on food-borne illnesses. (http://www.fsis.usda.gov/)

U.S. Food & Drug Administration Food Labeling Publications Page. (http://www.fda.gov/opacom/campaigns/3foodlbl.html)

U.S. Food & Drug Administration Center for Food Safety & Applied Nutrition. Includes dietary supplements warnings and safety information. (http://vm.cfsan.fda.gov/~dms/ds-warn.html)

U.S. Food & Drug Administration Center for Food Safety & Applied Nutrition. Provides information on food safety, food additives, dietary supplements, and food biotechnology. (http://vm.cfsan.fda.gov/)

Learning Objectives

1. Describe the extent and causes of overweight in American society.
2. Describe the significance of body mass index (BMI) to health.
3. Explain the concept of fatness set point.
4. Explain why calorie-restricting weight-loss programs fail.
5. Discuss why exercise (and *not* calorie restriction) is the key to healthy weight maintenance.
6. List the psychological factors that contribute to weight problems.
7. Discuss the advantages and disadvantages of the medical treatments for overweight.
8. Describe the signs of anorexia nervosa and bulimia.

Study Guide and Self Assessment

What Are Your Weight Statistics?
Watching Your Weight
Body Image

Health and Wellness Online

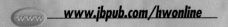 **www.jbpub.com/hwonline**

Chapter 6

Managing a Healthy Weight

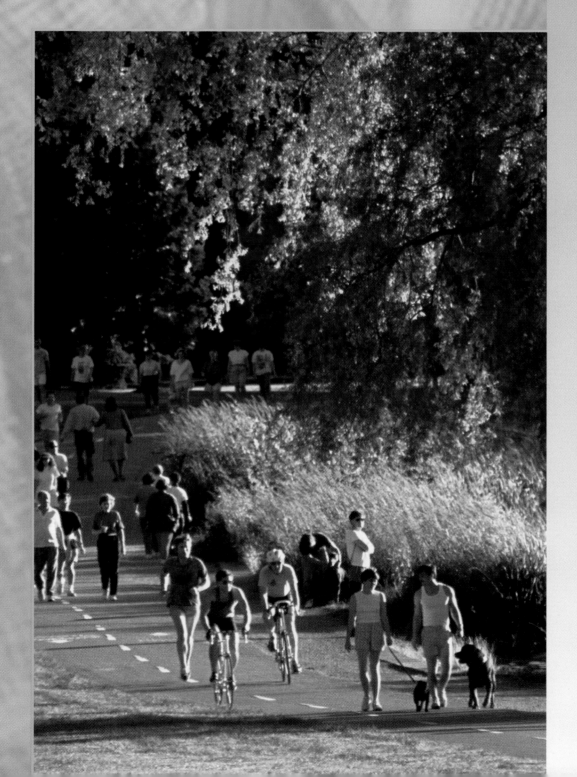

Judging from the number of books and magazine articles extolling various "surefire" weight loss programs and TV "infomercials" peddling exercise gear, it would appear that the U.S. national pastime is weight control. Indeed, about two-thirds of adult women and one-third of adult men are on so-called reducing diets ("so-called" because they invariably fail to reduce body size). About 54% of American adults are overweight (Figure 6.1); this puts them at risk for a variety of diseases (Figure 6.2). Annual health care costs related to overweight in the U.S. are approximately $120 billion.

Never eat more than you can lift.

MISS PIGGY

Many people whose body weight does not predispose them to health problems are still weight conscious, primarily for cosmetic reasons. Their goal is to achieve a body size and shape that meets society's standards of "perfection" (generated by the fashion and advertising industries). These individuals seem to be in a continual battle with the same 5, 10, or 20 pounds, which they struggle to shed to look youthful and attractive. Concern about body weight (more typically, body *fatness*) fuels a $40 billion industry of weight-reduction machines and programs, special foods, and dietary supplements, most of which are useless and costly in the long run.

With all the passion for being slim, it is no wonder that many people view any amount of visible fat on the body as something to get rid of. However, the human body has evolved over time in environments of food scarcity; hence, the ability to store fat easily and efficiently is a valuable physiological function that served our ancestors well for thousands of years. Only in the last few decades, and only in the wealthiest economies, has food become so plentiful and easy to obtain as to cause fat-related health problems. People

TABLE 6.1   Percentage of Daily Calories Provided by Typical Fast-Food Meals

Meal	Percentage of daily calories for three different daily calorie levels		
	1600 calories/day	2000 calories/day	2500 calories/day
Quarter Pounder French fries Milkshake	73	58	47
Whopper French fries Diet soft drink	66	54	43
Two slices of pizza Diet soft drink	33	25	20

no longer have to spend most of their time and energy gathering berries and seeds and hoping that a hunting party will return with meat. All we have to do nowadays is drive to the supermarket or the fast-food restaurant, where for a very low cost we can obtain nearly all of our daily calories (Table 6.1).

Body weight issues are not solely about food intake, but are about food intake in relation to a number of other factors: a sedentary lifestyle, heredity, advertising that promotes food products, lack of guidance regarding proper nutrition, confusing information about the effects of food on health and well-being, the custom of using body shape as a measure of social desirability, and a hectic, stressful lifestyle. In such a complex environment, the overavailability of food allows it to be used for a variety of reasons other than to provide nutrients and energy for life.

What Is Desirable Weight?

In most instances, concerns about being overweight are really concerns about being *overfat*. There is a difference. Some professional male athletes, for example, weigh much more than the recommended weight standards for persons of similar height. Yet as little as 1% of their body weight may be fat. Most of the body weight of a well-conditioned athlete is muscle and

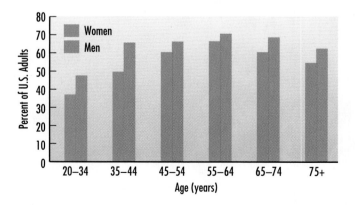

FIGURE 6.1   Prevalence of Overweight in the United States   Overweight is defined as a body mass index (BMI) greater than 25.0.
Source: Centers for Disease Control and Prevention, National Center for Health Statistics

Terms

essential fat: necessary bodyfat required for normal physiological functioning

storage fat: also called depot fat; energy stored as fat in various parts of the body

body mass index: a measure of body fatness, calculated by dividing body weight (in kilograms) by the square of height (in meters)

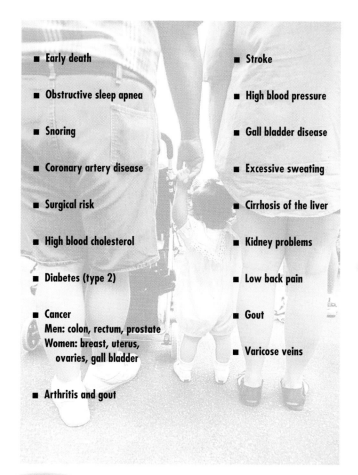

- Early death
- Obstructive sleep apnea
- Snoring
- Coronary artery disease
- Surgical risk
- High blood cholesterol
- Diabetes (type 2)
- Cancer
  Men: colon, rectum, prostate
  Women: breast, uterus,
  ovaries, gall bladder
- Arthritis and gout

- Stroke
- High blood pressure
- Gall bladder disease
- Excessive sweating
- Cirrhosis of the liver
- Kidney problems
- Low back pain
- Gout
- Varicose veins

FIGURE 6.2 Overweight and obese people have a greater likelihood of developing certain health problems than do people of normal weight.

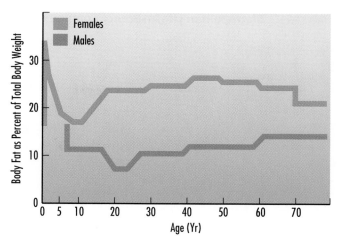

FIGURE 6.3 **Body Fat Percentage** The average percentage of total body weight that is body fat for U.S. men and women, by age.

bone. Female body builders, who are the leanest of all female athletes, have about 8% to 13% of their total body weight as fat. This probably represents the lower limit of fat for a healthy woman.

Body fat is composed of two parts: **essential fat**—fat necessary for normal physiological functioning, such as nerve conduction—and **storage fat.** Essential fat comprises about 3% to 7% of body weight in men and about 10% to 12% of body weight in women. This gender difference, which is presumably caused by hormones, is due to the deposition of greater amounts of fat on the hips, thighs, and breasts in females. Storage fat, also called depot fat, constitutes only a small percentage of the total body weight of lean individuals and 5% to 25% of the body weight of the majority of the population (Figure 6.3). However, storage fat can account for 40% to 50% of the body weight of some overweight persons.

Standards for the most "desirable" or "ideal" body weight or body composition (fat percentage) vary. For example, in some cultures, women with significant storage fat are considered physically attractive and sexually desirable, and fatness in children is considered a sign of robust health. In the United States, attitudes about desirable body configuration fluctuate and are often keyed to fashion trends. During the 1950s, for example, large body size, characterized by "full-figured" women and "he-men," was considered desirable, whereas today "slim is in."

Indexes of desirable body weight are given in tables of "ideal weight for height" issued by both government agencies and insurance companies and are based on statistics for longevity (Table 6.2) and the **body mass index** (BMI), which is calculated by dividing a person's weight in kilograms by his or her height in meters squared (Figure 6.4). Studies show that good health is associated with weighing no more than 5% below or 20% (for men) and 30% (for women) above the weight-for-height standards, or having a BMI between 19 and 25 (Willett et al., 1999) (Figure 6.5). Above the upper limits of these measures, people have higher risks for diabetes, gallbladder disease, varicose veins, arthritis, heart disease, stroke, high blood pressure, breathing problems, and accident proneness (because of a large body). People who are extremely overweight often face stigmas, such as job discrimination, lower social acceptance, and lower self-esteem.

Another health-related index of body size is the waist-to-hip ratio, which is calculated by dividing the circumference of the waist by the circumference of the hips. For example, someone with a 28-inch waist and 37-inch hips would have a waist-to-hip ratio of 0.75. Health problems are less likely in women whose waist-to-hip ratio is less than 0.8 and in men whose waist-to-hip ratio is less than 0.95. In other words, it is healthier for a body to be pear-shaped than apple-shaped, and it's healthier *not* to have a beer belly (Figure 6.6). Doctors sometimes use only the waist circumference as an indicator of health risks associated with being overweight. A waist circumference greater than 40 inches in men and 35 inches in women is associated with greater health risk.

TABLE 6.2   Metropolitan Life Insurance Company Weight-for-Height Tables

Women (with clothing)				Men (with clothing)			
Height (with shoes, 2-inch heels)	Small frame	Medium frame	Large frame	Height (with shoes, 1-inch heels)	Small frame	Medium frame	Large frame
4'10"	92–98	96–107	104–119	5'2"	112–120	118–129	126–141
4'11"	94–101	98–110	106–122	3"	115–123	121–133	129–144
5'0"	96–104	101–113	109–125	4"	118–126	124–136	142–148
1"	99–107	104–116	112–128	5"	121–129	127–139	135–152
2"	102–110	107–119	115–131	6"	124–133	130–143	138–156
3"	105–113	110–122	118–134	7"	128–137	134–147	142–161
4"	108–116	113–126	121–138	8"	132–141	138–152	147–166
5"	111–119	116–130	125–142	9"	136–145	142–156	151–170
6"	114–123	120–135	129–146	10"	140–150	146–160	155–174
7"	118–127	124–139	133–150	11"	144–154	150–165	159–179
8"	122–131	128–143	137–154	6'0"	148–158	154–170	164–184
9"	126–135	132–147	141–158	1"	152–162	158–175	168–189
10"	130–140	136–151	145–163	2"	156–167	162–180	173–194
11"	134–144	140–155	149–168	3"	160–171	167–185	178–199
6'0"	138–148	144–159	153–173	4"	164–175	172–190	182–204

Source: Metropolitan Life Insurance Company. Used by permission.

Managing Stress

Self-Esteem and Weight Control

Experts agree that for weight control to be effective it must begin in the mind, not the body. And two mental factors are crucial for a weight-control program to be effective: high self-esteem and will power.

One of the most effective ways to build self-esteem is positive self-talk, which in turn helps boost will power. Our minds, like frequency bands on a radio tuner, have many voices or stations. The one frequency people typically tune into is the voice of the *critic*—a negative voice who constantly tells us that we are not good enough; we are too fat, too skinny, too short, badly proportioned, or just plain ugly. But we have a choice. We don't have to listen to this voice of the critic. Like pushing a button of a car radio, we can tune out the critic's voice and find another station—one that gives better feedback. Like a distant radio station with much static, the reception may not come in clearly at first, but with

concentration, the voice that honors your being will come in much clearer. With practice, the message of choice will provide positive feedback.

One way you can tune into this frequency is to program your mind with positive affirmations: words, phrases, or expressions that you say to yourself to raise your self-esteem and confidence. These words of encouragement stroke the ego and enhance your sense of well-being. While this notion of giving yourself positive strokes may sound silly, it works. Many Olympic athletes, actors, and successful achievers use positive self-talk to accomplish their goals.

It is important to use the present tense, and even though the statement may not be true, say it as if it is, so "as if" becomes "as is." The following are some examples of positive affirmations that can help you raise your self-esteem, increase your will power, and help you control your weight. If you like

one of these, use it regularly three or four times per day (especially near meal times), or create your own statement. When you use an affirmation statement, say it to yourself and feel it at the gut level.

- I am at the right weight for my body size
- I am happy with my weight and body composition
- I am coming closer to my ideal body weight and composition
- I have the will power to eat only the amount of food I need to sustain optimal wellness
- I enjoy both high-quality food and high-quality exercise

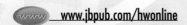
www.jbpub.com/hwonline

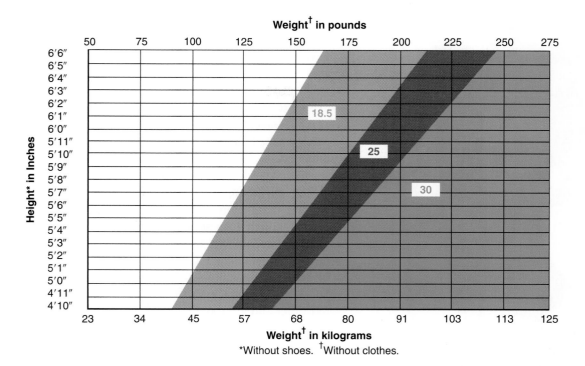

Directions: Find your weight on the bottom of the graph. Go straight up from that point until you come to the line that matches your height. Then look to find your weight group.

▓ **Healthy weight** BMI from 18.5 up to 25 indicates a healthy weight.
▓ **Overweight** BMI from 25 up to 30 indicates overweight.
▓ **Obese** BMI 30 or higher indicates obesity.

FIGURE 6.4   **Body Mass Index Chart**

The Regulation of Body Fat

The main principle of healthy weight maintenance is that you will store fat if you take in more calories than you expend. Calories enter the body as food: four calories per gram of protein or carbohydrate, seven calories per gram of alcohol, and nine calories per gram of fat. Calories leave the body as energy expended: to fuel basal (resting) metabolism, physical activity, growth, injury repair, and maintain body temperature. Calories from food that are not used right away are stored either as **glycogen,** a carbohydrate that is found in liver and muscle, or as **triglyceride,** a fat that is found in adipose tissue located on the body in all-too-familiar places. At nine calories per gram, fat is the most efficient form of energy storage (one pound of fat will fuel a 40-mile walk), and fat has other biological advantages: it's lightweight, compact, spongy, and a good thermal insulator.

The Fatness Set Point

The body has an extremely complex fatness-control mechanism called the **fatness set point,** which maintains fatness within narrow limits. Just as house tem-

perature is maintained by a thermostat, the amount of body fat is maintained by the nervous system and a particular group of hormones. In your house, when the temperature drops below the "set point" on the thermostat, the heater starts to return the house to the pre-set temperature. When the house temperature rises, the air conditioner starts.

The same feedback principle applies to body fatness. If the amount of body fat decreases below the fatness set point (perhaps because an individual goes on a calorie-restricting diet), the nervous and hormone systems counter the loss by increasing appetite and conserving energy. If the amount of body fat exceeds the fatness set point (perhaps because an individual overeats), the nervous and hormone systems counter the gain by decreasing appetite and increasing energy use.

Terms

glycogen: a storage form of carbohydrate

triglyceride: a storage form of fat

fatness set point: the physiologically regulated amount of fat on the body

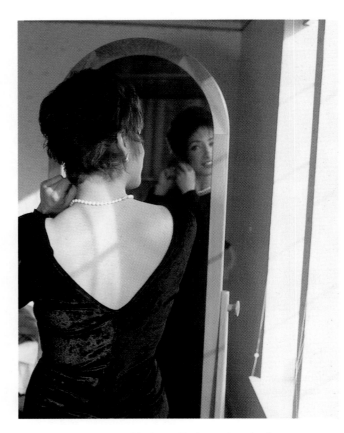

Most people want to "feel good" about their bodies.

The fatness set point is controlled in a region of the hypothalamus of the brain referred to as the **appestat,** because it controls appetite and eating behavior. When your body needs calories, nerves and hormones signal the appestat and you feel hungry. When the body has sufficient calories, nerves and hormones signal the appestat and you feel full. Many situations and factors influence the appestat.

Appestat Turn-Ons

- *The amount of available energy in your body:* You haven't eaten in several hours and your blood glucose level is low.
- *Eating habits:* It's your usual dinner time and you expect to eat whether or not you are hungry.
- *Food triggers:* You walk into the mall and smell freshly baked chocolate chip cookies and can't resist one.

Appestat Turn-Offs

- *Gastric distention:* You've just overeaten and you feel as though your stomach is going to explode.
- *Food palatability:* A friend orders a pizza with toppings that you don't like and suddenly you're not hungry.
- *Social circumstances:* You invite a new love interest to dinner and are too distracted by your emotions to eat.

As long as you are generally healthy, the appestat is working properly, *and you are paying attention to it,* you are unlikely to develop a weight (fat) problem since your calorie intake will pretty much equal your calorie output; this is called being in a state of **energy balance.** However, you only have to exceed energy balance a little bit to develop a weight problem over time. Consider this example:

Marci is a 26-year-old woman of normal weight with a BMI of 23 who recently changed jobs. Previously the office manager in a small real estate company, she now works as an executive assistant in a much larger firm. Two consequences of this change are: (a) Marci now spends more time sitting at her desk typing and answering the phone than in her former job, where she moved around for *every* office

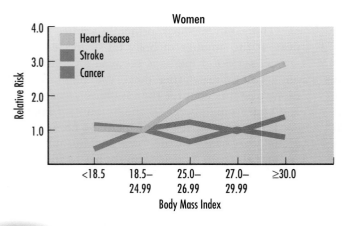

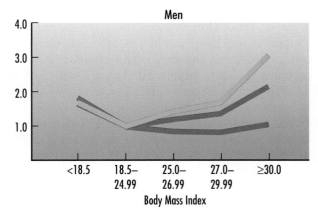

FIGURE 6.5   Relative Health Risks of Various Body Mass Indexes (BMIs)   The relative risks for persons with various BMIs of death from coronary heart disease, cardiovascular disease, and cancer, as well as death from accidents, suicides, and other causes have been standardized to the BMI range 18.5 to 24.99. The higher relative risk of a BMI of < 18.5 is possibly related to smoking and weight loss from poor mental health.

Source: Data from Seidell, J. C., et al., (1996). Overweight, underweight, and mortality. *Archives of Internal Medicine, 156,* 958–963.

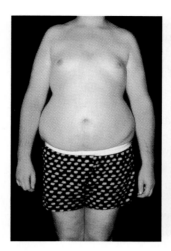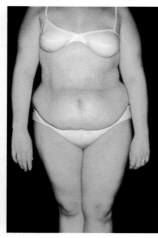

FIGURE 6.6 **Apple or Pear?** Apple-shaped people carry much of their body fat above the waist. Pear-shaped people carry their body fat on the hips and thighs. Studies show that it's healthier to be pear-shaped than apple-shaped.

task, and (b) she now goes to lunch with office mates. The combination of less movement and fast-food lunches has increased Marci's daily calorie intake over expenditure an average of 10%.

What's 10%? That's about 160 calories per working day, or 3200 calories a month. At 3500 calories per pound, that's enough for Marci to gain about 10 pounds per year. You can see what a few years at this job might do to Marci's waistline. When the office crew goes to lunch, often their intention is to socialize and get away from the stress of the office; they don't intend to consume a big lunch. However, the desire to be social, the smell of food, and the size of the portions make it easy to ignore satiety signals from the appestat and to overeat.

Of course, Marci could prevent gaining those 10 pounds a year by being more mindful of her lunchtime eating behaviors and walking an extra 20 minutes every day (four calories per minute). If she doesn't, however, her body is likely to store those excess calories as fat, and in a couple of years she is likely to find herself with a BMI near 30 and in need of a new wardrobe. And if that happens and she decides to lose that extra fat, she's likely to discover—as many of us do—that it will take effort to slim down, and without a permanent change in exercise and eating habits, it will be very difficult to keep the lost weight (fat) from returning.

That's because the body doesn't like to let go of fat it has accumulated, or as scientists say, the body defends against fat loss. Remember that the body is designed to store fat easily, in case you ever have to go without food for several days as your ancient ancestors did. Of course, that almost never happens to modern people, but those built-in, efficient fat-storage mechanisms are still present. So once fat is deposited, it's very hard to lose.

Another reason it is hard to lose fat is that a decrease in body fat triggers an increase in the efficiency with which the body uses energy. The resting metabolic rate decreases, and the efficiency with which muscles do work increases (Leibel et al., 1995).

Another way the body defends against fat loss is through the action of a hormone called **leptin,** which is manufactured by fat cells. When fat cells are laden with triglyceride, they secrete leptin into the bloodstream, where it finds it way to the appestat, causing a decrease in appetite and an increase in energy use. When fat cells are relatively devoid of triglyceride, leptin secretion diminishes, and appetite increases. If someone does not produce sufficient leptin, or if someone's appestat does not respond to leptin, then that person may be susceptible to becoming overfat. Genetic (inherited) variations in the leptin regulatory system may explain the susceptibility of some people to overfatness (Schwartz and Seeley, 1997).

That the body defends against weight loss explains why many a dieter's most ardent attempts to lose weight (fat) by lessening the intake of food result in failure. Calorie restriction puts a person in a state of semi-starvation, which triggers the array of biological mechanisms designed to conserve both body fat and energy expenditure. Moreover, calorie restriction is no fun. Often people become bored eating the same required foods or frustrated with not being able to eat the kinds and quantities of food they want. They become obsessed with food, and after a time they give up their diet and return to their former eating habits. And when they gain weight, they blame themselves for being weak-willed failures.

 ## Sensible Weight Maintenance

Many advertisements suggest that a healthy body is one that is slim and muscular. However, research shows that a variety of body sizes, shapes, and fat compositions are healthy. For example, a woman who is 5 feet 4 inches tall can weigh between 110 pounds (BMI = 19) and 148 pounds (BMI = 25) and still have a healthy body weight. What would be unhealthy is striving for an unattainable body weight and shape and then criticizing oneself for failing to attain it. This

Terms

appestat: region of the hypothalamus that controls appetite and eating behavior

energy balance: when energy consumed as food equals the energy expended in living

leptin: a hormone that controls appetite

is not good for self-esteem or mental health, and it defeats a sensible weight maintenance program.

It is true that individuals with BMIs of 30 or more should reduce their body fat percentage to avoid a variety of health problems. But instead of setting the unrealistic goal of slimming to a BMI of 20 and harshly criticizing themselves when that goal is not met, they should try to reduce their body weight by 10%, which often puts them in the range of good health.

> *The trouble with Italian cooking is that after five or six days you're hungry again.*
>
> HENRY MILLER

Those who are not clinically overfat but wish to slim down for cosmetic reasons should realize that stereotypes of attractiveness are often very difficult to attain without a predisposing genetic makeup or a visit to the cosmetic surgeon. Sensible weight management begins with being aware of social pressures toward unattainable goals and not succumbing to advertising and fashion trends.

No calorie-restricting weight-loss program has ever been shown to be effective over the medium-to-long term, regardless of advertising claims to the contrary. Programs lasting 2, 6, 12, or 24 weeks that are based on particular foods and portions can produce considerable weight loss, but 67% of people regain that weight within 1 year, and 95% regain it within 5 years. Improved nutrition, regular exercise, and a desire to feel good are the ways people who lose considerable weight are able to maintain the new, healthful body weight for many years (Klem, et al., 1997).

Since calorie-restricting diets by themselves don't work, what does? Unless you have a fat-storage disease, you can do it by living healthfully and letting your body find the weight that's natural for it, which involves:

- *Eat only when hungry.* Pay attention to hunger and satiety signals from your appestat. Be aware of habits and customs that influence your eating behavior: Do you eat at predetermined times of day (mealtime, between classes, on the way to work) regardless of your state of hunger? Do you eat *everything* on your plate? Do you work or study while eating?

- *Eat low on the food pyramid.* Base your diet on breads, pasta, vegetables, fresh fruits, and grains. This will keep you from overconsumption of calories, because you will more easily feel full. Also, you are less likely to consume fat calories that are "hidden" in manufactured foods to make them palatable.

- *Exercise.* Move your body around for at least 20 minutes per day, three to four times a week. And don't subscribe to the myth that exercising will increase appetite and food consumption. In fact, except for individuals who expend enormous amounts of energy (e.g., lumberjacks, football players), the opposite is true. Appetite and food consumption tend to decrease as physical activity increases.

- *Limit mindless snacking.* Mindless snacking is the kind we do when we are ravenously hungry, stressed, or zoned-out watching TV. We wish that bag of chips were bottomless. TV advertisers encourage mindless snacking. They know that when you're watching TV you're in a state of autohypnosis, and they bank on your susceptibility to their images of beer, snack foods, candy, and soft drinks. Instead of mindless snacking, it's better to focus on the food you are eating. Be aware of satiety signals from your appestat. Ask yourself if you really want that candy bar or would you rather have a piece of fruit. Say to yourself, "That's enough for now."

- *Consume little or no alcohol.* Alcohol contains seven calories per gram (about 100 calories per 12-ounce beer, 4-ounce glass of wine, or one shot of distilled liquor). A couple of beers per day without a compensatory reduction in food intake or increase in exercise could lead to an excess of body fat rather quickly.

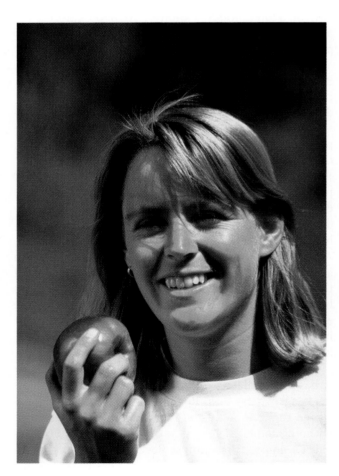

If you have to snack, choose healthy foods such as fruits and vegetables.

- *Be aware of eating triggers.* Many of us are susceptible to environmental cues that trigger eating. For example, some people cannot pass a candy or soft-drink machine without feeding it money in exchange for it feeding them. At some worksites, well-meaning supervisors provide pastries and candy for their staff members, who may have a difficult time resisting, especially when stressed or fatigued.

- *Don't feed your feelings.* Stress, anxiety, loneliness, boredom, and anger can motivate overeating. Many people derive emotional comfort from food. One possible explanation is that, as children, we learn to associate eating (particularly nursing as infants) with receiving love, affection, and comfort. Another possibility is when we consume certain foods, particularly those containing sugar and fat, they contribute to feelings of calm.

The energy equivalent of 1 pound of body fat is 3500 calories. If you want to adopt a weight-reducing program that results in a loss of 1 pound a month, plan your dietary and physical activities so you can produce a net daily deficit of 120 calories. Walk a little more each day or cut out a soft drink or a couple of cookies (Table 6.3). If you want to lose one pound a week, plan for a net daily deficit of 500 calories that includes at least a 300-calorie expenditure per day of exercise (Table 6.4). The number of calories is not nearly as important as *making a plan to which you can realistically adhere over the long haul.* Here are some other suggestions:

- Keep a diary of your weight-loss activities and modify things in your plan that do not work.

- Keep faith with your intention to attain a healthful weight. Don't let the inevitable setbacks demoralize you.

TABLE 6.3	**Activity Equivalents of Calories in Some Foods (in Minutes)**				
Food	*Walking*	*Cycling*	*Swimming*	*Running*	*Yoga*
Apple	20	12	9	5	20
Can of beer	30	18	13	8	30
Piece of cake	70	45	35	20	70
Two cookies	20	12	9	5	20
One doughnut	30	18	13	8	30
Double-scoop ice cream cone	40	25	18	11	40
Piece of pie	70	45	35	20	70
Piece of pizza	35	22	16	10	35
20 french fries	60	40	30	17	60
10 potato chips	20	12	9	5	20
8-oz. soft drink	25	15	11	7	25
Hamburger	70	45	35	20	70

- Don't count calories or constantly weigh yourself; focus on feeling good.

- Ignore weight loss and exercise-machine advertising.

 ## The Medical Management of Overweight

Managing body weight is principally a matter of adopting healthful living habits: eating foods low on the food pyramid, limiting consumption of fast foods and other fatty foods, and increasing exercise. Still, some people cannot successfully manage weight on their own, and they may benefit by seeking the help of

Wellness Guide

Mindful Eating

Eating should be a relaxed, pleasurable activity but is rarely that in our daily, hectic lives. We "eat on the run" or take only enough time to "just grab a bite." Most teenagers polish off a full plate of food in a couple of minutes. Just as taking time for physical activity is important for your body, so is taking time with your meals. You can begin to break the habit of wolfing down your food by practicing "mindful eating."

Start by choosing a very small piece of food,

perhaps a grape, slice of carrot, or a piece of dried fruit. Sit quietly and slowly place the food in your mouth. Pay attention to its texture and flavor.

Begin to chew it very slowly and notice the response in your mouth—how your saliva starts to flow and how your jaw is moving. Chew until you feel ready to swallow; pay attention to the process of swallowing. Practice this mindful eating exercise every day until you feel that you have become more aware of your food and the nourishment you receive from it.

When you eat a meal focus all of your attention on the food and the satisfaction of eating. Do not read or watch TV while eating. Make eating a quiet, pleasurable occasion. Do not bring problems or arguments to the table. By eating slowly and quietly you also will hear the message from your stomach when it is full. Listen to the message and stop eating.

Mindful eating can be a powerful technique in weight control and limiting food consumption that your body does not need.

Wellness Guide

Weight-Management Suggestions

Control your home environment in these ways:

1. Do all at-home eating at the kitchen or dining room table.

2. Eat without reading or watching TV.

3. Keep tempting foods out of sight, hard to reach, and bothersome to prepare.

4. If you must snack, have low-calorie foods accessible, visible, easy to reach, and ready to eat.

5. Store tempting foods in containers that are opaque or difficult to open.

6. Give other family members their own snack-food storage areas.

7. Don't do non–food-related activities in the kitchen; stay out of the kitchen as much as possible.

Control your work environment in these ways:

1. Do not eat at your desk or while working. Eat at some place designated (by you) for eating only.

2. Do not keep tempting food near your workplace.

3. Prepackage low-calorie snacks and take them with you to work.

4. Carry no change to use at vending machines.

5. Use exercise instead of food when you need to take a break from work.

6. If you eat in a cafeteria, plan your order in advance and bring only enough money to cover your order.

Manage your daily food sources:

1. Do not shop when hungry.

2. Shop from a list prepared beforehand.

3. Shop quickly.

4. Avoid buying large sizes of hard-to-resist high-calorie foods.

5. Prepare foods during periods when your control is highest.

6. Try to prepare several meals at once (lunches with dinners).

7. Remove leftovers from sight as soon after mealtime as possible (use opaque storage devices).

Control your mealtime environment:

1. Do not keep serving bowls at the table.

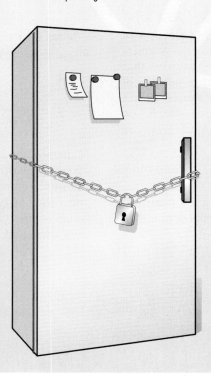

2. Use smaller plates, bowls, glasses, and serving spoons.

3. Remove the plate from the table as soon as you finish eating.

4. Practice polite refusal when extra food is offered to you.

Eat slowly:

1. Put down the eating utensil, sandwich, drink, or chicken leg between bites.

2. Swallow what is in your mouth before preparing the next bite.

3. Cut food as it is needed rather than all at once.

4. Stop eating a few times during the meal to control your eating rhythm.

5. Make each second serving only half as large as the usual amount.

Control snacking:

1. Instead of snacking, do an activity incompatible with eating.

2. Instead of snacking, do something you like to do or a small task around the house or office.

3. Instead of snacking, do a short burst of intense activity or a relaxation exercise.

4. Brush your teeth or use mouthwash to curb the urge to eat.

5. Make snacks difficult to get.

6. Drink a large glass of water before snacking.

7. Have low-calorie snack foods on hand rather than high-calorie foods.

Source: J. Waltz, *Food Habit Management* (Seattle, WA: Northwest Learning Associates, Inc., 1978).

---

a health professional. Methods that health professionals employ to help people reduce and maintain body weight include psychological counseling, hypnotherapy, medications, and surgery.

Counseling and Hypnosis

Counseling for weight loss using cognitive behavioral therapy involves helping patients examine the reasons for their unhealthful eating and exercise behaviors and develop ways to behave more healthfully. Hypnosis has been shown to increase the benefits of counseling (Kirsch, 1996).

Psychological Counseling

Psychological counseling for weight loss and maintenance focuses on:

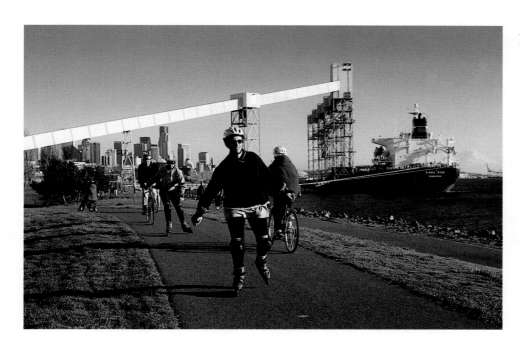

Exercise is essential to effective weight management.

- increasing one's self-awareness of the inner dialogue that contributes to the weight problem

- education about nutrition and physical activity

- setting realistic weight management goals and adopting feasible plans for accomplishing them

- teaching about "feeding one's feelings" and the tendency to eat when feeling stressed

- providing social support for weight management activities

- identifying and managing mental health issues, such as depression and anxiety, that may be associated with weight issues

Psychological counseling is generally effective in facilitating weight loss of about a pound a week and a significant percentage of the initial body weight, and it

promotes weight loss maintenance for several months after treatment ends (Poston and Foreyt, 2000).

Medications

Medications to produce weight loss include appetite suppressants, agents that alter certain neurotransmitters in the brain (norepinephrine or serotonin) to make one feel less hungry, and a drug that blocks the absorption of fat from the intestines (orlistat). Drugs alone cannot produce significant weight loss, and generally any weight lost is regained when the drug is no longer taken. This is why health professionals consider medications to be an adjunct to lifestyle modification (diet, exercise, and greater awareness of eating habits) and not to be used alone to achieve weight loss.

Surgery

Surgery may be indicated for people with a BMI over 40 or people with a BMI between 35 and 40 who have severe weight-related medical conditions, such as heart problems or diabetes, and who have not responded to supervised diet and exercise regimes or drug therapy. The rationale of surgical treatments for obesity is to alter the anatomy of the gastrointestinal tract so that only a fraction of food ingested in a meal is absorbed into the body.

One such operation, called *gastroplasty*, involves using surgical staples to close the stomach into two pouches. Ingested food goes into the first pouch, which is small, and then passes through a tube into the larger second pouch and on into the digestive system. When the small pouch is full of food, nerve signals are sent to the appestat and the person feels full and presumably stops eating.

TABLE 6.4	**Approximate Energy Expenditures During Various Activities**

Light exercise (4 calories per minute)

Cycling 5 mph	Slow dancing	Ping-pong
Walking 3 mph	Volleyball	Yoga
Canoeing	Softball	T'ai chi ch'uan
Housecleaning	Golf	

Moderate exercise (7 calories per minute)

Tennis	Basketball	Snowshoeing
Fast dancing	Swimming 30 m/min	Walking 4.5 mph
Cycling 9 mph	Heavy gardening	Roller skating

Heavy exercise (10 calories per minute)

Jogging	Mountain climbing	Skiing
Climbing stairs	Cycling 12 mph	Ice skating
Football	Handball and racquetball	

Dollars and Health Sense

The Marketing of Weight-Loss Drugs

With as much as one-half of the U.S. adult population classified as overweight and one-fourth as obese, it doesn't take much imagination to see that inventing a pill that would "melt away fat" would make a lot of money. So far, despite claims to the contrary, no such pill exists. This does not stop pharmaceutical companies from putting out drugs for weight loss and backing them up with extensive marketing campaigns.

Sibutramine, an appetite suppressant that increases brain levels of both norepinephrine and serotonin, is one such drug. In clinical trials with very overweight people, sibutramine alone contributed to a 5% reduction in body weight, or about 10 pounds, after six months of use. When used in conjunction with lifestyle changes, counseling, and a low-calorie liquid diet, however, weight loss increased to 15%. The amount of weight lost due to taking the drug was about one-half pound a month, which could have been achieved by walking an additional 15 minutes per day.

Appetite suppressants have a long and checkered history. In the 1960s, amphetamine (before it was made illegal) was often prescribed for weight loss. A disastrous side effect of treatment, however, was physical dependency and many negative physical and psychological effects of the drug (see Chapter 16). In the mid-1990s, people were prescribed the combination of phentermine and fenfluramine ("phen/fen"), a regimen that caused pulmonary hypertension (a fatal condition) and damaged heart valves. In 1997, "phen/fen" was banned by the FDA.

Orlistat (Xenical) is a drug that prevents the absorption of fat from the digestive tract. In 1998, the FDA approved its use for weight loss, even though pre-approval tests of this drug's effectiveness showed that after one year, very overweight users lost, on average, only seven pounds—the same result could be achieved by walking 20 minutes a day. Half of the experts on the FDA approval panel voted not to approve orlistat, but it was approved anyway. Orlistat has some awful side effects, such as bloating, flatulence, oily stool, diarrhea, and fecal incontinence. It also inhibits the absorption of esssential fat-soluble vitamins. Some proponents of the drug suggest that the uncomfortable side effects are part of the treatment, because they act as a deterrent to eating fatty foods.

Despite the fact that drugs like sibutramine and orlistat are minimally effective, they are marketed with considerable vigor by both the pharmaceutical companies that make them and a variety of businesses (most of them on the Internet) that make exaggerated promises about their effectiveness. However, because they are only marginally effective, these drugs may create false expectations for overweight people, leading to further discouragement. Drug companies reap considerable profit from weight-loss pills; users get little benefit and often suffer great disappointment, discomfort, and expense.

Another procedure, called *gastric bypass*, reduces the stomach volume by creating two unconnected pouches, and it shunts food from the upper pouch directly to the upper bowel, thus bypassing the lower part of the stomach and the duodenum. This operation works by preventing the ingestion of large meals and reducing the absorption of ingested sugars and fats. Patients lose significant amounts of body fat, although they do not become fashionably thin.

Liposuction

Liposuction is the surgical removal by suction of fat stored under the skin and is not recommended as a substitute for proper diet, exercise, and counseling for weight loss and weight management. It is for shaping the body. Indeed, after the surgery, without attention to diet and exercise, fat may appear on other parts of the body. In 1998, approximately 218,000 liposuction procedures were performed in the United States by plastic surgeons, dermatologists, and other physicians. Liposuction is currently the most common cosmetic surgical procedure performed (Matarasso and Hutchinson, 2001). Liposuction is surgically risky, and anyone considering it should investigate the procedure thoroughly. Although rare, deaths have occurred from liposuction (Rao, Ely and Hoffman, 1999).

Weight-Control Fads and Fallacies

"Lose weight effortlessly, even as you sleep!" "New diet discovery lets you lose excess pounds in just one week!" So claim advertisements for products and eating regimens that are directed to chronic dieters and others concerned about being overfat. Some products, like "diet rings" and weight-loss soaps, are clearly worthless, but some overweight people are so desperate they will try anything.

Unfortunately for consumers, nearly all of the claims made by heavily advertised weight-control regimens and products are exaggerated and misleading. By themselves, these programs are not likely to produce a significant reduction in body fat over any long-term period. The only way to reduce body fat and maintain healthy body weight is by lifestyle modifications that include changing eating behaviors and increasing the level of physical activity.

Three ineffective, weight-control products or schemes are: (a) body wraps, (b) chemicals, and (c) diet programs.

Body Wraps

Body wraps are plastic or rubber garments, ranging from waist belts to entire body suits, that are worn during exercise, routine daily activity, or sleep in order to produce weight loss. A wrap designed for just one part of the body (such as the waist or hips) is supposed to reduce the size of just that body region ("spot reducing").

Body wraps do result in weight loss and a reduction in body size. The catch is that the weight lost is body water and not body fat. These garments increase perspiration; they do not diminish the body's fat stores. The lost body water is quickly regained and so is the lost body weight. Because these products cause a loss of body water, they make dehydration a potential danger. Some athletes have died from exercising while using body wraps.

The appeal of body wraps stems from the common misconception that fat can be eliminated from the body by heat. The phrase "burning off fat" is part of the professional physiologist's jargon and contributes to this false notion. The process by which body fat is reduced does not involve heat. (Human body temperature is uniformly maintained at 37°C.) The "burning" that physiologists speak of is a chemical breakdown of fat molecules requiring oxygen, not the liquefaction and evaporation that one would expect from high temperatures. Hence, the claim that body wraps reduce body size by "melting away fat" is quite misleading.

Chemicals

A number of products that contain drugs and "natural" substances are sold as weight-loss remedies. Often these products are used in conjunction with dieting, modification in eating behavior, and exercise programs, so they appear effective to the naive consumer. However, no single product by itself has been shown to reduce weight safely and permanently.

Benzocaine, an anesthetic, is found in candies, lozenges, and chewing gums sold as aids to weight reduction. Benzocaine is supposed to help produce weight loss by numbing the sense of taste and thereby reducing the desire for food. There is no scientific evidence, however, that temporarily reducing the sense of taste leads to weight loss. Because benzocaine is intended as

Terms

liposuction: surgery used to remove fat under the skin in order to reshape parts of the body

appetite suppressants: drugs that diminish the sense of hunger

benzocaine: an anesthetic sometimes used in over-the-counter weight-control products to numb the sense of taste

Managing Stress

Treating the Underlying Emotional Causes of Obesity

Mrs. Johnson made an appointment with a psychologist to discuss being overweight. She is 40 years old, 5 feet 5 inches tall, and weighs 180 pounds. She works as a nurse at a community hospital and has no serious medical problems. She is married, her husband is unemployed, and she has three teenage children at home. Her take-home pay is modest, and the family never has enough money to pay bills. She eats mostly "junk food" from fast-food restaurants and does not exercise.

Since appropriate weight depends on *both* a healthy diet *and* exercise, the counselor must look for barriers to those two goals (Foreyt, 1997). The counselor must help the patient discover the causes of stress and negative emotions that underlie the weight problem. These generally include job or family stressors, depression, anger, loneliness, or boredom. Sometimes adult obesity has its roots in childhood sexual abuse (i.e., having a large body makes one sexually unattractive and is therefore protective).

Social aspects of being overweight also have to be explored. What are the barriers to obtaining healthy food? Does the job require a lot of travel time or sitting for extended periods? How can exercise be incorporated into the daily lifestyle?

In Mrs. Johnson's case, she has a high-stress, low-paying job, a bad marriage, and children at a difficult stage of development. Her lifestyle is out of control. With the counselor's help, Mrs. Johnson adopted a low-fat diet and began jogging in the morning before work. Later, she added weight training to her exercise program. After a few months she obtained a better-paying job with regular hours. She and her husband went to a marriage counselor and eventually decided to divorce. After about a year, Mrs. Johnson's weight stabilized at 130 pounds. She has maintained her low-fat diet and continues to exercise. She has found new friends and has begun going out on dates with men.

Many overweight people have problems similar to Mrs. Johnson's. Counseling, diet changes, exercise, and social support can help most overweight people who are willing to make the effort to change their lives.

a topical anesthetic, these products are useful (if at all) only if they are not swallowed.

Bulk-producing agents, such as methylcellulose, psyllium, and agar, are supposed to produce a sense of fullness in the gastrointestinal tract, thus suppressing appetite. These agents swell when mixed with water and are much more effective as laxatives than as weight reducers. Glucomannan, a bulk-producing starch derived from konjac tubers, is often touted by health food enthusiasts as a "natural" weight-loss method. There is no evidence that glucomannan or any other bulk producer aids weight loss.

Hormones, such as human chorionic gonadotropin (HCG) and thyroid hormone, and chemicals with thyroid hormone activity are occasionally offered by unscrupulous clinics and on the Internet as aids for weight loss. None of these is effective as a weight reducer. Moreover, because hormones are regulators of the body's homeostatic mechanisms, it is never wise to take them unless monitored closely by a well-trained clinician.

Vitamins, minerals, and some amino acids (including arginine, ornithine, tryptophan, and phenylalanine) are occasionally sold as weight-loss agents. For example, spirulina, a product made from blue-green algae, is claimed to be effective in reducing weight because it contains the amino acid phenylalanine, which supposedly regulates the body's appetite. Vitamins, minerals, and amino acids have not been shown to be effective in causing weight loss. And in very high doses, some of these substances, although "natural," can be harmful.

Diet Programs

If you want to make some money, get involved in publishing a book that describes a "revolutionary" new diet for weight loss. So many people make a hobby of trying fad diets that the book is virtually guaranteed to sell many copies. Be sure that the diet you invent requires no exercise, is based on some "new" dietary or nutritional discovery, carries an air of authoritativeness, and promises a rapid reduction in body weight, although not necessarily a reduction in body fat. It doesn't matter a bit if the lost weight is regained in a short time. In fact, it's probably better for the weight-loss industry if your diet does not produce permanent weight loss, since that would reduce the sales of the next crop of diet books.

Many of the weight-loss diets that have come and gone have been based on altering the usual proportions of the three basic types of foods—protein, fat, and carbohydrate. Hence, the high-fat, low-fat, high-carbohydrate, low-carbohydrate, high-protein, and low-protein diets have all had their day. Occasionally diet regimens require the ingestion of only certain kinds of foods, such as fruits (grapefruit or papaya), cottage

cheese, or steak. Fortunately, most of these unusual diets are too expensive, too boring, or too fatiguing to maintain for long, and people give them up before the nutritional deficiencies they can produce cause irreparable harm. In 2001, the U.S. Department of Agriculture summarized all of the research on the efficacy of popular weight-loss diets (USDA, 2001). The summary noted than any diet that reduces the number of calories a person consumes (e.g., 1400–1500 calories per day) results in weight loss. High-fat low-carbohydrate diets, low-fat, and very-low-fat diets were found not to be as nutritionally adequate as diets containing moderate amounts of fat, carbohydrate, and protein.

A variety of weight-loss programs not only tell clients how to lose weight, but also supply packaged foods and, sometimes, social support to bolster the weight-loser's efforts. Many of these programs are based on severely calorie-restricted regimens. Some plans use "real" food but control the portion size and others are based on liquid diets containing sufficient protein, vitamins, and minerals to prevent the loss of lean body tissue. As with other special efforts to lose weight, the dietary plans often fail because they are difficult or expensive to maintain, and also because they often do not include lifestyle changes that promote maintaining a healthy body weight.

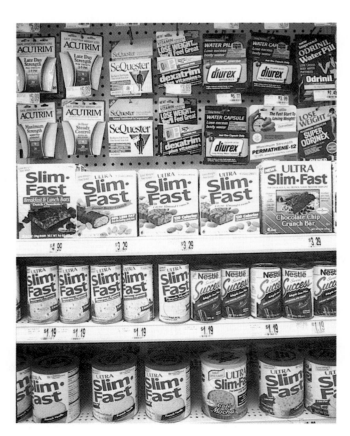

People take hundreds of different herbs, supplements and other pills to lose weight.

Body Image

Body image is a person's mental "picture" of her or his body. Nearly everyone has a body image. Nearly everyone judges that image as good, or less good, by comparing her or his body image to a standard of the "ideal body" communicated to individuals by their culture and people who are important to them, such as lovers, family, and friends. The judgment a person makes about her or his body image is called *body esteem.* Individuals with a positive body image tend to have higher body esteem than do individuals with a less positive body image.

Many women are excessively concerned about their body image and tend to have low body esteem because they believe themselves to be overweight. Books, films, TV, and popular magazines (especially women's magazines) consistently send messages that our society esteems thin women and disdains heavy ones. Whereas maintaining appropriate body size is associated with good health, attempting to achieve an unrealistic ideal of slimness is oppressive to many women. Failure to meet unrealistic standards leads many women to judge themselves as unattractive and lowers their self-esteem.

The current emphasis on slimness is partly fad—there have been times when thinness was associated with being sickly and a full body was a sign of health and sexual attractiveness—and partly desire to be healthy and fit. A lean body is associated with high status, sexual attractiveness, youthfulness, and a demonstration of the personal power to be trim and fit in a culture in which sedentary habits and overeating are common.

For the most part, standards of attractiveness and a healthful appearance are set by companies seeking to sell products and increase profits. Advertisements try to convince women that they fall short of an ideal and that, by purchasing a product, dieting, or exercising to change their body size and shape, they can improve themselves and their lives. These messages cause many women to judge themselves on how they look and cause many men to judge women largely by their physical appearance. Overconcern about body image and weight can have adverse health consequences, including:

- Depression from low body esteem and low self-worth
- Poor nutrition from extensive dieting
- Inadequate calcium and iron intake from under-nutrition
- Anorexia or bulimia
- Musculoskeletal injuries from overexercising
- Risks associated with cosmetic surgery
- Cigarette smoking to reduce body weight

Eating Disorders

For women, a slim body reflects the current trend toward gender equality: it represents a rejection of the traditional woman's role as homemaker and child-bearer and emphasizes a new femininity characterized by individualism, athleticism, and nonreproductive sexuality.

Whereas freedom from traditional sex-role behavior may be praiseworthy, using slimness as a measure of social achievement has become an oppressive standard for many, particularly for young people. In some instances, individuals develop such a morbid fear of becoming fat that they adopt unusual (and very unhealthy) eating behaviors.

Young athletes, who are often obsessed with high achievement in sports, may also be susceptible to an inordinate fear of fatness. Most serious athletes are encouraged to be as lean as possible, and some overreact to the expectations of parents and coaches by restricting their food intake to excessively low amounts. This behavior, called **anorexia athletica,** affects both males and females. According to Nathan J. Smith, an expert in sports medicine, "losing fat becomes a challenge in which the athlete promises himself uncompromised success. Hunger pains become gratifying signals of accomplishment, and food becomes the opponent in a contest that he is dedicated to win by an overwhelming score" (Smith, 1980). Counseling and reassurance that athletic goals can be met without such drastic eating behavior usually alleviate the condition.

He who doesn't mind his belly will hardly mind anything else.
SAMUEL JOHNSON

Although abnormal eating behavior can be caused solely by the fear of becoming fat, there are instances when a compulsive desire to be slim is a manifestation of more complex psychological stress. Increasing demands on school health services for help with abnormal eating behavior indicate that many young people, especially young women, have problems associated with eating. Three of the most common eating

Terms

bulk-producing agents: agents used to promote a sense of fullness in the gastrointestinal tract, thus suppressing appetite

hormones: complex chemicals, produced and secreted by endocrine glands, that travel through the bloodstream

body image: a person's mental image of his or her body

anorexia athletica: athletes who restrict their food intake to stay slim or lean

disorders are anorexia nervosa, a voluntary refusal to eat, bulimia, binge eating and immediate purging of the ingested food either by vomiting or by using laxatives, and binge eating disorder, episodes of binge eating without subsequent purging.

Anorexia Nervosa

Anorexia nervosa is characterized by a relentless pursuit of thinness resulting in progressive weight loss and metabolic disturbances. Most of those affected are young women. Anorexia is not caused by any known disease-causing agent but by self-induced starvation, which can lead to serious illness and even death.

Elizabeth Barrett Browning (1806–1861), one of England's most famed poets, is thought to have had anorexia nervosa. As a teenager, Elizabeth was nagged by her parents to eat and gain weight, yet she stubbornly refused to eat much more than toast. When she met her future husband, poet Robert Browning, she weighed only 87 pounds. Apparently the Barrett family possessed characteristics found in other families with an anorectic member: overprotectiveness, overinvolvement with each other, and inability to express or resolve intrafamilial conflict.

Stubbornness and irony are characteristics of anorexia nervosa. For example, persons with anorexia nervosa are likely to defend their emaciated appearance as normal and will insist that weight gain makes them feel fat. Besides distortions in normal body image, anorectic people tend to have a fanatical preoccupation with food. They may spend an inordinate amount of time planning and preparing elaborate meals for others, while they themselves eat only a few bites and claim to be full. Often they will not eat in the presence of others; when they do, they may dawdle over their food. Some anorectic persons resort to self-induced vomiting or frequent use of diuretics or laxatives to reduce their body weight. These practices may lead to severe depletion of body minerals, which can precipitate abnormal heart rhythms and even cardiac arrest. Despite the low intake of calories, anorectic persons are remarkably energetic and tend to be hyperactive.

Another characteristic of anorexia nervosa is a paralyzing sense of powerlessness. Persons with anorexia see themself as responding to demands of others rather than taking initiative in life. Children with anorexia tend to be obedient, dutiful, helpful, and excellent students. Some psychologists interpret the intense preoccupation with weight loss as an expression of an underlying fear of incompetence. Control of eating and body weight becomes a way of demonstrating general control and competence.

One theory seeks to explain anorexia as a preoccupation with extreme slimness (and associated absence of menstruation) in an attempt to remain a child who is cared for and fed by others, who can be stubborn and obstinate, and who has no sexual identity or desires. Another theory suggests that anorexia is the manifestation of a struggle for a sense of identity and personal effectiveness through controlling the environment; the resulting stubborn, rejecting behavior then becomes reinforced by the attention received from others. Yet another theory sees anorexia as a manifestation of impaired family interaction. The family of the anorectic person becomes so engrossed with the symptoms that they avoid dealing with conflicts among themselves.

Three goals characterize the treatment of anorexia nervosa: (a) weight gain, (b) changed attitudes toward food and eating, and (c) resolution of underlying personal and family conflicts. Unfortunately, therapeutic intervention is not always successful and the condition may persist for years. Anorexia nervosa has a 15% to 20% mortality rate.

Bulimia

Bulimia is marked by a voluntary restriction of food intake followed by a binge-purge cycle: extreme overeating, usually of high-calorie junk foods, immediately followed by self-induced vomiting, use of diuretics or laxatives, or intense exercise. Like anorexia nervosa, bulimia occurs primarily in young women with a morbid fear of becoming fat, who pursue thinness relentlessly. Most bulimic persons are model individuals: good students, athletes, extremely sociable, and pleasant. Fearing discovery of their bulimic behavior, they frequently carry out their binge-purge episodes in private. Bulimic persons usually are aware that their binge-purge behavior is abnormal; however, they are unable to control it. Many feel guilty and depressed about their problem, which leads to a tendency to hide the behavior. Bulimia can pose a serious risk to health for many of the same reasons that anorexia does.

Several theories have been proposed to explain bulimia. One is that bulimia is a maladaptive way of dealing with anxiety, loneliness, and anger. Another suggests that bulimia is a manifestation of the drive to become the "ideal" woman, achieving the societal

Terms

anorexia nervosa: emotional disorder occurring most commonly in adolescent females, characterized by abnormal body image, fear of obesity, and prolonged refusal to eat, sometimes resulting in death

bulimia: serious disorder, especially common in adolescents and young women, marked by excessive eating, often followed by self-induced vomiting, purging, or fasting

binge eating disorder: an uncontrolled consumption of large quantities of food in a short period of time, even if the person does not feel hungry

Global Wellness

Eating Disorders Are a Worldwide Concern

Eating disorders among women are becoming a worldwide problem. They used to be common only in North American and Europe, but now have spread to other regions of the world, including Saudi Arabia, China, Russia, Latin America, and Asia.

The growing prevalence of eating disorders is caused, experts say, by young women trying to emulate advertising models and actors that they see on TV, in films and magazines, and on the Internet. These media present images of "ideal" women as unrealistically thin, which causes some women to lose social and psychological confidence in themselves; they attempt to regain it by disordered eating behaviors. For example, after the introduction of TV to the island of Fiji in 1995, the number of teenage girls with eating disorders rose from 3% to 15%. Fiji has only one TV station, which broadcasts shows from the United States, Australia, and the United Kingdom. Whereas the increase might be attributable to something other than TV, researchers believe that the dramatic jump in the prevalence of eating disorders after the introduction of TV is the most plausible explanation.

In Argentina, aggressive advertising by the diet and cosmetic industries is generally recognized as contributing to an epidemic of eating disorders. Major newspapers distribute discount coupons for diet and liposuction clinics. And Argentine clothing manufacturers—out of step with international standards—size women's clothes much too small (e.g., a "medium" T-shirt that is more suitable for a pre-adolescent rather than an adult), reinforcing the idea that a woman must be extremely thin to be normal. The Argentine government and health establishment have begun a large media campaign of their own to educate young women on the dangers of believing what they see on TV, in the movies, and in magazines with respect to eating, body size, and cosmetic surgery.

---

norm of slimness. Bulimic persons tend to have low self-esteem and a weak sense of identity.

Recovering from bulimia includes stopping binge-purge cycles and regaining control over eating behavior. Persons with bulimia must also establish more appropriate ways to handle unpleasant feelings and discomfort with close relationships, and their self-esteem must be improved. Often psychological counseling is helpful.

Binge Eating Disorder

Binge eating disorder is characterized by an uncontrolled consumption of large quantities of food in a short period of time, even if the person does not feel hungry. During binge episodes, food is consumed much faster than usual, and frequently the person is alone to avoid embarrassment about the amount of food eaten. A binge episode is often followed by feelings of disgust, depression, and guilt.

About 2% of adults in the United States (about 4 million people) have binge eating disorder, and most of them are overweight. About 10% to 15% of people who are mildly obese and who try to lose weight on their own or through commercial weight-loss programs have binge eating disorder. The disorder is even more common in people who are very overweight.

Many people with binge eating disorder have a history of depression and impulsive behavior (acting quickly without thinking). Many people who are binge eaters say that being angry, sad, bored, or worried can cause them to binge eat. People with binge eating disorder tend to be malnourished because they consume large amounts of fat and sugar, which have few essential nutrients.

Most people with binge eating disorder have tried to control it on their own, but are unable to control it for very long. People with binge eating disorder should get help from a health professional, which could include instruction in how to keep track of and change unhealthy eating behaviors, identifying social factors that contribute to the problem, psychological counseling, and medications.

It's in Your Hands

Successful weight control involves reducing intake of calories (often by recognizing the social and psychological reasons that cause overeating) and increasing the level of physical activity. Heavily advertised reducing schemes, such as body wraps, diet pills, and fad diets, are almost totally ineffective in producing permanent fat reduction and weight loss.

The primary reason that people are overfat is that their lifestyles do not include sufficient physical activity to use up the calories ingested in food. You can begin today to consciously watch what you eat and how much you exercise. You need not start out with an all-out diet or exercise regime; start slowly. When offered a cookie, decline. When you have the choice between the elevator and stairs, take the stairs. These efforts, which appear to be small, can make a difference when made daily and over an extended period of time.

Wellness Guide

Elite Athletes Are at Risk for Eating Disorders

In 1988, at age 16, Christie Henrich missed making the U.S. Olympic team in women's gymnastics by less than two-tenths of a point. At her performance peak, Christie weighed 93 pounds. During one of the international competitions in 1988, a judge told her that she needed to watch her weight if she wanted to be a champion. According to her coach, Christie perceived herself as being too fat to be an Olympic competitor, so she began to starve herself (anorexia) and to vomit when she did eat (bulimia). By 1990, she was too weak to compete, even though she was ranked among the top 10 women gymnasts in the U.S. In 1994, Christie Henrich died; she weighed less than 60 pounds.

If someone you know seems to have an eating problem, here are some ways to help.

- Express your concern about any apparent weight loss. Even if the person denies that anything is wrong, your concern may alert him or her that something is wrong.

- Encourage the person to talk about his or her feelings concerning problems or worries, even if they are not food-related. Listen without making judgments.

- Suggest that the person see a health counselor, physician, or mental health professional.

- Express your own concerns to a professional counselor who may be able to intervene and help.

While eating disorders are estimated to occur in 1% to 3% of the general population, they occur in 15% to 62% of female athletes (Tofler, et. al., 1996). Many ambitious female athletes suffer from what is called the "female-athlete triad," which is characterized by eating disorders, menstrual dysfunction, and osteoporosis. Coaches, parents, and athletes themselves need to pay much more attention to their health and to make sure that athletic goals do not lead to severe illness and even death.

Anorexia and bulimia are very serious disorders and require professional help.

Critical Thinking About Health

1. Jordana couldn't stand herself anymore, so she went to the campus health center's peer nutrition counseling program for help.

   "I disgust myself," she told her counselor. "I'm fat, fat, fat and no matter what I do I can't change it. I jog, I don't eat ice cream. I suck."

   While not ready for a starring role on "Baywatch," Jordana wasn't fat, according to her counselor. Her BMI calculated out to 28.4. "It's a little on the high side," said the counselor, "but you're not in the danger zone."

   "Tell that to my Dad," Jordana snapped. "And my boyfriend. When they look at me, their eyes go right to my stomach. It's like that's all I am—a stomach on legs!"

   a. What expectations regarding body size and shape do you experience as a member of your sex?

   b. How were these expectations transmitted to you and by whom (or by what social institution)?

   c. How are these expectations enforced in your peer group, and what are the social penalties for not meeting such expectations?

   d. To what lengths do people go to meet these expectations? Are any of these practices extreme or unhealthy?

2. Sam: Oh, man, not Roni. She's too wide!
   Mick: No, she's not. She's real nice. Call her.
   Sam: Nah.
   Mick: You're a dweeb, sucker. You didn't like Nan because her face was too round. You didn't like Carla because she was too tall. You didn't like Evy because . . . why didn't you like Evy, anyway? I forget.
   Sam: Thunder thighs.
   Mick: You're going to wind up one lonely dude, dude.

   a. Is Sam really destined to be lonely or is he being smart to wait for someone who matches his ideal of the perfect body?

   b. In your peer group, are there examples of people being attracted to people who *do not* resemble the ideal? Can you explain that discrepancy?

   c. What is the social purpose of an ideal body size and shape?

3. It is likely that in the near future there will be many drugs that are moderately effective in producing weight (fat) loss. It is also likely that these drugs will carry some risks to health.

   a. Do you think that such drugs should be made available to anyone who wants them, or should such medications be restricted to people whose weight puts them at serious risk for health problems and premature death?

b. Besides potential harm from side effects, is it appropriate for people to depend on drugs for weight maintenance instead of modifying dietary and exercise habits and learning to reduce stress?

4. How have eating disorders touched your life?

Health in Review

- Approximately one-third of the U.S. population is overfat and at risk for a variety of illnesses, including heart disease, diabetes, hypertension, and gallbladder disease.
- Obesity is defined as having a body weight 20% (for men) and 30% (for women) over recommended weight for height or a body mass index greater than 30.
- Health problems are less likely when the waist-to-hip ratio is less than 0.8 (women) or 0.95 (men).
- Body fatness is maintained around a set point, which is maintained by neural and hormonal signals acting on the "appestat" in the brain, which controls feelings of hunger and satiety. Many physiological, psychological, social, and environmental factors affect the appestat and thus body weight.
- Healthy body weight corresponds to having a body mass index between 19 and 25. There are a variety of ways to achieve a healthy body weight. Starvation dieting is *not* one of them.
- Counseling, surgery, and medications can help some overweight people lose body fat and maintain a healthy body weight.
- People eat for reasons other than hunger, such as social interaction, recreation, and relief from stress.
- Successful weight control involves changing eating and exercise habits.
- There are three major ineffective weight control schemes: body wraps, diet pills, and diet programs.
- Three common eating disorders are anorexia nervosa, bulimia, and binge eating disorder.

Health and Wellness Online

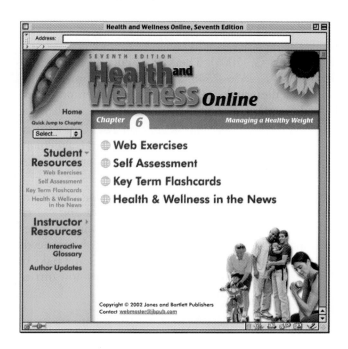

The World Wide Web contains a wealth of information about health and wellness. By accessing the Internet using Web browser software, such as Netscape Navigator or Microsoft's Internet Explorer, you can gain a new perspective on many topics presented in *Health and Wellness, Seventh Edition.* Access the Jones and Bartlett Publishers Web site at http://www.jbpub.com/hwonline.

References

Foreyt, J. P. (1997, August 15). An etiological approach to obesity. *Hospital Practice*, 123–148.

Kirsch, I. (1996). Hypnotic enhancement of cognitive-behavioral weight loss treatments. *Journal of Consulting and Clinical Psychology, 64(3)*, 517–519.

Klem, M. L., Wing, R. R., McGuire, M. T., Seagle, H. M., and Hill, J. O. (1997). A descriptive study of individuals successful at long-term maintenance of substantial weight loss. *American Journal of Clinical Nutrition, 66*, 239–246.

Leibel, R. L., Rosenbaum, M., and Hirsch J. (1995). Changes in energy expenditure resulting from altered body weight. *New England Journal of Medicine, 332*, 621–8.

Matarasso, A. and Hutchinson, O. H. Z. (2001). Liposuction. *Journal of the American Medical Association, 285*, 266–268.

Poston, W. S. and Foreyt, J. P. (2000). Successful management of the obese patient. *American Family Physician, 61*, 3615–3622.

Rao, R. B., Ely, S. F., and Hoffman, R. S. (1999). Deaths related to liposuction. *New England Journal of Medicine, 340*, 1471–1475.

Schwartz, M. E., and Seeley, R. J. (1997). Neuroendocrine responses to starvation and weight loss. *New England Journal of Medicine, 336*, 1802–1811.

Seidell, J. C., Verschuren, W. M. M., van Leer, E. M., and Kromhout, D. (1996). Overweight, underweight and mortality. *Archives of Internal Medicine, 156*, 958–963.

Smith, N. J. (1980). Excessive weight loss and food aversion in athletes simulating anorexia nervosa. *Pediatrics, 66*, 139–142.

Tofler, I. R., et al. (1996). Physical and emotional problems of elite female athletes. *New England Journal of Medicine, 335*, 281–83.

Wickelgren, I. (1998). Obesity: How big a problem? *Science, 280*, 1364–1367.

Willett, W. C., Dietz, W. H., and Colditz, G. A. (1999). Guidelines for healthy weight. *New England Journal of Medicine, 341*, 427–434.

Suggested Readings

Becker, A. E. et al. (1999). Eating disorders. *New England Journal of Medicine, 340*, 1092–1098. An up-to-date review of the topic.

Brownell, K. D. (2000). *The LEARN Program for Weight Management* (10th Ed.) New York: American Health Publishing. This is the most widely used weight control manual in the world.

Kassirer, J. P., and Angell, M. (1998). Losing weight—An ill-fated New Year's resolution. *New England Journal of Medicine, 338*, 52–54. Puts the issue of weight loss for health reasons in perspective and cautions against overconcern about body size.

Must, A. et al. (2000). The disease burden associated with overweight and obesity. *Journal of the American Medical Association, 282*, 1523–1529. Examines the prevalence of obesity-related diseases in the United States.

Regulation of body weight. (1998, May 29). *Science*, 1363–1390. This issue contains a series of up-to-date articles on the causes of obesity, treatment options, and research strategies for finding ways to prevent or treat obesity.

Rosenbaum, M., Leibel, R. L., and Hirsch J. (1997). Obesity. *New England Journal of Medicine, 337*, 396–406. This is a thorough discussion of research on the causes and treatment of obesity.

Taubes, G. (2001). The soft science of dietary fat. *Science, 291*, 2536–2545. An analysis of how fat has become a dietary demon but has never been proved to be bad for otherwise healthy people.

Vogel, S. (1999). *The Skinny on Fat: Our Obsession with Weight Control*. New York: W. H. Freeman. An examination of biological, medical, and cultural aspects of weight control.

Weil, Andrew (2000). *Eating Well for Optimum Health: The Essential Guide to Food, Diet and Nutrition*. NY: Knopf. The well-known physician describes his nutritional formula for supplying the basic needs of the body for calories and nutrients, reducing risks of disease, and fortifying the body's defenses and intrinsic mechanisms of healing.

Learning Objectives

1. Define physical activity.
2. Describe the health benefits of physical activity.
3. Describe the psychological benefits of physical activity.
4. Define aerobic training and strength training.
5. Make a plan for incorporating physical activity into your life.
6. Describe common overuse syndromes.

Study Guide
and
Self Assessment

Determine Your Fitness Index
Determine Your Flexibility Index

Health
and Wellness
Online

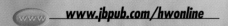 *www.jbpub.com/hwonline*

Chapter 7

Physical Activity for Health and Well-Being

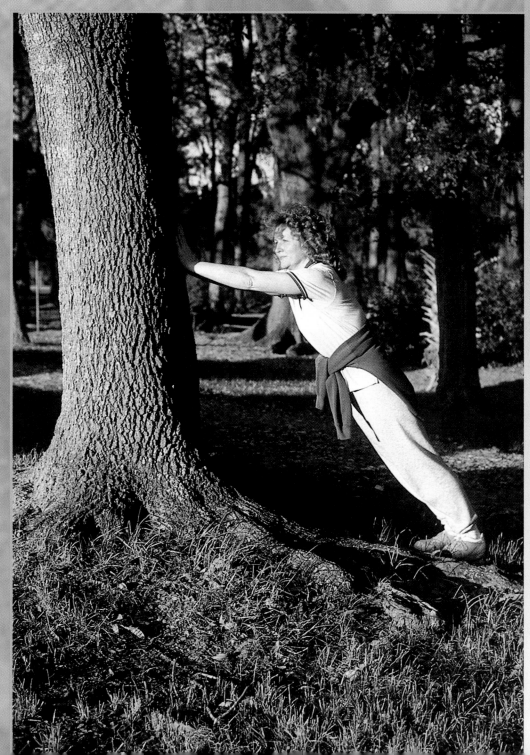

Industrial society depends on an enormous variety of machines that free people from an equally enormous number of physical tasks. Some of these tasks, such as heavy construction work or large-scale farming, would be almost impossible without the help of machines. Others, such as traveling to work or school, getting to the seventh floor of a building, or washing clothes, could be accomplished without the aid of machines (and some people argue they ought to be), but few of us are likely to give up the use of cars, elevators, and washers. They simply make the tasks of daily living easier. But as a result, many of us get little exercise in the work we do. Furthermore, much of our leisure time is spent in sedentary activities, such as watching TV. Only 25% of the U.S. population engages in regular, leisure-time physical activities (Surgeon General's Report, 1999).

> *Beware all enterprises that require new clothes.*
> HENRY DAVID THOREAU
> *WALDEN*

Many studies indicate that regular physical activity, whether it is work-related or recreational, contributes to health and well-being and lowers the risk of many diseases, including heart disease, high blood pressure, stroke, diabetes, osteoporosis, obesity, and colon cancer. Also, regular physical activity increases your ability to overcome fatigue, cope effectively with stress, and fight off colds and other infections by boosting the immune system. Furthermore, regular physical activity puts into life the good feelings and enjoyment that come from movement.

What Is Physical Activity?

The health club and exercise equipment industries and the advertising and TV infomercials that support them can easily lead people to think that exercising for health requires considerable time, energy, equipment, special clothing, and money. These investments can seem so overwhelming that some people forego exercising altogether.

Fortunately, physical activity does not require special equipment or spending a lot of money. Physical activity is anything you do when you are not sitting or lying down. Besides jogging, swimming, cycling, and aerobic dancing, physical activity includes yoga, tai chi ch'uan, martial arts training, gardening, and walking. For instance, regular walking strengthens muscles, increases aerobic capacity, clears and quiets the mind, reduces stress, expends calories, and causes few injuries, if any. Other than appropriate shoes, walking requires no special clothing, equipment, or money, and it can be worked into a busy schedule.

An ongoing study has shown that walking two miles a day reduced the risk of heart disease and can-

cer by half (Hakim et. al., 1998). So, instead of eating at breaks at work or between classes, take a walk to release mental and physical tensions. When you drive somewhere, park far enough away that you walk the last 10 minutes to your destination. Walk up stairs instead of using the elevator.

When you have physical activity in your life, other healthy behaviors often follow, such as improved eating habits and a reduction in alcohol consumption. Also, physical activity may lessen stress so that undesirable stress-reducing behaviors, such as cigarette smoking, overeating, or drug consumption, stop.

If none of these points convinces you of the many benefits of exercise, think of it as setting aside time and attention for *you*. Many people feel overwhelmed by the demands of school, job, and family. Just taking a few minutes several days a week to exercise can give you the chance to relax, reflect, and indulge your imagination.

Physiological Benefits of Physical Activity

Research shows that moderate, and not necessarily extensive, exercise is sufficient for good health (Figure 7.1). A daily brisk walk of 30 to 60 minutes will do. Running several miles or working out for an hour or two in the gym every day is unnecessary. In fact, high levels of exercise often increase the risk of injury.

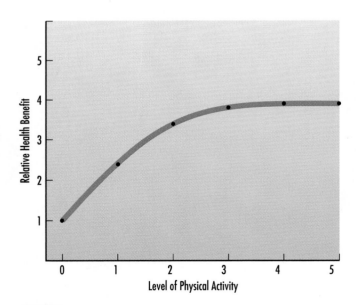

FIGURE 7.1   Health Benefit of Physical Activity   The graph is a composite from many studies that demonstrate the positive effect of physical activity on health. Notice that the graph is not linear; the largest benefit comes from changing from a sedentary lifestyle to one with low-to-moderate levels of physical activity. High levels of physical activity do not produce corresponding gains in health. Health benefits include lessened risk of morbidity and mortality from cardiovascular disease, cancer, hypertension, and type 2 diabetes. Each level of physical activity (e.g., walking, running, cycling) corresponds to between 500 and 1000 calories per week of activity.
Source: Adapted from Blair et al., 1992.

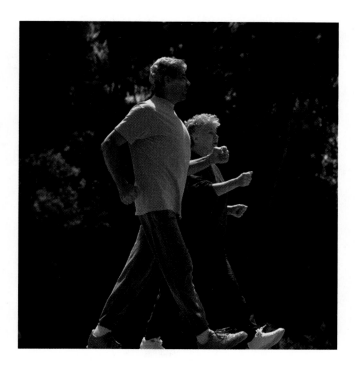

Walking is an excellent form of exercise at any age.

The Health Benefits of Physical Activity

In the 1950s, researchers found that 30% fewer conductors on London's double-decker buses had heart disease as compared to their co-workers who drove the buses. The proposed reason for this difference was that the conductors were much more active than the drivers because they continually moved between the decks of the buses taking passengers' tickets. Studies in the early 1980s showed that American men who exercised regularly (expending more than 2,000 calories a week by walking, climbing stairs, or sports activity) had a much lower risk than nonexercisers of developing cardiovascular disease or experiencing a heart attack.

Those pioneering studies and hundreds of subsequent ones have uncovered many health benefits of physical activity. Among them are: Increased strength of the heart muscle; increased flow of blood to the heart; increased bone mass and resistance to osteoporosis; decreased amount of fat in the blood; decreased heart rate; increased longevity; maintenance of normal blood pressure and reduction in blood pressure in people with hypertension; maintenance of body weight within generally accepted normal limits; prevention and alleviation of chronic low-back pain; improved sleep; greater energy reserve for work and recreation; improved posture, which leads to improved physical appearance and the ability to withstand fatigue; greater ability of the body to cope with illness or accidents.

If you exercise regularly, your overall risk of a heart attack is about 50% less than if you are inactive.

With routine exercise you can reach a level of physical fitness comparable to an inactive person 10 to 20 years younger. Exercise increases the size of your coronary arteries and reduces clogging due to atherosclerosis (see chapter 14). Exercise also increases the efficiency of your blood's oxygen-carrying capacity and your muscles' uptake of oxygen.

Exercise has been linked to increased levels of high-density lipoprotein (good) cholesterol and decreases low-density lipoprotein (bad) cholesterol and triglyceride levels (see Chapter 14). After exercising regularly for 6 to 12 months, lowered cholesterol levels can mean as much as a 30% reduction in the risk of coronary artery disease. The Centers for Disease Control and Prevention and the American College of Sports Medicine recommend 30 minutes of physical activity at least 5 days a week. They define physical activity as anything from running to raking leaves to playing with the kids. Also you don't have to do all your activity at once. You can break up those 30 minutes into smaller segments; say, three 10-minute walks. Or, you can mix a little walking with taking the stairs instead of the elevator, doing a little gardening, or washing the car (Table 7.1).

TABLE 7.1   Calories Used by Everyday Activities
Use an average of 200 calories a day by doing these activities and decrease your risk of disease and live longer, without ever going near a gym or treadmill.

Activities	Calories used in 10 minutes*	
	Women	Men
Walking fast	45	60
Painting	45	60
Weeding	45	60
Washing a car	45	60
Playing tag with a child	50	67
Mowing the lawn	55	73
Square dancing	55	73
Scrubbing floors	55	73
Hiking off-trail	60	80
Biking to work	60	80
Shoveling snow	60	80
Moving furniture	60	80
Walking upstairs	70	93
Cross-country skiing	80	106
Backpacking	80	106
Running upstairs	150	200

*Figures are for a 132-pound woman and a 176-pound man. All values are approximate and will vary from person to person.

Psychological Benefits of Physical Activity

Regular physical activity can result in periods of relaxed concentration, characterized by reduced physical and psychic tensions, regular breathing rhythms, and increased self-awareness. This effect is often compared to meditation and is the aim of all Eastern body work, including hatha yoga (Figure 7.2), t'ai chi ch'uan, and many martial arts practices. This effect also results from any physical activity in which one focuses the mind to produce a loss of self-consciousness through

FIGURE 7.2 **The Sun Salute** This hatha yoga exercise is a series of twelve postures or asanas, intended to be done in one flowing routine. Each of the twelve postures is held three seconds.

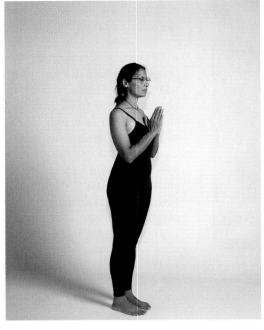

Position 1 Stand erect with your feet hip-width apart and palms together in front of your chest. Inhale and exhale slowly and calmly.

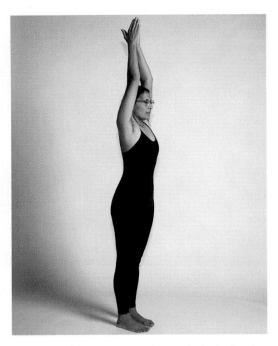

Position 2 Inhaling, raise your arms above your head, palms facing in. Lengthen through the spine, but do not arch your back.

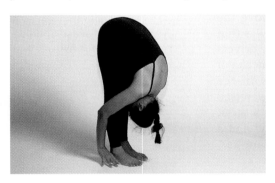

Position 3 Exhaling, bend forward from the hips, keeping your arms extended and your head hanging loosely between them. Keep your legs slightly bent and relax your neck and shoulders.

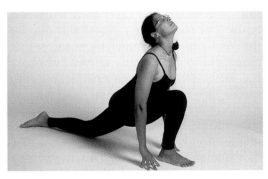

Position 4 Inhaling, bend both knees and place your palms flat on the floor by the outsides of your feet. Extend your left leg back. Stretch your chin toward the ceiling.

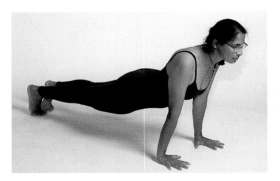

Position 5 Continue while holding the breath if you can—don't strain. Reach your forward leg back next to the other leg. Hold your body straight, supported by your hands and toes, with ankles, hips, and shoulders in a straight plane.

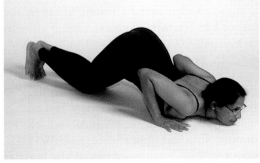

Position 6 Exhaling, lower your knees, chest, and chin or forehead to the floor, keeping your hips up and toes curled under.

total concentration on various body movements. T'ai chi ch'uan instructor Sophia Delza (1996) explains:

The goal of t'ai chi ch'uan is the achievement of health and tranquillity by means of a "way of movement," characterized by a technique of moving slowly and continuously, without strain, through a varied sequence of contrasting forms that create stable vitality with calmness, balances strength with flexibility, controlled energy with awareness. The

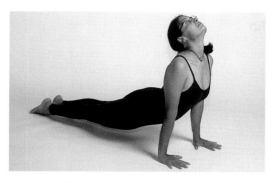

Position 7 Inhaling, bring the tops of your feet to the floor, straighten your legs, and come up to straight arms, opening the chest and stretching your chin toward the ceiling. Be careful not to overarch your lower back.

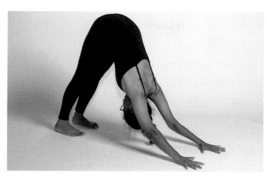

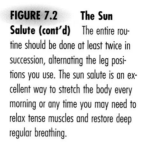

FIGURE 7.2 **The Sun Salute (cont'd)** The entire routine should be done at least twice in succession, alternating the leg positions you use. The sun salute is an excellent way to stretch the body every morning or any time you may need to relax tense muscles and restore deep regular breathing.

Position 8 Exhaling, curl your toes under and raise your hips into an inverted "V." Push back with your hands and lengthen your spine by reaching your hips upward. Keep your head hanging loosely.

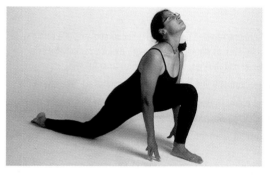

Position 9 Inhaling, lift your head and bring your left leg between your hands, keeping the right leg back. Raise your chin toward the ceiling.

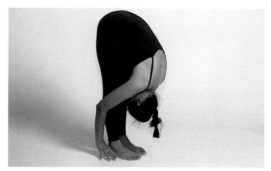

Position 10 Exhaling, bring your left foot forward so your feet are together. Bend forward from the hips, keeping your legs slightly bent and your upper body relaxed. If you can, touch your head to your knees and place your palms beside your feet.

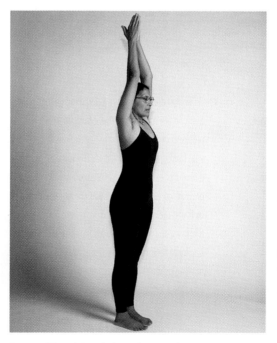

Position 11 Inhaling, slowly straighten up with your arms extended above your head. If you have any lower back pain, be sure to bend your knees.

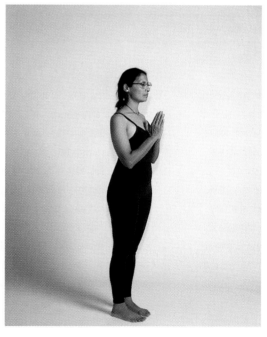

Position 12 Exhaling, bring your hands together in front of you. Close your eyes for a moment and feel the sensations in your body.

calmness that comes from harmonious physical activity and mental perception, and the composure that comes from deep feeling and comprehension are at the very heart of this exercise.

Several hypotheses have been offered to explain the psychological benefits of exercise:

1. Exercise becomes a means for autohypnosis, which increases the tendency for creative visualization.
2. Exercise increases the body's output of **epinephrine,** which produces feelings of euphoria.
3. Exercise changes the pattern of the secretion of brain neurotransmitters, particularly **norepinephrine,** which produces changes in mood.
4. Exercise increases the secretion of **endorphins** and **enkephalins,** hormone-like substances that can facilitate feelings of inner peace.

 ## Fitness and Conditioning

A major outcome of regular physical activity is fitness. However, **fitness** is an elusive concept, not easily defined. For some, fitness means a lean, svelte, muscular body. For others, fitness means being in "top shape"—the capacity for strenuous exercise, such as hiking, swimming, running, or skiing long distances. But a lean, muscular body or exceptional physical endurance probably represents the extreme of the concept of fitness. Sports physiologists usually define fitness as (a) adequate muscular strength and endurance to accomplish one's individual goals, (b) reasonable

joint flexibility, (c) an efficient cardiovascular system, and (d) body weight and percent body fat within the normal range.

Because modern lifestyles do not require much physical movement, few adults in industrial societies are naturally fit. Rather, achieving fitness requires a commitment of time and energy to regular activities other than school, work (particularly sedentary work), and family responsibilities. To be fit, you must engage in activities that challenge the mind and body beyond what is required by a sedentary lifestyle.

There are a wide variety of conditioning programs or training regimens to improve fitness, but they tend to fall into two major categories: **aerobic training,** which increases the body's ability to use oxygen and

Terms

epinephrine: hormone secreted principally by the adrenal medulla with a wide variety of functions, such as stimulating the heart, making carbohydrates available in the liver and muscles, and releasing fat from fat cells

norepinephrine: hormone that has many of the same effects as epinephrine

endorphins and **enkephalins:** morphine-like substances that are secreted by the brain that mitigate pain; produced during strenuous exercise and childbirth

fitness: the extent to which the body can respond to the demands of physical effort

aerobic training: exercise that increases the body's capacity to use oxygen

strength training: the use of resistance to increase one's ability to exert or resist force for the purpose of improving performance

training effect: beneficial physiological changes as a result of exercise

Managing Stress

Walking in Balance

Native Americans have an expression that helps when trying to understand our place in the physical world. The expression "walking in balance" means becoming aware of engaging your body with your mind in the natural world, feeling a sense of connectedness rather than separation from nature. Many people speak of a runner's high when they exercise, referring to the mind-body integration in which there is also a sense of oneness. Walking in balance suggests that we combine the powers of the mind and body to become more aware of ourselves in our environment.

During your next workout try one of these exercises.

1. While you dress and warm up, think of a problem you are dealing with (e.g., term paper topic, roommate difficulties, finding a job). Identify the problem and name it. Once you begin exercising, think of the problem and at least three ways to solve it. The best type of activity for this thinking is rhythmical, like running, walking, or swimming. Before you shower and change, write down your solutions and put the paper aside for a few hours. Then refer back to it and see how clearing your mind by exercising can really help to solve everyday life issues.

2. While you dress and warm up, remind yourself that you are taking time away from your problems and worries—a mini-vacation, if you will, from daily responsibilities. The mission during this exercise period (preferably walking or running) is to see where you are exercising as if you are seeing it for the first time. Notice the trees, the birds, the clouds in the sky, and so on. Try to feel that you are a part of nature by noticing as much about the natural world as you can.

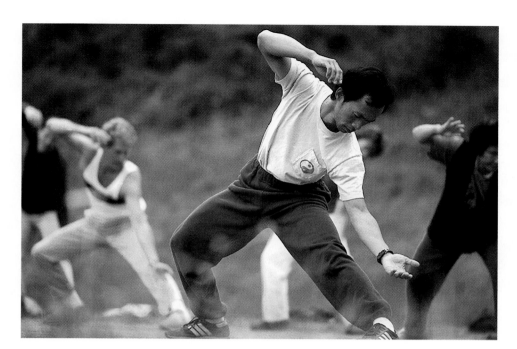

T'ai chi exercises help maintain physical fitness and mind-body harmony.

improves endurance, and **strength training,** which enhances the size and strength of particular muscles and body regions.

Aerobic Training

Aerobic exercise involves stimulating heart and lungs for a period sufficient to increase the amount of oxygen that the body can process within a given time. Changes in physiology resulting from aerobic exercise are collectively called the **training effect.** Inducing the training effect involves exercising so that heart rate increases to between 60% and 80% of its theoretical maximum.

Three to four days of exercise per week is sufficient to produce a training effect. Two days per week may suffice for people already in good condition. One day a week does little to improve fitness and may increase the chances for injury. Also, exercise more than 5 days a week does little to increase fitness. It does expend calories, but it also makes one susceptible to injuries.

To obtain optimal training benefits you should exercise within your training heart-rate zone. The simplest method of computing this is to subtract your age from 220 to determine your maximum heart rate (MHR) and then multiply by 60% and 80%. While you exercise, your heart rate per minute should fall between these two values. For a 21-year-old, the target heart rate range would be 120 to 160 beats per minute (Table 7.2).

To measure your exercise heart rate, you should stop about 5 minutes into the aerobic part of your exercise to check your heart rate. Your heart rate should

TABLE 7.2   Maximum and Target Heart Rates Predicted from Age
Take your pulse for 15 seconds immediately after exercising, and multiply by four. If heart rate is in the target range for your age, optimal training benefits have been obtained. If below target range, step up activity. If above the maximum, take it easier during workouts and gradually increase intensity.

Age (in years)	Predicted maximum heart rate (in beats per minute)	Target heart rate range (in beats per minute)
20	200	120–160
25	200	117–156
30	194	114–152
35	188	111–148
40	182	108–144
45	176	105–140
50	171	102–136
55	165	99–132
60	159	96–128
65	153	93–124

gradually increase during your warm-up, reach maximum level during your aerobic exercise, and gradually decrease during your cool-down exercises (Figure 7.3). Many activities can provide aerobic conditioning, including walking, running, bicycling, swimming, cross-country skiing, rowing, basketball, racquetball, and soccer.

Managing Stress

Stages of Exercise-Induced Relaxed Concentration

Exercise is a great way to relieve stress. It reduces muscle tension; stimulates regular, deep breathing; increases blood levels of endorphins; and creates an opportunity to free the mind from worries. The next time you exercise, see if you can become aware of these four stages of *stress relief through exercise:*

Stage 1: Paying Attention

At the beginning of an exercise session, you focus your mind on the activity and allow any thoughts that arise to pass out of your mind. When you notice them, simply say to yourself, "Oh, I have a thought," and bring yourself back to focusing on your activity.

Stage 2: Interested Attention

After a period of concentrating and letting go, you no longer have to concentrate on eliminating distractions, and you sense a flowing with the activity.

Stage 3: Absorbed Attention

Absorption with the activity is so great that it is very difficult for you to be distracted by what is going on around you. You may experience altered perceptions of space and time, and your mind may move through thoughts and images without your direction. The experience can be dreamlike, except you are entirely awake and attentive.

Stage 4: Merging

You no longer are aware of any separation between you and what you are doing. The experience of union is complete: physical, mental, and spiritual. You attain a complete loss of self-consciousness, and even though you may be working your body very hard, mentally and spiritually you feel very calm.

Strength Training

Strength training involves repetitively moving muscles against resistance, commonly applied by weights, such as barbells, dumbbells, and exercise machines, but also by simple pushing against an immovable object (**isometric training**). A stronger body is better able to combat fatigue; in sports, strength can improve athletic performance and reduce the likelihood of injury. For some, "pumping iron" helps release stress-induced muscle tensions.

Many people are drawn to strength training for cosmetic reasons. In their desire to look good, individuals may not receive adequate instruction in strength-training methods and may injure themselves. It is essential to build strength gradually with proper techniques.

Compared to most aerobic exercise, strength training produces only a modest improvement in cardiovascular fitness. The time spent exercising is insufficient to increase the heart rate long enough to produce a training effect. The energy expended during strength training is about four calories per minute, nearly the same as for walking or swimming at a comfortable pace.

A common myth associated with strength training is that consuming high-protein foods and special vitamin supplements will increase muscle mass. This assumption is incorrect. Muscle tissue responds to the demands of work, not to food. In a progressive strength-training regime, sufficient protein to build new muscle tissue will be obtained in a well-balanced diet. Excess protein and vitamins are simply excreted.

Drugs and Athletic Training

The saying "better living through chemistry" has invaded the gymnasium and practice field as some athletes turn to drugs (so-called "ergogenic" aids) to bulk up, increase strength and endurance, and enhance athletic performance. **Anabolic steroids** (testosterone and testosterone-like substances such as "Andro") are among the most abused substances by athletes. These drugs, however, are extremely dangerous. While they do increase muscle strength in both women and men, they also increase the risks of heart attack, stroke, liver damage, and cancer. Human growth hormone is another drug used by some athletes to increase muscle strength. Studies show, however, that this hormone is ineffective in increasing muscle mass. Any drug taken by injection carries the risk of transmitting HIV and hepatitis virus.

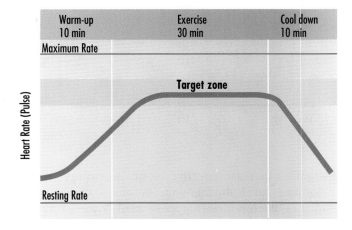

FIGURE 7.3   Heart Rate Pattern for a Typical Exercise Routine A diagram of heart rate during warm-up, aerobic exercise, and cool-down.

Source: A. L. Thygerson, *Fitness and Health* (Boston: Jones and Bartlett, 1989), p. 38.

Dollars and Health Sense

The Business of Sports Supplements

Americans spend between $1 billion and $2 billion annually on sports supplements that they hope will improve their strength, endurance, or performance in some physical activity (Consumer Reports, 2001). World-class athletes, hoping to gain a slight edge in competition, often resort to taking prescription drugs and hormones. In a world where winning is everything, anything goes. Banned substances have been detected in athletes in all world-class sporting events from the Olympics to swimming to cycling races.

The average athlete may not want to take prescription drugs that usually must be obtained illegally, but he or she may seek out sports supplements assuming that they are safe. However, many of these over-the-counter sports supplements contain substances that potentially are harmful. The three most common ingredients in sports supplements are:

androstenedione, a hormone that upsets sex hormone balances and may result in premature puberty or stunted growth in adolescents;

creatine, a substance in muscle used to store energy and to increase short-term strength, but which may cause kidney problems;

ephedra, a Chinese herbal that acts as a stimulant, affects the cardiovascular system, and the use of which has been fatal in some instances.

In general, young people are the ones most attracted to the use of sports stimulants so that they can become bigger, faster, and stronger. They also are the ones most susceptible to harm by the use of sports supplements. More than a million athletes, most of them young, take sports supplements and are encouraged to do so by company advertising. Often the labels on sports supplements do not indicate what substances they contain or the amount of each substance in a dose. As long as our society places so much emphasis on winning, on trim bodies, and on good looks, companies are eager to provide substances that promise quick physical changes. Sports supplements can be harmful, are not necessary to enjoy physical activities, and should be avoided by everyone.

Creatine, a natural substance in muscle tissue required for muscle contraction, can be purchased as a nutritional supplement. Because creatine supplementation can delay the onset of fatigue in skeletal muscles and increases work capacity, many athletes use it to increase muscle mass and stamina. Laboratory studies show that creatine supplementation is more effective on untrained individuals than on trained athletes, perhaps because the muscles of trained individuals are already working near peak efficiency without the supplement (Mujika and Padilla, 1997). In doses commonly used (3 to 5 g/day), creatine apparently is not harmful.

 ### Making Physical Activity a Priority

For many people, the mere mention of physical activity conjures up unpleasant images of painfully boring exercises or rough competitive sports whose proposed beneficial effects on health and character development rarely seem to meet the promises made by enthusiastic players and coaches.

Part of the idea of physical activity is to incorporate a playful or joyful activity into your life for its own sake. Americans are highly product-oriented; we tend to value what we do on the basis of outcome. With physical activity the *process of doing* is itself the reward. So choose activities that you will enjoy. If you like to be around people, join an exercise class or organize some friends to be active with you. After you have accomplished a difficult task, reward yourself with praise. And remember, physical activity, even active sports, does not have to involve competition unless you want it to.

Choosing the Right Exercise

Once you have decided to begin exercising, it is tempting to do what others are doing (e.g., roller blading, jogging, racquetball). But before you go out and buy expensive running shoes and that new outfit, you must decide what exercise is right for you. First you may want to ask yourself what your goals are in an exercise program. Some goals may be: stress reduction; a healthy heart; weight control or weight reduction; greater strength; building muscles; greater stamina; or relaxation.

After you have determined your goals, you want to make sure that the activities you adopt go along

Terms

isometric training: a type of strength training

anabolic steroids: synthetic male hormones used to increase muscle size and strength

creatine: a natural substance in skeletal muscle tissue, which also can be taken in dietary supplement to enhance muscle performance

with your goals. You may choose swimming as your main exercise. Swimming is good for weight maintenance, but not for body building. Other important factors when selecting your exercise of choice are: motivation; realistic expectations; comfort; convenience; and cost factors.

To be sure you can commit to an exercise class, take a trial class before signing up for several months. Make sure you enjoy the exercise. You should be able to enjoy working out and getting in shape at the same time. The more you enjoy what you are doing, the more likely you will stay motivated and continue to exercise and meet your fitness goals.

If you have never exercised or are not in good shape, do not expect to see results overnight. Achieving physical fitness takes time and consistency. Changes will most likely be seen in the first month; however, achieving total physical fitness will take months of constant exercise.

When I feel a desire to exercise, I lie down until the thought passes.
W. C. FIELDS

For some people, a fitness club or recreation center can be intimidating if everyone else is in good shape. Some find more informal "shaping-up" classes better for them. However, for others, being surrounded by a lot of physically fit people in a fitness club is motivating. Some may wish to stay at home and exercise.

You need to decide in what environment you feel comfortable exercising.

Make sure whatever activity you choose is convenient. Don't choose one that requires you to drive 30 minutes, because before you know it you will be saying "it's too far." Choose an activity within a convenient distance.

Decide how much money you can afford to spend. Remember to include the cost of equipment, proper clothing, and transportation. Look into exercise classes that allow you to pay as you go; or find a fitness club that will allow you to join for a one-month trial program. Both options are good if you are still unsure about which exercise program is right for you.

Types of Beneficial Exercises

Different kinds of exercises provide different benefits. After you have determined your goal(s) and your method of exercise, you must make sure the exercise provides the type of benefit you wish to achieve. There are exercises that help relieve stress, aid the heart, control weight, define muscles, improve strength, increase power and **endurance,** and maintain **flexibility.** You may choose one or more of these; you decide.

Exercising for Stress Reduction   Exercise is a form of positive stress; one of its effects is to cancel the negative emotional stresses that accumulate daily. Almost

Wellness Guide

Getting into Shape

Undertake a program to increase aerobic conditioning by following these guidelines:

1. Frequency: you should exercise three to five times a week.

2. Intensity: you should exercise within 60% to 80% of your exercise heart rate.

3. Duration: you should exercise within your target zone for 20 to 60 minutes each time.

4. Type of exercise: appropriate exercises are rhythmic and continuous and use the large muscles of the legs and hips. Such exercises include walking, jogging, bicycling, swimming, cross-country skiing, and aerobic dancing.

5. Warm up and cool down. It is optimal to raise the body's core temperature about 1°F to 3°F by doing the warm up and stretching activities before the aerobic workout. After the aerobic workout, you should slow your heart rate and cool down for 30 to 60 minutes. Optimal time to stretch is when the muscles are warmed (i.e., after aerobic exercise).

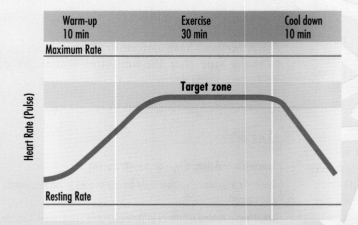

any exercise where you work out for at least one-half hour is effective. Pleasant surroundings also help in relieving stress. Swimming is soothing and relaxing for many people; others enjoy jogging.

Exercising for Your Heart Aerobic exercises are considered the most effective in terms of increasing heart capacity. Thirty minutes is what most studies believe is the magic number to produce maximum benefits from aerobics (this 30 minutes does not include the **warm-up** or **cool-down** periods).

Exercising to Maintain Weight Regular physical activity carried out consistently over many months (indeed, for life) is the key to weight management and weight reduction (see chapter 6). When you exercise regularly, not only do you expend calories, but you also tend not to use food to relieve stress-related mental tension: you tend to eat less in general. It requires the expenditure of 3500 calories to lose one pound of body fat. That is the equivalent of walking for about 14.6 hours (walking expends 4 calories per minute) or jogging about 8 hours (jogging expends about 7 calories per minute). Anyone on a weight-loss program needs both to reduce the consumption of needless calories and increase significantly the time devoted to physical activity. This is why achieving *and maintaining* weight loss takes time and perseverance.

Exercising for Strength Body building generally means weight training with light barbells, dumbbells, and weight machines. In strength training, you use many of the same techniques as those for building muscles. The difference between muscle building and strength building is that less weight and more repetitions are used with strength building. In other words, instead of lifting 100 pounds 10 times, you might lift 10-pound weights 50 times: the same amount of body work builds strength instead of bulk muscle.

Exercising for Endurance and Power Endurance is your body's ability to withstand stress over a period of time, and power is your muscles' ability to perform over an extended period of time. Endurance is built by gradually increasing the length of time of strenuous activity, whereas power is achieved by short bursts of strenuous activity followed by rest periods. Sports not suitable for strength and endurance are softball and golf.

Exercising for Flexibility Calisthenics and yoga are great for flexibility. Keep in mind that flexibility should not be confused with fitness; flexibility is part of fitness, but flexibility exercises alone do not make a person physically fit. Almost all sports and exercises will increase flexibility. Stretching exercises should be incorporated into all sports activities and workouts (Figure 7.4).

Terms

endurance: the ability to work out over a period of time without fatigue

flexibility: the ability of a joint to move through its range of motion

warm-up: low-intensity exercise done before full-effort physical activity to improve muscle and joint performance, prevent injury, reinforce motor skills, and maximize blood flow to the muscles and heart

cool-down: light or mild exercise immediately following competition or a training session; the primary purpose is to speed the removal of lactic acid from the muscles and allow the body to gradually return to a resting state

Wellness Guide

What's Your Excuse? Changing the Attitudes That Block Exercising

Excuse	New Attitude
Exercise is work.	I'm going to do something active that I enjoy and that makes me feel good.
I don't have time.	I can always find 5 or 10 minutes here and there to move my body, even if it's just for a short walk.
I'm too tired.	I don't feel like it now, but I know that after I exercise I always feel better.
I'll fail.	If I start slowly and do what I can, that is success enough. Being healthy and well is not a contest.
I'm too old.	Too old for what? I just want to enjoy myself.
I'm too heavy.	I always feel better after I move my body.
Exercise is boring.	I can make exercise interesting by choosing an activity I like, and doing it with a friend or while listening to the radio.
It's too cold (icy, rainy, hot, etc.).	I'll exercise at home by stretching out, or maybe I'll take a walk at the mall.

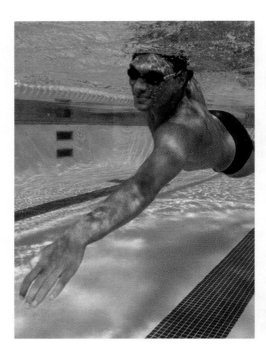

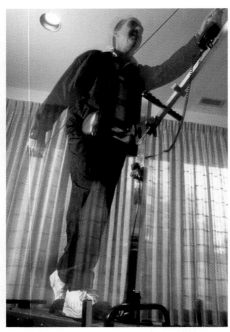

When choosing an exercise, pick one that's fun and convenient for you.

Don't ask your muscles to do more than they can. Relishing the pain of overexertion—"going for the burn"—is dangerous. This pain is the body's message that something is wrong, not that the exerciser is lazy. If you want to increase your performance, build muscle strength slowly, following a supervised regime. Also, preactivity and postactivity stretching helps to prevent damage to muscles and joints. Injuries are more likely if equipment such as weights and other kinds of apparatus are improperly used or are in disrepair.

Wellness Guide

A Plan for Fitness

Here are some guidelines to keep in mind when incorporating any kind of physical activity into your life:

1. **Have a plan.** Before beginning any body work program, you need to develop a plan and commit yourself to it for a reasonable amount of time. To make a plan that will help you achieve your personal goals, you can consult a high school or college coach, attend an exercise class, or follow the plan in one of the "how to" books that have been written for almost every activity.

2. **Get a physical checkup.** If you have been inactive for many months or have concerns about your body's ability to perform at the level you would like, you may want to have a physician check you over.

3. **Accomplish goals.** The goal of any body work program is attainment of complete mind-body harmony. This can be done by progressively attaining higher and higher goals. It is customary in our culture to measure progress by "how far" and "how fast." Such goals might be suitable for competitive athletes, but they are unsuitable for people who engage in body work activities for the purpose of receiving greater enjoyment from living. For most of us, personal goals based on such questions as "Does this level of activity make me feel good?" or "Does this help me toward my goal of losing weight?" make more sense than blind adherence to a stopwatch.

4. **Progress slowly.** Slow, deliberate progress gives you the opportunity to integrate your body work activity into your normal life routine. Begin slowly; don't impulsively try to run a long distance the first day.

5. **Warm up and cool down.** All body work activity should be preceded by a brief period of stretching, breathing, and relaxation to prepare your mind and body to receive the utmost benefit and pleasure from body work. This is a good time to focus attention on how your body feels. When you have finished your body work activity, it is a good idea to let your body cool down slowly. If you have been involved in strenuous aerobic exercise, slowly reduce the pace of your activity until your heart rate and breathing return to almost normal. By slowly reducing your activity level you help prevent muscle cramps that sometimes occur when strenuous activity is suddenly stopped. You can prevent later muscle stiffness by doing a few stretching exercises to loosen the muscles that have worked hard during exercise. While cooling down, try to focus your attention on the sensations that your body work has brought you.

Most people participate in physical activity because (a) they want to have fun, (b) they want to gain a sense of accomplishment by doing something well, and (c) they want to feel physically and psychologically better. While pursuing these goals, no one wants to be hurt. It turns out that maximizing the "have fun, do well, feel good" aspects of exercise and minimizing the potential for injury go together. Physical activity is most satisfying when you are totally absorbed in it, when your body responds readily to your commands, when you run or play with confidence, and when your equipment and conditions are optimal. Take sports seriously enough to enjoy them, while minimizing the likelihood of injuries.

Walking and Health

If jogging, swimming, cycling, aerobic dancing, and other strenuous activities aren't for you, try walking. Regular walking contributes many of the health benefits of other activities. And walking has advantages that other activities do not: other than appropriate shoes, no special clothing or equipment is required, and walking can be fit easily into a busy schedule.

Walking contributes the most to health when it is done regularly (about four times a week) for a minimum of 20 minutes each day. How strenuous the walk should be depends on the desires and physical abilities of the walker. Most of the benefits can be derived by walking between two and four miles per hour. Aerobic capacity can be increased by walking briskly enough to increase the heart rate.

Exercise Abuse

Although few would argue that being fashionably healthy and attractive are desirable goals, many people are so zealous in pursuing these goals that they harm themselves. For example, some individuals place higher priority on running or other fitness activities than they do on work, family, interpersonal relationships, and even their own health. Some are unwilling to stop exercising (even for a day!) to attend to other matters in life or to allow an exercise injury

to heal properly. In their attempts to attain the "perfect body," a large number of women exercise and lose weight to such extremes that they stop menstruating (**athletic amenorrhea**) or develop anorexia or bulimia (see chapter 6).

The most common form of exercise abuse is exercising a body part or the entire body beyond its biological limit, to the point of injury. Such injuries are referred to as **overuse syndromes.** Between 25% and 50% of athletes visiting sports medicine clinics may have sustained

It's true that hard work never killed anybody, but I figure, why take a chance?
RONALD REAGAN

an overuse injury. Commonly, overuse injuries affect the skin and muscles, tendons, ligaments, and joints, which are constructed of fibrous bands of protein. These fibers can be torn if they are overloaded, as when lifting a heavy weight or running at top speed, or when forced to perform when fatigued. Damage can also occur by repeated small injuries that lead over time to a more serious problem. The common causes of overuse injuries are excessive exercising, faulty technique, and poor equipment.

All bodies are not anatomically capable of the same degree of physical exertion, especially the high performance exhibited by marathon runners or triathletes. The architecture of the body, the alignment of the legs, the capacity of the lungs, the size and strength of the bones and muscles, and other anatomical factors set limits on an individual's physical ability. Few people have the biological endowment to perform at championship levels. Physical activity can be much more enjoyable when you respect, accept, and appreciate your body's biological limits.

Terms

athletic amenorrhea: irregular or cessation of menstruation due to excessive participation in athletics

overuse syndromes: injuries to muscles, tendons, ligaments, and joints resulting from too much exercise

Wellness Guide

Common Overuse Injuries

Strain: Commonly referred to as "pulled muscles" or "pulled tendons." Caused by overstretching, tearing, or ripping of a muscle and/or its tendon

Tendonitis: Inflammation of a tendon caused by

chronic, low-grade strain of a muscle-tendon unit

Bursitis: Inflammation of the lubricating sac (*bursa*) that surrounds a joint caused by repeated low-grade strain of the joint's supporting tissues

Sprain: Overstretching or tearing of ligaments

Blisters: Fluid-filled swellings on the skin caused by friction from the rubbing of skin against shoes, clothing, and equipment

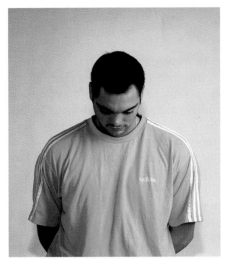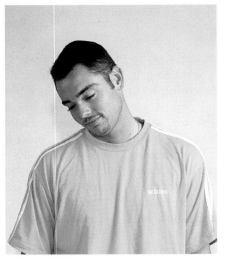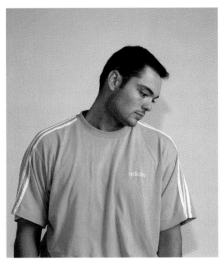

Neck   Drop your chin to your chest. Turn your head as far right as you can without moving your shoulders and hold. Repeat to the left. Tilt your head toward the left ear without bending your torso or hunching your shoulders and hold. Repeat to the right.

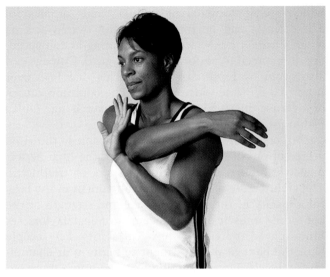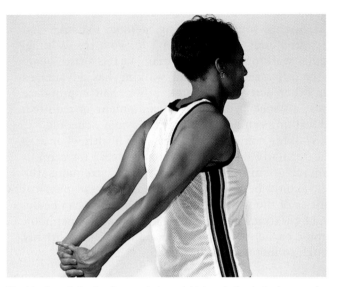

Shoulder Stretch 1   With your left hand, grasp your right elbow and pull your arm across your chest, keeping it bent at a 90° angle. Alternate arms.

Shoulder Stretch 2   Standing, grasp both arms behind your back and raise them up as far as you can.

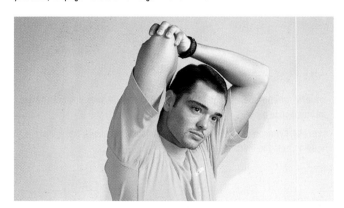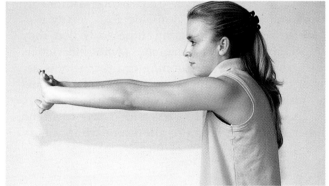

Triceps Stretch   Grasp the opposite elbow and pull the arm behind the head and down until a stretch is felt in the back of the arm. Hold and then repeat for the other arm.

Upper-back Stretch   Clasp your hands in front of your body, and press your palms forward.

FIGURE 7.4   **Flexibility Exercises**   It is best to do stretching exercises when the muscles are warm. You should stretch to the point of *mild* discomfort, but stop immediately if you experience pain—particularly in the lower back or knees. Hold all stretches for 15–30 seconds, rest for 30–60 seconds, and then repeat the stretch, trying to go a little further. For all standing stretches, legs should be hip-width apart, with knees slightly bent, back straight, and weight evenly distributed from the front to the back of the feet. To view a video of the exercises visit

  www.jbpub.com/hwonline

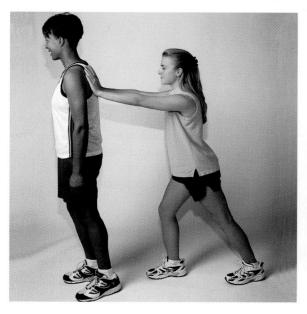

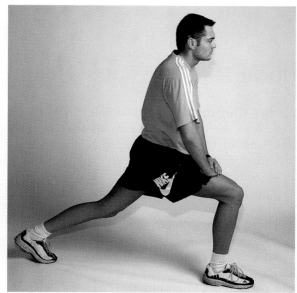

Calf Stretch   Stand approximately 2 to 3 feet away from a wall, tree, or stretching partner. Move one foot in close to the wall, while keeping the back leg straight behind you with the foot and heel flat on the ground. Slowly move your hips forward, bending the forward knee and keeping the back foot on the ground. You should feel a slight stretch in your calf muscles. Repeat with the opposite leg.

Lunge Stretch   Step forward and bend your forward knee, keeping it directly above your ankle. Stretch your other leg back behind you but don't lock your knee. Press your hips forward and down to stretch. Your arms can be at your sides, on top of your knee, or on the ground for balance. Repeat on the other side.

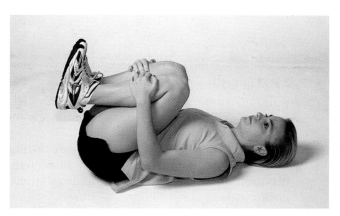

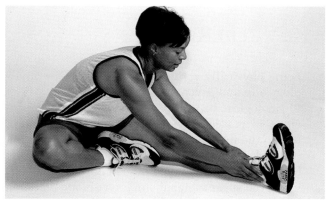

Low Back Stretch   Lie on your back and pull both knees in to the chest. Keep your lower back on the floor.

Modified Hurdler   Sit with your right leg straight out in front of you and your left leg tucked close to your body. Reach toward your right foot as far as possible. Do not curve your back. Go only as far as you can with a straight back. Repeat for the other leg.

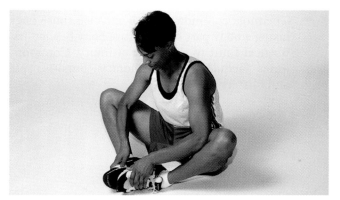

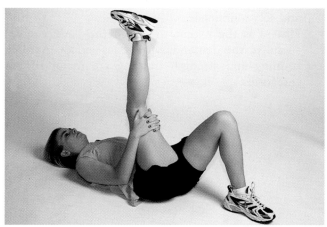

Groin Stretch   Sit with your back straight (don't slouch; you may want to put your back against a wall) and bend your legs, with the soles of your feet together. Try to get your heels as close to your groin as is comfortably possible. For a passive stretch, push your knees to the floor as far as you can (you may use your hands to assist but do not resist with the knees) and hold them there. This can be hard on the knees so please be careful. Now, keep your knees where they are, and then exhale as you bend over, trying to get your chest as close to the floor as possible.

Supine Hamstring Stretch   Lie on your back and pull one leg up to a stretched position. The leg should remain as straight as possible. The opposite leg should be bent with the heel on the floor; keep your lower back on the floor. Alternate legs.

Critical Thinking About Health

1. Another Christmas Day at Grandma's. Well, almost. After everyone had eaten all they possibly could and all the children had ripped open their Christmas gifts, Suzanne's Uncle Ron sat next to her on the couch.

    "I understand that you're taking a health class at school," he said.

    "That's right," Suzanne replied.

    "Then tell me," Uncle Ron continued, "What's the best exercise? My New Year's resolution is to get back in shape, and I want to do it right this time. I'm joining the gym on January 2. What workouts do you recommend?"

    a. What advice should Suzanne give her uncle? Take into account that Uncle Ron has tried working out before, apparently without success. Uncle Ron is a 39-year-old telecommunications engineer who works long hours at a computer terminal when he's at his office. His job also requires him to travel, so he eats a lot of fast food. He is married and has three young children.

2. What are the effects on society and on organized sports of athletes using performance-enhancing drugs, even when such substances are legal?

3. How far? How fast? How much? How might questions such as these affect a person's attitude and approach to physical activity for health (i.e., not competition)? List a new set of questions that illustrate a noncompetitive perspective on physical activity for health.

Health in Review

- Being physically active helps us to be both physiologically and psychologically well.
- Physiological benefits from physical activity include increased efficiency and strength of heart, lungs, and muscles; more effective weight control; reduced fatigue and increased energy; a higher level of immunity; lower blood cholesterol levels; improved sugar metabolism; lower blood pressure; and improved posture.
- Psychological benefits from physical activity include: reduced fatigue and better sleep patterns; a more positive mental outlook; less stress; release of tension and anxiety; and improved self-image and self-confidence.
- Fitness is the extent to which the body can respond to the demands of physical effort. Aerobic training and strength training are major fitness categories.

- Aerobic conditioning may be achieved through walking, running, bicycling, swimming, cross-country skiing, rowing, basketball, racquetball, and soccer.
- Aerobic exercise strengthens the heart. Strength training produces only a modest improvement in cardiovascular fitness, but builds muscle strength, unlike aerobic conditioning.
- Goals for an exercise program may include stress reduction; a healthy heart; weight control or maintenance; greater strength; muscle-building; greater stamina; or relaxation.
- The most common form of exercise abuse is exercising a body part or the entire body beyond its biological limit to the point of injury. Common injuries include strain, tendonitis, bursitis, sprain, and blisters.

Health and Wellness Online

The World Wide Web contains a wealth of information about health and wellness. By accessing the Internet using Web browser software, such as Netscape Navigator or Microsoft's Internet Explorer, you can gain a new perspective on many topics presented in *Health and Wellness, Seventh Edition*. Access the Jones and Bartlett Publishers Web site at http://www.jbpub.com/hwonline.

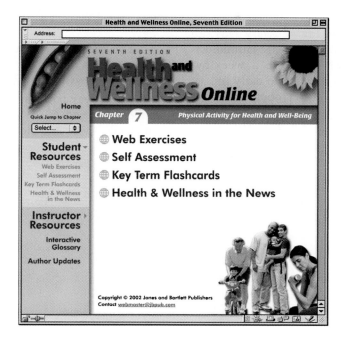

References

Blair, S. N., Kohl, H. W., Gordon, N. F., and Paffenbarger, Jr, R. S. (1992). How much physical activity is good for health? *Annual Review of Public Health, 13,* 99–126.

Consumer Reports (2001 June). Sports-Supplement-dangers, 40–42.

Delza, Sophia (1996). *The tai chi chuan experience: Reflections and perceptions on body-mind harmony.* New York: State University of New York Press.

Hakim, A., Petrovitch, H., Burchfiel, C. M., Ross, G. W., Rodriguez, B. L., White, L. R., Yano, K., Curb, J. D., and Abbott, R. D. (1998). Effects of walking on mortality among nonsmoking retired men. *The New England Journal of Medicine, 338,* 94–9.

Mujika, I., and Padilla, S. (1997). Creatine supplementation as an ergogenic aid for sports performance in highly trained athletes. *International Journal of Sports Medicine, 18,* 491–496.

U.S. Department of Health and Human Services, Centers for Disease Control and Prevention, National Center for Chronic Disease Prevention and Health Promotion, and President's Council on Physical Fitness and Sports. (1999). *Physical activity and health: A report of the Surgeon General* (http://www.cdc.gov/nccdphp/sgr/sgr.htm).

Suggested Readings

American Heart Association. *Just Move*. A website offering fitness news, a virtual personal trainer, and exercise tips. (http://www.justmove.org/home.cfm)

Anderson, B. (2000). *Stretching*. New York: Shelter Publications. Easy-to-follow exercises and drawings.

Blair, S. (ed) (2001). *Active Living Every Day: 20 Weeks to Lifelong Vitality*. Champaign, IL: Human Kinetics. Several exercise experts provide a week-by-week guide to adding physical activity to daily life.

Feuerstein, G. and Payne, L. (1999). *Yoga for Dummies*. Foster City, CA: Hungry Minds. Two world-renowned yoga instructors tell how to practice this ancient mind-body method.

How fit are you? (1997). *Consumer Reports on Health, 9(7)*, 27–31. How to improve your strength, aerobic capacity, flexibility, and balance.

Optimal workouts. (1997). *UC Berkeley Wellness Letter, 13(7)*, 6–7. Advice on the best workout programs.

The President's Council on Physical Fitness. Information on dozens of exercise topics for people of all ages. (http://www.fitness.gov/)

Walk away pounds. (1997). *Weight Watchers Magazine, 30(2)*, 64–66. Walking instructions and advice on proper shoes and clothing.

Building Healthy Relationships

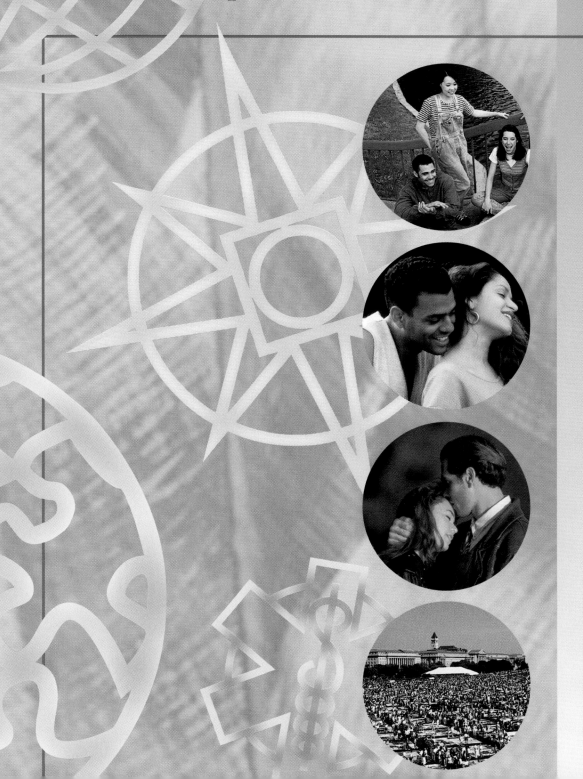

1. Define the terms sex, sexuality, sexual, menopause, masturbation, gender role, gender identity, sexual orientation, heterosexual, homosexual, bisexual.
2. Compare and contrast traditional gender roles for males and females.
3. Describe the male reproductive system.
4. Describe the female reproductive system.
5. Explain the menstrual cycle.
6. Explain the sexual response cycle.
7. Identify and discuss several different sexual difficulties.
8. Describe an intimate relationship.
9. Identify and describe the essential components of good communication.

Study Guide
and
Self Assessment

How Realistic Are Your Attitudes About Love?
An Assessment of Sexual Communication
Gender Roles in Society

Health
and Wellness
Online

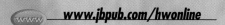 **www.jbpub.com/hwonline**

Chapter 8

Developing Healthy Intimate and Sexual Relationships

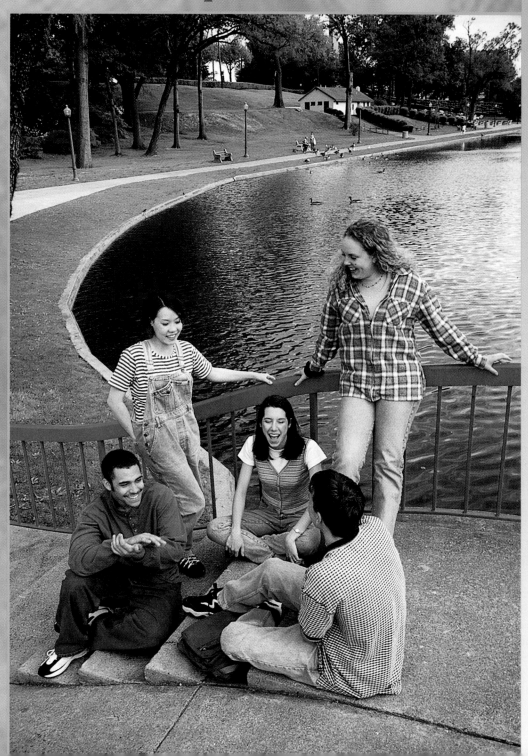

Sexuality represents a truly holistic aspect of living, for it involves the simultaneous expression of mind, body, and spirit—the whole self. Although sexuality is commonly represented in advertising and other media as having to do solely with physical gratification, most people are aware that sexuality involves much more than the stimulation of the body's sex organs. Sexuality involves thoughts, feelings, and identity. Sexuality is also a powerful form of communication between people.

> *Marrying a woman for her beauty makes no more sense than eating a bird for its singing. But it's a common mistake, nevertheless.*
>
> CHARLES FRAZIER
> *COLD MOUNTAIN*

From the standpoint of personal health, sexuality is an area over which you have considerable individual control. You choose when and with whom you wish to have sex, and which feelings you wish to express in sexual ways. With some fundamental knowledge of sexual biology, you can conduct your sexual life responsibly, thus avoiding unnecessary illness and exercising a choice of whether and when to have children. This chapter introduces the topic of sexuality and discusses the nature of the sexual self and of sexual expression.

Defining Sex and Sexuality

Sex

Sex can refer to (a) an individual's classification as male or female as determined by the presence of certain anatomical and physiological characteristics, (b) a set of behaviors, and (c) the experience of erotic pleasure.

At the most fundamental biological level, sex refers to the mating of two anatomically distinct individuals, a male and a female, each of which manufactures specific cells, or **gametes,** which fuse to become the first cell of a new individual. To facilitate the fusion process (called **fertilization**), males and females possess specific organs and display certain behaviors that are intended to bring about the union of gametes.

Often the word *sex* is used to denote aspects of an individual's personal characteristics that are thought to derive from her or his biological classification. Thus, the biological property of "femaleness" is associated with the social quality of "femininity," and the biological property of "maleness" is associated with the social quality of "masculinity." Although most modern dictionaries still define sex as having to do with personality characteristics, this concept is more accurately referred to as *gender* to distinguish its origins in culture rather than biology.

Besides biological classification, sex is also associated with certain behaviors that are defined as **sexual.**

These activities usually involve touching in various ways certain anatomical regions of the body, such as the genitalia and breasts, and sexual intercourse.

Sex can also mean erotic pleasure, a certain kind of experience with unique and identifiable qualities that distinguish it from other kinds of pleasure, such as the satisfaction of hunger or the enjoyment of music. A variety of circumstances and events has the potential to activate the erotic pleasure centers, including certain kinds of tactile stimulation (e.g., touching, kissing) of certain body regions (e.g., mouth, breasts, genitals); certain kinds of visual, olfactory, and auditory stimulation; and fantasy. Potentially erotic stimuli become actual erotic stimuli when other centers in the brain interpret them as erotic. That is why not every touch, kiss, or potentially sexual situation is erotically arousing.

Identical behaviors may be erotically pleasurable in some instances but not in others. Kissing a child or a grandparent can be very different from kissing a spouse. The touching of the genitals in a medical examination is not the same as the touching of the genitals when expressing love and affection to a sexual partner.

Defining sex in terms of what is experienced makes no reference to any particular outcome other than the experience itself. Sex is not defined by certain genital responses, such as erection of the penis, nor is it defined in terms of a variety of changes in physiology, such as increased heart rate, blood pressure, and muscle tension. Nor is sex defined in terms of experiencing orgasm. Although it is true that sexual pleasure is usually associated with certain genital and physiological responses and sometimes orgasm, these outcomes are not sufficient to define sex because they can occur without the experience of erotic pleasure.

Defining sex in terms of the experience makes no reference to interaction with any particular person. Sexual pleasure can be experienced by oneself through masturbation or fantasy. It can be experienced with someone of the same or the other sex. It can be experienced in a variety of social contexts.

Sexuality

Sexuality, as distinct from sex, consists of the aspects of a person's sense of self that are used to create sexual experiences. Another term for sexuality is the sexual self, which has several dimensions:

1. The *physical dimension* refers to any region of the body to which an individual gives sexual meaning, including the organs and organ systems that one employs to create erotic experiences (e.g., the skin, genitals). It also includes the physical features that define oneself to oneself and to others as a sexual being.

2. The *psychological dimension* refers to emotions and conscious and unconscious beliefs that guide

the interpretation of experience. This aspect of sexuality generates strategies for actions that are intended to satisfy the individual's wants and needs.

3. The *social dimension* refers to sexual attitudes and behaviors that affect an individual's interactions with members of the social groups to which she or he belongs.

4. The *orientation dimension* refers to the tendency to feel most "naturally" sexually attracted to, and the ability to emotionally bond with, members of a particular gender. About 85% to 90% of Americans are oriented to members of the opposite sex; the rest of the population orients to individuals of either sex (bisexuals) or, more often, exclusively to members of the same sex (homosexuals). Individuals do not choose their sexual orientation; it develops as a fundamental aspect of a person's personality. Scientific studies are being undertaken to determine any genetic, hormonal, metabolic, or psychological mechanisms underlying sexual orientation.

5. The *developmental dimension* is the evolution of oneself throughout a lifetime. This evolution includes the body, belief systems, and the ways sex is employed to create and maintain intimacy.

6. The *skill dimension* speaks to the physical and social skills that affect how well one meets one's sexual wants and needs.

Gender Identity and Gender Role

Although anatomy and physiology explain the biological bases of human sexuality, most people's sexual experiences also involve beliefs, thoughts, feelings, and social behaviors. How individuals come to think and behave sexually is almost entirely a product of what they learn as children about the kinds of behaviors that are expected of members of one sex or the other. Studies of psychosexual development indicate that the development of gender identity and the subsequent expression of sex-specific behaviors begins with the sex typing of

Terms

sex: has several definitions: (a) an individual's classification as male or female based on anatomical characteristics; (b) a set of behaviors; (c) the experience of erotic pleasure

gametes: sex cells, either sperm or ova, that fuse at fertilization; gametes carry a complete set of genetic information from each parent that is passed on to the child

fertilization: the fusion of a sperm cell and an ovum

sexual: characterized by or having the qualities of sex; the opposite is asexual

sexuality: a person's sense of self that is used to create sexual experiences

gender identity: awareness of being male or female

gender role: behaviors specific to a gender

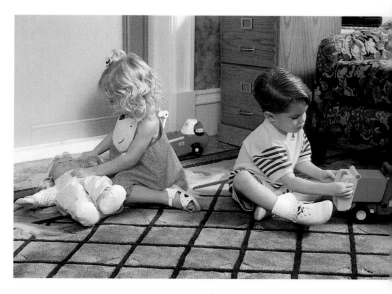

Often, children are taught early on how to "act" female or male.

newborn infants. When a child is born, almost the first thing noticed is its biological sex as determined by the appearance of its external genitals. If the infant is born with a penis, those attending the birth will exclaim "It's a boy!" Similarly, "It's a girl!" follows the observation of a newborn female's external genitals.

Having been sex typed at birth, the infant is thereafter treated by adults in a manner they think is appropriate for a child of that sex, and eventually the infant incorporates into his or her self-image the awareness of being a male or a female. This awareness, called **gender identity,** refers to our own personal, subjective sense that "I am a male" or "I am a female." **Gender role** refers to a collection of attitudes and behaviors that are considered normal and appropriate in a culture. Gender roles establish sex-related behavioral expectations that people are expected to fulfill.

By about the age of two, a child's gender identity is fixed for life. How the child comes to act on the self-knowledge of its maleness or femaleness depends on the interrelationship of a variety of factors. Children learn attitudes and behaviors by modeling after adults, such as parents, teachers, celebrities, and fictional characters, and they are also trained by reward and punishment. Whatever the sources of information and influence, children learn early which attitudes and behaviors are appropriate for males and which are appropriate for females. By the age of three, children are capable of citing a long list of behaviors that are expected of one sex and not the other.

Exactly which attitudes and behaviors are deemed appropriate for both sexes depends on the culture in which people live. In some societies, gender role behaviors are strictly defined, and little deviance from the stereotype is allowed. Our culture possesses a set of traditional stereotypic gender role expectations that include economic role, dominance or submissiveness in social relationships, responsibilities for home and child care, mode of dress, personal appearance, and mode of expression of emotions.

Defining Sexual Orientation

A person's **sexual orientation** is his or her attraction toward and interest in members of one or both genders. A **heterosexual** is a person who is attracted to someone of the opposite gender. A **homosexual** is attracted to someone of the same gender. Therefore, a homosexual's gender identity agrees with his or her biological sex. That is, a homosexual person perceives himself or herself as male or female, respectively, and feels attraction toward a person of the same sex. A **bisexual** is someone who is attracted to members of both genders. The terms heterosexual and homosexual do not imply normalcy or a type of sexual act; they simply describe a person's preference with regard to one gender or another. The concept of sexual orientation and identity has evolved over time, as views of masculinity and femininity have changed. Today we view masculinity and femininity as a set of characteristics, which vary among both men and women.

Alfred Kinsey, a sex researcher in the mid-1900s, developed a seven-category sexual behavior rating scale to study the sexual behaviors of people (Figure 8.1). The scale ranges from 0 to 6, with 6 representing exclusively homosexual behavior, and 0 representing exclusively heterosexual behavior. Values 1 through 5 showed predominately heterosexual or homosexual behavior, respectively, but also indicate some of the other type of sexual behavior.

> *In love, as in nearly all human affairs, a satisfactory relationship is the result of a misunderstanding.*
>
> CHARLES BAUDELAIRE
> *MY HEART LAID BARE*

While this continuum represented the best approach at the time for classifying sexual behavior, it did not adequately reflect the sexual interests and needs of individuals. The scale indicated the type of sexual activity in which people participated, but it did not measure a person's degree of heterosexual or homosexual attractions. It did not take into account that some persons might be having heterosexual experi-

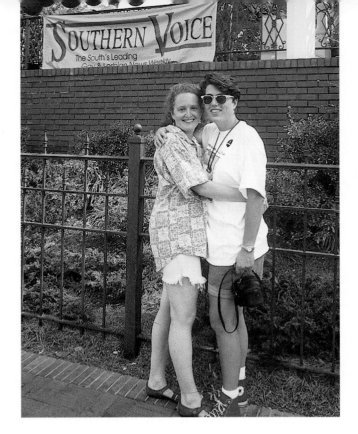

Intimate relationships between couples of the same sex are increasingly accepted in our society.

ences, but really were attracted to others of the same gender. This scale only looked at behavior. Later research has shown the greater complexity of human sexuality.

Researchers asked a sample across the United States to self-report whether they considered themselves homosexual or heterosexual. About 1.4% of women and 2.8% of men reported same-gender sexuality. However, 6.2% of the heterosexual men reported being somewhat attracted to men, and 4.5% indicated the idea of sex with another man was appealing. Of the women, 5.6% reported finding the idea of sex with a woman appealing, and 4.4% reported sexual attraction to women.

The researchers concluded: "Put simply, we contend there is no single answer to questions about the prevalence of homosexuality. Rather, homosexuality is a complex, multidimensional phenomenon whose salient features are related to one another in highly contingent and diverse ways" (Lauman et al., 1994).

0	1	2	3	4	5	6
Exclusive heterosexual experience	Heterosexual with incidental homosexual experience	Heterosexual with substantial homosexual experience	Equal heterosexual and homosexual experience	Homosexual with substantial heterosexual experience	Homosexual with incidental heterosexual experience	Exclusively homosexual experience

FIGURE 8.1   Kinsey Scale of Sexual Behavior   Kinsey believed that some people did not fit into strict same-gender or opposite-gender sexual behavior. His scale of sexual behavior reflects this belief.

Sexual Biology

One of the fundamental roles of sexuality is biological reproduction. The reproductive role of the male is to produce reproductively capable sperm and to deposit them in the female reproductive tract during sexual intercourse. The reproductive role of the female is to provide reproductively capable eggs, called **ova,** and to provide a safe, nutrient-filled environment in which the fetus develops for the 9 months of pregnancy.

Male or female reproductive biology is genetically determined at conception. The fusion of an X-bearing egg with the X-bearing sperm produces a female (XX); fusion with the Y-bearing sperm produces a male (XY). Once the chromosome pattern is set, the development of the sexual anatomy follows from the precise instructions of the genes contained in the chromosomes. A particular chromosome set determines whether the as yet immature sex cells that appear at about the fifth week of development will eventually produce sperm or ova. The sex chromosomes determine whether the fetus will ultimately develop the male sex organs—

testes, sperm ducts, semen-producing glands, and penis; or the female organs—ovaries, fallopian tubes, uterus, vagina, and external female genitals.

The genetic determination of sexual anatomy also specifies the pattern of male or female steroid hormone production, which in turn affects the **secondary sex characteristics** that distinguish males and females: the extent and distribution of facial and body hair; body build and stature; and appearance of breasts (Figure 8.2).

Terms

sexual orientation: attraction toward and interest in members of one or both genders

heterosexual: someone who is attracted to people of the opposite gender

homosexual: someone who is attracted to people of the same gender

bisexual: someone who is attracted to members of both genders

ova: a term for female eggs (singular, *ovum*)

secondary sex characteristics: anatomical features appearing at puberty that distinguish males from females

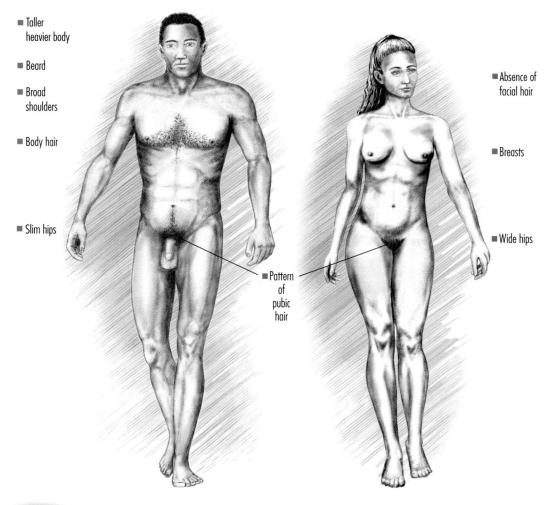

- Taller heavier body
- Beard
- Broad shoulders
- Body hair
- Slim hips
- Pattern of pubic hair
- Absence of facial hair
- Breasts
- Wide hips

FIGURE 8.2   **Secondary Sexual Characteristics of Men and Women**

FIGURE 8.3 **A Cross-section of the Female Sexual-Reproductive System**

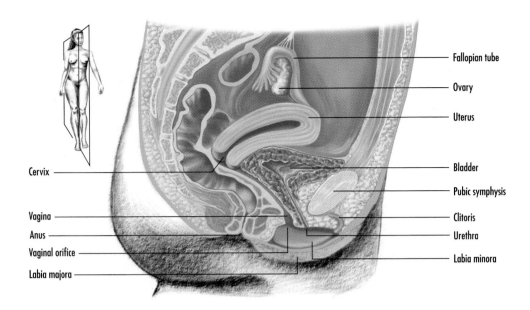

Fallopian tube

Ovary

Uterus

Bladder

Pubic symphysis

Clitoris

Urethra

Labia minora

Cervix

Vagina

Anus

Vaginal orifice

Labia majora

Female Sexual Anatomy

A woman's internal sexual organs consist of two **ovaries,** which lie on either side of the abdominal cavity, the **fallopian tubes,** the **uterus,** and the **vagina;** together these structures make up a specialized tube that goes from each ovary to the outside of the body (Figure 8.3). The function of the ovaries, which are about the size and shape of almonds, is to produce fertilizable ova as well as sex hormones, which control the development of the female body type, maintain normal female sexual physiology, and help regulate the course of a normal pregnancy. The fallopian tubes gather and transport the ova that are released from the ovaries (about one each month). The two fallopian tubes connect to the uterus, an organ about the size of a woman's fist, which is situated just behind the pelvic bone and the bladder (Figure 8.4). The uterus is part of the passageway for sperm as they move from the vagina to the fallopian tubes to effect fertilization; after fertilization, it provides the environment in which the fetus grows. It is the inner lining of the uterus that is shed each month in menstruation.

The lower part of the uterus is the **cervix,** and the cavity of the uterus is connected to the vagina by means of a small opening called the cervical os. The cervix secretes mucus, which changes in consistency depending on the phase of the menstrual cycle. Some women learn to estimate the time of **ovulation** (ovum release) by examining their cervical mucus.

The vagina is a hollow tube that leads from the cervix to the outside of the body. The nonaroused vagina is approximately three to five inches long. Normally, the vaginal tube is rather narrow, but it can readily widen to accommodate the penis during intercourse, a tampon during menstruation, the passage of a baby during childbirth, or a pelvic examination. The vagina possesses a unique physiology that is maintained by the secretions that continually emanate from the vaginal walls. These secretions help control the growth of microorganisms that normally inhabit the vagina, and they also help to cleanse the vagina. Because the vagina is a self-cleansing organ, it is usually unnecessary to employ any extraordinary cleansing measures, such as douching. Very often douching merely upsets the natural chemical balance of the vagina and increases the risk of developing vaginal in-

Terms

ovaries: a pair of almond-shaped organs in the female abdomen that produce egg cells (ova) and female sex hormones

fallopian tubes: the usual site of fertilization; a pair of tube-like structures that transport ova from the ovaries to the uterus

uterus: the female organ in which a fetus develops

vagina: a woman's organ of copulation and the exit pathway for the fetus at birth

cervix: the lower, narrow end of the uterus

ovulation: release of an egg (ovum) from the ovary

vaginitis: an infection of the vagina

vulva: the female external genital structures

clitoris: small, sensitive organ located above the vaginal opening; center of sexual pleasuring

labia minora: a pair of fleshy folds that cover the vagina

labia majora: a pair of fleshy folds that cover the labia minora

urethra: a tube that carries urine from the bladder to the outside

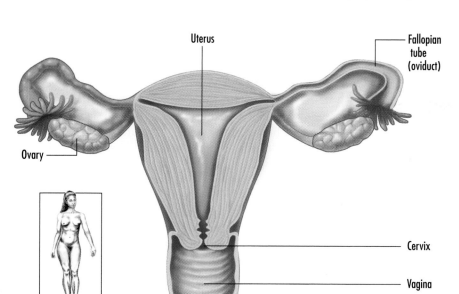

Uterus

Fallopian tube (oviduct)

Ovary

Cervix

Vagina

FIGURE 8.4   **Female Reproductive System**

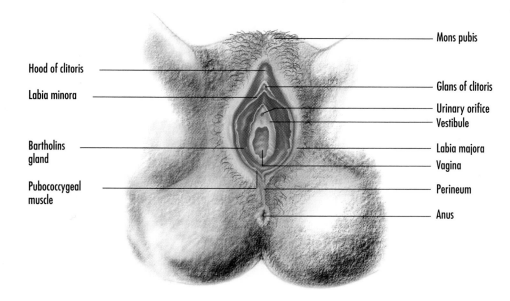

Hood of clitoris

Labia minora

Bartholins gland

Pubococcygeal muscle

Mons pubis

Glans of clitoris

Urinary orifice

Vestibule

Labia majora

Vagina

Perineum

Anus

FIGURE 8.5   **External Female Sexual Reproductive Organs**

fections, called **vaginitis.** Symptoms of vaginitis include irritation or itching of the vagina and vulva, unusual discharge, and sometimes, a disagreeable odor.

A number of factors increase susceptibility to vaginitis, including the use of antibiotics, emotional stress, a diet high in carbohydrates, hormonal changes caused by pregnancy or birth control pills, chemical irritants, intercourse without adequate lubrication, and heat and moisture retained by nylon underwear and pantyhose.

Vaginitis must be treated and cured. Chronic irritation resulting from long-term infections may predispose women to cervical cell changes that could lead to cervical cancer.

The **vulva** encompasses all female external genital structures—the hair, the folds of skin, the **clitoris,** and the urinary and vaginal openings (Figure 8.5). The smaller, inner pair of folds are called the **labia minora,** and the larger, outer pair are called the **labia majora.** The clitoris, a highly sensitive sexual organ, is situated above the vaginal opening. The external part of the clitoris, although tiny, has about the same number of nerve endings as the head of the penis. Although other sexual organs have additional functions of reproduction or the elimination of waste material, the only purpose of the clitoris is sexual arousal.

The opening of the **urethra,** which is the exit tube for urine, is located at the vaginal region just below the clitoris. The fact that the urethra is only about one-half inch long and located so close to the vagina makes it susceptible to irritation and infection, called **urethritis,** characterized by a burning sensation during urination and usually by the frequent urge to urinate. Occasionally, bacteria introduced into the urethra migrate the short distance to the bladder and produce a bladder infection called **cystitis.** The symptoms of cystitis are similar to those of urethritis.

The most frequent causes of urethritis and cystitis are irritation from sexual intercourse and the introduction of bacteria from the anal region into the vaginal region and into the urethra. To prevent urethritis and cystitis, care should be taken not to introduce anal bacteria into the vaginal region during sexual activity (manually or with the penis). It is recommended that a woman urinate immediately after having sex, wear absorbent cotton underpants or underpants with a cotton crotch, and wipe the urethra in the front-to-back direction after urinating.

A mild case of urethritis or cystitis can be helped by drinking a lot of fluids to wash the bacteria from the urinary tract and by making the urine more acidic, either by high doses of vitamin C or acidic fruit juices. It is also advisable not to drink alcohol and ingest caffeine or spices, for these substances may irritate an already inflamed urinary tract. If pain is severe or if there is blood in the urine, consult a physician.

In addition to the primary sex organs, women have secondary sex characteristics, including the **breasts.** The breasts consist of a network of milk glands and milk ducts embedded in fatty tissue, and are influenced by pregnancy, nursing, or birth control pills, as well as the different phases of the menstrual cycle. The variation in breast size among women is due to differing amounts of fatty tissue within the breasts. There is little variation among women in the amount of milk-producing tissue; thus, a woman's ability to breast feed is unrelated to the size of her breasts.

The breasts are supplied with numerous nerve endings, which are important in the delivery of milk

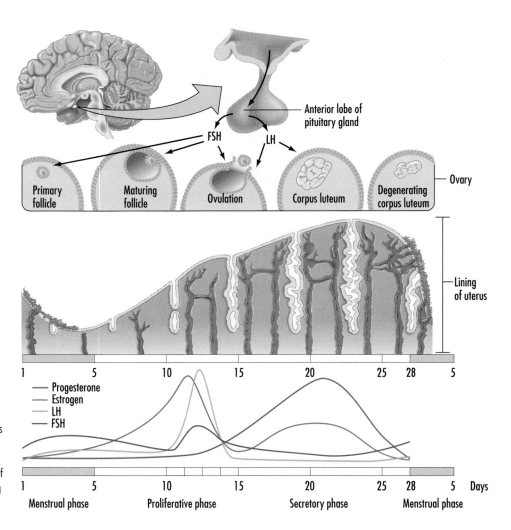

FIGURE 8.6   Hormonal Control of Menstrual Cycle Hormones from hypothalamus control release of hormones from pituitary gland, which in turn regulates production of ovum and sex hormones from ovaries. Note how the rise and fall of the hormones is related to building up and sloughing off of the uterine lining.

to a nursing baby. These nerves also make the breast highly sensitive to touch, and many women find certain forms of tactile stimulation to be sexually pleasurable. Sexual arousal, tactile stimulation, and cold temperatures can cause small muscles in the nipples to contract, resulting in erection of the nipples.

The Menstrual Cycle

Each month or so, women usually produce one ovum that is able to be fertilized. During each period of this ovum production—the menstrual cycle—a woman's body undergoes several hormonally induced changes that prepare her body for pregnancy if the ovum is fertilized. One of these changes involves the thickening of the lining of the uterus, the **endometrium,** to support the first stages of pregnancy. If conception does not occur, the lining sloughs off and is discharged as menstrual flow. In addition, certain blood vessels in the uterus increase in size. Their role is to bring the maternal nutrients to the fetus via the placenta if pregnancy occurs. This produces a loss of about 15 to 45 milliliters (about two or three tablespoons) of blood, mucus, and endometrial membranes, which leaves the body through the vagina over the course of 3 to 6 days. This discharge is **menstruation.**

The length and regularity of the menstrual cycle vary from woman to woman. Most women experience cycles of approximately 28 days, with cycle lengths between 24 and 35 days being the most common. Shorter and longer cycles are possible, but they are regarded as irregular cycles. Irregular cycles can occur monthly, with the number of days between menstruations varying from cycle to cycle. Irregular cycles are common when females first begin to menstruate and also when they stop producing ova later in life.

The menstrual cycle is controlled by a number of hormones (Figure 8.6). Hormones from the hypothalamus in the brain are secreted and influence the release of other hormones from the pituitary gland. The pituitary gland produces two gonad-stimulating hormones, **follicle-stimulating hormone** (FSH) and **luteinizing hormone** (LH). These hormones circulate throughout the woman's bloodstream and induce the secretion of estrogen and progesterone from the ovaries (Table 8.1). The menstrual cycle is regulated so that if fertilization does not occur, the hormonal support of tissue growth in the uterus stops, and the uterine tissue is lost in a menstrual discharge.

Menopause

Menarche is the first menstruation a young woman experiences. The average age for menarche is between 12 and 13 years of age, although it can occur as early as 10 years of age or as late as 19 years of age. **Menopause** is the gradual cessation of ovulation and menstruation.

Terms

urethritis: an irritation or infection of the urethra caused by bacteria

cystitis: inflammation of the bladder

breasts: secondary sex characteristics; a network of milk glands and ducts in fatty tissue

endometrium: the inner lining of the uterus

menstruation: the regular sloughing of the uterine lining via the vagina

follicle-stimulating hormone: stimulates ovaries to develop mature follicles (with eggs); the follicle produces estrogen

luteinizing hormone: stimulates the release of the ovum (egg) by the follicle; the follicle produces progesterone

menarche: the beginning of menstruation

menopause: the cessation of menstruation in mid-life

TABLE 8.1   Functions of Estrogen and Progesterone

Organ	Effect of estrogen	Effect of progesterone
Ovary	Increases sensitivity to gonadotropins; stimulates growth in ovarian cells	
Fallopian tubes	Increases motility and secretion	Decreases motility
Uterus	Stimulates proliferation of blood vessels; increases size of muscle cells; stimulates production of cervical mucus	Increases secretory activity of endometrium; decreases contractions in uterine muscle; causes changes in viscosity of cervical mucus
Vagina	Stimulates growth and changes in vaginal cells; maintains vaginal secretions	Causes changes in cells of vagina
Breasts	Stimulates growth and development of nipple and milk ducts	
Secondary sex characteristics	Stimulates feminine pattern of hair growth; stimulates feminine pattern of fat distribution	

Menopause is a time when the ovaries stop producing ova and the ovaries' production of hormones wanes considerably. Therefore, the two principal biological consequences of menopause are: a woman no longer is capable of becoming pregnant, and her body may undergo some changes from the diminished production of ovarian hormones, like estrogen. There is a wide range of age for menopause. Many women experience menopause between ages 50 and 52; however, it can occur as early as age 35 and as late as age 55. The age at which menopause occurs may be affected by hereditary, social, and nutritional factors. There is no relation between the age at which menopause occurs and the age at which a woman first begins to menstruate.

Some people see menopause as a time of rapid degeneration of a woman's body and the onset of emotional instability. They also may have the mistaken idea that because menopause signifies the end of reproductive capacity that it necessarily means the end of a woman's sexual interest and abilities. None of these beliefs has a factual basis, but what people believe may have a powerful effect on changes in physiology. We have ample evidence all around us that age is no barrier to living a fulfilled and enjoyable life. Women who accept menopause as a natural part of their life process need not slow down. They can continue to be active and healthy and can continue to enjoy sex.

Male Sexual Anatomy

The principal reproductive role of male sexual organs is to make numerous viable sperm cells and to deliver them into the female reproductive tract during sexual intercourse. The male sexual and reproductive system consists of two **testes,** the sites of sperm and sex hormone production; a series of connected sperm ducts that originate at the testes, course through the pelvis, and terminate at the urethra of the penis; glands that produce seminal fluid; and the **penis,** the organ of **copulation** (Figure 8.7).

The penis consists of nerves, blood vessels, fibrous tissue, and three parallel cylinders of spongy tissue. It does not contain bone, nor does it possess an abundance of muscular tissue, contrary to some people's beliefs. However, there is an extensive network of muscles around the base of the penis that help to eject both semen and urine through the urethra.

The testes are located in a flesh-covered sac, the **scrotum,** that hangs outside the man's body. In the embryo, the testes develop inside the body, but just before birth they descend into the scrotum. Inside the scrotum, the testes are kept at a temperature a few de-

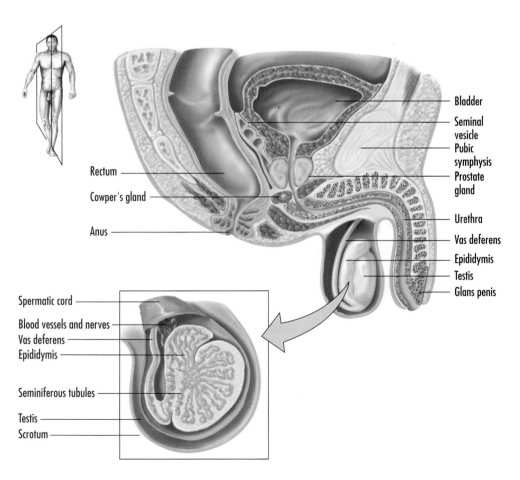

Rectum

Cowper's gland

Anus

Bladder

Seminal vesicle

Pubic symphysis

Prostate gland

Urethra

Vas deferens

Epididymis

Testis

Glans penis

Spermatic cord

Blood vessels and nerves

Vas deferens

Epididymis

Seminiferous tubules

Testis

Scrotum

FIGURE 8.7   *Male Reproductive Organs*

grees cooler than the internal body temperature, a condition that is apparently necessary for the production of reproductively capable sperm. Normally, the scrotum hangs loosely from the body wall, although influences such as cold temperatures or sexual stimulation may cause it to move closer to the body. One testis is usually a little higher than the other.

When a man ejaculates, sperm are propelled through the sperm ducts and out of the penis by contractions of the smooth muscles that line the ducts and the muscles of the pelvis. As they move out of the male body, the sperm mix with secretions of seminal fluid from the **seminal vesicles, prostate gland,** and **Cowper's glands** to form **semen.** The semen, which is the gelatinous milky fluid emitted at ejaculation, contains a mixture of about 300 million sperm cells and about 3 to 6 milliliters of seminal fluid. The seminal fluid contributes 95% or more of the entire volume of semen.

The penis is normally soft, but when a man becomes sexually aroused, its internal tissues fill with blood and the penis enlarges and becomes erect. An erection is a process coordinated by the autonomic nervous system. When a male becomes sexually aroused, the nervous system transmits messages that induce expansion of the arteries leading to the three erectile cylinders of spongy tissue in the penis. All men are born with a fold of skin, the **foreskin,** that covers the end of the penis. For centuries, Jewish and Moslem families have surgically removed the foreskin from male children for religious reasons. This procedure is called **circumcision.** Although there is no clear medical indication that circumcision is beneficial, removal of the foreskin does eliminate the buildup of **smegma,** a white, cheesy substance that can accumulate under the foreskin. The belief that circumcision

leads to an increase in sexual arousal because it exposes the glans and the related belief that circumcision produces an inability to delay ejaculation are myths. For most men, circumcision has no effect on sexual arousal and sexual activity.

Sexual Arousal and Response

Sexual arousal and response are often thought of in terms of genital stimulation, genital responses, and orgasm. But in reality, sexual experience is a holistic process involving one's body, mind, emotions, spirit, and relationship with the partner.

Sexual Arousal

Because sex is a whole-person experience, sexual interaction involves a change from a nonerotic to an erotic state of being, one in which erotic experience—for whatever reasons—is expected and sought. The change from a nonerotic to an erotic state usually involves these elements:

1. *Sexual interest:* openness to erotic arousal
2. *Desire or motivation:* energizing oneself toward creating an erotic experience
3. *Decision:* offering or accepting invitations for sex
4. *Participation:* engaging in behaviors that produce erotic arousal

Studies indicate that in both men and women sexual interest is influenced strongly and possibly maintained completely by androgens (principally testosterone), which are hormones manufactured in the testes, ovaries, and adrenal glands. For example, men with very low levels of androgen because of illness or disease usually report a loss of interest in sex. However, testosterone-replacement therapy in such men tends to restore sexual interest.

Similarly, women who have had their ovaries and adrenal glands surgically removed for treatment of cervical or breast cancer (to prevent production of hormones that might stimulate the growth of the cancer) often report a loss of interest in sex. Interest can be restored with replacement testosterone, but not estrogen or progesterone. Also, women's sexual interest does not change predictably when estrogen levels fall during the menstrual cycle or after menopause.

Although in our society people are expected to be highly and frequently interested in sex, in reality the desire for sexual activity varies among individuals and couples, changes over time, and is influenced by interpersonal and psychological factors. For example, many couples report a higher degree of sexual desire at the beginning of their relationship than after the relationship has matured. Alternatively, couples who have

---

Terms

testes: a pair of male reproductive organs that produce sperm cells and male sex hormones

penis: the male's organ of copulation and urination

copulation: sexual intercourse

scrotum: the sac of skin that contains the testes

seminal vesicles: sac-like structures that secrete a fluid that activates the sperm

prostate gland: gland at the base of the bladder providing seminal fluid

Cowper's glands: small glands secreting drops of alkalinizing fluid into the urethra

semen: a whitish, creamy fluid containing sperm

foreskin: a fold of skin over the end of the penis

circumcision: a surgical procedure to remove the foreskin from the penis

smegma: a white, cheesy substance that accumulates under the foreskin of the penis

been together for many years may experience an increase in sexual interest when the childrearing phase of the family life cycle is completed. Various physical and psychological situations can affect sexual interest as well. For example, many women report a transient loss of sexual interest during the first few weeks after childbirth. And depression is sometimes associated with loss of interest in sex.

Having sexual desire does not necessarily mean that a person will behave sexually. Human sexual behavior is not "reflexive"; activity does not occur automatically whenever one feels "horny" or one is presented with a sexual opportunity. Instead, sexual activity is the result of a decision (except in instances of sexual coercion and assault) that is based on desire to conform to social norms, personal values, and physical and psychological needs.

Creating a sexual experience involves two kinds of decision. The first concerns context, that is, the social situation in which sexual activity takes place. Societies have rules and norms that govern sexual activity. Individuals are not permitted to have sex with just anyone or in any social setting. For example, most people have sex only in the bedroom, not in the living room or kitchen or dining room.

The second type of decision concerns participation in a sexual episode. Even in a situation or relationship in which sexual activity is acceptable, and opportunities to have sex are present, a person can decide "yes," "no," "not yet," or "maybe" whenever a sexual opportunity occurs. The decision is made by evaluating how one feels physically and emotionally at the time, one's personal criteria for being sexual within the presenting situation, and one's expectation of how having sex at that time will affect one's self-esteem and the relationship.

There is no formula for creating sexual arousal. Everyone has preferences. In situations and circumstances that they deem appropriate for sex, most people respond sexually to being touched in certain ways. Certain regions of the body are highly sexually sensitive in nearly all people. These are the classic erogenous zones—the genitals, the breasts, the anus, the lips, the inner thighs, and the mouth.

The Sexual Response Cycle

When a person becomes sexually aroused, the brain and nervous system prepare the body for sexual activity. Impulses from the brain are transmitted by the spinal nerves to various parts of the body and cause physiological changes. These changes include: the tightening of many skeletal muscles (**myotonia**); changes in the pattern of blood flow or **vasocongestion** (especially an increase in blood flow in the pelvis); increases in heart rate, blood pressure, and respiratory

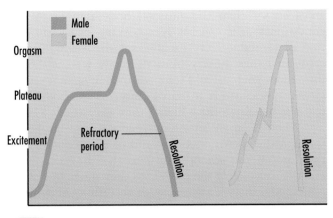

FIGURE 8.8   **Sexual Response Cycle as Identified by Masters and Johnson**

rate; increase in the general level of excitement; and increase in erotic feelings.

Increased pelvic blood flow in the male produces erection of the penis. The penis enlarges because the spongy tissues within it fill with blood. In the female, increased pelvic blood flow produces lubrication of the vagina and swelling of the clitoris and vaginal lips. Vaginal lubrication is produced by the release of fluids from the walls of the vagina. Swelling of the clitoris and vaginal lips is due to the filling with blood of spongy tissues within them. In some women the changes in blood flow due to sexual arousal also produce a swelling of the breasts.

Regardless of the type of sexual stimulation, the physiological response in both men and women is similar and follows a pattern called the **sexual response cycle**, which consists of four phases as identified by Masters and Johnson (Figure 8.8):

- *Phase 1:* Excitement, in which the person experiences sexual arousal from any source and the body responds with specific changes: erection of the penis in males; vaginal lubrication and swelling of the clitoris and genitalia in females; and sex flush in both males and females.
- *Phase 2:* Plateau, in which the physiological changes of the excitement phase level off, although subjective feelings of sexual arousal may increase.
- *Phase 3:* Orgasm, in which the tensions that build up during excitement and plateau are released.
- *Phase 4:* Resolution, in which the body returns to the physiologically nonstimulated state. In addition, Masters and Johnson include a refractory period (a recovery stage in which there is a temporary inability to reach orgasm) in the male resolution phase.

There is considerable variation in the extent and duration of the sexual response cycle among individuals of either sex. There is even variation in the nature of the response in the same person, for each sexual encounter is different. Masters and Johnson (1966) found more variation in the sexual response cycle for women than for men.

Orgasm

When sexual arousal builds to a certain point, the associated sexual tensions are released in an **orgasm.** The orgasmic response in both women and men frequently is associated with rhythmic contractions of the pelvic muscles; tightening of the muscles of the face, hands, and feet; and feelings of pleasure. Most commonly, men ejaculate during orgasm, although it is possible for males to experience orgasm without ejaculation and vice versa. The media have perpetuated the myth that during male or female orgasm, bells ring, the earth shakes, lights flash, and moans and groans are elicited. But often orgasms are quiet.

Orgasmic experiences vary greatly from person to person and from one encounter to another. For all persons there are "big orgasms" and "little orgasms" depending on the level of arousal. Sometimes, if a person is not sufficiently aroused, or too tired, tense or ill, there may be no orgasm.

Our society is oriented toward achievement, and it has become common to apply measures of success to sex, especially orgasm. For example, many people believe that "success" is determined by the number of orgasms a woman has during a sexual episode. By this standard, a successful male is someone who can delay ejaculation until his partner has experienced at least one orgasm and preferably more, whereas a successful female is someone who can have several explosive orgasms in every sexual encounter. Men and women who cannot "manufacture" the appropriate number of orgasms may be erroneously labeled "inadequate" by themselves and others. When people become overly concerned with "succeeding" or "performing well," they can become psychologically detached from the activity. Rather than abandon themselves completely to sexual experience, they withdraw their attention and observe their actions. This is called **spectatoring.**

Couples are likely to enjoy sex more if they allow for different kinds of orgasm experience:

- Either partner may reach orgasm through manual, oral, or other means of sexual stimulation before or after intercourse.
- Sexual activity need not stop after one partner reaches orgasm. If a couple chooses, lovemaking can continue until both wish to stop.
- Neither individual may desire an orgasm during a particular sexual episode. Physically expressing love and caring does not require orgasm.

Masturbation

Masturbation is self-stimulation to produce erotic arousal, usually to the point of orgasm. While social and religious attitudes in many cultures consider it improper, immoral, or perverse, masturbation is nevertheless practiced widely throughout the world and even among other animal species.

Many people find masturbation a rewarding variation in their sex lives. People masturbate for many of the same reasons that they have partner sex: to experience erotic pleasure; to relieve physical tensions; to produce a sense of relaxation; to induce sleep; and when done with a partner, to create feelings of intimacy and bonding. Often, people find masturbation to be valuable as a means of self-exploration so they can better understand what pleases them sexually.

A number of personal harmful effects have long been rumored to result from masturbation. Among them are hair loss, insanity, pimples, warts, unhappy personal relations, and the inability to have children. There is no evidence that any of these claims are true. Physically, masturbation is harmless as long as it is not injurious to the stimulated organs.

Sexual Abstinence

Although for most people interest in and desire for sex is relatively constant, some people choose to abstain from sexual activity. For religious reasons certain people practice lifelong sexual abstinence (sometimes called **celibacy,** which literally means remaining unmarried). Some individuals refrain from sexual intercourse until they marry. Still others avoid sexual interaction because they fear the closeness and intimacy implied by sex or they have strong negative feelings regarding sex.

Individuals not wishing to practice lifelong sexual abstinence may nevertheless benefit from a sex "time

Terms

myotonia: muscle tension

vasocongestion: the engorgement of blood vessels in particular body parts in response to sexual arousal

sexual response cycle: the physiological response in both men and women as described in four phases

orgasm: the climax of sexual responses and the release of physiological and sexual tensions

spectatoring: observing one's own sexual experience rather than fully taking part in it

masturbation: self-induced sexual stimulation

celibacy: sexual abstinence

out." For example, recovery from a physical or emotional illness may include sexual abstinence. No sex is a sure way to avoid an unintended pregnancy or a sexually transmitted disease. Some people find abstaining helpful while recovering from the break-up of a love relationship. The healing of the emotional wound seems to proceed more smoothly without the emotional intensity that often accompanies sexual interaction.

Sexual abstinence can also provide an opportunity to develop a new set of personal and relational experiences. By avoiding the intimacy that accompanies a lot of sex, abstinence provides a way to discover new dimensions in interpersonal relationships. Without the diversion of sex (or the search for sex partners) an individual can focus on self-development, career, or school and put energy into long-time friendships. New romantic relationships can develop without the pressure for sex early in the relationship, thus permitting the partners to develop trust and caring before becoming sexual.

For some, sexual abstinence seems like a hardship because their sexual needs and their needs for touching, physical contact, and emotional closeness may not be met. During a period of sexual abstinence, the need for touching and physical contact can be met through professional (nonsexual) massage, or hugging among friends and between parents and children. Masturbation can relieve sexual tensions. And intimacy needs can be met by deepening one's ongoing friendships, giving oneself to others through volunteer work, increasing one's level of self-awareness and self-development, or involving oneself in spiritual and religious activity.

Sexual Difficulties

Many individuals expect sex always to be exciting and satisfying; anything less is cause for concern. Life is full of changes, however, and the demands of career or parenting or occasional physical illness can sometimes produce a temporary loss in interest in sex or the ability to engage in sex (Table 8.2). Such changes in sexual interest and ability are normal and usually resolve themselves eventually. Persistent difficulties with sex may signal that consulting a therapist would be helpful. Lack of interest in sex may be connected to many factors, including failure to communicate likes and dislikes; boredom; stress, fatigue, and depression; alcohol and drugs; pregnancy and children; hostility and anger; change in physical appearance; and physical illness.

Lack of Interest   Therapists and counselors refer to the lack of interest in sex as hypoactive sexual desire or sexual aversion, and note that it can result from:

1. *Underlying sexual difficulty.* One or both partners may have some physical difficulty engaging in sex: a man may be unable to gain or maintain an erection or a woman experiences pain during intercourse. Such problems can make sexual activity unpleasant for either or both partners, and they eventually lose sexual interest in each other.

2. *Failure to communicate likes and dislikes.* One partner may find some aspects of sex unsatisfying and not communicate this information to the partner. Resentment and displeasure may subsequently build up to the point that interest in sex is lost.

3. *Boredom.* Like anything else that becomes predictable and routine, sex can become boring if it is always done in the same way and at the same time. As with other activities, the old cliché is true: "Variety is the spice of life."

4. *Stress, fatigue, and depression.* Being emotionally drained by work or other responsibilities or being "low" or "blue" can interfere with sexual desire.

5. *Alcohol and other drugs.* Frequent ingestion of alcohol and other drugs can lower sexual desire. Drug use can also turn off a partner who does not want to make love to someone who is drunk or on drugs. Some medications can also lessen interest in sex.

6. *Pregnancy and children.* During pregnancy and child raising the increase in responsibilities and the decrease in private time can lower interest in sex.

TABLE 8.2   Factors Contributing to Sexual Difficulties

Types of factors	*Examples*
Organic factors	Illness of any kind Hormonal, vascular, and neurological illness Fatigue or psychoendocrine stress Medications and recreational drugs
Values, beliefs, and attitudes	*Negative values about sex:* Sex is dirty; sex is sinful Genitals (especially female) are dirty Women are not supposed to enjoy sex Men are supposed to always be interested in sex Men are supposed to always be capable of sex *Narrow definition of sex:* Sex = penis-in-vagina intercourse Goal orientation (sex = orgasm) Performance expectations
Personality and experiences	Low self-esteem Emotional difficulties (anxiety, depression, grief) Prior incidence of sexual abuse Poor body image
Relationship factors	Discomfort with intimacy Relationship problems Fear of pregnancy or sexually transmitted disease Sexual orientation

Wellness Guide

Tips for Enhancing Sexual Experience

- Create pleasure by stimulating the whole body, not just the genitals.
- Vary the manner and intensity of stimulation. Allow sensations to build and wane.
- Try not to make sex = work.
- Set aside time that is free of intrusions and distractions. Disconnect the phone; lock the door to ensure privacy.
- Make yourself an open, effective channel for sexual arousal before sexual activity begins.

Satisfying sex is not a mechanical activity involving only bodies, but a blending of mind-body energies. Remove sex-negative energies such as hunger, fatigue, and anger, and focus your energy on sex through deep breathing or other relaxing activity.

- Be aware of differences between you and your partner in the state of readiness for sexual activity. Try to synchronize both partners' states of sexual arousal through talking, light touching,

dance, massage, and so on, before sexual activity begins.

- Address concerns about birth control and STDs prior to sexual experience.
- Take your time. Go slowly.
- Communicate likes and dislikes to your partner either verbally or nonverbally.
- Do not focus just on orgasms. Learn to appreciate the many sexual sensations from touching all parts of the body.

Busy couples must make an effort to schedule time to be together (for sex and other activities).

7. *Hostility and anger.* Unresolved conflicts are a common cause of lost sexual interest. It may be difficult to feel intimate with someone with whom you are angry.

8. *Change in physical appearance.* Once they are in a relationship, some people stop caring about their appearance, which may lessen a partner's sexual interest.

9. *Physical illness.* Physical illnesses can cause some people to believe they shouldn't have sex. For example, the man who has a heart attack may be afraid to have sex because he fears another heart attack.

Erection Problems Difficulty in achieving or maintaining an erection can be the result of an injury or disease. It can also be due to alcohol, heroin, and other recreational drugs and some medications for high blood pressure. More often, however, erection problems are the result of fear of sexual performance (including anxiety about one's ability to get an erection) or the wish not to be sexual with a particular partner.

Ejaculation Control It is impossible to define "rapid" or "premature" ejaculation in terms of minutes; however, some therapists define it as absence of voluntary control of ejaculation. Ejaculation is a reflex activity that a man can learn to control just as he does bladder function. The key to controlling ejaculation is awareness of the bodily sensations that signal the onset of ejaculation, followed by modulating arousal according to one's desires.

Painful Intercourse In women, painful intercourse can be caused by vaginal infections, insufficient vaginal lubrication before intercourse (usually the result of not being sufficiently sexually aroused), and anxiety-produced spasms of the muscles surrounding the vagina, which makes vaginal penetration painful. Another source of pain associated with intercourse, which can affect both women and men, is a deep, aching sensation in the pelvis for women or scrotum ("blue balls") for men occurring during sex. This condition is caused by the congestion of blood in the pelvic region brought about by sexual arousal. Orgasm often reverses the congestion, but lack of orgasm can cause blood to remain and cause discomfort and pain.

Orgasm Difficulties Both men and women can have difficulty experiencing orgasm. Most often this difficulty is the result of insufficient sexual arousal, perhaps because of aversion to a particular partner, fear of pregnancy or sexually transmitted diseases, fear of letting go, lack of trust, or negative attitudes about sexual pleasure.

Developing Positive Sexual Relationships

We all need intimacy—that feeling of closeness, trust, and openness with another person that tells us that our innermost self can be shared without fear of attack or emotional hurt and that we are understood in the deepest sense possible.

Intimate relationships can have an enormous impact on one's sense of vitality and well-being. When an intimate relationship is flowing smoothly, it can produce rich emotional satisfaction unparalleled by any other experience. Those who are involved in genuinely supportive and caring relationships tend to feel confident about the potential of life to be harmonious and beautiful. On the other hand, when an intimate relationship is not going well, those involved can be overwhelmed by moroseness, and unable to think of anything but their misery. They can be angry, depressed, anxious, or distraught, sometimes to the point of being unable to function at work or at school.

A lack of intimacy in life can adversely affect physical health as well as emotions and feelings. Studies indicate that married people are in better physical health than divorced, separated, and widowed people. The association between intimacy and physical health is suggested by the finding that recently widowed people suffer increased mortality during the first few months after the death of their spouse. Apparently these people do indeed die of a "broken heart." Such evidence demonstrates the substantial link between emotions and physical health that is so fundamental to the holistic health philosophy.

What Is Intimacy?

Many people mistakenly equate genuine intimacy with sexual intercourse. This happens because love and affection are feelings associated with intimacy, and in our culture there is much confusion about love and sex. But intimacy is a feeling, not an act. It is the *quality* of a relationship between two people—a shared experiencing of their personal lives. People who have an intimate relationship may or may not choose to express their closeness with sex.

Many kinds of intimacies are possible. There are intimacies between other-sex peers, same-sex peers, children and parents, members of a family, neighbors, close friends, and even co-workers. Each intimacy has its unique and distinctive quality depending on the people involved, on the extent to which their personal histories are similar, and on the facets of themselves they choose to share with each other.

Yet intimacies possess certain common characteristics. They are relationships of mutual consent. One person cannot be intimate with another unless both agree that that is what they want. Intimacies tend to grow deeper and richer over time; partners need to share meaningful experiences in order to establish genuine trust and caring. Intimacies also carry the feeling that the personalities of the intimates are interconnected in some complex way. This is not the same as the feeling of having their identities merge so they become "one," but rather that they feel both joined and separate at the same time in some way.

The Life Cycle of Intimate Relationships

Intimate relationships tend to develop through the stages of (a) selecting a partner, (b) developing intimacy, and (c) establishing commitment. Before an intimate relationship can develop, however, the partners have to be psychologically open to entering and maintaining it. Some individuals choose not to be involved in an intimate relationship, perhaps because they wish to devote energies to school, work, or self-development or they find intimate relationships to be distracting or psychologically threatening. In some instances, previous life experiences can leave an individual fearful of emotional closeness, which can block the establishment of intimacy. In some of these instances, there are repeated attempts to form relationships; however, without the element of intimacy, these relationships often fail.

Factors that influence the choice of intimate partners include:

- *Proximity.* People are most likely to become intimate with someone with whom they are in physical proximity.
- *Similarity.* Similar age, religion, race, education, social background, attitudes, values, and interests affect the possibility for intimacy in two ways: (1) they influence proximity and (2) they reflect social norms for permissible peer intimacies. Note, for example, biases against interracial and older-younger intimacies. Colleges and universities provide students with

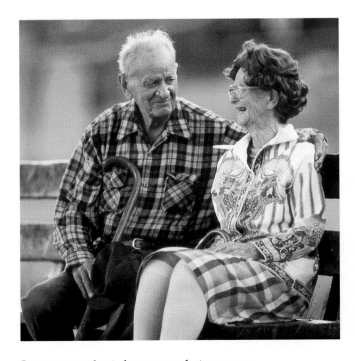

Intimacy is a basic human need at every age.

relatively easy access to a "pool of eligibles" because they bring together individuals of similar age, religion, intelligence, expectations, and values.

- *Physical appearance.* Physical appearance provides cues that indicate who among the pool of eligibles is a desirable intimate partner. Those who are judged "attractive" tend to be thought of as kind, understanding, and affectionate ("what is beautiful is good"). Pairing with someone who is considered physically attractive enhances one's social status and self-esteem.

Developing Intimacy

Most people want their intimate relationships to develop feelings of closeness, positive regard, warmth, and familiarity with the other's innermost thoughts and feelings. This deep knowledge of each other comes from sharing the most important and often secret aspects of one's personality—one's goals, aspirations, strengths, weaknesses, and physical and sexual desires. The sharing of such private information is called **self-disclosure.**

When relationships begin, little intimate information is usually disclosed. People talk about the weather, the stock market, or politics. They gossip about professors, students, or other people they know. And they ask each other the classic leading questions: Where are you from? What do you do? What's your major? People face these questions so many times that they become adept at revealing as much or as little about themselves as feels comfortable. It is when they begin to talk about their personal history, current life problems, hopes and aspirations, and fears and personal failures that they begin to disclose important information—important because disclosing it makes them feel vulnerable. Most people discuss their deepest feelings only with those in whom they have developed considerable trust.

Intimacy develops through a progressive, mutual revealing of innermost thoughts. Psychologists compare people's personalities to onions—having many layers from an outer surface to an inner core. As acquaintances gain more and more knowledge about each other, they penetrate deeper and deeper through the layers of the other's personality, which establishes their intimacy. Another view compares intimate development to the peeling of an artichoke. Resistance and barriers to sharing information about oneself are like the leaves of the artichoke; as intimacy progresses, intimates peel away the leaves to get to the other's "heart."

Self-disclosure leads to the development of intimacy in two ways. First, you tend to be affected either positively or negatively by the information that is disclosed. If you make a positive judgment, you are likely to want to continue interacting with that person, for you believe that future interactions will be equally or even more positive. The same logic applies to negative assessments. If your reaction is unfavorable, you are likely to terminate the relationship, or perhaps maintain it on a lesser level of intimacy.

The second way that self-disclosure leads to intimacy is the *act* of self-disclosure, which, regardless of the information offered, often leads to reciprocal self-disclosure. By sharing important information, you communicate that you trust the other person, and usually that person accepts your trust and becomes more willing to disclose information. In this way intimacy progresses by a cycle of self-disclosure leading to trust, which brings about self-disclosure, which leads to more trust, and so on.

Establishing Commitment

After a period of self-disclosure, individuals may sense that their relationship has progressed to a state of "us-ness," that it has become a special friendship, a love relationship, or a marital-type relationship. This state of "us-ness" is one of commitment, which has three aspects.

- *An action, pledge, or promise.* One makes a promise and thus announces one's intention explicitly, even if it is only to the partner. Various social values and norms regarding keeping promises and the guilt and loss of self-esteem that come with breaking promises are among the "push" factors that keep a person committed. If the promise involves a social ritual (i.e., marriage ceremony, getting pinned), then family, friends, and the state become additional "push" factors.
- *A state of being obligated or emotionally compelled.* This state involves a cluster of emotions such as love, comfort, caring, and relief from separation anxiety and loneliness.
- *An unwillingness to consider any partner other than the current one.* The rewards of the current relationship outweigh the costs of exploring other opportunities for intimacy.

Endings

Everything in the universe (even the universe itself!) has a beginning and an end. Close relationships have a

Intimacy begins by doing fun things together.

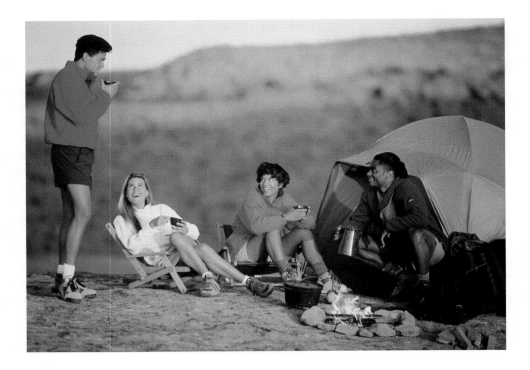

beginning and an end also. Sometimes a relationship lasts for only a few minutes; sometimes it lasts until one of the partners dies (and even then the relationship may still be "alive" in the imagination of the surviving partner). Sometimes the structure of a close relationship persists but the closeness and the dynamism wane, creating a "shell" relationship without vitality. Sometimes a relationship goes through cycles of birth and death within the structure of its ongoingness. When a close relationship ends, some or all of its structure, exchange of resources (e.g., love, caring, financial support), and feelings of attachment and emotional bondedness end also.

Endings occur for a variety of reasons. Partners' feelings of attachment and bondedness may be absent or weak. Life goals, values, or interests may no longer be shared. One or both partners may be unwilling or unable to invest personal resources such as greater time shared with the partner, or to commit to an exclusive relationship. Whether partners continue in a relationship also is affected by their assessment of other options such as another potential partner or singlehood. Without suitable alternatives, leaving a relationship may seem difficult, unwise, or impossible.

Another reason ongoingness stops is that the partners, either individually or as a dyadic unit, are unable to move the relationship into its next stage. For example, some couples cannot navigate the transition from being idealistic, passionate lovers to realistic, companionate lovers. In nonmarital close relationships, a partner may not be considered suitable as a

potential marital partner, even in the presence of considerable love, attachment, and liking.

Another factor associated with endings is lack of support, or even hostility, from the partners' social network. Families may not accept a son's or daughter's choice of a dating or marital partner. Interracial, disabled, and same-sex relationships are still heavily stigmatized in our society.

Occasionally the seeds of an ending are sown into a relationship at its beginning. For example, partners may seek closeness as a way to cope with or avoid personal problems. They may feel rejected and lonely because of the break-up of a previous relationship. They may feel that they cannot take care of themselves. They may be afraid of leaving home or school. If, as often happens, a partner or relationship does not turn out to be the solution to a personal problem, a disappointed, angry, or frustrated partner may seek alternative ways of coping. These alternatives, such as drug or alcohol abuse, extra-relationship affairs, or physically or emotionally abusing the partner (or other family members) (see chapter 23), may very well be destructive to the relationship.

When a break-up does occur, individuals may feel tired, lethargic, lonely, sad, depressed, angry, resentful, and guilty. They may be unable to sleep or eat, may miss class, or be unable to work. They may withdraw from friends. They may find concentrating difficult, because they are continually thinking about the partner and what happened in the relationship. They may feel helpless ("what will become of me?") and hopeless ("I'll never find a true love") or skeptical and cynical ("love can never work out").

Some partners feel relaxed, hopeful, and relieved that what they identify as a bad or going-nowhere relationship has ended, and they are free to pursue personal goals or find a relationship partner who is better suited to them. Sometimes individuals feel euphoric and self-confident. They say that the separation was for the best, and they become more active and outgoing. This positive outlook may alternate with emotional distress.

When a person is emotionally (and sometimes physically) wracked with the pain of an ending, he or she may have difficulty seeing any good in that experience, but often endings mark the start of a new and better future. A study of remarried people showed that many had learned a lot about themselves and the nature of close relationships from a previous marriage(s) and found that their current marriage was much more satisfying. Guiding principles for enhanced relationships are patience and experience.

Communicating in Intimate Relationships

Communication is a symbolic process of creating and sharing meaning. At the heart of communication is an individual act, which involves imparting a message to another person to share information or feelings, to coordinate behavior with an individual or group of people, or to persuade someone to do something.

A communication act begins as a mental image; an idea, a wish, or a feeling (or some combination of all three). If humans were capable of mind reading, senders could impart mental images directly to receivers. Few people can read minds, however, so communication requires that thoughts be transformed into symbols that can carry information. Those symbols make up the message. The most common symbols in communication are:

- *Words:* spoken, printed, or shouted
- *Visual images:* paintings, sculpture
- *Posture or body language:* gaze, touch, smile, physical proximity, folding arms, frowning, turning away
- *Objects:* flowers, gifts, food
- *Behaviors:* doing a favor, giving a kiss, ignoring an appointment

Terms

literal message: a message that is conveyed by symbols

metamessage: how the message is interpreted between sender and receiver

The sender's encoding of her or his mental images into the symbols that make up the message is only half of a communication act. The other half is the receiver's reactions: this involves taking in the symbols that make up the message and decoding them into her or his own mental images. Thus, a communication act requires two transformations: in the sender, the transformation of mental images into symbols; in the receiver, the transformation of symbols into mental images.

Consider this example of a communication act between Beth and Ron one rainy morning. Beth doesn't want Ron to get wet in the rain, so she decides to use spoken words as the symbols to encode her thoughts. Beth says, "Ron, it's raining." Ron hears Beth's words, and decodes them into a mental image of the weather that day, and he picks up his umbrella.

In this communication act Beth accomplished her goal. But a different outcome could have occurred if one or more of the steps in the communication act had been distorted, weakened, or blocked completely. For example, if Beth had said "it's raining" in a tone of voice that Ron didn't appreciate, or if her words had been misunderstood, the communication process would have been distorted.

> *Start every day with a smile and get it over with.*
> W. C. FIELDS

Every communication act carries two types of message or potential meaning. The first is the **literal message,** which is the message conveyed by the symbols themselves, as in the words "it's raining." The second is the **metamessage** ("meta" is the Greek word for "beyond," "additional," or "transcendent"), which carries implicit messages about the reason for the communication, how the message is to be interpreted, and the nature of the relationship of the sender and receiver. Most metacommunication occurs unconsciously.

When Beth said to Ron, "it's raining," not only did she send a literal message about the weather, but she also sent several metamessages, including "I care about you" and "an expectation in our relationship is that we help each other out."

After Beth had told Ron that it was raining, if Ron had kissed Beth and said, "Thanks, honey, for looking out for me," he would have been responding to one of the metamessages in the communication. If Ron had interpreted the metamessage as, "Ron, you're terribly childlike and I have to make decisions for you"—even though Beth didn't intend to impart that message—Ron might have responded angrily with something like, "Beth, I can look out for myself!" Her feelings may then have been hurt and possibly they would have had an argument. Acknowledging and responding to metamessages can sometimes be much more important than dealing with the literal ones.

The basis for effective sexual communication is **mutual empathy**—the underlying knowledge that each partner in a relationship cares for the other and knows that the care is reciprocated.

Sending Clear Messages

A clear message is one in which the symbols represent as closely as possible the sender's intent. Clear messages are best delivered with **I-statements;** these are sentences that begin with (or have as the subject) the pronoun "I." I-statements clearly identify the sender as the source of a thought, emotion, desire, or act: I think . . . . I feel . . . . I want (need) . . . . I did (will do) . . . .

If I could tell you what it meant, there would be no point in dancing it.
ISADORA DUNCAN, dancer

You-statements, which begin with (or have as the subject) the pronoun "you," as in "You always . . . ," "You never . . . ," "You are . . . ," or the interrogatives, "Why don't you . . . ?" or "How could you . . . ?" often are put-downs or character assassinations. They imply that the receiver is not-OK. Very often the not-OK message is explicit, as in "You're incompetent" or "You're stupid"—just about any negative adjective will do. People often respond to the metamessage in a you-statement, which is "I think you're no good," by feeling attacked, which can lead to hurt feelings and counterattacks or withdrawal.

Effective Listening

Effective communication requires both sending and receiving, both talking and listening. Effective listening is important because the receiver not only takes in the sender's message, but also helps establish the physical and emotional context for the communication. The listener also must communicate to the sender that the sender's message was received. This is called **feedback.** Some techniques for effective receiving are: giving the sender your full attention; making eye contact; listening; being empathic; being open for receiving the message; giving verbal feedback; acknowledging the sender's feelings; praising the sender's efforts; and being unconditional.

Give the Sender Your Full Attention Don't fake it. If you can't pay attention because you are tired, hungry, distracted, angry, or whatever, tell the sender how you feel and ask if it's OK to talk after you rest, or eat, or go to the bathroom, or just talk at another time. The sender is likely to grant your request if immediacy is not an issue, because he or she wants your full attention.

Make Eye Contact Try to assume similar postures (i.e., both sitting or both standing) to create a sense of equal status. Making eye-to-eye contact allows the sender to feel comfortable as well as conveying that you are listening to her and taking in the complete message.

Just Listen Don't interrupt until you have a signal that the sender is finished or until the sender has asked for a response, unless you don't understand what is being communicated. You can acknowledge that you are actively listening with gestures, nods, and vocalizations like "uh-huh," "yes," "go on," "I see," and so forth.

Be Empathic Try to "hear" the sender's feelings as well as the words. Be open to the sender's intentions and motivations as well as her or his ideas. Ask yourself, "What is this person feeling right now?"

When communication breaks down, stress and tension ensue.

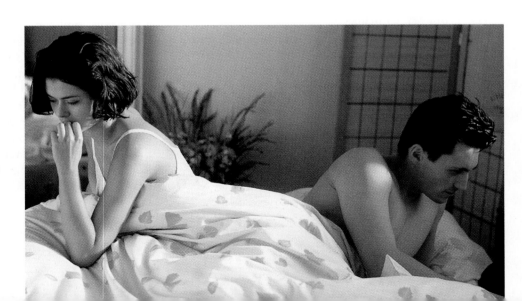

Managing Stress

<u>Pillow Talk</u>

When problems arise among intimate couples, virtually every incident can be traced back to some misinterpretation in communication. "I thought you said this!" "I thought you meant that." Although not all communication styles are verbal, the amount of communication expressed through words leads to most of the difficulty in relationships. Poor communication in any relationship, and in particular sexual relationships, can lead to stress.

There are many issues involving sexual intercourse that can act as stressors. These include, but are not limited to, contraception, fertility control, risk of pregnancy, infertility, STDs, vaginismus, molestation, celibacy, guilt, rape, self-respect, abortion, impotency, premature ejaculation, intimacy, ability to reach orgasm, homosexuality, and sexual satisfaction. This incomplete list is quite long and each item weighs heavy as a stressor for those who experience it. In addition, problems of this nature do not go away once a couple has initiated sexual relations. To the contrary, if communications are poor at the start of a relationship, they tend to get worse as the relationship continues. Sex counselors advocate that *before* and *after* each and every act of sexual intimacy there should be a thorough conversation airing these and other issues. As any AIDS patient or women with an unwanted pregnancy will tell you, the short-term pleasures of sex are surely not worth risking your life, nor are they worth the days, months, and years of agony that may follow unresolved sex-related problems. The stakes of sexual encounters are high. Make it a point to include a healthy conversation as a requirement in all sexually intimate encounters.

Here are some suggestions for conversation with someone you become intimate with.

- Learn to become comfortable with words about sexual intimacy, such as erection, penis, orgasm, and condom. The inability to articulate your feelings and preferences creates additional stress in relationships.

- If you are anxious about explaining your feelings, rehearse a conversation in which you ask your partner how he or she feels about you, where he or she likes to be touched, or tell him or her that you wish to date him or her exclusively (specific aspects of this degree of intimacy).

- Learn to ask your partner what pleases him or her and what they don't like. Conversely, feel assertive enough to make known your preferences to your partner. Don't assume that he or she knows.

Open channels of communication are vital to the health of intimate relationships, whereas poor communication only adds to the stress of a relationship. In uncomfortable moments, your first reaction may be to avoid confronting issues of intimacy. At these times, rather than giving in to reactions of avoidance or silence, we must respond with an open heart.

Be an Open Channel for Receiving the Message Don't judge or evaluate the sender or the message while the sender is talking. Try not to correct the sender or, if the sender is being critical of you, to think of a defense.

Give Verbal Feedback Don't mind read. Summarize in your own words your understanding of the sender's thoughts and emotions. This way the sender can find out if the message that was intended was actually received. If so, then you can respond. If not, then the sender can try again. Ask for clarification if there's something you don't understand. You can say something like, "I don't think I understand everything you were saying about your mother. Can you tell me again, maybe in a different way?"

Acknowledge the Sender's Emotions "It seems to me that you're feeling . . ." and if you're not sure, add "do I have that right?" By acknowledging or providing feedback, you are sharing what you believe are the sender's emotions. If you are incorrect, the sender can relay that to you.

Praise the Sender's Effort Acknowledge the sender's efforts for investing the time, energy, and care to communicate with you, especially if the communication was a difficult one.

Be Unconditional Let the sender know that you respect him or her even if you are uncomfortable with the messages that are being communicated. Assure the sender that even though things may be difficult, you are willing to continue talking and working through difficult feelings.

Terms

mutual empathy: both partners care about and understand each other

I-statements: statements beginning with "I"; positive communication skill

you-statements: statements beginning with "You"; negative communication skill

feedback: response of the receiver of a message to let the sender know the message was received

Expressing Anger Constructively

Disagreements and conflicts are inevitable in any close relationship. The notion that people in intimate relationships shouldn't have to fight because love makes them see eye to eye on everything and the idea that you can't possibly be angry with someone you love are romantic myths. By expressing anger constructively, intimates fight for the success of their relationship as well as for their individual needs.

In constructive fighting, there should be no "winner" and no "loser." Good fights are efforts of individuals to be heard and to improve the relationship. The best fights occur when the people involved feel that they have gained something.

Here are some suggestions for expressing anger constructively:

- Try not to let anger and resentment build up over time. Express feelings when you become aware of them.

- Agree on a time, a place, and the content for fights. It is certainly acceptable to get mad spontaneously if that is how you feel, but it is better to set aside a specific time for the resolution of an issue rather than trying to deal with it when you or your partner may not be psychologically or physically ready to argue. Be sure that the person you are angry with knows what the issue is before the fight.

- Be specific as to what you are angry about and stick to the issue. Don't bring up old hurts. Try not to discuss second and third topics, especially as a means of retaliation.

- Attack the problem, not each other. Don't denigrate the other's personal qualities. Use I-statements to communicate resentments. I-statements tell how you feel. You-statements are often received as personal attacks. At the same time, express appreciation for your partner as a person. This acknowledges that we can be angered by our partners' behaviors and feel loving toward them as people at the same time.

- Try to resolve the issue with an air of compromise and respect. Try to understand the other's point of view.

- Know when it is time to stop. Sometimes you can sense that the argument isn't getting resolved. It is okay to acknowledge that and to take a few hours or days to reconsider things and to discuss the issue again. Sometimes emotions are too high and it is not possible to think clearly. That may be the time to stop the fight until tempers cool.

- Engaging in sex or any other affectionate behavior before an issue is resolved should not be taken as a sign that everything is forgotten. Such behavior shows that the fight fits into what is believed to be healthy relationship.

- Don't hold grudges.

Critical Thinking About Health

1. Think about the small children in your immediate or extended family. How did your family gender-type these children (e.g., clothes, toys, decoration of rooms, playmates)? How does the media contribute to gender-typing of children? Does gender-typing continue as we grow older? (Give examples to back up your answer.)

2. In the United States when a boy is born, the parents are faced with the decision of whether to have him circumcised. Proponents of circumcision have any number of reasons for supporting it: religion, culture, health, or hygiene. Opponents of circumcision say that it is unnecessary surgery that brings with it unnecessary risk and pain to the child. What are your beliefs on circumcision? On what do you base your beliefs? Talk to someone who disagrees with you and see if your beliefs change or soften.

3. Communication is critical to negotiating condom use, whether for birth control or prevention of sexually transmitted diseases. There are many reasons why men and women do not want to use a condom, but you must be prepared in advance to respond thoughtfully and respectfully to ensure a condom will be used. Describe how you would respond to the statements below:

    Condoms are too expensive.
    Sex isn't pleasurable with a condom.
    I'm Catholic; I'm not allowed to use a condom.
    I can't believe that you think I have an STD.
    If you really loved me, you wouldn't ask me to use a condom.

4. Masturbation is a natural and common part of people's sex lives. Why do you think people are so embarrassed to talk about it? Have you ever discussed it in a serious way with a friend or lover? How do you think the myths about masturbation affect our reactions to it?

5. List all the people (e.g., parents, siblings, friends, boyfriends or girlfriends, spouses) that you are currently "intimate" with. (Remember that "being intimate" does not mean "having sex.") Describe what each of those relationships means to you and discuss how they all contribute to your health and happiness.

Health in Review

- Sex refers to one's biological classification as male or female and to the experience of creating erotic pleasure.
- Sexuality consists of the aspects of oneself that affect sexual experience: the physical, psychological, social, orientational, developmental, and sexual skill dimensions of the whole self.
- One's sexual biology is determined by genetic makeup, which in turn determines the nature of sex organs: the testes, sperm ducts, semen-producing glands, and penis in the male; and the ovaries, fallopian tubes, uterus, vagina, and external genitalia in the female.

- One's sexual psychology is rooted in gender identity, which guides gender role behaviors.
- Sexual arousal and response involves four phases: excitement, plateau, orgasm, and resolution.
- Sexual difficulties include lack of interest in sex, lack of erection, lack of ejaculatory control, painful intercourse, and difficulties with orgasm.
- Intimate relationships involve sharing one's innermost self. They develop through three stages: selecting a partner, developing intimacy through self-disclosure, and commitment.
- Effective communication is crucial for developing and maintaining relationships.

Health and Wellness Online

The World Wide Web contains a wealth of information about health and wellness. By accessing the Internet using Web browser software, such as Netscape Navigator or Microsoft's Internet Explorer, you can gain a new perspective on many topics presented in *Health and Wellness, Seventh Edition*. Access the Jones and Bartlett Publishers Web site at http://www.jbpub.com/hwonline.

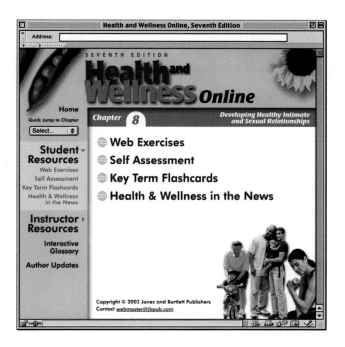

References

Laumann, E. O., Gagnon, J. H., Michael, R. T., and Michaels, S. (1994). *The social organization of sexuality: Sexual practices in the United States.* Chicago: The University of Chicago Press.

Masters, W., and Johnson, V. (1966). *Human sexual response.* Boston: Little, Brown.

Suggested Readings

Boone, L. (1998, February 15). Love is a story: A new theory of relationships. *Library Journal, 123(3),* 162. The article analyzes romantic relationships.

Gattuso, J. (1997). *A course in love: Powerful teachings on love, sex, and personal fulfillment.* NY: HarperCollins Publishers. The book is written by a well-known speaker on relationships. It provides guidelines for developing healthy relationships.

Michael, R. T., Gagnon, J. H., Laumann, E. O., and Kolata, G. (1994). *Sex in America.* Boston: Little, Brown. Findings from a national study of adult sexual behavior. Book is intended for the general audience.

Schnarch, D. (1998). *Passionate marriage.* NY: Henry Holt and Co. This respectful, erotic, uplifting, and spiritual guide shares how couples can—and must—simultaneously break through the sexual and emotional blocks that hold them back from total satisfaction.

The Boston Women's Health Book Collective (1998). *Our bodies, ourselves for the new century: A book by and for women.* NY: Touchstone. This book reflects the vital health concerns of women of diverse ages, ethnic and racial backgrounds, and sexual orientation—a must read for every woman.

Zilbergeld, B. (2000). *The new male sexuality.* NY: Bantam/Dell. The most comprehensive coverage of male sexuality available.

Study Guide and Self Assessment

To Be or Not To Be Parents

Health and Wellness Online

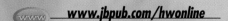 **www.jbpub.com/hwonline**

Understanding Pregnancy and Parenthood

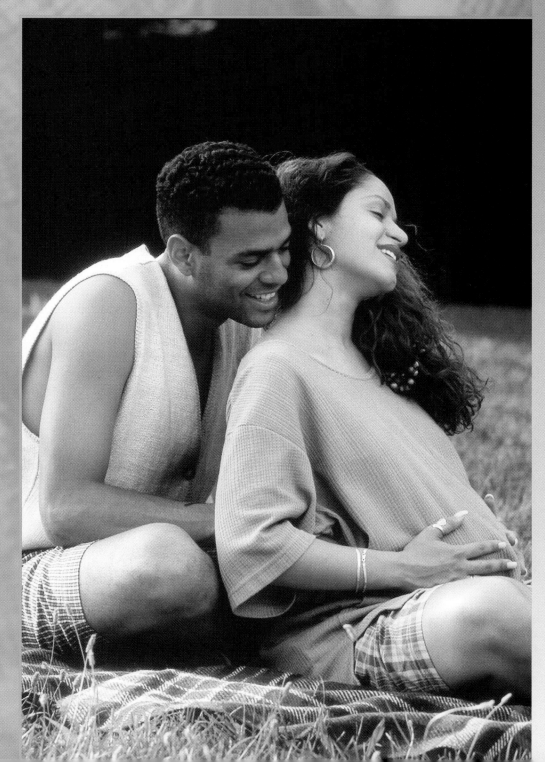

This chapter is about one of the most profound life experiences: creating a child. Many people are awed by the idea that the union of one of their body's cells with a cell from their mate can bring forth a unique human being whose well-being is highly dependent on the physical and emotional foundations they provide. There is a tremendous responsibility in being the best kind of parent so that both the child and society benefit.

People want children for a variety of reasons. A couple may believe that a child is an expression of their love and that having children adds to their sense of bonding. Some see a child as a way to leave a legacy to the world or to carry on the family name. Some couples may feel pressured by their families or by societal or religious expectations to have children, and others may hope that having children will improve their marriage. Being a parent can make some people feel important, needed, or proud. Parenthood may reinforce the ideals of feminine and masculine roles (see chapter 8). Prospective parents may also see children as adding fun, excitement, love, and companionship to their lives.

A man spoke frantically into the phone. "My wife is nine months pregnant and her contractions are only two minutes apart."
"Is this her first child?" the doctor asked.
"No!" the man screamed, "This is her husband!"

Choosing Whether or Not to Be a Parent

Not everyone chooses to become a parent. About 5% of fertile American married couples do not become parents. Some see parenthood as infringing on their career goals or as an unnecessary or unwanted addition to their intimate partnership. Some may have doubts about their psychological or economic abilities to nurture or support children. Others may know or suspect that their children might inherit a genetic disease. Still others may feel that they do not want to contribute more children to an already overpopulated world.

Giving birth to and raising a child requires major adjustments in the parents' lives. The career plans of one or both parents and the distribution of family resources—time, energy, physical space, and money—may change. First-time parents may feel overwhelmed by their responsibilities. The decision to parent should not be taken lightly. The years of parenting are often intense. However, you will never experience such responsibility, hard work, and intimacy as that involved in the growth and development of another human being.

Children do not ask to be born. Parents make that decision. Therefore, before committing to this decision, potential parents must be as certain as they can that their decision is appropriate for their life goals and that they have the means to care for their children.

Becoming Pregnant

For most people, becoming a parent involves pregnancy—a 40-week period, during which a fetus grows inside the mother's uterus and the mother's body undergoes important changes to nurture the developing child. Every pregnancy begins with **fertilization,** which is the fusion of a father's sperm cell with a mother's ovum to form the first cell of their child, called the fertilized egg, or **zygote.** When a man ejaculates during sexual intercourse, hundreds of millions of sperm cells are released into the vagina. Propelled by the swimming motion of their long tails, these tadpole-like cells make their way through the uterus and into the fallopian tubes, the usual site of fertilization

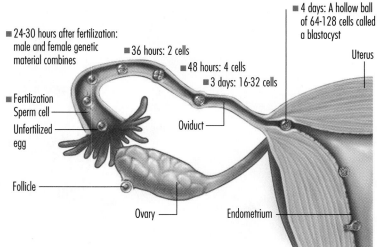

FIGURE 9.1   Fertilization and Early Development of the Embryo   Joining of sperm and egg in fertilization. After fertilization, zygote travels down fallopian tube to uterus. Implantation of zygote begins approximately 6 days after fertilization.

- 24-30 hours after fertilization: male and female genetic material combines
- 36 hours: 2 cells
- 48 hours: 4 cells
- 3 days: 16-32 cells
- 4 days: A hollow ball of 64-128 cells called a blastocyst
- Uterus
- Fertilization
- Sperm cell
- Unfertilized egg
- Oviduct
- Follicle
- Ovary
- Endometrium
- 6 or 7 days: Blastocyst attaches itself to the uterine wall
- 11 or 12 days: Implantation of the embryo

(Figure 9.1). Only one of the many sperm cells actually fertilizes the egg. After fertilization, the zygote moves to the uterus, where it implants in the inner lining and proceeds to develop as an **embryo.**

During each of a woman's menstrual cycles usually one ovum, but sometimes two or more, are able to be fertilized. Once freed from the ovary at ovulation, these eggs can survive for about 24 hours. After ovulation, the lining of the uterus thickens, its glands become filled with nutrients, and small blood vessels enlarge to bring maternal nutrients to the embryo, should pregnancy occur.

Sperm are produced in the testes in narrow, highly coiled, tube-like structures called **seminiferous tubules** (see chapter 8). It takes about 70 days for an immature sperm cell to develop into a mature sperm. Once in the vagina, sperm must travel about 30 centimeters to the site of fertilization in the fallopian tube, which, on a comparative basis, is equivalent to a person traveling nearly 6 miles.

The cervix is the gateway for passage from the vagina to the uterus (see chapter 8). For most of the month, fluid produced by glands in the cervix is dense. This thick cervical mucus keeps sperm from penetrating as readily as they do at the woman's most fertile time. It also prevents some microorganisms from entering the uterus. Near the time of ovulation, the cervical mucus becomes more fluid and has the consistency of egg white, and becomes organized into channels that orient sperm movement toward the uterus. A woman can learn to "read" her cervical mucus to determine the days on which she is fertile, either as a way to increase the probability of conception or as a form of birth control (see chapter 10).

Within seconds following ejaculation in the vagina, some sperm move through the cervix and uterus and into the fallopian tubes. The majority of sperm, however, become trapped in coagulated semen in the upper portion of the vagina. After about 20 minutes, the coagulated semen liquefies and sperm move into microscopic folds in the cervix. Weak or abnormal sperm are unlikely to move beyond the cervix. Healthy, motile sperm tend to be released into the uterus continuously throughout the ensuing 48 hours. Several hundred sperm capable of fertilization ap-

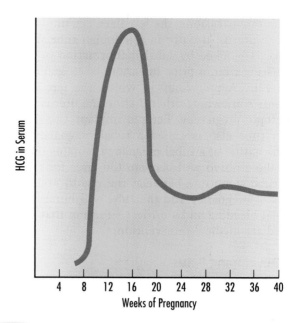

FIGURE 9.2   Pattern of Human Chorionic Gonadotropin (HCG) Secretion during Pregnancy

proach an ovum, but only one succeeds in penetrating the ovum's outer membrane.

During the first 3 days after fertilization, the cells of the embryo replicate at about daily intervals, and the embryo moves along the fallopian tube toward the uterus. By about the fourth day after fertilization, the embryo, now comprised of between 50 and 100 cells, arranged as a fluid-filled sphere, enters the uterus. On about the sixth day after fertilization, the embryo attaches to the lining of the uterus; shortly thereafter, it implants in the uterus by eroding the uterine lining.

 Pregnancy

Soon after the embryo implants in the uterus, it secretes a hormone unique to pregnancy, called **human chorionic gonadotropin (HCG)** into the maternal bloodstream (Figure 9.2). Under the influence of HCG, the mother's ovaries are stimulated to increase the production of estrogen and progesterone, which in turn forestalls the next menstrual period and permits the pregnancy to continue. Increases in the levels of estrogen and progesterone bring about the first noticeable signs of pregnancy: absence of the next menstrual period, occasional nausea and vomiting referred to as "morning sickness," enlarged and tender breasts, increased frequency of urination, fatigue, and enlargement of the uterus. Both clinical and home pregnancy tests are based on analyzing a woman's urine for the presence of HCG. Such tests are about 80–90% accurate. The most frequent type of inaccuracy is a false negative result—reporting no pregnancy when one actually exists.

Terms

fertilization: the fusion of a sperm cell and an ovum

zygote: the first cell of a new person, formed at fertilization

embryo: the developing infant during the first two months of conception

seminiferous tubules: convoluted tubules in the testicles that produce sperm

human chorionic gonadotropin (HCG): a hormone produced furing the first stages of pregnancy; it is used as a basis for pregnancy tests

On rare occasions, the fertilized egg implants outside the uterus, usually in a fallopian tube where its passage is blocked by tubal malformation or scarring or twisting from a prior infection, often gonorrhea or chlamydia. A pregnancy in which the fertilized egg implants somewhere other than in the uterus is called an **ectopic pregnancy.** Ectopic implantation in a fallopian tube also is called a tubal pregnancy. If the ectopic nature of a tubal pregnancy remains undiscovered, the embryo will become too large for the fallopian tube sometime between the eighth and twelfth weeks of pregnancy and the tube will burst, creating internal bleeding and a critical situation that requires immediate medical intervention.

The Developing Fetus

The 9-month span of pregnancy is customarily divided into three 3-month segments called trimesters. Characteristic changes occur in each trimester.

First Trimester

Day 1: The sperm joins with the ovum (egg) to form one cell, which is smaller than the head of a pin. The embryo has inherited 23 chromosomes from each parent, 46 total, which contain the complex genetic blueprint for every detail of development.

Days 3 to 4: The fertilized egg journeys down the fallopian tube to the uterus, where the lining is now prepared for implantation.

Days 5 to 9: During this time, the fertilized egg implants itself in the rich lining of the uterus and begins to draw nourishment.

Days 10 to 14: The developing embryo signals its presence through placental chemicals and hormones, preventing the mother from menstruating.

Day 20: An early brain, spinal cord, and nervous system have already developed.

Day 21: The heart begins to beat.

Day 35: Five fingers are visible on the hand. The eyes darken as pigment is produced.

Day 40: Brain waves can be detected and recorded.

Week 6: The embryo's liver is producing its own blood cells, and the brain controls movements of muscles and organs. The mother has missed her second period and has probably confirmed that she is pregnant.

Week 7: Teeth buds can be seen on the newly formed jaws. New eyelids close to protect the sensitive developing eyes. The eyes will not reopen until the end of the sixth month and beginning of the seventh month.

Week 8: The embryo is now officially called a fetus (Latin for *young one* or *offspring*). Everything that can be found in a human adult is now present in the fetus. The stomach produces digestive juices and the kidneys have begun to function. Forty separate sets of muscles are operating. Testicles begin to form in the male; ovary formation occurs a little bit later in the female. The fetus responds to touch, but the body is so small (about 1½ inches long) that the mother is not yet able to feel any movement.

Week 9: Fingerprints are already evident on the skin. The fetus will curl its fingers around an object placed in the palm of its hand.

Week 10: The uterus has now doubled in size. The fetus can squint, swallow, and wrinkle its forehead.

Wellness Guide

Home Pregnancy Testing

When a woman wants to know if she is pregnant, she can consult a health care provider or go to a family planning or public health clinic. Or, she can administer a pregnancy test herself. Several home pregnancy testing kits are now available without prescription at low cost, and they are relatively easy to use.

Virtually all chemical tests for pregnancy—those carried out in clinics and the self-test kind—analyze a woman's blood or urine for the hormone of pregnancy, human chorionic gonadotropin, HCG.

The home pregnancy tests are not 100% accurate. Only rarely (about 3 times in 100) does the test indicate pregnancy when the woman is not pregnant. A "false positive" result is likely to be discovered when the woman seeks prenatal care.

The home test for pregnancy is wrong about 20% of the time when it indicates that a woman is not pregnant when in fact she is. About half of these "false negative" results occur because the test has been administered too early in the pregnancy. About half of the "false negatives" are corrected if the test is re-administered in about a week. However, about 10% of women who are pregnant still get the inaccurate test result that they are not pregnant. This is one of the most serious drawbacks of home

pregnancy tests, because the risk of complications in pregnancy and abortion rise the longer in pregnancy a woman waits to obtain professional care.

In spite of the possibility of inaccuracy, many physicians and family planning consultants believe home pregnancy testing to be useful. It enables women to take a more active part in their own health care, and it may help women who "would rather not think about it" confront the possibility that they are pregnant.

Week 11: The fetus now sleeps, wakes, and exercises its muscles energetically—turning its head, curling its toes, and opening and closing its mouth. The fetus breathes amniotic fluid to help strengthen its respiratory system.

Second Trimester

Month 4: The ears are functioning, and the fetus hears the mother's voice and heartbeat as well as external noises. The eyebrows and eyelashes become visible. The fetus' entire body structure is formed, and the skin is covered with fine down-like hair. The sex of the fetus can be identified by ultrasonography, which uses high-frequency sound waves to create a visual image (sonogram).

Month 5: The mother can feel movement now, often referred to as the *"quickening."* If a sound is especially loud or startling, the fetus may jump in reaction to it. The scalp hair is visible. The skin is covered by a cheese-like substance that will remain until after birth. The fetus is now 8 inches long and weighs about 11 ounces.

Month 6: Oil and sweat glands are functioning. Eyelids have separated and are open and skin is wrinkled. The fetus is 10 to 12 inches long and weighs 1 to 1½ pounds. About 4 out of 10 babies born now will survive.

Third Trimester

Month 7: The baby uses four senses, all but touch, and can recognize the mother's voice. By the end of this month, the head and body are more proportionate, and the eyes are open. The testes of the male have descended into the scrotum. The baby has rotated and repositioned with the head downward toward the cervix of the uterus and now weights 2½ pounds and is about 11 to 13 inches long. About 9 out of 10 babies born now will survive.

Month 8: By the end of this month, the baby weighs 3½ to 4 pounds and is 14 to 16 inches long. Almost all babies born now will survive.

Month 9: The skin has lost its wrinkled appearance as a result of the accumulation of body fat. Toward the end of this month, the baby is ready for birth. Healthy fetuses born after the normal 266-day gestation period weigh between 5 and 10 pounds (The First 9 Months Fetal Development, 1998).

Fetal development and growth take place with the fetus enclosed in a fluid-filled membranous sac called the **amnion,** which forms during the second week of development. As it develops in the **amniotic fluid,** the fetus is able to grow unimpeded by the mother's internal organs. The amniotic fluid also protects the fetus from potentially damaging jolts when the mother changes her body position. The amnion ruptures just before birth, sometimes called "breaking of the bag of waters."

The growth and development of the fetus are supported by the **placenta,** an organ unique to pregnancy. The placenta manufactures many hormones needed to sustain pregnancy and is responsible for transporting oxygen and nutrients from the mother to the fetus and waste products from the fetus to the mother.

A number of changes occur in a pregnant woman's physiology (Figure 9.3). For example, the blood plasma increases in volume as much as 50% over her nonpregnant levels; the heart beats 10% faster and with 20% to 30% greater output per minute; the number of red blood cells increases; and breathing becomes deeper and slightly faster. One of the most striking changes during pregnancy is the growth of the uterus. The nonpregnant uterus is approximately 7 to 8 centimeters long (2¾ to 3½ inches) and weighs about 60 to 100 grams (2 to 3½ ounces). By the end of pregnancy, the uterus is approximately 30 centimeters long (12 inches) and weighs nearly 1,000 grams (2.2 pounds).

Sexual Interactions During Pregnancy

A woman's sexual interest and responsiveness may change throughout the course of her pregnancy because of the many psychological, emotional, and physical changes that influence her attitude toward and enjoyment of sex. Some of the most common reasons women give for decreasing sexual activity during pregnancy include physical discomfort, feelings of physical unattractiveness, and fear of injuring the unborn child.

It is now generally accepted that, in pregnancies where there are no risk factors, sexual activity and orgasm may be continued, as desired, until the onset of labor. Unless her health care provider counsels a pregnant woman to the contrary, there is no physical reason to forgo sex during pregnancy.

Some couples find that pregnancy is a good time to explore new lovemaking positions—side by side, rear entry, or woman above are generally more comfortable at this time. Even if intercourse is not desired, pregnancy can also be a time to try other sensual and sexual pleasures, such as oral sex, mutual masturbation, massage, or just total body touching and holding.

Terms

ectopic pregnancy: a pregnancy occurring outside the uterus, usually in a fallopian tube

amnion: the inner membrane that forms a fluid-filled sac surrounding and protecting the embryo and fetus

amniotic fluid: fluid in the amniotic sac

placenta: the flat circular vascular structure within the pregnant uterus that provides nourishment to and eliminates wastes from the developing embryo and fetus and is passed as afterbirth after the baby is born

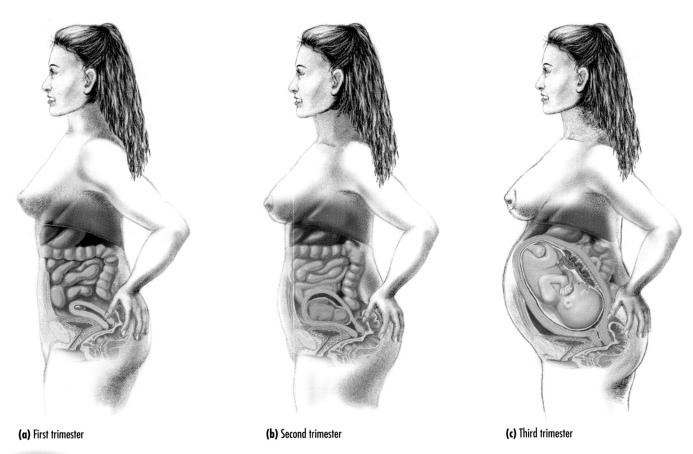

(a) First trimester   **(b)** Second trimester   **(c)** Third trimester

FIGURE 9.3   Changes in Woman's Body During Pregnancy   Through the three trimesters, the shape of the pregnant woman's body changes dramatically.

Health Habits During Pregnancy

Every child deserves to be born as healthy as possible. It is only fair to the unborn child—who did not ask to be conceived—that all the genetic potential to develop a healthy body and mind be given the opportunity to be fully expressed. Few of us are as careful about maintaining proper health habits as we could be. Most people live with whatever risk might be associated with nonhealthy behaviors and are presumably willing to accept the consequences of those behaviors. But when a woman is pregnant, disregarding fundamental health practices endangers her child as well as herself, and perhaps more so, because the developing baby's body and mind are extremely vulnerable to damage. A mother-to-be must make every effort to practice good health habits. If her developing baby could talk, he or she might say, "Mom, my lifelong health and well-being are in your hands now. I know nine months is a long time to have to be concerned about what you eat and drink, but it's important to me that you do the right things for both of us. Not only will that give me the chance to become the best person I can be, but will also keep you healthy so we can share a lot of good times after I'm born." The

factors that deserve a pregnant woman's attention to ensure her own health and that of her baby are proper nutrition, obtaining professional prenatal care, getting enough exercise, refraining from smoking and consuming alcohol or other drugs while pregnant, and accepting and dealing with emotional and sexual feelings that may be different from those experienced when not pregnant.

Nutrition

Throughout pregnancy, the fetus' cells and physiological capacities are developing. Perhaps more than at any other time of life, an ample supply of nutrients is required so that the formation of new cells and the development of organs proceeds optimally. All fetal nutrients come from the mother via the placenta. Therefore, a pregnant woman directly influences the nutritional status of her baby, and she must be aware that she must "eat for two," meaning that she must be sure her diet contains adequate nutrients for herself and for her baby. Mothers-to-be who eat highly nutritious diets during pregnancy are more likely to give birth to healthy babies than are mothers whose diets are nutritionally poor. Pregnant women should increase their intake of essential nutrients and calories

(Table 9.1). For some women it is advisable to supplement a generally well-balanced diet with extra iron and folic acid. Remember that early in the pregnancy, the developing fetus inside of the mother is tiny and only requires about 300 calories a day. Later, as the mother's metabolism speeds up, she may need more than the 300 calories for her baby.

Many pregnant women are concerned with the amount of weight they gain. Not long ago, some doctors restricted weight gain by pregnant women because they believed that gaining too much weight may contribute to **toxemia,** characterized by high blood pressure (sometimes referred to as pregnancy-induced hypertension—PIH) and fluid retention (edema). The early stage of toxemia is known as **preeclampsia,** which is characterized by protein in the urine and swelling of the face, hands, and feet. In the later stage of toxemia, referred to as **eclampsia,** the woman will experience blurred vision and headaches leading to convulsions, coma, and possibly death. Toxemia is not common and the signs typically occur after the twentieth week. Toxemia can be controlled through a well-balanced diet, exercise, and regular blood pressure checks during prenatal visits. While it is never good to weigh too much, current obstetric practice allows a mother-to-be to gain a reasonable amount of weight, about 28 to 30 pounds by the end of pregnancy, most of which comes in the last two-thirds of pregnancy. About 7 of these pounds are contributed by the fetus. The enlarged uterus accounts for another 2 pounds, and the placenta and amniotic fluid contribute 1 pound each. About 4 to 8 pounds of fluid are added to the maternal system as extra blood and extracellular fluid. And the mother may gain about 4 pounds of body fat.

Physical Activity and Exercise

There are benefits to being physically active during pregnancy. Some women feel lethargic during pregnancy. In just a few weeks, their bodies take on unfamiliar proportions and they have to carry up to 20% more weight than when they are not pregnant. They may feel uncomfortable, unattractive, and clumsy. Through movement and exercise, a pregnant woman can become accustomed to the

TABLE 9.1   Recommended Daily Dietary Allowances for Nonpregnant, Pregnant, and Lactating Women, Ages 25–50

	Nonpregnant	Pregnant	Lactating
Protein (g)	50	60	64
Vitamin A (μg)	800	800	1300
Vitamin D (μg)	5	10	10
Vitamin E (mg)	8	10	12
Vitamin C (mg)	60	70	95
Thiamine (mg)	1.1	1.5	1.6
Riboflavin (mg)	1.2	1.6	1.8
Niacin (mg)	13	20	20
Vitamin B_6 (mg)	1.6	2.2	2.1
Folacin (mg)	180	400	280
Vitamin B_{12} (μg)	2	2.2	2.6
Calcium (mg)	800	1200	1200
Phosphorus (mg)	800	1200	1200
Magnesium (mg)	280	320	355
Iron (mg)	10	15	15
Zinc (mg)	12	19	16
Iodine (μg)	150	200	200

Source: Food and Nutrition Board, *Recommended Dietary Allowances* (Washington, D.C.: National Academy of Sciences National Research Council, 1989).

temporary changes in her body and accept pregnancy as a positive and fulfilling time of her life. Physical activity also helps prepare the mother's body for childbirth, which is often physically demanding. By keeping active, a pregnant woman can improve her circulation and thereby reduce swelling and formation of varicose veins in the lower legs, which can be common in pregnancy. Well-conditioned women who engage in aerobics or run regularly have (as a group) shorter labors and fewer cesarean deliveries. Exercise during pregnancy can tone a woman's muscles so that her body returns more quickly to its original shape after delivery. Perhaps the greatest benefit from physical activity during pregnancy is maintaining the habit of being active. That way, after the baby is born, the mother can lose body fat gained during pregnancy and return her body to a firm nonpregnant state.

The degree of physical activity a pregnant woman engages in depends on her desires and abilities. Some athletic women engage in sports almost to the day of delivery. Women who are not routinely athletic are wise to begin a program early in pregnancy that involves exercises to maintain correct posture, strengthen abdominal muscles, and improve their breathing and ability to relax.

Terms

toxemia: an infrequent complication of pregnancy characterized by high blood pressure and fluid retention

preeclampsia: an early stage of toxemia characterized by protein in the urine, high blood pressure, and edema

eclampsia: A late stage of toxemia characterized by blurred vision, headaches, convulsions, coma, and possibly death

Emotional Well-Being

Pregnancy can be a time of intense feelings, not only for the mother-to-be but also for her partner and others who are close to her. Enthusiasm, excitement, anticipation, fear about the baby's condition, uncertainties about one's suitability as a parent, and a desire for more (or less) love, affection, and sex are all natural. Recognizing that intense feelings are normal in pregnancy and accepting them with patience and understanding are the keys to a rewarding experience.

Perhaps the best way to deal with intense feelings at any time in life, including pregnancy, is to take time each day to quiet the mind and body with meditation, yoga, or other relaxation methods. Massage is also beneficial, and it fulfills some of the desires of those who feel more sensual during pregnancy. Some couples feel increased desire for sexual intercourse during pregnancy, which is all right unless the woman has a medical problem that would be worsened by sex. In that event couples can engage in the many forms of pleasuring that do not involve sexual intercourse.

Prenatal Care

Pregnancy involves several profound biological changes. Not only does the fetus develop from a single cell to a 7- or 8-pound newborn infant (composed of many millions of cells) but the mother's body also undergoes a number of anatomical and physiological changes in order to support fetal development. Moreover, the fetal-maternal relationship is maintained by the placenta, an organ that develops only during pregnancy and is expelled from the mother's uterus after the baby is born. Any rapidly changing system is vulnerable to errors and problems, and so it is with pregnancy and fetal development. That is why it is recommended that mothers-to-be receive professional prenatal care. A number of studies have shown that the more prenatal care a woman receives, the fewer problems she will have during pregnancy and childbirth and the more likely that her infant will be born healthy. Professional prenatal care can help a mother-to-be avoid the consequences of a number of pregnancy-specific illnesses, such as toxemia, pregnancy-induced diabetes, and infection. These illnesses can threaten both the mother's health and the proper development and delivery of her baby. Professional prenatal care can also help manage problems resulting from a malfunctioning placenta and can educate a mother about proper nutrition and advise her on how smoking at any time during pregnancy can adversely affect her baby's development, as can consumption of alcohol. Maternal infections that are harmful to the fetus, such as rubella (German measles), syphilis, gonorrhea, toxoplasmosis, herpes, and the HIV infection, can be detected and managed. Another reason for prenatal care is to be sure the maternal and fetal blood cells are immunologically (Rh factor) compatible.

Risks to Fetal Development

The subject of birth defects is one for special consideration. The causes for some birth defects are unknown. Other birth defects may be caused by known factors or agents that adversely affect an embryo or fetus during development. The rapidly developing fetus is dependent on the mother for nutrients, oxygen, and waste elimination because all of these substances pass through the placenta. Although the placenta prevents some kinds of

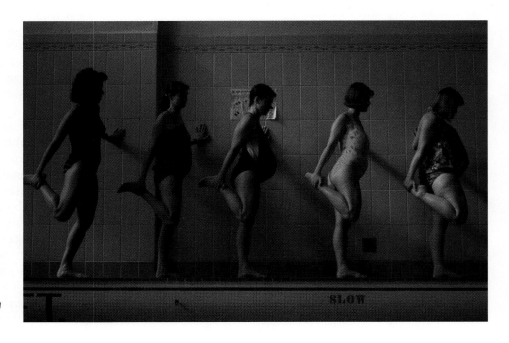

Staying physically active during pregnancy has many benefits.

bacteria and viruses from passing into the fetal blood system, many others are able to cross through the placenta, including the AIDS virus. Furthermore, many substances ingested by the mother, such as drugs, alcohol, and nicotine from tobacco, easily cross through the placenta and damage the developing fetus.

Drugs

Any drugs or medication taken by a pregnant woman can significantly affect the fetus. Especially critical are drugs that, if taken during the embryonic period (from week 2 through week 8), can cause developmental malformations.

Aspirin and other drugs that contain salicylate are not recommended for use during the last 3 months of pregnancy unless under a physician's supervision. Acetylsalicylate, found in many painkillers, can prolong pregnancy and cause excessive bleeding before and after delivery.

Alcohol

When alcohol crosses the placental barrier, it reaches a level in the fetus equal to that in the body of the woman. Because the body of the fetus is small and its detoxification system immature, alcohol remains in fetal blood long after it has disappeared in the woman's blood. The relationship between fetal alcohol exposure and occurrence of birth defects is complex. However, scientists agree that drinking alcohol can harm the fetus, and that the risk of damage increases as the quantity and frequency of maternal alcohol consumption increases. The fetus is at risk of developing fetal alcohol syndrome (FAS) if the mother drinks six or more drinks per day during her pregnancy. The symptoms of FAS include growth retardation, facial malformations, and central nervous system dysfunctions, including mental retardation and behavioral dysfunctions. FAS is the third most common cause of mental retardation in the western world, after Down syndrome and malformations of the nervous system. This is particularly distressing because FAS can be prevented!

Cigarette Smoking

Another serious health hazard for the fetus is cigarette smoking. Maternal smoking increases the chances of spontaneous abortion and of complications that can result in fetal or infant death. Smoking reduces the amount of oxygen in the bloodstream, and this can adversely affect the fetus by slowing its growth. Infants of mothers who smoked during pregnancy often weigh less and are in poorer general condition than are infants of nonsmoking mothers. Smoking may be teratogenic, causing cardiac abnormalities and anencephaly (absence of a cerebrum). Maternal smoking appears to be a significant factor in the development of cleft lip and palate, and a positive relationship has been shown between both cigarette smoking and inhalation of passive (secondhand) smoke and the occurrence of sudden infant death syndrome (SIDS).

How to Detect Birth Defects

Tests such as amniocentesis and chorionic villus sampling may be performed if there is reason to suspect that there may be fetal abnormalities. Other circumstances in which tests may be beneficial include pregnant women over age 35, parents who have previously given birth to a child with birth defects, and parents

> *When I was a kid my parents moved a lot . . . but I always found them.*
> RODNEY DANGERFIELD

with a history of genetic or chromosomal disorders who may want to confirm the absence of birth defects in an unborn child (see Chapter 15).

Amniocentesis

A reliable and accurate test, known as an **amniocentesis,** can be performed between the fourteenth and eighteenth week of pregnancy. The procedure consists of inserting a hollow needle with the assistance of ultrasonographic imagery through the woman's abdominal wall and into the uterine cavity to draw out a sample of the amniotic fluid (fluid surrounding the fetus). Fetal cells are cultured for chromosomal analysis and analyzed under a microscope. The procedure can detect several hundred fetal abnormalities and biochemical defects.

The test can be performed during any trimester if enough fluid is present. If done during the first trimester, it is usually for genetic studies; in the second trimester, for Rh isoimmunization studies; and in the third trimester, for assessing fetal lung maturity.

Chorionic Villus Sampling

Chorionic villus sampling (CVS) is used during the first trimester of pregnancy to detect biochemical disorders and chromosomal abnormalities. Chorionic

Terms

amniocentesis: a procedure that involves aspiration of amniotic fluid from the uterus to detect certain abnormalities in the fetus

chorionic villus sampling (CVS): a method to detect biochemical disorders and chromosomal abnormalities in the fetus

Dollars and Health Sense

The Dark Side of Ultrasound

Ultrasound scans detect diseases and defects by visualizing organs and tissues in the body. They are used most frequently to detect developmental abnormalities in a fetus during pregnancy. Because the organs of a fetus can be observed, sex determination of the fetus is also possible although it is considered unethical to use ultrasound solely for this purpose. In many countries, however, this is its primary purpose.

In India, China, South Korea, and other Asian countries, male babies are much more highly prized by parents than female babies because of cultural customs and because boys are expected to take care of their parents in old age. Girls also require the payment of an expensive dowry when they marry. As a result of centuries of cultural customs,

newborn females are often abandoned or allowed to die. Now, however, a pregnant woman can use ultrasound to determine the sex of her fetus with the object of aborting the pregnancy if it is a girl. (Women are often just as adamant about having a boy as are their husbands.) India passed a law against sex determination in 1994, but no one has ever been convicted of violating the law, and the use of ultrasound is not monitored. Although the normal ratio of male to female pregnancies is approximately one to one in all populations at conception, in some areas of India the ratio is now 1000 newborn males to 770 newborn females.

Even remote villages have access to ultrasound. Portable machines are carried from village to village, and an abortion may be obtained at clinics

for less than $50. Continued use of ultrasound around the world for sex determination and the elimination of female fetuses will have serious social consequences in the future, not the least being the shortage of marriageable women.

Number of Females to 1,000 Males (Total Population) in Some Countries	
India	933
China	944
Indonesia	1,004
United States	1,029
Japan	1,041
Russia	1,140
World	986

villi are threadlike protrusions on a membrane surrounding the fetus that are comprised of fetal cells. This test involves inserting a thin catheter with the assistance of ultrasonographic imagery through the abdomen or vagina and cervix into the uterus, where a small sample of chorionic villi is removed for analysis. This procedure has an advantage over amniocentesis because it can be done as early as the eighth week after the last menstrual period.

Problems During Pregnancy

Most women have uneventful pregnancies, but others encounter complications along the way. Spontaneous abortion, stillbirth, preeclampsia, and premature birth are some of the problems that pregnant women may face.

Spontaneous Abortion and Stillbirth

Spontaneous abortion, or miscarriage, occurs in the first 20 weeks of pregnancy when the fetus cannot live outside the uterus. A stillbirth is one in which there are no signs of life in the fetus at birth or after.

The majority of miscarriages occur in the first 12 weeks of pregnancy and may appear as a heavier than usual menstrual flow; miscarriages that occur later may involve uncomfortable cramping and heavy bleeding. Miscarriages increase in frequency with

maternal and paternal age. An early miscarriage might be the result of an embryonic or fetal problem, such as a chromosomal or developmental abnormality. It is estimated that 10% of all pregnancies end in spontaneous abortion.

Miscarriage or stillbirth can be a significant loss for the woman or couple. She may experience feelings of anger, grief, despair, guilt, jealousy, and isolation. A woman's adjustment after a loss through miscarriage or stillbirth is not only emotional but also physical. Her body experiences the sudden withdrawal of pregnancy hormones. Friends and family can be helpful in acknowledging the loss and asking what the experience has been like for the person.

Childbirth

For the parents, the moment of childbirth can bring a mixture of feelings that might include great joy, relief that the 9 months of waiting are over, and surprise at the baby's appearance. All in attendance may experience concern for the condition of the mother and baby and awe and wonder at the miracle of new life.

Childbirth Preparation

A variety of programs and organizations provide education for parents-to-be in preparation for the childbirth experience and parenthood. These are usually

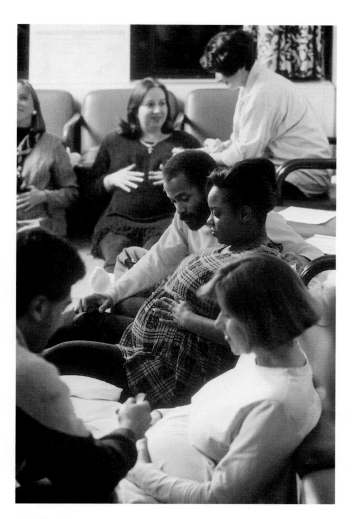

Childbirth preparation classes help ensure a healthy baby.

6- to 8-week courses, sometimes called "natural childbirth," "Lamaze," or simply childbirth preparation. Childbirth preparation classes can enhance the intimate relationship of the expectant couple and increase their confidence and self-esteem. In addition, women who participate in childbirth preparation are likely to have less pain and discomfort in childbirth, to require less medication, and to have fewer complications. Prepared women are also more likely to have positive attitudes toward childbirth and parenting. Fathers who attend childbirth preparation classes tend to feel more comfortable about sharing the birth experience with their partners and about helping them during it. They are also more likely to be interested and involved in parenting after the baby is born.

Almost all childbirth preparation courses teach prospective parents the basic biology of pregnancy and childbirth. They also teach breathing and relaxation exercises, and some teach imagery and affirmations, all intended to make the delivery of the baby proceed more smoothly and comfortably. While attending these courses, parents-to-be meet other expectant couples with whom they can share their feelings and experiences. The classes also address birthing options. Since childbirth preparation courses reflect the biases of those who teach them, prospective parents are likely to gain more complete information about birthing options by consulting additional sources (e.g., books, other parents).

Studies have shown that continuous emotional support during labor can shorten labor time, give the woman in labor greater perception of control, decrease her need for pain medication, and, overall, lead to fewer complications that affect the baby. On the other hand, labor can be slowed or stopped if the woman feels uncomfortable, anxious, frightened, or experiences performance pressure because of others' expectations about how the labor should be proceeding.

Giving Birth

A few weeks before the onset of childbirth, or **labor,** the fetus becomes positioned for birth by descending in the uterus, a process called **lightening.** When this happens the pressure on some of the mother's internal organs is relieved and she may find it easier to breathe, stand, and digest food. In about 95% of all births the fetus is in a head-down position. When not head-down, the fetus may be head-up, referred to as a breech position. In nearly all instances, the fetus' legs are tucked up against its abdomen in the "fetal position."

Throughout much of pregnancy, the uterus contracts intermittently, tightening in waves that sometimes are so gentle that the woman is unaware of them. During the last half of pregnancy, a woman may at times feel her abdomen becoming hard or otherwise perceive the uterine contractions as they prepare her body for the true labor. Health professionals refer to these as **Braxton-Hicks contractions.** They can be distinguished from true labor by their occurrence at irregular intervals and their rather short duration.

There are three generally recognizable stages in the process of childbirth (Figure 9.4). Before the first stage begins, the cervix has already effaced (flattened and thinned) and dilated slightly. The **first stage** of labor starts with the beginning of uterine contractions and lasts until the cervix is fully dilated. Another indication of first-stage labor may be the "bloody show,"

Terms

labor: the process of childbirth

lightening: the positioning of the fetus for birth by descent in the uterus

Braxton-Hicks contractions: normal uterine contractions that occur periodically throughout pregnancy

first-stage labor: the beginning of labor during which there are regular contractions of the uterus

the discharge of the mucous plug from the cervix. The first stage is the longest of the three stages, usually lasting 10 to 16 hours for the first childbirth and 4 to 8 hours in subsequent deliveries. This stage lasts until the cervix is dilated 10 centimeters.

The **second stage** of labor begins when the cervix is fully dilated and the infant descends farther into the vaginal birth canal (normally, head first). This stage lasts from 30 minutes to 2 hours. During this time the woman can actively push with each contraction until the infant is expelled. The remaining amniotic fluid gushes out. The infant is cleaned and its vital signs, such as breathing and color, are quickly checked. The umbilical cord is clamped off several inches from the navel, and the baby soon begins to breathe.

The **third stage** of labor lasts from the time of birth until the delivery of the placenta, or **afterbirth.** With one or two more uterine contractions, the placenta usually separates from the uterine wall and is expelled from the vagina, generally within 30 minutes after the baby is born. During this time, the uterus begins returning to its original size.

Medical Interventions

Options for Controlling Discomfort

Intense discomfort or pain can accompany labor, especially in the later phases of the first stage and the early stages of the second. The intensity of feeling is caused by stretches and strains on the uterine muscle tissue, effacement of the cervix, and stretching of the perineum. Pain relief methods include relaxation techniques, deep breathing, acupuncture, hypnosis, massaging and supporting of the perineum by the birth attendant, medications that block pain awareness (analgesia), and medications that block the pain sensations (anesthesia). The most common anesthesia used during labor is a regional anesthetic to diminish sensation only in the pelvic region. This leaves the mother conscious during labor so that she can actively "bear down" to help push the baby out. General anesthesia (complete unconsciousness) is used only in cases of difficult births and interventions, such as cesarean sections.

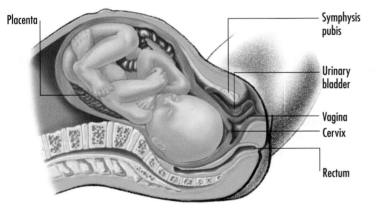

Placenta · Symphysis pubis · Urinary bladder · Vagina · Cervix · Rectum

(a) Early first-stage labor

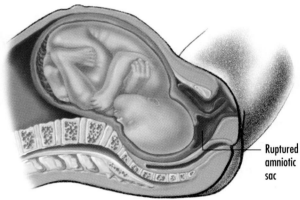

Ruptured amniotic sac

(b) Later first-stage labor: the transition

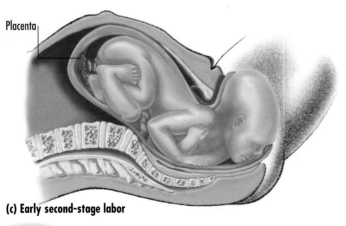

Placenta

(c) Early second-stage labor

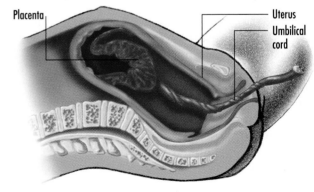

Placenta · Uterus · Umbilical cord

(d) Third-stage labor: delivery of afterbirth

FIGURE 9.4   Childbirth   The stages of labor. **(a)** First stage: The cervix is dilating. **(b)** Late first stage (transition stage): The cervix is fully dilated, and the amniotic sac has ruptured, releasing amniotic fluid. **(c)** Second stage: The birth of the infant. **(d)** Third stage: Delivery of the placenta (afterbirth).

Managing Stress

Pregnancy and Childbirth: Belly Breathing Exercise

In Lamaze classes expectant mothers (and fathers) are taught to place the emphasis of their breathing on the lower stomach or diaphragm. During the several hours of labor and the actual delivery, this breathing skill is employed to ease the pain of childbirth. What is taught and practiced in the stressful event of childbirth is now taught and practiced in several other stressful situations as well.

Each breathing cycle is comprised of four distinct phases:

Phase I: Inspiration, taking the air into your lungs through the passage of your nose or mouth

Phase II: A very slight pause before exhaling the air out of your lungs

Phase III: Exhalation, releasing the air from your lungs and through the passage it entered

Phase IV: A very slight pause after exhalation before the next inhalation is initiated.

These phases can be enhanced when the breathing cycle is exaggerated by taking a very slow and comfortable deep breath. When trying this technique, try to isolate and recognize these four phases by identifying them as they occur. Remember not to hold your breath at any one time during each phase. Rather, learn to regulate your breathing by controlling the pace of each phase in the breathing cycle. Remember that diaphragmatic breathing is not the same as hyperventilation: this style of breathing is slow, relaxed, and as deep as feels comfortable. The most relaxing phase of breathing is the third phase, exhalation. In this phase the chest and abdominal areas relax, producing a relaxing effect throughout the body. When focusing on your breathing, feel how relaxed your whole body becomes during exhalation, especially your chest, shoulders, and abdominal region.

An Energy Breathing Exercise

There are three phases to this exercise and you can use this technique either sitting or lying down.

1. First get comfortable, allowing your shoulders to relax. If you choose to sit, try to keep your legs straight. As you breathe in, imagine that there is a circular hole at the top of your head. As the air enters your lungs, visualize energy in the form of a beam of light entering the top of your head. Bring the energy down, from the crown of your head to your abdomen as you inhale. As you exhale, allow the energy to leave through the top of your head. Repeat this 5 to 10 times, trying to coordinate your breathing with the visual flow of energy. As you continue to bring the energy down to your stomach area, allow the light to reach all the inner parts of your upper body. When you feel comfortable with this first phase, you are ready to move on to the second phase.

2. Now, imagine that in the center of each foot, there is a circular hole through which energy can flow in and out. Again think of energy as a beam of light. Concentrating on only your lower extremities, allow the flow of energy to move up from your feet into your abdomen as you inhale from your diaphragm. Repeat this 5 to 10 times, trying to coordinate your breathing with the flow of energy. As you continue to bring the energy up into your stomach area, allow the light to reach all the inner parts of your lower body.

3. Once you have coordinated your breathing with the visual flow of energy through your lower extremities, begin to combine the movement of energy from the top of your head and your feet, bringing the energy to the center of your body as you inhale air from your diaphragm. Then, as you exhale, allow the flow of energy to reverse. Repeat this 10 to 20 times. Each time you move the energy through your body, feel each body region—each muscle, organ, and cell—become energized. At first it may be difficult to visually coordinate the movement of energy coming from opposite ends of your body, but this will become very easy with practice.

Occasionally the course of labor may slow to a degree that may be harmful to both mother and fetus. Because the hormone oxytocin stimulates uterine contractions, modern obstetric practice often calls for administering oxytocin during difficult childbirth. For centuries, midwives and birth attendants in many countries have stimulated the breasts of laboring mothers to augment labor, as breast stimulation causes the natural release of oxytocin from the mother's posterior pituitary gland.

Episiotomy

Besides the administration of medications, an **episiotomy,** an incision in the perineum from the vagina to the anus, can be performed late in the first stage of labor before the head of the infant emerges. The procedure may be necessary when the infant's head is too large for the opening, when the infant is

Terms

second-stage labor: the stage during which the baby moves out through the vagina and is delivered

third-stage labor: the stage during which the afterbirth is expelled

afterbirth: placenta and fetal membranes

episiotomy: an incision in the perineum to facilitate passage of the baby's head during childbirth, while minimizing injury to the woman

in distress or in an irregular position, when there is need for a forceps delivery, or when the perineum has not stretched sufficiently.

The benefits of episiotomies are that they speed up birth time, prevent tearing, protect against incontinence, protect against pelvic floor elevations, and heal more easily than tears. Although these are valid reasons for an episiotomy, the procedure can result in infection, increased pain, increase in third- and fourth-degree vaginal lacerations, slower healing, and increased discomfort when intercourse is resumed.

If a woman is concerned about having an episiotomy, she should talk to her doctor, because much of the time episiotomies are not necessary. However, to avoid an episiotomy, the woman must have a good understanding of labor and be willing to go through the entire process, which means being able to control pushing so the perineum has adequate time to stretch completely to reduce the likelihood of tearing.

Cesarean Section

When a normal vaginal delivery is considered dangerous or impossible, a fetus is removed through an incision made in the abdominal wall and uterus, in a surgical procedure called a **cesarean section,** or **C-section.** Cesarean births may be recommended in a variety of situations, including a fetal head that is too large for the mother's pelvic structure, maternal illness, active herpes infection in the vaginal tract, fetal distress during labor, birth complications such as breech-fetal presentation (feet or bottom coming out of the uterus first), or previous C-section (Greene, 2001).

The Postpartum Transition

After the child is born, the mother goes through several weeks of postpartum transition called the **puerperium.** During this time, the physiological changes of pregnancy slowly reverse and the vagina and the surrounding structures recuperate from labor. Uterine tissue that is no longer needed is discharged for the first month or so after childbirth. The discharge, called lochia, at first resembles a heavy menstrual flow, then typically tapers off after a week or two. Following delivery, estrogen and progesterone levels, which were high during pregnancy, drop rapidly, reaching almost zero about 72 hours after birth.

During this period the mother and her partner begin to adjust to their often demanding new life situation. Childbirth and infant care are exhausting. Many women experience the "baby blues," which are transitory mood changes involving tiredness, depression, loneliness, or fear. These feelings usually abate in the weeks following childbirth, but a minority of women experience postpartum depression severe enough to be disabling and require professional help. Postpartum mood changes are so common that experts suggest they may be related to the massive changes in hormone levels that accompany childbirth. Others, while not denying the effects of hormonal changes, point out that childbirth is a life transition that brings many changes and psychological adjustments for the woman, her partner, and other family and household members.

It is recommended that couples refrain from intercourse for several weeks following childbirth to allow episiotomy incisions to heal and the uterus and vagina to return to prepregnancy states. Intercourse is usually physically safe within 3 to 4 weeks after delivery, but this all depends on the mother's desire and comfort.

Breast-Feeding

The preparation of the breasts for nursing begins in the early weeks of pregnancy with an increase in the number of milk ducts and the deposit of fat in the breast tissue. This growth causes breast tenderness early in pregnancy. In addition to the increase in breast size, the nipples enlarge and often deepen in color. About midway into pregnancy, the breasts begin to manufacture **colostrum,** a yellowish precursor to actual mother's milk. For the first few days after birth, colostrum is the major substance emitted from the breasts. As the newborn nurses, colostrum is drained from the breasts and is replaced by mother's milk. Colostrum contains nutrients and is especially high in antibodies that protect the infant against infection. Mother's milk contains specific milk proteins, antibodies, lactose, fat, and water. The synthesis of milk is controlled by the pituitary hormone **prolactin,** the levels of which rise tremendously during pregnancy and are maintained as long as the mother continues to nurse.

Milk is delivered from the breast through the coordinated activity of the mother and infant. Inserting the nipple into the baby's mouth activates the baby's sucking reflex. When the baby sucks, nerve impulses which stimulate the release of the hormone oxytocin

---

Terms

cesarean section: delivery of the fetus through a surgical opening in the abdomen and uterus

puerperium: the 6 weeks after childbirth, also called postpartum period

colostrum: yellowish liquid secreted from the breasts; contains antibodies and protein

prolactin: a hormone produced by the anterior lobe of the pituitary gland that stimulates milk secretion

weaned: to discontinue breast-feeding, using other means to provide nutrients

infertile: unable to become pregnant or to impregnate

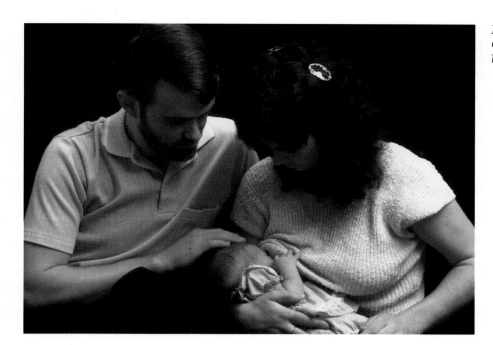

Breast milk provides a baby with essential nutrients and helps prevent infections.

are transmitted from the breast to the mother's brain. Oxytocin circulates through the mother's bloodstream to the breasts, where it causes the muscle cells that line the milk ducts to contract and eject milk from the nipple. Oxytocin also stimulates contractions of the uterus, so breast-feeding helps return the uterus to its prepregnant size.

A mother can nurse for many months. As long as the baby is sucking and the breasts are regularly drained of milk, the hormonal stimulation of milk production will continue. Without such stimuli, milk production stops. The many advantages of breast-feeding include:

- It is economical, readily available, and eliminates the effort involved in purchasing, preparing, and heating bottles and formula.

- It transfers immunity (protection against infections) from the mother to the infant, and breast milk itself and the act of nursing stimulate the development of the infant's own immune defenses.

- Breast milk promotes development of the infant's digestive system.

- Breast-fed babies have fewer allergies, less diarrhea, fewer dental problems, and less colic (stomachache).

- Breast milk is nutritionally balanced for human infants; formulas containing cow's milk are not nutritionally identical to human milk, although they are nutritionally adequate.

- Breast-feeding may increase the psychological attachment between mother and infant.

- The hormones involved in the production and release of milk cause uterine contractions, which help the uterus return to its normal size. During the first week or so after childbirth these contractions may be intense and even painful. Thereafter some women describe them as pleasurable, sensual, or erotic.

Many women find that breast-feeding offers them a relaxing, pleasurable experience with their babies. Often the pleasurable feelings of breast-feeding will have an erotic tone, possibly producing genital sensations and even occasionally orgasm. These feelings and responses are normal and natural, and a women need not feel guilty or distressed by them.

The many advantages of breast-feeding do not mean that bottle feeding is not wholesome. Many healthy, well-adjusted people were bottle-fed infants. Some women are physically unable to breast-feed. Some mothers choose not to breast-feed because work, family, and other responsibilities make it inconvenient. Breast-feeding in public or at work is, unfortunately, still not acceptable in many communities or places of employment. Some women choose not to breast-feed because they fear that changes in the shape of their breasts will decrease their sexual attractiveness.

Some women breast-feed their infants for several weeks or months and then gradually substitute bottle feedings for breast feedings until the child is completely **weaned,** that is, has stopped nursing altogether. More important than whether the milk comes from the breast or a bottle is the physical contact and loving the infant receives while being fed.

Infertility

Approximately one in five of all American married couples of childbearing age are **infertile,** which means that they are unable to become pregnant after a year of trying. Male factors are responsible for infertility in about 40% of infertile couples; female factors in another 40% to 50%. In about 10% of infertile couples, no cause can be determined. With professional help, about half of all infertile couples can eventually have children. A significant percentage of couples medically determined to be infertile eventually have children without medical interventions.

In both sexes, infertility can be caused by a variety of conditions that adversely affect the functioning of an otherwise normal reproductive system. For example, ill health, cigarette smoking, chronic alcohol use, marijuana and other drug abuse, exposure to radiation or toxic chemicals, malnutrition, anxiety, stress, and fatigue can lessen a person's reproductive capabilities. Medical treatments or changes in lifestyle can often restore fertility.

> *The reason grandparents and grandchildren get along so well is that they have a common enemy.*
> SAM LEVENSON

Obstacles to Fertility

Because sperm and ovum production and the functions of the male and female reproductive tracts are absolutely dependent on adequate hormone production, hormonal problems are a common cause of infertility in both men and women. Infertility can also be caused by anatomical abnormalities or damage to the male or female reproductive systems (see chapter 8). A common cause of damage is scarring and subsequent blocking of the fallopian tubes and, less frequently, the epididymis, by gonorrhea or chlamydia infections (see chapter 11). The scar tissue from such diseases blocks the tubes and prevents the passage of sperm and ova. Growths and tumors in the reproductive tract can also block the passage of sperm and ova. Sometimes surgical repair of blocked or damaged tubes can restore fertility.

Problems with **insemination** and sperm transport can also cause infertility. For example, a man may have difficulty getting and maintaining an erection or ejaculating into the vagina. A woman may produce very thick or voluminous cervical mucus, which can block entry of sperm into the uterus. Sometimes a couple has trouble conceiving because they are not having intercourse near the time of ovulation.

Enhancing Fertility Options

A variety of medical interventions are available to help infertile couples become pregnant. For example, if a male partner produces too few sperm, but those he does produce are healthy, conception is unlikely to oc-

cur. For conception to occur, more than 20 million healthy sperm need to be deposited in the vagina. Fertilization can be facilitated by introducing semen obtained from the man directly into the cervix with a syringe. This is called **artificial insemination.** If the male partner cannot produce sufficient numbers of healthy sperm even for artificial insemination, the couple may become pregnant by artificial insemination with semen from a donor.

Another way to overcome infertility is *in vitro* **fertilization (IVF),** which involves obtaining several ova from the ovaries and fertilizing them in a laboratory dish. The resultant embryo is placed into the woman's uterus. *In vitro* fertilization is employed when a woman's fallopian tubes do not function correctly. GIFT (gamete intrafallopian transfer) and ZIFT (zygote intrafallopian transfer) are similar to *in vitro* fertilization. With GIFT, the ova are placed in equal numbers in each of the fallopian tubes and semen is introduced directly into the tubes. With ZIFT, eggs are fertilized *in vitro* and an embryo is placed in the fallopian tube. These procedures are successful between 10% and 20% of the time.

For some couples, the prospect of not being able to have a child is devastating. Many of these couples embark on lengthy efforts, which may cost thousands of dollars and consume much of their emotional energy, to become pregnant and have a healthy baby. Such couples may be asked to keep careful records of the woman's fertility cycle and to time intercourse for maximum likelihood of conception. They may be counseled to have intercourse at certain times after hormone treatments. They may make repeated visits to fertility clinics to undergo IVF or other medical interventions.

About 40,000 infertile couples in the United States attempt to have a child using IVF techniques each year. However, for most of these couples repeated attempts to conceive end in failure. For women under age 35, the success rate is approximately 20%; for women over age 40, the success rate is under 10%. In addition to the poor success rate, couples can pay several thousand dollars for each attempt to become pregnant and health insurance generally does not cover any IVF costs.

Terms

insemination: introduction of semen into the uterus or oviduct

artificial insemination: introduction of semen into the uterus or oviduct by other than natural means

***in vitro* fertilization (IVF):** a procedure in which an egg is removed from a ripe follicle and fertilized by a sperm cell outside the human body; the fertilized egg is allowed to divide in a protected environment for about 2 days and then is inserted back into the uterus

Adoption

There are many reasons why adults may want to raise children who are not biologically their own. They may be partially motivated by a concern with overpopulation and a desire to give homeless children love and security. Another common reason is that a couple is unable to have children because of infertility. One alternative for couples, or even single people and gay couples, is adoption. Many adoptions bring the happiness anticipated to otherwise childless couples.

There are three avenues to pursue when couples would like to adopt a child. Most commonly, adoptions are handled through state-licensed *private* or *public adoption agencies*, usually nonprofit social services, which handle approximately 70% of all adoptions. An agency adoption may be the best option for adopting an older child, a minority child, or a child with special needs, although agencies also help in the adoption of infants and foreign children. Signing up with an adoption agency can be a lengthy process, often lasting several years.

Another way to adopt a child is through an *independent* or *private adoption*. The individuals wishing to adopt a child make arrangements with a woman who wants to give up custody of her child, often with an attorney, physician, or cleric serving as an intermediary. Every state has its own laws concerning independent adoption, and the prospective parents should know the laws in their state as well as the state of the birth mother. In all independent adoptions, the birth parents can give consent for adoption only after the birth of the child.

A third avenue to pursue is an *international adoption*. This is becoming an increasingly popular avenue for prospective parents. Both state and federal requirements must be met in international adoptions; however, the waiting period is not as lengthy as it is in private or public adoptions.

Critical Thinking About Health

1. There is controversy about the use of oxytocin to augment labor. Critics of its use charge that some hospital staff administer oxytocin to force the birth to occur when the staff is most available rather than letting the mother deliver on her own schedule. Also, there is no consensus regarding what conditions should signal the use of oxytocin. Labor augmentation is needed when uterine contractions are weak or absent or when the fetus is in distress (not breathing). Studies fail to show that oxytocin is required in the majority of normal births.
   a. Would you request that no oxytocin be used during the birth of your child?
   b. Under what circumstances would you request oxytocin?

2. You have recently found out you are 6 weeks pregnant (or that your girlfriend is pregnant). You have been dating for 6 months and have discussed marriage. But neither of you has finished college and you both want to go to graduate school.
   a. List the options available to you. Identify the pros and cons for each option.
   b. Of the options listed, which would you do given the above circumstances? Why?

3. We know that drugs, alcohol, and smoking are dangerous to a developing fetus. Imagine that you are working as a server in a restaurant.
   a. What would you do if a customer who was pregnant ordered a glass of wine? Would you serve her?
   b. What would you do if a customer who was pregnant was smoking a cigarette? Would you say something?
   c. How do the woman's rights compare to the fetus' rights?

4. You and your spouse recently found out that you are pregnant for the first time. Already you are getting lots of information and "advice" from your family and friends. You've even had to suffer through some pregnancy horror stories.
   a. Where can you go to get your own sound and impartial advice?
   b. Are you prepared to make some of the important decisions about your pregnancy? For instance, have you thought about the following:
      • Will you take childbirth classes? What method will you follow (Lamaze, Bradley, etc.) or will you use a doula (a trained labor-support person)?
      • Will you use natural childbirth?
      • Will you use any painkilling drugs during labor?
      • Will you allow the doctor to give you an episiotomy?
      • Will you talk to your doctor about using oxytocin to augment labor?
      • Will you circumcise your male child?
      • Will you use a conventional doctor and deliver at a hospital or will you use a midwife and deliver at home?

Health in Review

- Conception, pregnancy, and childbirth are important and meaningful life experiences. The decision to become a parent requires psychological and physical preparation so every child can have parents prepared to meet its needs.
- Fertilization is followed by cleavages of the embryo as it moves into the uterus. About the sixth day after fertilization the embryo implants in the lining of the uterus, and for the next 266 days or so the fetus develops. After 40 weeks of pregnancy a baby is born.
- Health habits during pregnancy, such as good nutrition, seeking prenatal care, exercise and physical activity, and emotional well-being are particularly important for the development of a healthy fetus.
- Taking drugs, consuming alcohol, and smoking cigarettes during pregnancy can cause fetal damage or birth defects. Tests, such as amniocentesis or chorionic villus sampling, are available to determine whether or not birth defects are present.

- Optimal childbirth can be achieved by attending childbirth preparation classes, ensuring emotional support for the mother during childbirth, and making wise choices about medical interventions, such as episiotomy and pain management.
- Childbirth is divided into three stages. The first stage starts with the beginning of labor and lasts until the cervix is fully dilated. The second stage is the birth of the baby. The third stage is the delivery of the placenta.
- The period after childbirth may involve breastfeeding and resumption of sexual activities.
- Approximately 20% of American married couples are infertile. Some of these couples can be medically assisted to become pregnant; pregnancy also may occur with *in vitro* fertilization or artificial insemination.
- Adoption is an alternative for childless couples. Children can be adopted through a private or public adoption agency or in an independent or private adoption or an international adoption.

Health and Wellness Online

The World Wide Web contains a wealth of information about health and wellness. By accessing the Internet using Web browser software, such as Netscape Navigator or Microsoft's Internet Explorer, you can gain a new perspective on many topics presented in *Health and Wellness, Seventh Edition*. Access the Jones and Bartlett Publishers Web site at http://www.jbpub.com/hwonline.

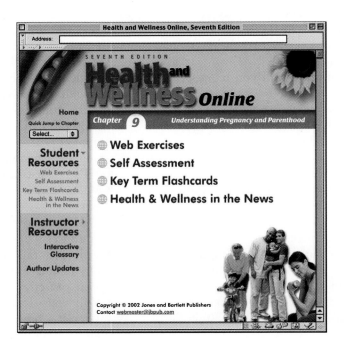

References

Greene, M. F. (2001). Vaginal delivery after caesarean section—Is the risk acceptable? *New England Journal of Medicine, 345,* 54–55.

Suggested Readings

Balaskas, J. (1997, April). *Easy exercises for pregnancy.* New York: Macmillan General Reference. Guide helps pregnant women to alleviate the aches and pains normally associated with pregnancy and prepares them to make the childbirth experience as easy as possible.

Conti, J., Abraham, S., and Taylor, A. (1998). Eating behavior and pregnancy outcome—What do we know? *Journal of Psychosomatic Research, 44*(3–4), 465–477. The article studies the relationships among clinical eating disorders, maternal body weight, shape, eating concerns, and pregnancy outcomes. Certain pregnancy outcomes of concern include low-birth-weight infants.

Eisenberg, A., Hathaway, S., and Murkoff, H. (1997). *What to expect when you're expecting.* NY: Workman. This popular guide to pregnancy covers every aspect of the prenatal period from developmental stages to nutrition.

Harris, A. C. (1997). *The pregnancy journal: A day to day guide to a healthy and happy pregnancy.* San Francisco: Chronicle Books. A practical, informal guide covering medical, emotional, and spiritual information for a woman or couple who are expecting a baby.

Jones, M. (1998). *Motherhood after 35: Choices, decisions, options.* Tucson, AZ: Fisher Books. For women between 35 and 45 who are trying to have a baby or who have already conceived, this book evaluates the advantages and the risks of later motherhood.

Study Guide
and
Self Assessment

Contraceptive Comfort and Confidence Scale

Health
and Wellness
Online

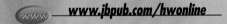 **www.jbpub.com/hwonline**

Chapter 10

Choosing a Fertility Control Method

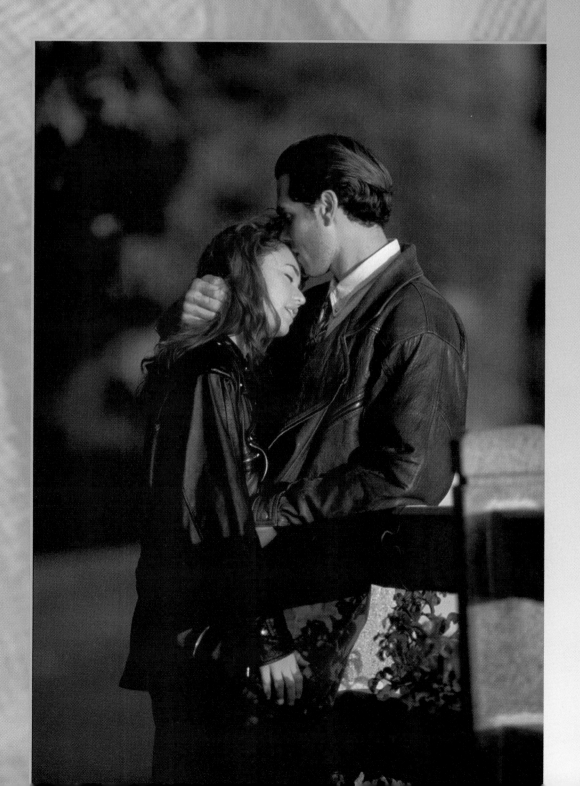

To be aware of the many facets of human sexuality—sexual values, the structure of sexual anatomy, aspects of sexual identity and sexual behavior, and sexual responsiveness—is the first step toward attaining a healthy and fulfilling sexual life. Because sexual activities nearly always involve others, our sexual decisions must also involve concern for the health and well-being of the partner. In this chapter, we discuss responsible sexual decision making as it pertains to the avoidance or termination of unintended pregnancy and the prevention of sexually transmitted (venereal) diseases.

 ## Fertility Control

Approximately 70 million Americans engage in between 1 billion and 6 billion acts of sexual intercourse each year for reasons other than to produce children. Instead of procreation, people often have sex because it is pleasurable and a way to express love and affection. Given the choice, most persons would prefer to separate nearly all of their sexual experiences from conception. People have many reasons for practicing fertility control (Table 10.1) and, fortunately, modern biotechnology has produced highly effective aids for preventing unintended pregnancies. Thirty-five million women in the United States practice contraception. Among them, 39% rely on sterilization, 31% on birth control pills, 20% on barrier methods, and 2% on intrauterine devices.

> *It's better to know some of the questions than all of the answers.*
> JAMES THURBER

Throughout history, hundreds of methods of fertility control have been advocated; however, at no time in the past have people had available to them as many safe, reliable methods of fertility control as they have today. Unlike the ancient methods, which were often based on observing animals, their own trial and error, or rooted in superstition and folklore, today's fertility control methods are based on scientific knowledge of human reproductive biology. Some of the modern fertility control techniques are preconception methods (contraceptives). They work by preventing the development or union of sperm and ova. Other techniques are postconception methods. They inhibit in various ways the development of the fertilized ovum or embryo.

When you consider the several methods of fertility control, keep in mind that sex without intercourse is a highly effective way to prevent pregnancy. Genital (penis-in-vagina) intercourse is not the only way to give and receive sexual pleasure. Touching, kissing, and stroking can bring intense sexual enjoyment and even orgasm to both partners.

There is no fertility control method that is perfect for everyone. Except for abstinence from sexual intercourse, no single method is 100% effective, 100% free of side effects, absolutely safe, financially available to everyone, and 100% reversible. Without a perfect contraceptive, avoiding an unintended pregnancy requires weighing the benefits and drawbacks of the various methods and choosing the one(s) that both partners are comfortable using and that they will use properly each time sexual intercourse takes place. Even the most technologically perfect contraceptive would fail if it were not used properly and consistently.

A fertility control method's effectiveness is measured in terms of its **failure rate,** which is the percentage of women who, on average, are likely to become pregnant using a particular method for a year. Each method has two failure rates: the **lowest observed failure rate,** a measure of how a method performs when used consistently and as intended, and the **typical**

TABLE 10.1   Some Common Reasons for Fertility Control

Reason	Explanation
Enhancing sexual pleasure	Anxiety about the possibility of pregnancy can divert a person's attention from the sexual experience and interfere with the flow of sexual feelings. Also, worry during intercourse can cause difficulties with erection and ejaculation in men and with vaginal lubrication and orgasm in women.
Family planning	Safe, reliable fertility control affords couples the opportunity to plan the size of their family and the timing of their children's births. Couples can have children when the family's financial resources are sound and the parents' relationship is ready for raising a child or children.
Increasing women's life choices	Fertility control allows women to choose when to devote time and energy to various life pursuits, including parenthood. In the not-too-distant past, when fertility control methods were unreliable, it was difficult for a woman to integrate her personal goals with parenthood because she had little control over the timing of the births of her children.
Health considerations	Fertility control helps couples reduce the risk of passing a hereditary disease to children. Fertility control also is advantageous to women for whom pregnancy and childbirth may be a significant health risk. Fertility control can prevent pregnancy in teenagers, who experience more pregnancy-related problems than older women.
World overpopulation	Some couples keep their families small because they want to take some responsibility for limiting the growth of the human population. Some people fear that overpopulation will create pressures for food, water, living space, energy, and other resources.

Global Wellness

Fertility Control and Management in Different Countries

The United Nations predicts that the world population will range between 8 and 12 billion by the middle of this century. A global view on the issue of fertility management and control can give us insights on personal decisions made by others.

Japan

In Japan, the government bans the use of oral contraceptives, and physicians discourage sterilization as a fertility control method. Japan uses more condoms than any other country. Condoms are widely available, and homemakers can purchase them from door-to-door saleswomen. Japan also has one of the highest abortion rates among

industrialized nations. Abortions are legal and actively promoted by the government; however, for the most part, the general public does not approve of them.

Brazil

Brazil's population has been on a steep rise for several decades; despite this rise, the country does not have a national family planning policy. Brazil's traditional attitudes toward gender, sexuality, and fertility provide a challenge for those concerned about overpopulation. Recently, Brazil has been testing NoFertil, the first contraceptive pill for men.

This pill is made from gossypol, a substance produced from cotton plants.

India

Less than 50% of the couples in India—the second most populous country on Earth—use any type of fertility control. At one time the government promoted family planning; however, this effort was discredited after thousands of Indian teenagers were sterilized. The government has developed policies that prohibit civil service workers from receiving promotions or tax benefits if they have more than two children.

---

failure rate, a measure of how a method performs allowing for all of the errors and problems typically associated with a method (Table 10.2).

 ### Withdrawal

The withdrawal method of fertility control (**coitus interruptus**) requires that the man withdraw his penis from the vagina before ejaculation. In theory, withdrawal prevents sperm from being deposited in the vagina and subsequently fertilizing an ovum. The male must exercise great control and restraint in order to withdraw the penis in time. Withdrawal is risky because a small emission may occur before ejaculation (pre-ejaculate), which may contain HIV or other STD bacteria or viruses. Even if no sperm are actually deposited in the vagina, pregnancy is possible if sperm are released near the vagina and enter later, perhaps inadvertently, through body-to-body contact.

Withdrawal can diminish a couple's sexual pleasure. When the man must concentrate on withdrawing and the woman is concerned about whether he will withdraw in time, neither is free to fully experience the pleasure of sexual intercourse.

 ### Douching

Douching (rinsing of the vagina with fluid) after sexual intercourse is a method of birth control that is almost totally ineffective. After ejaculation in the vagina, thousands of sperm move through the cervix and enter the uterus within a few seconds. There simply isn't time to flush out sperm from the vagina before a significant number enter the uterus. Furthermore, the force from the spray of the douche may propel sperm into the uterus, aiding conception rather than preventing it. Douching is unnecessary for most women because the vagina is constantly cleansing itself.

 ### Hormonal Contraception: The Pill

In 1960, the U.S. Food and Drug Administration (FDA) approved the use of oral hormonal contraceptive agents for women. Today millions of women in the United States are "on the pill." Worldwide, the number of users is thought to exceed 150 million.

Terms

failure rate: likelihood of becoming pregnant if using a birth control method for one year

lowest observed failure rate: likelihood of becoming pregnant if using a birth control method consistently and as intended

typical failure rate: likelihood of becoming pregnant considering all the potential problems associated with a birth control method

coitus interruptus: removing the penis from the vagina just prior to ejaculation; also called withdrawal or pulling out

douching: rinsing the vaginal canal with a liquid; not an effective means of birth control or STD prevention

TABLE 10.2   Effectiveness Rates of Birth Control Methods

Method	Typical failure rate (%)	Lowest observed failure rate (%)
No Method (chance)	85	85
Withdrawal	19	4
Combination Birth Control Pill	5	0.1
Progestin-only Pill	5	0.5
Depo-Provera	0.3	0.3
Norplant	0.09	0.09
Copper T IUD	0.8	0.6
Male Latex Condom	14	3
Female Latex Condom	21	5
Diaphragm	20	6
Cervical Cap	20	9
Spermicide Alone	26	6
Fertility Awareness	25	1–9
Female Sterilization	0.5	0.5
Male Sterilization	0.5	0.5

Data are percent of women becoming pregnant using a method for one year. Typical failure rate means that the method was not always used correctly and with every act of sexual intercourse. Lowest observed failure rate means the method was used correctly and with every act of sexual intercourse.

Source: U.S. Food and Drug Administration, 1998

The reasons for the pill's popularity include its convenience, low cost, reversibility, tolerable side effects (for most users), and, most significantly, its effectiveness. The pill is 95% to 99.9% effective in preventing conception, when used correctly.

Combination Birth Control Pills

The most common hormonal contraceptives contain a combination of two synthetic hormones that in many ways mimic the actions of a woman's natural ovarian hormones. One of the synthetic hormones is similar to the natural hormone estrogen, and the other is similar to the natural hormone progesterone. The progesterone-like compound is called a progestogen or progestin. In addition to combination oral contraceptives, a progestin-only pill (minipill) is available. The mechanisms by which the synthetic hormones are thought to prevent pregnancy are shown in Table 10.3.

More than 40 brands of birth control pills are available. Many have similar ingredients in identical dosages, but are produced by different manufacturers. Today, combination pills generally contain between 20 and 35 micrograms of estrogen and 0.5 and 1.5 milligrams of progestin, compared with 100 to 175 micrograms of estrogen and 10 milligrams of progestin in

the pills of the 1960s. Progestin-only minipills contain 0.35 milligrams of progestin or less. Some combination pills also have an iron supplement to help prevent iron-deficiency anemia. Combination pills vary from one brand to the next in the potency of estrogen and progestin.

Regardless of brand or dose of synthetic hormones, the method of taking the combination oral contraceptives is the same. The pills come in packages of 21 or 28 pills. In the 21-pill packets, all the pills contain a prescribed mixture of the two synthetic hormones. In the 28-pill packets, 21 of the pills contain hormones; the other seven pills are inert or contain iron and serve as a way to keep track of the days that no hormone is to be taken. The pills with the hormones are usually a different color from the inert, or iron-containing tablets. The first pill in a packet is taken on a predetermined day, and one pill is taken each day. Approximately two days after the last active pill is taken, a menstrual period should occur. Minipills come in 28-day packets; each pill contains active hormone. One pill is taken each day for an entire cycle, even during menstruation.

Those using pills are encouraged to take their daily pill with some routine activity, such as eating a meal, brushing their teeth, or going to bed. Taking the pill at the same time each day increases its effectiveness and decreases the likelihood of forgetting to take it. The hormones in today's birth control pills only prevent ovulation for approximately 24 hours. This is why the timing of taking the pill is important. It takes up to 1 month for the pill to become effective; thus, it is important to use a back-up method until the first packet is completed.

If you forget to take one pill, take it as soon as you remember. Take the next pill at your regular time. This means that you take two pills in one day. You

TABLE 10.3   Mechanisms of Action of Estrogens and Progestogens Used in Oral Contraceptives

Hormone	Mechanisms of action
Estrogens	1. Inhibition of ovulation by suppressing the release of pituitary hormones FSH and LH 2. Inhibition of implantation of the fertilized egg 3. Acceleration of transport of the ovum in the fallopian tube 4. Accelerated degeneration of the corpus luteum, which secretes progesterone, and consequent prevention of normal implantation of the fertilized ovum
Progestogens	1. Production of thick cervical mucus, which blocks sperm transport from the vagina to the uterus 2. Change in the character of cervical mucus such that sperm are less able to effect fertilization 3. Deceleration of ovum transport in the fallopian tubes 4. Inhibition of implantation 5. Interruption of the hormonal regulation of ovulation

Wellness Guide

A Comparison of Various Contraceptive Methods

Method	How it works	Effectiveness	Advantages	Disadvantages
Withdrawal	Man withdraws penis from vagina before ejaculation	Low	Causes no health problems	Requires considerable control on the part of the male; may decrease sexual satisfaction
Fertility awareness	Intercourse only on a woman's "safe" days	Moderate, if used consistently and conscientiously	Causes no health problems	Sometimes difficult to predict "safe" days May require long periods of abstention from sexual intercourse
Hormonal contraceptives	Prevents the release of eggs from the ovaries	High	Easy to use Does not interfere with sexual activity	May cause unintended physiological effects (weight gain, breast tenderness) May cause serious health problems
IUD	Prevents implantation and first stages of pregnancy	High	Always available when needed Does not interfere with sexual activity	May cause heavy menstrual bleeding and cramps May increase the chance of pelvic infection
Diaphragm	Blocks sperm from reaching egg; kills sperm	High, if used consistently and correctly	Causes no health problems	Must be used with each incidence of intercourse Must be fitted by a clinician
Cervical cap	Blocks sperm from reaching egg; kills sperm	Moderate	Can remain in place for up to 24 hours	Must be fitted by a clinician May cause cervical irritation
Vaginal foam or creams	Kills sperm	Moderate, if used consistently and correctly	Causes no health problems Can be obtained without a doctor's prescription Protects against sexually transmitted diseases	Must be used before each incidence of intercourse Found messy by some couples
Condom	Prevents sperm from entering vagina	High, if used consistently and correctly	Causes no health problems Can be obtained without a doctor's prescription Helps prevent spread of sexually transmitted diseases	May detract from sexual pleasure May break or tear
Vaginal foam and condom together	Prevents sperm from entering vagina and kills any sperm that accidentally enter	High	Causes no health problems Can be obtained without a doctor's prescription Helps prevent spread of sexually transmitted diseases	Same as for condom alone and foam alone

need not use a back-up birth control method. If you forget to take two pills in a row during week one or week two, you need to take two pills on the day you remember and two pills the next day. Then take one pill a day until you finish the package. You may become pregnant if you have sex in the 7 days after you miss your pills. You must use another birth control method (such as condoms, foam) as a backup for those 7 days. If you forget to take two pills in a row during the third week, throw out the rest of the pill pack and start a new pack that same day, unless you start your pills on a Sunday. Then you should keep taking one pill a day until Sunday and on Sunday throw out the rest of the pack and start a new pack of pills that same day. As before, you may become pregnant if you have sex in the 7 days after you miss your pills. You must use a back-up fertility control method for those 7 days.

The effectiveness of birth control pills may be lessened when they are taken simultaneously with certain other medications, such as antibiotics, anticonvulsants, and a variety of pain relievers and anti-inflammatory drugs. Pill users should continue birth control pill use and consult their health professional about this possibility when taking other medications.

Approximately half the women using oral contraceptives experience unwanted and unintended side effects. Most of the time the side effects present little long-term risk to health, and often they disappear after several cycles on the pill. The more common of the less serious side effects are nausea, weight gain, breast tenderness, mild headaches, spotty bleeding between periods, decreased menstrual flow, increased frequency of vaginitis, increased depression, and lowering of the sex drive. Some other frequent side effects of the pill are considered beneficial by many women. Among these are lessening of acne outbreaks, diminution and even absence of menstrual cramps, decreased number of menstrual bleeding days, and absolute regulation of the menstrual cycle, which can be important for travelers and athletes.

Studies indicate that pill use may help prevent certain diseases. Women who take combination birth control pills have about one-third the chance of developing pelvic inflammatory disease, one-half the chance of developing benign (noncancerous) breast disease and ovarian cysts, nearly complete protection against ectopic pregnancy, and one-half the risk of developing iron-deficiency anemia in comparison to the general population. Data also indicate that combination birth control pills may protect against rheumatoid arthritis, endometrial cancer, and ovarian cancer.

There is no evidence that fertility is affected by taking the pill, even after many years of use. Some women, however, experience menstrual irregularities after discontinuing the pill. Despite the myth, after discontinuing the pill, women can become pregnant immediately. Studies indicate that there is no association between pill use and the possibility of birth defects in children born to pill users.

> It's been so long since I made love, I can't remember who gets tied up.
>
> JOAN RIVERS

For a small percentage of women, oral contraceptives present a severe health risk. Several studies have shown that the risk of fatal blood clots and heart attack is greater for some women who take oral contraceptives than for those who do not. Women most at risk are those who are over age 35 and those who smoke cigarettes. These women should consider using a birth control method other than the pill. Any pill user who experiences severe abdominal pain, chest pain, headaches, unusual eye problems (blurred vision, flashing lights, temporary blindness), or severe calf and thigh pain should consult a physician or family planning agency immediately. The risk of developing liver disease, gallbladder disease, high blood pressure, and stroke is also slightly greater for pill users. Recent studies show that pill use carries no increased risk of developing breast cancer.

Progestin-Only Contraceptives

Progestin-only contraceptives are available as pills, injections, and implants. Progestin-only contraceptives work by inhibiting ovulation and thickening the cervical mucus, making it more difficult for sperm to reach the egg. Side effects may include menstrual irregularities, weight gain, depression, fatigue, decreased sex drive, acne or oily skin, and headaches. Progestin-only contraceptives are completely reversible. A woman returns to her previous level of fertility when she stops using any of the methods.

Depo-Provera is a 12-week supply of a hormone similar to progesterone, one of the hormones that regulate the menstrual cycle. It is called depo-medroxyprogesterone acetate (DMPA) and is injected intramuscularly by a health care provider. The hormone is released at a steady rate. At the end of the 12 weeks, a replacement injection or another contraceptive must be obtained.

Depo-Provera acts by preventing the egg cells from ripening. If an egg is not released from the ovaries during the menstrual cycle, it cannot become fertilized by sperm and result in pregnancy. Depo-Provera also causes changes in the lining of the uterus that make it less likely for pregnancy to occur. Depo-Provera is over 99.7% effective.

To stop using Depo-Provera, the woman does not get the next injection. Most women who get pregnant do so within 12 to 18 months of the last injection. This method can be used while breast-feeding, starting 6 weeks after delivery. The most common side effects include: irregular menstrual bleeding, amenorrhea, weight gain, headache, nervousness, stomach pain or cramps, dizziness, weakness or fatigue, and decreased sex drive. Depo-Provera is intended to prevent pregnancy only, and does not protect against the transmission of sexually transmitted diseases (STDs). Therefore, another method needs to be used in conjunction with Depo-Provera to prevent STD transmission.

Norplant consists of six thin, hormone-containing (levonorgestrel) capsules made of soft flexible material, which are placed in a fan-like pattern under the skin on the inside surface of the upper arm. After insertion, the hormone is released into the body continuously, keeping the ovaries from releasing eggs. One insertion is effective for up to 5 years. Norplant is nearly 100% effective in preventing pregnancy; however, it is not effective in protecting against STDs. Norplant is inserted by a trained medical professional in an office or clinic; the procedure takes about 10 to 15 minutes. Once under the skin, the capsules are invisible, but the outline of the capsules can be felt and sometimes seen. For some women, discoloration over the placement site occurs, which usually reverses when the capsules are removed, and irregular menstrual bleeding and weight gain may also occur. The removal procedure (or replacement with fresh hormone-filled capsules) is supposed to be simple. In some women, however, fibrous scar tissue builds up around the capsules, making their removal difficult and painful.

The Intrauterine Device

The **intrauterine device (IUD)** is a small device, containing copper or the hormone progesterone, implanted by a health care professional inside the uterus. A short string hangs into the vagina where it cannot be seen but where a woman can reach up and feel for its placement once a month after menses (Figure 10.1).

The possible mechanisms by which IUDs work include: (a) killing or weakening sperm; (b) altering the timing of the ovum's or embryo's movement through the fallopian tube; or (c) inhibiting implantation of the embryo in the uterine lining. Although IUDs have been available for many years, the exact mechanism of action of IUDs is not completely understood. IUDs seem to affect the way the sperm or egg moves.

During the 1960s and 1970s, several kinds of IUD were available. Early in 1986, however, all but one of the major types of IUD had been withdrawn from the U.S. market because hundreds of IUD current and former users claimed that they were harmed by the device. These users sued the manufacturers of IUDs, and manufacturers chose to withdraw the devices from the U.S. market rather than face the enormous costs of both legal defense and large financial settlements. So costly were the damages assessed against one IUD, the Dalkon Shield—the use of which was associated with pelvic infections, ectopic pregnancies, and several deaths—that its manufacturer declared bankruptcy.

Currently, two types of IUD are available in the United States: the Progestasert, and the ParaGard Copper T 380A. Both are plastic devices shaped like a "T."

Progestasert continuously releases a small amount of progestin and must be replaced every year. The Para-Gard contains copper and can be left in place for 10 years.

Research indicates that IUD use increases the risk for pelvic inflammatory diseases, uterine perforations, and increased risk of **ectopic pregnancy,** if a pregnancy occurs with the device in place. **Pelvic inflammatory disease (PID)** can damage the fallopian tubes sufficiently to make a woman infertile or to increase the likelihood of ectopic pregnancy.

Barrier Methods

Barrier methods of fertility control involve devices that physically block the path of sperm movement in the female reproductive tract and usually bring sperm in contact with a sperm-killing (spermicidal) chemical, most often nonoxynol-9. Several contraceptive methods work on this principle, including the diaphragm; the cervical cap; spermicidal foams, jellies, and creams; and the condom.

The Diaphragm

The **diaphragm** is a dome-shaped latex cup, which is placed in the vagina to cover the cervix (Figure 10.2). A metal spring in the rim of the diaphragm holds the device snugly in place between the back wall of the vagina and the pubic bone in the front of the pelvis. In this position the diaphragm blocks the movement of sperm from the vagina to the uterus, although it does not fit snugly enough to keep all of the sperm out. Its primary purpose is to hold a spermicide in place next to the cervix. Correct usage requires that the rim and

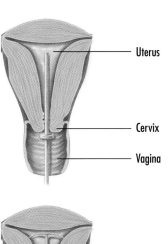

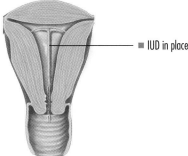

FIGURE 10.1   The IUD is inserted past the cervix into the uterus. Prior to insertion the length of the uterus is measured with an instrument called a sound. Upon insertion the arms of the IUD gradually unfold. Once the inserter is removed the threads attached to the IUD will be clipped to extend into the vagina through the cervical opening.

Labels: Uterus, Cervix, Vagina, IUD in place

Terms

progestin-only contraceptives: work by inhibiting ovulation and thickening of the cervical mucus; completely reversible

Depo-Provera: injectable form of medroxyprogesterone acetate

Norplant: hormone-containing capsule inserted under the skin

intrauterine device (IUD): a flexible, usually plastic, device inserted into the uterus to prevent pregnancy

ectopic pregnancy: implanting of the embryo outside the uterus, usually in the fallopian tubes

pelvic inflammatory disease (PID): inflammation of the pelvic structures, especially the uterus and fallopian tubes; often caused by a sexually transmitted disease

diaphragm: a soft, rubber, dome-shaped contraceptive device worn over the cervix and used with spermicidal jelly or cream

cup of the diaphragm be coated with a tablespoon or two of a spermicidal jelly or cream. The diaphragm should be left in place 6 to 8 hours after intercourse. The spermicides used with the diaphragm also help prevent the transmission of some microorganisms responsible for genital infections.

One major advantage of the diaphragm is the absence of major medical problems associated with its use. A very few women or their partners may be allergic to the latex or the spermicide and some develop urinary tract infections. Some women may experience discomfort with the diaphragm in place. Changing brands or getting a better-fitting diaphragm often solves these problems.

Another advantage is that the diaphragm can be inserted up to 6 hours before intercourse, so a couple does not have to interrupt sexual pleasuring to insert the device. If a diaphragm is inserted several hours before sexual activity, however, it is advisable to put an additional amount of spermicidal jelly or cream into the vagina before intercourse. The diaphragm must be left in place 6 to 8 hours after last intercourse, but should not be used longer than 24 hours because of the possible risk of toxic shock syndrome.

Each woman must be fitted (by a family planning professional or a physician) with a diaphragm that is the correct size for her. The need for proper fitting is one reason that diaphragms are available only by prescription. Any change in a woman's body size—a gain or loss of several pounds, pregnancy, or pelvic surgery—is reason to check the fit and have a new diaphragm prescribed if necessary. A woman should not use another woman's diaphragm because the fit might be wrong, lowering the device's effectiveness.

After each use the diaphragm should be washed with mild soap and water, rinsed thoroughly, and dried in the air or with a towel. Perfumed talcum powders, petroleum jelly, or scented creams should not be used with the diaphragm. Occasionally the rubber darkens, but this generally does not impair effectiveness.

One disadvantage of the diaphragm is the possibility of dislodgment during intercourse. Only rarely will a man feel the diaphragm during sexual intercourse if the device is inserted properly. If either the man or the woman experiences unusual sensations or discomfort during intercourse, then the diaphragm may not be inserted correctly, it may have become dislodged during intercourse, or it may be the wrong size. Other disadvantages of the diaphragm are that spermicides can be messy to use, and the diaphragm should not be used during menstruation or vaginal infection.

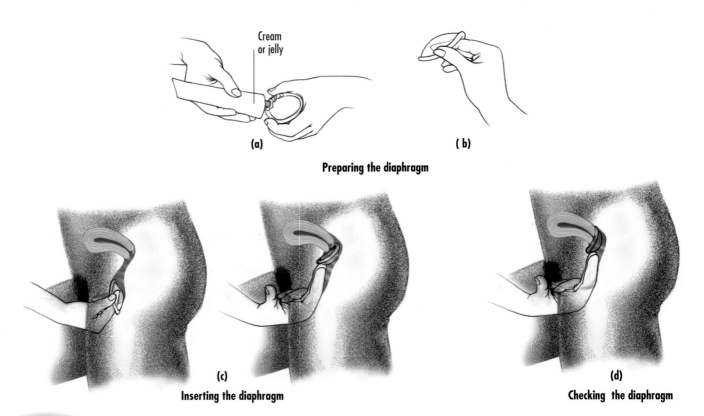

Preparing the diaphragm

(a)   (b)

Inserting the diaphragm   (c)   (d)   **Checking the diaphragm**

FIGURE 10.2   **Procedure for Inserting a Diaphragm**   (a) Before inserting the diaphragm coat the rim and cup with a spermicidal cream or jelly. (b) Squeeze the rim of the diaphragm together between your thumb and index finger. (c) Insert the diaphragm into the vagina with the rim facing up and push it toward the small of your back. As you let go of the diaphragm it will spring open, continue to guide it to your cervix with the tips of your fingers. (d) Be sure to check that the diaphragm completely covers the cervix.

Periodically the diaphragm should be held against a light to check for tiny holes and weak spots (where the rubber buckles). With proper care a diaphragm will last a year or two.

The Cervical Cap

The **cervical cap** is a cup-shaped rubber device that snugly covers the cervix similar to the way a thimble fits on a finger (Figure 10.3). Like a diaphragm, a cervical cap needs to be coated with spermicide to be as effective as possible and remain in place for 8 hours after last intercourse. Cervical caps come in several sizes and must be fitted for each woman. One distinct difference between the diaphragm and the cervical cap is the fact that the cervical cap can be inserted up to 24 hours before intercourse.

The principal advantages of the cervical cap are:

- Low cost and convenience
- Can be inserted any time of the day intercourse is anticipated
- Sexual activity can take place spontaneously during the ensuing 24 hours without concern about fertility control.

The major disadvantages of the cervical cap are difficulty with insertion and removal, occasional discomfort during intercourse, dislodgment during intercourse, and possibly irritation of the cervix. The cervical cap should not be left in place for more than 48 hours at a time.

Vaginal Spermicides

A variety of fertility control methods consist solely of a spermicidal chemical (nonoxynol-9 or octoxynol) and an inert substance that transports and retains the **spermicide** in the vagina, which kill sperm and help inactivate viruses and bacteria. Specific directions in the packages tell you how to insert the spermicide and what timing recommendations and repeat applications are necessary. These agents include foams, gels, creams, and vaginal **suppositories.** Although often displayed in stores with other feminine hygiene products, vaginal spermicides should not be confused with douches, deodorant products, or lubricants, none of which are effective fertility control methods.

The effectiveness of all of the vaginal spermicides depends on a sufficient quantity of sperm-killing chemical bathing the cervix at the time of ejaculation. Among typical users, however, the failure rate is about eighteen pregnancies per 100 women per year. Using vaginal spermicides requires dedication and competence. Users must put the spermicide in the vagina immediately before every act of intercourse and before each subsequent intercourse in the same sexual encounter.

Users of foam should be sure that the foam is frothy and bubbly, which is achieved by shaking the container about twenty times before filling the applicator. Because there is no way to know how much foam remains in a container, a spare container should be kept on hand.

Suppositories should be placed as far back in the vagina as possible so that the dissolved spermicide covers the cervix. It is important to allow enough time (from 10 to 30 minutes, depending on the product) for the suppository to dissolve completely before each act of intercourse. Vaginal suppositories have the disadvantage of the waiting period to allow the tablet to melt.

Major advantages of vaginal spermicides are:

- They are available without a doctor's prescription.
- They can be purchased in pharmacies and many supermarkets.
- The spermicidal chemicals give some added protection against STDs.
- The effectiveness of spermicidal agents increases to nearly 100% when they are used simultaneously with a condom.

Vaginal spermicides tend to be slippery, which occasionally can be a nuisance, but the moisture can augment a woman's natural vaginal lubrication and enhance sensation. These methods may also be a hindrance to oral-genital stimulation. In rare instances, someone may be allergic to a particular product. Changing brands may alleviate this problem. Some women experience irritation if the tablet has not

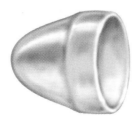

FIGURE 10.3   **Cervical Cap**

Terms

cervical cap: small latex cap that covers the cervix, used with spermicidal jelly or cream inside the cap

spermicide: a chemical that kills sperm; particularly foams, creams, gels, and suppositories used for contraception

suppositories: a medicine placed in a body orifice to dissolve and sometimes to be absorbed; birth control suppositories contain spermicidal chemicals

dissolved completely before intercourse takes place. Some erroneously believe that spermicides cause birth defects; this belief is a myth.

Male Condoms

The male **condom,** or rubber, is a membranous sheath that covers the erect penis and catches semen before it enters the vagina. About 99% of male condoms are made of latex; the rest, so-called "skin" condoms, which are not effective against STDs, are manufactured from lamb intestines.

Condoms can be obtained in pharmacies, supermarkets, vending machines, and through mail order advertisements in newspapers, magazines, and catalogs. When stored in a cool, dry place, condoms retain their effectiveness for up to 5 years. Kept in a warm environment, such as in a wallet in the back pocket of one's pants or in the glove compartment of a car, the latex will deteriorate. To be effective, condoms must be used with water-based lubricants, such as K-Y Jelly, because petroleum-based lubricants will cause the latex to deteriorate.

There are many advantages to using condoms. Condoms are:

- Easy to obtain
- Inexpensive
- Free of medical risk (rarely a man or a woman may be allergic to the latex, lubricant, or spermicide)
- Reliable
- Effective
- Proven protection against STDs

A primary reason for condom failure in preventing pregnancy is error in use. Used in conjunction with another barrier method, such as a diaphragm or spermicidal foam, condoms are nearly 100% effective. Another advantage is that condoms help prevent the transmission of chlamydia, gonorrhea, herpes, HIV infection, and other kinds of infections.

Some people complain that the condom diminishes pleasurable sensations, but the device does not totally block genital feeling, which, in any event, is only one of many factors that contribute to sexual arousal and pleasure. A negative attitude about condoms may diminish pleasure far more than a thin layer of latex ever could. Instead of thinking about how condoms block sensations, it might enhance lovemaking to think of them as a fun way to help

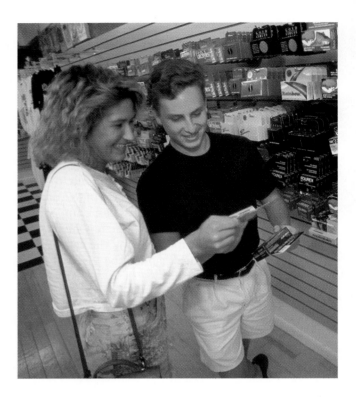

Condoms are an effective form of fertility control and provide protection against STDs. It's important that both partners take responsibility for using condoms.

make lovemaking more pleasurable because of the protection they provide.

When using a condom, consider ways to incorporate putting on the device without interrupting lovemaking. For example, having a condom available before sexual activity begins makes breaking off contact to obtain one unnecessary. Before intercourse begins, either partner can put the condom on the erect penis while the couple continues to fondle, talk, or play.

Female Condoms

The female condom, the brand name of which is Reality, is a thin, loose-fitting polyurethane plastic pouch that lines the vagina. It has two flexible rings: an inner ring at the closed end, used to insert the device inside the vagina and hold it in place, and an outer ring which remains outside the vagina and covers the external genitalia. Figure 10.4 shows the insertion and positioning of the female condom. Because the device is made from polyurethane, which is 40% stronger than latex, the female condom can be used with any type of lubricant without compromising the integrity of the device.

Two advantages of the female condom are that (a) it warms up instantly to body temperature once it is inserted, thus enhancing sensation for both partners and (b) it provides protection from STDs (by covering

Terms

condom: a latex or polyurethane sheath worn over the penis (male condom) or inside the vagina (female condom); can be both a barrier method and act as a prophylactic against sexually transmitted diseases

both internal and external genitalia), including HIV, and prevents pregnancy. Also, the female condom is easy to buy in drugstores and supermarkets, an erection is unnecessary to keep the female condom in place, and it can be used by people allergic to latex or spermicide.

Some disadvantages of the female condom are that it cannot be used with a male condom, and is not as effective as a male condom. Its pregnancy failure rate was 5% for those who used it correctly every time compared with 3% for the male condom. The typical failure rate, for those who did not use it correctly every time they had sex was 21% compared to 12% for the male latex condom. Occasionally, the outer ring may be pushed inside the vagina. Other problems include (a) difficulties in insertion and removal; (b) minor irritation; (c) discomfort or breakage, which can be decreased by using enough lubrication; (d) it is not aesthetically pleasing; and (e) it costs more than male condoms.

Wellness Guide

Putting On a Condom

For pleasure, ease, and effectiveness, both partners should know how to put on and use a condom. To learn without feeling pressured or embarrassed, practice on your penis or a penis-shaped object, such as a ketchup bottle, banana, cucumber, or squash.

Remember: Practice Makes Perfect

- Put the condom on before the penis touches the vulva. Men leak fluids from their penises before and after ejaculation. Pre-ejaculate ("pre-cum") can carry enough sperm to cause pregnancy and enough germs to cause STDs.

- Use a condom only once. Use a fresh one for each erection ("hard-on"). Have a good supply on hand.

- Condoms usually come rolled into a ring shape. They are individually sealed in aluminum foil or plastic. Be careful—don't tear the condom while unwrapping it. If it is brittle, stiff, or sticky, throw it away and use another.

- Put a drop or two of lubricant inside the condom.

- Place the rolled condom over the tip of the hard penis.

- Leave one-half inch of space at the tip to collect semen.

- If the penis is not circumcised, pull back the foreskin before rolling on the condom.

- Pinch the air out of the tip with one hand. (Friction against air bubbles causes most condom breaks.)

- Unroll the condom over the penis with the other hand.

- Roll it all the way down to the base of the penis.

- Smooth out any air bubbles.

- Lubricate the outside of the condom.

Taking Off a Condom

- Pull out before the penis softens.

- Don't spill the semen—hold the condom against the base of the penis while you pull out.

- Throw the condom away.

- Wash the penis with soap and water before embracing again.

Source: Planned Parenthood Federation of America, Inc. http://www.plannedparenthood.org/

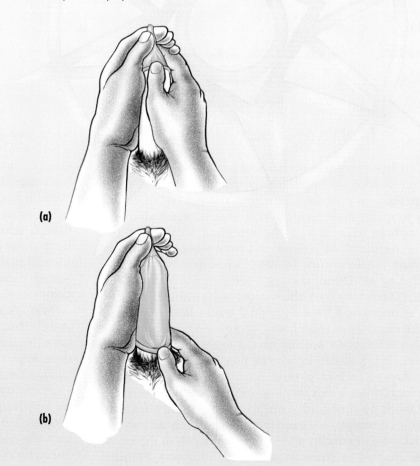

(a)

(b)

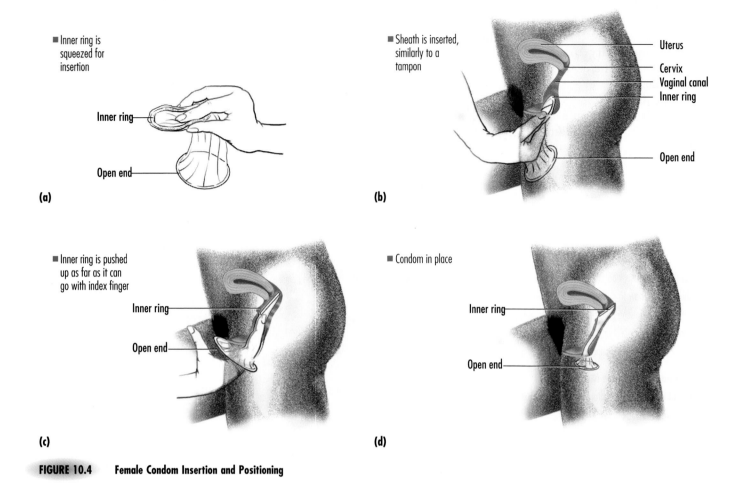

(a)
■ Inner ring is squeezed for insertion

Inner ring

Open end

(b)
■ Sheath is inserted, similarly to a tampon

Uterus
Cervix
Vaginal canal
Inner ring

Open end

(c)
■ Inner ring is pushed up as far as it can go with index finger

Inner ring

Open end

(d)
■ Condom in place

Inner ring

Open end

FIGURE 10.4   **Female Condom Insertion and Positioning**

Fertility Awareness Methods

Fertility awareness methods of fertility control (sometimes called natural family planning, the rhythm method, or periodic abstinence) attempt to determine a woman's most fertile period; that is, when an ovum has been released from the ovary and is capable of being fertilized. In general, the time when a woman is most fertile occurs 14 days before her next period. During ovulation, the egg lives only 24 hours. If the egg is not fertilized, the woman will shed the lining of the uterus and have a period 2 weeks later. Although the egg lives only 24 hours, sperm can live 3 to 5 days inside the body waiting for the egg to mature. Therefore, it is possible to become pregnant during the 5 to 6 days of each menstrual cycle. In women who cycle every 28 days, this fertility occurs mid-cycle. Fertility cannot be predicted with absolute certainty because no two women are exactly alike and even an individual woman's cycles may vary from month to month or be affected by stress, lack of sleep, or illness. Fertility awareness methods of birth control either estimate

when ovulation is most likely to occur or indicate when ovulation has already taken place, thereby telling a couple the days in the menstrual cycle not to have unprotected intercourse. Those are referred to as "unsafe days." The days when a woman is not likely to be fertile are referred to as "safe days." On unsafe days, a couple should use an alternative method of birth control, such as condoms, a diaphragm, or spermicidal foam. Other options include enjoying ways of sexual pleasuring other than genital intercourse, or complete sexual abstinence.

Couples using fertility awareness methods should realize that, even on safe days, fertilization is still possible because of natural variations in a woman's reproductive processes. Therefore, safe days are really *relatively* safe days.

Fertility awareness offers the advantages of posing no health risks and being cost-free; furthermore, some people's religious convictions make fertility awareness the only acceptable method of birth control. The effectiveness of fertility awareness is among the lowest of the common methods, about twenty pregnancies per 100 women per year. Failures occur because people do not keep careful records, they find the intervals of abstinence during the unsafe days too long, and they find having to plan sex only for the safe days a hindrance to spontaneous lovemaking.

Calendar Rhythm

Calendar rhythm is a way to estimate the most likely fertile, or unsafe, days in a woman's menstrual cycle by assuming that:

1. Ovulation usually takes place 14 days (plus or minus 2 days) before the onset of the next menstrual flow.
2. An ovum is capable of being fertilized for 24 hours.
3. Sperm deposited in the vagina remain capable of fertilization for up to 3 days.

Using calendar rhythm effectively requires knowledge of the female fertility cycle and instruction in doing the calculations correctly (Figure 10.5). Family planning agencies, women's health clinics, and books on fertility awareness methods can be helpful in learning the method.

The Temperature Method

The **basal body temperature (BBT)** is the lowest temperature in a healthy person during waking hours. In 70% to 90% of women, the BBT rises approximately one degree after ovulation, presumably because of changes in hormone levels. By keeping a daily record of the BBT, a woman can determine when ovulation has occurred and therefore the unsafe and safe days for intercourse between ovulation and the beginning of the next menstrual cycle. Because the BBT method cannot predict when ovulation will occur, a woman must still estimate with another fertility awareness method (calendar method, mucus method) the safe and unsafe days before ovulation.

Temperature measurements should take at least 5 minutes. Temperature measurements should be taken at the same time each day, and a record should be kept on a graph (Figure 10.6). Once the BBT has risen for 3 consecutive days, a woman can assume that ovulation has taken place and that the rest of the days in that menstrual cycle are safe for unprotected intercourse.

The Mucus Method

Certain hormone-sensitive glands in the cervix produce mucus that changes in amount, color, and consistency during different phases of the menstrual cycle. Learning to recognize the changes in cervical

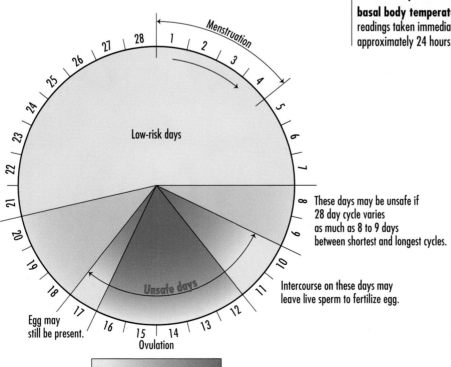

These days may be unsafe if 28 day cycle varies as much as 8 to 9 days between shortest and longest cycles.

Intercourse on these days may leave live sperm to fertilize egg.

Egg may still be present.

Low risk   Unsafe

FIGURE 10.5   Calendar Method The calendar method is based on avoiding intercourse when sperm can fertilize ovum. Unsafe days for intercourse in this chart are days 12 to 16.

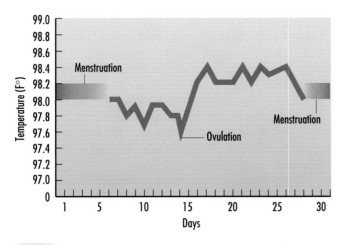

FIGURE 10.6   **Basal Body Temperature Method of Contraception**   A woman's body temperature rises about one degree during the days following ovulation. Once the BBT has risen for 3 consecutive days, assume that ovulation has taken place and that the rest of the days in that menstrual cycle are safe for unprotected intercourse. To use the BBT method, a woman must record her basal body temperature each morning before engaging in *any* activity. Thus, it is advisable to record the body temperature before going to sleep. Temperature measurement should last at least 5 minutes.

mucus can help determine when ovulation occurs, and safe and unsafe days for intercourse can be planned accordingly.

The mucus method requires that cervical mucus be examined frequently during the cycle. Samples of mucus may be obtained with a finger or on toilet tissue or discharge on underpants may be observed. Collection with a finger is best because it permits direct determination of the amount and consistency of mucus.

Because douching, vaginal infections, semen, contraceptive foams and jellies, vaginal lubricants, medications, and vaginal lubrication from sexual arousal can interfere with the recognition of mucus patterns, women wishing to use the mucus method should obtain instructions from an experienced user, a family planning clinic, or a health center. A woman should plan on charting her cervical mucus for at least a month to learn her individual pattern of mucus changes before relying on the method for fertility control.

The **sympto-thermal method** involves using the temperature and mucus methods simultaneously.

Chemical Methods

Chemical methods of fertility awareness measure the amount of **luteinizing hormone** in a woman's urine, which peaks at the time of ovulation. Ovulation predictor kits to measure the levels of LH can be purchased in pharmacies. Manufacturers claim that the kits have an accuracy rate of 85%.

 ## Sterilization

Sterility is being permanently unable to have children. For people who are certain that they do not want children, or, as is more often the case, no more children, surgical methods that render a person sterile but have no effect on sexual arousal or activities may be the most desirable form of birth control. Indeed, for married couples over age 30, "permanent fertility control" (sterilization of either the male or female partner) has become the most frequently chosen method of fertility control. The popularity of sterilization as a method of fertility control stems from its nearly 100% effectiveness, the relative safety of the procedure, and its relatively low one-time cost.

Male Sterilization

The sterilization of a man is called **vasectomy.** Approximately 500,000 men in the United States choose vasectomy every year. This procedure involves the cutting and tying of each of the two vas deferens, the tubes that connect the testes (where sperm are made) to the penis (Figure 10.7). When these tubes are cut, sperm are no longer emitted upon ejaculation because their passage is blocked. Because the cut is made "upstream" from the organs that produce seminal fluid, a man still ejaculates, but the semen contains no sperm cells. And because the sperm cells make up only a

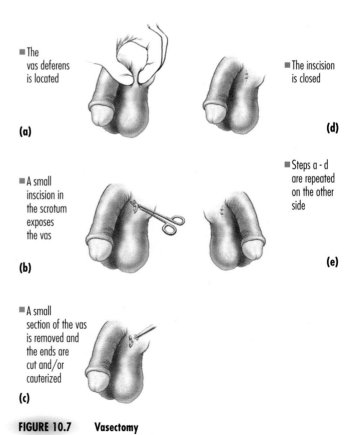

■ The vas deferens is located

(a)

■ A small inscision in the scrotum exposes the vas

(b)

■ A small section of the vas is removed and the ends are cut and/or cauterized

(c)

■ The inscision is closed

(d)

■ Steps a - d are repeated on the other side

(e)

FIGURE 10.7   **Vasectomy**

small percentage of the total volume of the semen, neither a man nor his partner is aware of any change in their sex life, except that no other form of contraception is needed.

Although vasectomy should be considered a permanent form of contraception, it is sometimes possible to reverse the condition by rejoining the cut ends of the vasa deferentia. The success of vasectomy reversal as measured by the ability to have children again is about 50% although some surgeons claim much higher reversal rates.

One of the reasons vasectomy is such a popular method of contraception is that it is uncomplicated and causes few problems. The procedure is usually carried out in a doctor's office with a local anesthetic in about 15 to 30 minutes. The incidence of postoperative complications is very low, and within a week most men can return to regular activities, including sex. About one-half to two-thirds of vasectomized men develop antibodies to sperm, but there is no evidence to suggest that this is harmful. A man can be fertile for several weeks, because the sperm pathway contains sperm present before the vasectomy. Once these are ejaculated the man is sterile.

Female Sterilization

The principal sterilization procedure for women is **tubal ligation,** which is the blocking of the fallopian tubes (Figure 10.8). Blocking can be accomplished by cutting and tying the tubes, by sealing the tubes (cautery), or by closing them with clips, bands, or rings. Most tubal ligations can be performed under local anesthesia in about 20 minutes in a clinic or a doctor's office, and the woman can usually go home the same day or the day after. The incidence of postoperative complications is low.

Most tubal ligations are "band-aid" surgeries, so-called because the operation requires only one or two inch-long incisions to be made. The incisions allow the surgeon to enter the abdominal cavity and locate and block the fallopian tubes. Entry to the abdominal cavity is generally through an incision just below the umbilicus. Vaginal tubal ligation is called **culpotomy.** There are two types of abdominal tubal ligations, **minilaparotomy** and **laparoscopy.** The main difference between the two is the way the fallopian tubes are visualized. In minilaparotomy, the doctor exposes the tubes to direct view; in laparoscopy, the tubes are visualized with a cylindrical viewing device (the laparoscope), which is placed in the abdominal cavity through a small surgical incision.

Although tubal ligation is intended to be a permanent form of birth control, accidental pregnancies occur because a blocked tube spontaneously reopens. Surgical reversal of tubal blocking may be possible if a

(a) Sagittal section

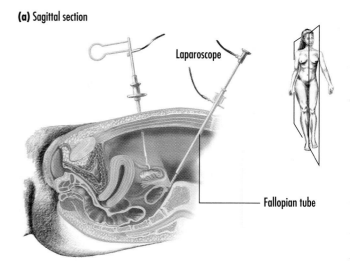

Laparoscope

Fallopian tube

(b) Front view

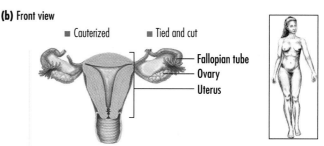

■ Cauterized   ■ Tied and cut

Fallopian tube
Ovary
Uterus

FIGURE 10.8   Tubal Ligation   Female sterilization by laparoscopic ligation. **(a)** Cross section: The tubes are located using a laparoscope and cut, tied, or cauterized through a second incision. **(b)** Front view: The tubes after ligation.

woman later decides that she wants to have children, with a success rate of 50% to 70%.

Another female sterilization technique is **hysterectomy,** the surgical removal of the uterus. Most experts do not recommend hysterectomy solely for

Terms

sympto-thermal method: using both the BBT and the mucus methods at the same time

luteinizing hormone: anterior pituitary hormone that causes a follicle to release a ripened ovum and become a corpus luteum; in the male, it stimulates testosterone production and the production of sperm cells

sterility: not being able to be impregnated or impregnate

vasectomy: a surgical procedure in men in which segments of the vas deferens are removed and the ends tied to prevent the passage of sperm

tubal ligation: a surgical procedure in women in which the fallopian tubes are cut, tied, or cauterized to prevent pregnancy; a form of sterilization

culpotomy: a female sterilization procedure

minilaparotomy: female sterilization procedure in which the fallopian tubes are ligated or cauterized through a small abdominal incision

laparoscopy: a surgical incision into the abdomen used to visualize internal organs

hysterectomy: surgical removal of the uterus

sterilization purposes because, when compared to tubal ligation, the chances for postoperative complications are 10 to 100 times greater, the operation is more expensive, and the negative psychological effect may be greater.

Choosing the Right Fertility Control Method

Most users of fertility control are principally concerned with two questions: How well does the method work, and is it safe? The efficacy of a fertility control method can be evaluated in terms of the lowest observed failure rate which is how well the method performs if it is used consistently and as intended and the typical failure rate which is a measure of how well a method performs in actual use in a population. The typical failure rate takes into account improper, inconsistent, and careless usage.

Considerations about the safety of fertility control methods must take into account the health risks of a particular method, such as serious illness, the possibility of infection and its consequences, the risk of death, the risk of being unable to have children in the future, any effects on unborn children, and undesirable and unhealthful changes in the body.

Evaluation of a fertility control method's safety should also assess the physical and psychological consequences of an unintended pregnancy. These include the risks associated with terminating the pregnancy by abortion and the risks associated with carrying the pregnancy to term. Factors such as a woman's age, her physical health, whether she has had previous children, and her capacity to care for another child also need to be evaluated. Of course, the most serious risk associated with the use of any contraceptive is the risk of death, which is rare except for older pill users who smoke heavily.

Responsibility for Fertility Control

Most people engage in sexual activity because they want a joyous, rewarding experience. Because an unintended pregnancy can cause enormous hardship, birth control is an important part of every sexual relationship. Denying the possibility of pregnancy by assuming "it can't happen to me" is just gambling against the odds.

> *If only one could tell true love from false love as one can tell mushrooms from toadstools.*
>
> KATHERINE MANSFIELD

The responsibility for fertility control has two components. First, a fertility control method must be chosen, taking into consideration the nature of an individual's sexual activities or a couple's sexual relationship, the frequency of intercourse, future plans regarding children, and personal and religious values. Second, the chosen method must be used consistently and correctly.

For both technological and sociological reasons, there has been a tendency to associate the responsibility for fertility control with the partner for whose body a particular method is designed. For example, in the late nineteenth century, when withdrawal and the condom were the principal methods of fertility control, and women were not supposed to be interested in sex, men were considered to be the ones responsible for fertility control (when it was used at all). In the late 1960s, when the pill and IUD were heralded as "perfect" contraceptives and women began to assert themselves socially and politically, the responsibility for fertility control shifted almost totally to women.

Today a large percentage of sexually active people believe that both partners in a sexual relationship should share the responsibility for fertility control. Yet, because so many methods are intended for use by the woman, in actual practice many women are left to

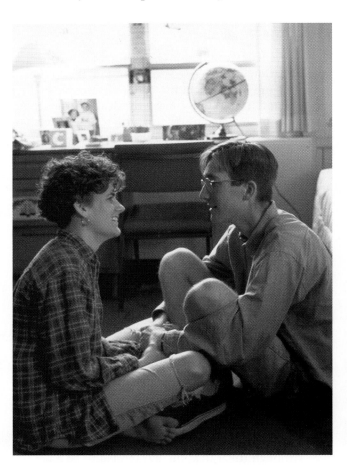

Choosing a fertility control method should be a decision made by both sexual partners and should be discussed before having sex.

manage fertility control on their own. Having to take total responsibility for fertility control can create resentment that blocks the feelings that many people wish to express with sex.

The responsibility for fertility control can be shared in a number of ways. The most important is to discuss it. In an ongoing relationship, there are many opportunities to talk about fertility control. Couples can go to fertility control clinics together, they can read and discuss information about the advantages and disadvantages of the different methods, and they can try out various methods to find out which are best suited for them. They can share the time and the financial costs of their chosen method, or they can divide responsibilities. For example, if a woman has to take time to go to a clinic or doctor, her partner could pay for the clinic visit and the contraceptives.

Partners can also share in using their chosen method. They can discuss any difficulties or concerns they have with their method of fertility control. Partners can even remind each other to use their chosen fertility control method. A man can learn how a diaphragm is used, a woman can learn about the condom, and they can incorporate into their lovemaking preparing to use these and other barrier methods. Furthermore, partners can share the responsibility of inserting, removing, and cleaning the woman's diaphragm or cervical cap. If a woman is using fertility awareness methods, a man can share the responsibility by helping to determine the safe and unsafe days and by sharing the responsibility for abstaining from sexual intercourse.

Partners who share the responsibility for fertility control are more likely to use their chosen method(s) properly, which makes fertility control more effective. And reducing the fear of pregnancy makes sex more enjoyable. Another benefit of sharing this responsibility is that it tends to enhance intimacy in a relationship. The discussion of fertility control and the mutual decision making involved in choosing and using a method lead to better communication.

It is always a good idea for you to have some method of fertility control with you if you anticipate that sexual intercourse might occur. For example, both men and women can carry a condom or spermicides with them on dates or to parties if they think that sexual activity is a possibility.

Discussing Fertility Control Responsibility

A couple shares the responsibility for fertility control because both partners are responsible if an unintended pregnancy occurs. This fact alone is the most important reason for discussing fertility control. Although it is important to discuss fertility control before having sex, many individuals are embarrassed to do so. Talking about contraception implies that sex is going to take place, which may force an individual to face internal conflicts about engaging in sex. Many individuals subscribe to the myth that good sex should be spontaneous rather than planned. Therefore, sex and fertility control remain undiscussed. First-time partners may not discuss fertility control before sex because they fear spoiling a romantic mood.

Still, the best time to discuss fertility control is *before* sexual intercourse. A partner might say, "I would really like to make love (have sex) with you, and I want to be sure we're protected." That kind of introduction can be followed by a statement of preference and personal responsibility, such as, "I prefer to use condoms" or "I'm on the pill" or, using a question, such as, "What birth control method do you prefer?" or "What are we going to do about control?"

In some cases, even if a man is concerned about an unintended pregnancy and sexual diseases, he may not feel comfortable bringing up the topic of control, fearing embarrassment or appearing ignorant or weak. Many women, however, welcome a man who initiates a discussion of control. Communication about control and other sexual matters, such as the role of sex in a relationship, likes and dislikes, and preventing STDs is vital to a healthy sexual relationship.

Why Sexually Active People Do Not Use Fertility Control

Despite a presumed and sometimes stated desire not to become pregnant, approximately 5% of married individuals and 15% of unmarried sexually active individuals use no fertility control. Some of the major reasons that people do not use fertility control, even if they wish to avoid pregnancy, include:

- *Low motivation.* People who have mixed feelings about avoiding pregnancy are less motivated to use fertility control. For example, a couple that has decided that they want to have a child "sometime in the near future" is less likely to be motivated to use fertility control than is a couple that is absolutely certain they do not want a child until some specified time, or at all.

- *Lack of knowledge.* Lack of knowledge about the process of conception and how to use fertility control effectively can lead to an incorrect perception of the risk of becoming pregnant. For example, some people believe the myths that pregnancy is not possible if a woman has an orgasm, if she urinates after intercourse, or if she is having sexual intercourse for the first time. Sometimes a method is believed to be more effective than it really is, or the chosen method is used incorrectly. For example, some people erroneously believe that a woman is most fertile during the bleeding days of the menstrual cycle and thus practice fertility awareness at the wrong time. Some couples lose, misplace, or run out of their primary method and do not have a back-up method available.

- *Negative attitudes about fertility control.* Some people believe that fertility control is immoral, a hassle, unromantic, or harmful. One's own negative attitudes or the perceived negative attitudes of others, such as peers or parents, can inhibit one from obtaining contraceptives. People use these as ex-

cuses not to visit doctors or clinics, or they may shy away from obtaining over-the-counter contraceptives.

- *Relationship issues.* Individuals in committed relationships are better contraceptors than individuals who are not in such relationships. Involvement with a committed partner tends to lessen guilt associated with sexual activity and hence improves attitudes about contraceptive practice. People in a committed relationship tend to have sexual intercourse more often and regularly, which gives the couple opportunities to talk about contraception and to become adept at using method(s). Individuals with irregular sexual contact, either because of geographi-

Wellness Guide

Birth Control Guide

	Male condom	Female condom	Spermicides used alone	Diaphragm with spermicide	Cervical cap with spermicide
Estimated effectiveness	86–98%	79–95%	72–94%	80–94%	80–90%
Risks	Rarely, irritation and allergic reactions	Rarely, irritation and allergic reactions	Rarely, irritation and allergic reactions	Rarely, irritation and allergic reactions; bladder infection; very rarely, toxic shock syndrome	Abnormal Pap test results; vaginal or cervical infections; very rarely, toxic shock syndrome
STD protection	Latex condoms help protect against STDs, including herpes and AIDS	May give some protection against STDs, including herpes and AIDS; not as effective as male latex condom	Unknown	None	None
Convenience	Applied immediately before intercourse; used only once and discarded	Applied immediately before intercourse; used only once and discarded	Applied no more than 1 hour before intercourse	Inserted before intercourse; can be left in place 24 hours, but additional spermicide must be inserted if intercourse is repeated	Can remain in place for 24 hours, not necessary to reapply spermicide upon repeated intercourse; may be difficult to insert
Availability	Nonprescription	Nonprescription	Nonprescription	Rx	Rx
Estimated cost*	$.25–2.50	$2.50	$8	$13–25	$13–25

STD, sexually transmitted disease; Rx, prescription only; PID, pelvic inflammatory disease.

cal separation or relationship problems, may have difficulties in establishing a birth control regime. In new or casual sexual relationships, there is a tendency to use no method or a poor method at first.

Emergency Contraception

Emergency contraception is designed to prevent pregnancy after unprotected vaginal intercourse. It is provided in two ways: (1) emergency IUD insertion within 5 days of unprotected intercourse; and (2) emergency hormonal contraception—two large doses of certain oral contraceptives taken 12 hours apart and

within 72 hours of unprotected intercourse. Side effects are infrequent. Nausea and vomiting are the most common, along with breast tenderness, irregular bleeding, cramping, and headache.

Emergency contraception is warranted if:

- The condom broke or slipped off, and the male ejaculated inside the vagina.
- A woman forgot to take her birth control pills.
- A diaphragm or cervical cap slipped out of place.
- The "safe" days are miscalculated.
- No birth control was used.
- A woman was forced to have unprotected vaginal intercourse.

Pills	Implant (Norplant)	Injection (Depo-Provera)	IUD	Periodic abstinence (NFP)	Surgical sterilization
95–99.9%	99.95%	99.7%	97.4–99.2%	Variable, perhaps 53–86%	>99%
Blood clots, heart attacks and strokes, gallbladder disease, liver tumors, water retention, hypertension, mood changes, dizziness, and nausea; not for smokers	Menstrual cycle irregularity; headaches, nervousness, depression, nausea, dizziness, change of appetite, breast tenderness, weight gain, enlargement of ovaries or fallopian tubes, and excessive growth of body and facial hair; may subside after first year	Amenorrhea, weight gain, and other side effects similar to those with Norplant	Cramps, PID, bleeding, infertility; rarely, perforation of the uterus	None	Pain, infection, and, for female tubal ligation, possible surgical complications
None	None	None	None	None	None
Pill must be taken on daily schedule, regardless of the frequency of intercourse	Effective 24 hours after implantation for approximately 5 years; can be removed by physician at any time	One injection every 3 months	After insertion, stays in place until physician removes it	Requires frequent monitoring of body functions and periods of abstinence	Vasectomy is a one-time procedure usually performed in a doctor's office; tubal ligation is a one-time procedure performed as outpatient surgery
Rx	Rx; minor outpatient surgical procedure	Rx	Rx	Instructions from physician or clinic	Surgery
$15–30/mo.	$500–600	$30–75/injection	$150–300	None	Men: $240–520 Women: $1,000–2,500

Source: Adapted from M. S. Goldberg, "Choosing a Contraceptive," *FDA Consumer* (1993): 18–25.

*Cost estimates from Planned Parenthood Federation of America, Inc.

Abortion

Abortion, in the form of the intentional, premature termination of pregnancy, is one of the oldest and most widely practiced methods of fertility control. Chinese medical writings from 2700 B.C. recommend abortion. A cross-cultural study found that all but one of 300 societies has used abortion to control the size of families. Currently, in the United States, approximately 1.5 million abortions are performed annually. This number represents about one-fourth of all pregnancies and about one-half of all unintended pregnancies.

Four types of abortions can be performed: medical abortions, early abortions, early second-trimester abortions, and abortion after 24 weeks of pregnancy. In very early abortion, the uterus is emptied with the gentle suction of a syringe; this type of abortion can be performed up to 49 days after the last menstrual period.

Medical Abortions

A medical abortion is done without entering the uterus. Either of two medications, methotrexate or mifepristone (RU 486) can be used for a medical abortion under the guidance of a health care provider. Each of these medications is taken together with another medication, misoprostol, and either combination will end a pregnancy. Medical abortions must take place within the first 6 weeks of pregnancy. If using the combination of methotrexate and misoprostol, an injection of methotrexate would be given and within 5 to 7 days a suppository of misoprostol would be inserted into the vagina. The pregnancy usually ends within a day or two.

With the RU 486 and misoprostol method, a woman swallows a dose of RU 486 and within several days inserts a misoprostol suppository into her vagina. The pregnancy usually ends within 4 hours. In both cases, the embryo and other tissue are eliminated through the vagina.

Early Abortions

The usual method for an early abortion is suction curettage. **Vacuum** or **suction curettage** is the safest and most commonly used abortion method; about 90% of all abortions are vacuum aspiration. The procedure takes about 10 minutes. Vacuum curettage is a two-part procedure. First, the woman is given general or (more often) local anesthesia and the cervix is gradually widened, either with a series of progressively tapered cylinders called dilators, or by insertion of slim rolls of **laminaria,** a seaweed product that expands when exposed to the liquid in cervical secretions. In the second part of the procedure, a narrow wand, called a **cannula,** is connected to a suction device, which is used to empty the uterus. Vacuum curettage is usually performed from 6 to 14 weeks after the woman's last period.

Dollars and Health Sense

U.S. Foreign Aid and Abortion

Through its Agency for International Development (AID), the U.S. government supplies money to organizations in other countries to implement programs in family planning and contraception. However, because of the pro-life views of Republican administrations, funds are denied to any country or organization unless it agrees to neither recommend nor perform abortions. (Democratic administrations generally have ignored or lifted the abortion restrictions by executive order.)

Public health experts believe that restricting the use of funds seriously reduces the use of contraceptives and family planning in countries that need it the most, especially those with devastating AIDS epidemics. It is estimated that approximately 78,000 women die each year from botched, illegal abortions (Holloway, 2001). In countries where abortion is legal, fewer abortions are performed and fewer women die during childbirth as compared to countries where abortion is illegal (see table below). Restricting how U.S. aid money can be used by health organizations in other countries harms women's health and results in many tragic deaths.

Countries Where Abortions Are Legal

	Abortions/ 1,000 women	Maternal deaths/ 100,000 births
United States	26	12
Australia	17	9
England/Wales	15	9
Japan	14	18
Netherlands	6	1

Source: Scientific American, April, 2001, pg. 20.

Countries Where Abortions Are Illegal

	Abortions/ 1,000 women	Maternal deaths/ 100,000 births
Peru	52	280
Chile	45	65
Brazil	38	220
Columbia	34	100
Mexico	23	110

Early Second-Trimester Abortion

Abortions performed early in the second trimester can be either **dilation and curettage (D and C)** or **dilation and evacuation (D and E).** These procedures can be performed up to the twenty-fourth week.

In a "D & C," the cervix is dilated as in the vacuum method, but instead of suction, the uterus is emptied by cleaning the inner lining with a spoon-shaped scraping-instrument (the curette).

If abortion is performed between the thirteenth and twentieth weeks of pregnancy, a procedure combining vacuum and surgical curettage, called dilation and extraction, or "D & E," is usually performed.

Surgical methods of abortion are relatively simple and safe. If done before the third month of pregnancy, they can be carried out in 30 minutes or less. The rate of major complications, such as excess bleeding, damage to the uterus, or infection, is low.

Abortion After 24 Weeks of Pregnancy

Only one out of every 10,000 abortions occurs after the twenty-fourth week of pregnancy. These are performed only when there is a serious threat to the woman's life or health or if the fetus is severely deformed. One procedure is called the induction method, which is usually done in the hospital and requires staying overnight.

The Legality and Morality of Abortion

The propriety of abortion as a socially sanctioned method of fertility control has been debated in Western societies for centuries. Over 2,000 years ago, the Greek philosophers Aristotle and Plato recommended abortion; whereas Hippocrates, the founder of modern medicine, forbade it. Throughout the Middle Ages and the Renaissance, abortion was common, although various religious leaders objected to the practice on ethical grounds.

When the U.S. Constitution was ratified, and for several decades after, abortion was legal if it took place before the time of "quickening"—when a woman could feel fetal movements. Quickening usually occurs near the sixteenth week of pregnancy. The first statutes regulating abortion were enacted in the 1820s in Connecticut and New York. These laws prohibited abortion before the time of quickening, principally to protect women from what by modern standards were primitive and dangerous surgical techniques. By the end of the Civil War, more states had enacted restrictive abortion legislation, not only to preserve the health and life of a pregnant woman, but also to encourage American-born women to have children and to discourage nonreproductive sex. By 1900, abortion was illegal in all U.S. jurisdictions, and it remained so for over 60 years.

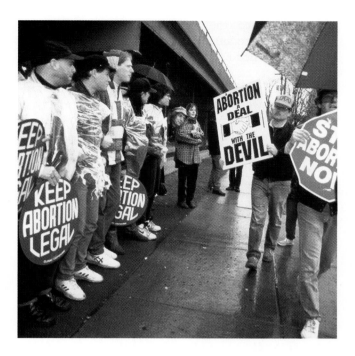

The option for abortion is a very controversial subject in our society.

Restrictive abortion laws did not stop women from having abortions, however. In the first decades of the twentieth century, millions of women obtained illegal abortions. Those with money could travel to other countries where abortion was legal and performed in a hospital with trained personnel, or they could obtain a clandestine abortion performed by an American physician who accepted the risk of prosecution in return for a high fee. Most women, however, had to obtain abortions from nonmedical people who

Terms

abortion: the expulsion or extraction of the products of conception from the uterus before the embryo or fetus is capable of independent life; abortions may be spontaneous or induced

vacuum (suction) curettage: removal of fetal tissue by suctioning off contents of the uterus

laminaria: a plug of sterile dried kelp (seaweed), which expands when in contact with water and can thus be placed in the cervical canal to dilate the cervix

cannula: a hollow tube for insertion into the body cavity

dilation and curettage (D and C): dilation of the cervix with use of a wand or laminaria and scraping the uterine lining; this procedure is often used during abortion

dilation and evacuation (D and E): dilation of the cervix and evacuation of the uterine contents using vacuum techniques

often performed the procedure using coathangers, spoons, disinfectant, or lye. Many women were maimed or killed by such procedures. The psychological trauma even of successful procedures was enormous. By the 1950s, an estimated 200,000 to one million women were getting illegal abortions annually.

By the 1960s, people began to take into account the social and psychological costs of illegal abortion, and on January 22, 1973 the U.S. Supreme Court declared that states could not make laws prohibiting abortion on the ground that they violated a woman's right to privacy, in this case, the right to decide about the outcome of a pregnancy. This decision, known as *Roe* v. *Wade*, declared (a) that the decision to have an abortion during the first trimester (12 weeks) of pregnancy should be left entirely to the woman and her physician, and (b) during the second trimester, indi-

vidual states could regulate the abortion procedure for only one purpose—to protect the woman's health.

Many people have mixed feelings about abortion. Because there is no universally accepted scientific definition of when a life begins, some individuals view abortion as murder. Some opponents of abortion believe that its availability encourages irresponsible sexual behavior or haphazard use of fertility control. Some see abortion as a threat to family life. Even the staunchest proponents of abortion rights would prefer that abortions never occur, but they argue that women must have the right to control their bodies. They believe that abortion is a necessary last resort if contraception fails, if a woman becomes pregnant because of rape or incest, if the child may suffer a birth defect, or if the woman's life and health are jeopardized by pregnancy or childbirth.

Critical Thinking About Health

1. Bill and Sandy have been dating for several months. One Friday evening they go out to dinner and then to a movie. After the movie they go back to Sandy's place. Bill and Sandy begin to kiss, and within 10 to 15 minutes they decide to have sexual intercourse. Neither of them has a condom or spermicide, and Sandy is not using any kind of fertility control method. Despite the fact that neither Sandy nor Bill is using fertility control or has a fertility control method with them, they have unprotected sexual intercourse that evening.
   a. What could they have done instead of having sexual intercourse?
   b. How could this situation have been avoided?
   c. Whose responsibility is it to plan for fertility control?

2. Compare and contrast the abortion laws in your state with those of adjacent states. How might the differences in state laws encourage or discourage young women to cross state lines to receive an abortion?
3. Go to your student health center and find out which fertility control options are available to students who attend your college or university.
   a. How does one go about obtaining the available methods and how much do they cost?
   b. If there are some methods that are not available, ask why and find out where in your community they are available.

Health in Review

- A variety of safe, reliable, and effective fertility control methods are available today. These include hormonal contraception (the birth control pill and progestin-only contraceptives); barrier methods (condom, diaphragm, cervical cap, and spermicides); fertility awareness methods; the IUD; sterilization; and withdrawal.
- A contraceptive's effectiveness is measured in terms of lowest observed and typical failure rates.
- Although most fertility control methods are designed for use in the woman's body, both partners share the responsibility for fertility control. Com-

munication and cooperation are keys to shared responsibility.
- People who say they do not want to have a baby, yet do not use fertility control methods, tend to have low motivation, lack of knowledge of human reproduction and fertility control methods, or negative attitudes toward fertility control or are in relationships that hinder correct fertility control practice.
- Medical and surgical abortions are available.
- Abortion became legal in the U.S. in 1973 with the Supreme Court's *Roe* v. *Wade* decision.

Health and Wellness Online

The World Wide Web contains a wealth of information about health and wellness. By accessing the Internet using Web browser software, such as Netscape Navigator or Microsoft's Internet Explorer, you can gain a new perspective on many topics presented in *Health and Wellness, Seventh Edition*. Access the Jones and Bartlett Publishers Web site at http://www.jbpub.com/hwonline.

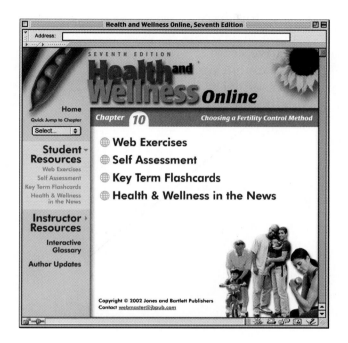

References

Hatcher, R. A., et al. (1998). *Contraceptive technology*. 17th ed. New York: Irvington Publishers.

Holloway, M. (2001, April). Aborted thinking. *Scientific American*, 19–20.

Suggested Readings

Hatcher, R. A., et al. (2000). *A personal guide to managing contraception for women and men*. NY: Bridging the Gap Communications. Accurate, up-to-date information on contraception and reproductive health.

Marrs, R., Bloch, L. F., and Silverman, K. K. (1998). *Dr. Marr's fertility book*. NY: Dell Publishing. America's leading infertility expert tells you everything you need to know about getting pregnant.

Nordenberg, T. (1998). Condoms—barriers to bad news. *FDA Consumer, 32*(2), 22–25. The article is an easy to understand and entertaining piece on the importance of using condoms during sexual encounters.

Planned Parenthood Federation of America (1998). *All about birth control: A complete guide*. NY: Three Rivers Press. A thorough, concise, and complete guide to all fertility control options available to women.

1. Describe the impact of sexually transmitted diseases (STDs) on society.
2. List the risk factors for contracting an STD.
3. Identify the causative agent, symptoms, and treatment for the following diseases: trichomonas vaginalis and gardnerella vaginalis, chlamydia, gonorrhea, syphilis, genital herpes, genital warts, pubic lice, scabies, and AIDS.
4. Understand the importance of testing for HIV infection and the proper testing procedures.
5. Identify several "safer sex" practices.
6. Describe the importance of effective communication in reducing the risk of STDs and AIDS.

Study Guide
and
Self Assessment

Home Test for HIV

Health
and Wellness
Online

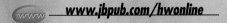 **www.jbpub.com/hwonline**

Chapter 11

Protecting against Sexually Transmitted Diseases and AIDS

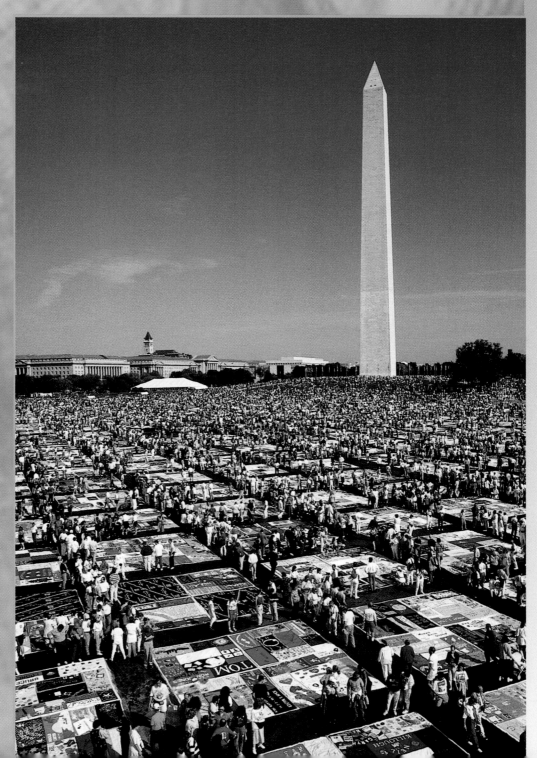

Throughout the world, about 25 different kinds of infectious organisms can be passed from person to person through sexual contact. The infections they cause are called **sexually transmitted diseases (STDs)** or sexually transmitted infections (STIs). The World Health Organization estimated that 360 million people in the world acquire an STD each year. Of the 25 kinds of STDs, only 12 are common in the United States (Table 11.1).

Sexually transmitted diseases have been afflicting humans for thousands of years. Ancient Chinese medical writings describe diseases of the genitalia that were probably syphilis. The ancient Egyptians described genital diseases that were probably gonorrhea. Old Testament and Talmudic writings describe a condition called "ziba," which was associated with the emission of fluid, referred to then as "issue," from the nonerect penis or the vagina. "Ziba" was probably gonorrhea, and "issue" was probably the discharge associated with gonorrhea. Many famous historical figures are thought to have had sexually transmitted diseases (Table 11.2).

> *Women need a reason to have sex. Men just need a place.*
> BILLY CRYSTAL

In the United States each year, approximately 15 million people acquire an STD—a rate of infection second only to the common cold (Figure 11.1). The majority of these cases are in people under age 25; two-thirds of the cases of gonorrhea and chlamydia are in people under age 24.

TABLE 11.2	**Famous People with an STD**

No one knows for sure, but historians say these famous people were infected with an STD.

Abraham	Job	Dürer	Gauguin
Sarah	King David	Schubert	Boswell
Julius Caesar	Cleopatra	Molière	Goethe
Charlemagne	Napoleon	Van Gogh	Oscar Wilde
Henry VIII	Columbus	Nietzsche	Goya
The Greats: Peter and Catherine			

The human and social costs of STDs are enormous. In the U.S., the direct and indirect economic costs of the major STDs and their complications total $20 billion a year. The human suffering and economic costs wrought by AIDS are also well known. Less well known are the disappointment and suffering of thousands of women who are left infertile after a serious STD-related pelvic infection. Women who acquire a human papillomavirus (HPV) infection (genital warts) are predisposed to cervical cancer. And the million people who acquire genital herpes each year will be potentially infectious for their entire lives.

STD Risk Factors

Several factors increase the risk of contracting an STD. Being aware of these factors can help you

TABLE 11.1	**Common Sexually Transmitted Diseases (STDs)**

STD	Symptoms	Treatment
AIDS	Flu-like symptoms followed by any of a number of diseases characteristic of immunodeficiency	New drugs may retard viral reproduction temporarily. Opportunistic infections can be treated to some degree.
Chlamydia	Usually occur within 3 weeks: infected men have a discharge from the penis and painful urination, women may have a vaginal discharge, but often are asymptomatic	Antibiotics
Gardnerella vaginalis	Yellow-green vaginal discharge with an unpleasant odor; painful urination; vaginal itching	Metronidazole
Genital warts	Usually occur within 1 to 3 months: small, dry growths on the genitals, anus, cervix, and possibly mouth	Podophyllin
Gonorrhea	Usually occur within 2 weeks: discharge from the penis, vagina, or anus; pain on urination or defecation or during sexual intercourse; pain and swelling in the pelvic region; genital and oral infections may be asymptomatic	Antibiotics
Hepatitis B	Low-grade fever, fatigue, headaches, loss of appetite, nausea, dark urine, jaundice	Rest, proper nutrition; vaccination for hepatitis B
Genital herpes	Usually occur within 2 weeks: painful blisters on site(s) of infection (genitals, anus, cervix); occasionally, itching, painful urination, and fever	None; acyclovir relieves symptoms
Molluscum contagiosum	Smooth, rounded, shiny, whitish growths on the skin of the trunk and anogenital region	Surgical
Pubic lice	Usually occur within 5 weeks: intense itching in the genital region; lice may be visible in pubic hair; small white eggs may be visible on pubic hair	Gamma benzene hexachloride
Syphilis	Usually occur within 3 weeks: a chancre (painless sore) on the genitals, anus, or mouth; secondary stage—skin rash—if left untreated; tertiary stage includes diseases of several body organs	Antibiotics
Trichomonas vaginalis	Yellowish-green vaginal discharge with an unpleasant odor; vaginal itching; occasionally painful intercourse	Metronidazole

decrease your risk of infection and help you to support STD prevention efforts in your community.

Multiple Sexual Partners

There is a large pool of unmarried sexually active people, because many individuals become sexually active in late adolescence and delay marriage until their mid-to-late 20s and early 30s. Approximately 20% of unmarried sexually active young adults report having more than one sexual partner in the previous three months (Santelli et al, 1998).

False Sense of Safety

Using birth control pills tends to decrease the use of condoms and spermicides, which help prevent transmission of STDs. The availability of antibiotics makes many people less afraid of sexually transmitted diseases. They erroneously believe that there is a cure for every STD.

Absence of Signs and Symptoms

Some STDs have very mild or no symptoms, so that the infection can worsen and may be unknowingly passed on to others. One study showed that approximately 8% of college students were infected with chlamydia and did not know it. Another 1.5% were infected with gonorrhea and did not know it. People infected with HIV can have mild or no symptoms for years, yet still be infectious.

Untreated Conditions

Some individuals lack sufficient knowledge of the signs and symptoms of STDs to know that they are infected. Those who are not accustomed to seeking health care, or who financially cannot afford it, are less likely to seek treatment for an infection. Furthermore, many individuals with STDs do not comply with treatment regimes. When medications are not taken for the required length of time, an infection may not be completely eradicated even though symptoms may disappear. People who do not complete treatment may still be infectious.

Impaired Judgment

The use of drugs, including alcohol, can increase the risk of transmitting STDs because people with alcohol-impaired judgment are less likely to use condoms. Also, people in a drugged condition may be more likely to have sex with someone they do not know; they may know nothing of their partner's past sexual and drug history (Graves and Hines, 1997).

Lack of Immunity

Some STD-causing organisms, such as HIV and herpesvirus, can escape the body's immune defenses, causing individuals to remain infected and transmit the infection. This may permit reinfection and also makes the development of effective vaccines difficult or impossible (see Chapter 12).

Body Piercing

Piercing of the body, particularly the genitals, increases the risk of transmission of STDs. The wound from piercing gives organisms direct access to the bloodstream, and pierced genitals may impede proper use of condoms. Moreover, people with nipple, tongue, and lip jewelry may have a higher risk of infection via oral sex. People who have their bodies pierced should follow after-care instructions faithfully to prevent infection and should abstain from sexual contact in the pierced region until the hole is completely healed, which takes 3 to 6 months.

Value Judgments

Unlike nearly all other kinds of infections, STDs are associated with sinfulness, dirtiness, condemnation, shame, guilt, and disgust. These negative attitudes keep people from getting check-ups, contacting partners when an STD has been diagnosed, and talking to new partners about previous exposures. In the nineteenth century, when syphilis was a scourge of

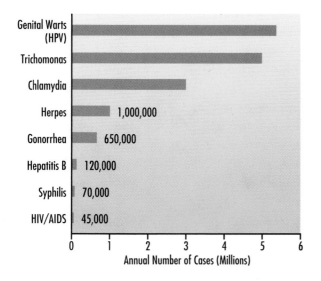

FIGURE 11.1 **Estimated Yearly Number of STDs in the United States**

Genital Warts (HPV)
Trichomonas
Chlamydia
Herpes — 1,000,000
Gonorrhea — 650,000
Hepatitis B — 120,000
Syphilis — 70,000
HIV/AIDS — 45,000

Annual Number of Cases (Millions)

Terms

sexually transmitted diseases (STDs): infections passed from person to person by sexual contact

Europe, rather than trying to prevent its spread (effective treatments had not yet been invented), countries blamed the disease on the weak character or immorality of their neighbors: the English referred to syphilis as the "French disease," and the French called it the "Spanish disease." Prejudice and scapegoating helped spread the disease.

Denial

With respect to contracting an STD, many people think, "It can't happen to me," or "He is too nice to have an STD," or "She isn't the type of person who would have an STD." Because there are no vaccinations against infectious agents that cause STDs, the only way to prevent them is for sexually active individuals, who are not in life-long single-partner (monogamous) sexual relationships, to assume responsibility for protecting themselves and their partners. This means becoming aware of the signs and symptoms of the common STDs and seeking treatment when such signs occur. It means that sexually active people who have more than one partner within a year should obtain periodic (about every 6 months) STD check-ups. It also means knowing about and practicing "safer sex."

> *If love is the answer, could you please rephrase the question?*
>
> LILY TOMLIN

 ## Common STDs

The most common STDs in the United States and Canada can be categorized according to the type of organism causing them (Table 11.3). Organisms that cause STDs are viruses, bacteria, protozoa, and insects. The distinction is important medically because there are no cures for viral diseases, whereas there are drugs that can eradicate bacteria, protozoa, and insects from the body.

Trichomonas and Gardnerella Vaginalis

Although not commonly thought of as sexually transmitted diseases, vaginal infections caused by the protozoan *Trichomonas vaginalis* and the bacterium *Gardnerella vaginalis* are transmitted during intercourse. Symptoms tend to occur only in women (vaginal itching and a cheesy, odorous discharge from the vagina), but the organisms can survive in the urethra of the penis and under the penile foreskin. A man who harbors these organisms can infect other partners or even reinfect the partner who transmitted the organisms to him. Medications can eliminate these infections, and it is essential for both partners to undergo treatment.

Chlamydia

Chlamydia is caused by the microorganism *Chlamydia trachomatis*, which specifically infects certain cells lining the mucous membranes of the genitals, mouth, anus, and rectum, the conjunctiva of the eyes, and occasionally other organs. The chlamydial microorganisms bind to surfaces and induce the host cells to engulf them. After gaining entrance to the cell, these organisms resist a host cell's defenses and eventually "steal" from the host cell the biochemical compounds required for their own survival. The chlamydial organisms use the stolen nutrients to reproduce and multiply, and ultimately the host cell dies.

In the United States and other Western countries, chlamydia is the most commonly reported STD. Each year approximately 3 million Americans are reported to contract chlamydia, which public health experts estimate represents only one-third of all actual cases. In as many as half of all cases, chlamydia occurs simultaneously with gonorrhea. Newborns also are susceptible to chlamydial infection if their mothers are infected at the time of delivery. The most common complications of chlamydial infection in newborns are conjunctivitis (eye infection) and pneumonia.

One reason that chlamydial infections are so common is that 75% of infected women and 50% of infected men often have extremely mild or no symptoms. Thus infected individuals can unknowingly transmit the infection to new sex partners. When symptoms do occur, they include pain during urination in both men

TABLE 11.3   Agents that Cause Common STDs

Infectious agent	Disease
Bacteria	
Chlamydia trachomatis	Chlamydia
Neisseria gonorrhea	Gonorrhea
Treponema pallidum	Syphilis
Gardnerella vaginalis	Vaginitis
Viruses	
Herpes simplex virus, types 1 and 2	Genital herpes
Human papillomavirus	Anogenital warts
Human immunodeficiency virus	AIDS
Hepatitis virus B	Hepatitis
Molluscum contagiosum virus	Molluscum contagiosum
Protozoa	
Trichomonas vaginalis	Vaginitis
Insects	
Phthirus pubis	Lice ("crabs")
Sarcoptes scabiei	Mites ("scabies")

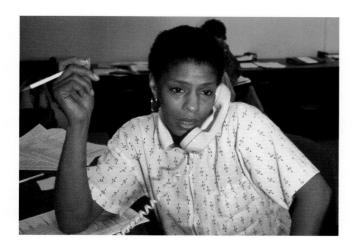

Getting help is the most important step in coping with an STD. There are many support groups and hotlines that can help you.

and women (dysuria) and a whitish discharge from the penis or vagina. Symptoms generally appear within 7 to 21 days after infection.

Chlamydia can be treated with antibiotics. Left untreated, the chlamydial bacteria can multiply and cause inflammation and damage of the reproductive organs in both sexes. In men, untreated chlamydia can result in inflammation of the epididymis (**epididymitis**), characterized by pain, swelling, and tenderness in the scrotum and sometimes by a mild fever. Damage to the tissues in the epididymis can eventually lead to sterility. In women, chlamydial infections affect the cervix, uterus, fallopian tubes, and peritoneum. Often chlamydial infections of the reproductive tract produce no symptoms until the infection is advanced. A woman may then experience chronic pelvic pain, vaginal discharge, intermittent vaginal bleeding, and pain during intercourse. Infection of the fallopian tubes can produce scar tissue that damages the tubes' lining and partially or completely blocks the tubes. These effects may increase the risk of ectopic pregnancy or render a woman infertile; in fact, about 10,000 cases of female infertility per year result from fallopian tube damage from chlamydia.

Terms

chlamydia: a sexually transmitted disease caused by the bacterium *Chlamydia trachomatis*

epididymitis: inflammation of the epididymis (a structure that connects the vas deferens and the testes)

gonorrhea: sexually transmitted disease caused by gonococcal bacteria (*Neisseria gonorrhea*)

syphilis: a sexually transmitted disease caused by spirochete bacteria (*Treponema pallidum*)

chancre: the primary lesion of syphilis, which appears as a hard, painless sore or ulcer often on the penis or vaginal tissue

Chlamydial infections induce an immune response in the host, but for unknown reasons infected individuals do not gain immunity to future chlamydial infections. This means that treated individuals can be reinfected upon exposure to chlamydia.

Gonorrhea

Gonorrhea, also known as "the clap," is caused by the bacterium *Neisseria gonorrheae.* Gonorrheal organisms specifically infect the mucous membranes of the body, most often the genitals, reproductive organs, mouth and throat, anus, and eyes. *N. gonorrheae* cannot survive on toilet seats, doorknobs, bedsheets, clothes, or towels. Transmission in adults almost always occurs by genital, oral, or anal sexual contact; infection of the eyes occurs by hand (often through self-infection). Each year, about 1 million American adults are infected with gonorrhea.

Newborn babies exposed to gonorrheal organisms in the mother's birth canal may develop gonorrhea of the eyes. Most states require that antibiotics or a few drops of silver nitrate be put into the eyes of babies immediately after birth to kill the gonorrhea bacteria and prevent possible blindness.

Although the bacteria causing them are different, the symptoms of gonorrheal and chlamydial infections are very similar. Like chlamydia, many people infected with gonorrheal organisms do not develop symptoms and their infections go unnoticed. If the infection progresses, men may develop epididymitis and women may develop infections of the uterus, fallopian tubes, and pelvic region. Such infections may cause sterility. When symptoms appear, they include painful urination in both sexes and a yellowish discharge from the penis or vagina. Occasionally there is pain in the groin, testes, or lower abdomen. The first symptoms of gonorrhea usually appear within 7 to 10 days after exposure.

Gonorrhea can be treated with antibiotics. However, new antibiotic-resistant strains of the organism are constantly evolving. In nearly half of all cases of gonorrhea, chlamydia also is present. Individuals undergoing diagnosis for gonorrhea should also be tested for chlamydia.

Syphilis

Syphilis is caused by a spiral-shaped bacterium called *Treponema pallidum.* These organisms are transmitted from person to person through genital, oral, and anal contact, as well as being acquired from infected blood. Syphilis can also be transmitted from a mother to her unborn fetus, perhaps as early as the ninth week of pregnancy.

The first noticeable sign of syphilis is a painless open sore called a **chancre** ("shanker"), which can appear any time between the first week and third month after infection. If the infection is not treated within that period, the chancre will heal and the disease will enter a secondary stage, characterized by a skin rash, hair loss, and the appearance of round, flat-topped growths on most areas of the body. Left untreated, the signs of the secondary stage also disappear, and the infection enters a symptomless (latency) period, during which the syphilis organisms multiply in many other regions of the body. In the final, tertiary stage, the disease eventually damages vital organs, such as the heart or brain, and can cause severe symptoms or death. Syphilis can be treated with antibiotics at any stage of the infection.

Genital Herpes

Herpes infections of the genital region are caused by either of two strains of *Herpes simplex virus* (HSV); HSV-1, which is associated primarily with cold sores on the mouth ("fever blisters"), and HSV-2, associated primarily with lesions on the penis, vagina, or rectum. As many as 40 million American adults have been infected with HSV-1 or HSV-2. Each year up to one million American adults acquire a genital herpes infection.

The major symptoms of a genital herpes infection are the presence of one or more blisters, which eventually break to become wet, painful sores that last about two or three weeks; fever; and occasionally pain in the lower abdomen. Eventually these initial symptoms disappear, but the herpes virus remains dormant in certain of the body's nerve cells, permitting periodic recurrences of symptoms at or near the site(s) of the initial infection. It is thought that stress, anxiety, poor nutrition, sunlight, and skin irritation can bring on recurrences.

Infections with HSV-2 are often asymptomatic. Indeed, 90% of people infected with HSV-2 do not know

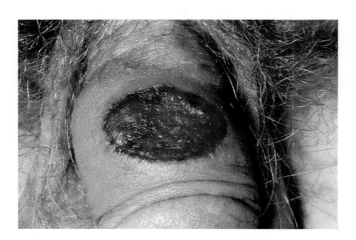

The first physical sign of a syphilis infection is an open lesion called a chancre.

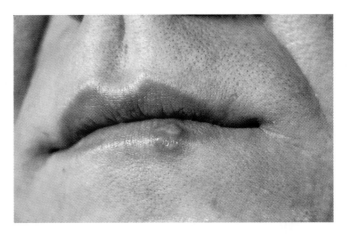

"Cold sores" on the lip or inside the mouth are a common occurrence in people who are infected by the herpes simplex virus. The sores usually heal in a week or so but can flare up again, because the viral infection is permanent.

it. Nevertheless, they are infectious and may contribute to the spread of the disease by having unprotected sex. If they appear, symptoms of a genital herpes infection are evident within two to 20 days after contact with the virus.

Recurrences are usually mild and last only about a week. They may be "telegraphed" by a tingling feeling or itching in the genital area, or pain in the buttocks or down the leg. For some people, these early symptoms can be the most painful and annoying part of an episode. Sometimes, only the tingling and itching are present, and no visible sores develop. At other times, blisters appear that may be very small and barely noticeable, or they may break into open sores that crust over and then disappear. Herpes is extremely contagious when a sore is present. People with open lesions should avoid sex with others until the lesions disappear. Even if no sore is present, transmission is possible, although much less likely, through the "shedding" of virus particles from the skin.

Whereas genital herpes infections are caused most frequently by HSV-2 and oral herpes infections are caused most frequently by HSV-1, both HSV-2 and HSV-1 can cause genital and oral infections with identical symptoms. Thus, people with oral herpes can transmit the infection to partners via oral sex. They can also transmit it to themselves through masturbation. Occasionally, sores also appear on other parts of the body where the virus has entered through broken skin.

Herpes simplex also can infect the eyes, leading to impaired vision and even blindness. If the virus is present in the birth canal, newborn babies can be infected, often resulting in brain damage and abnormal development. In the United States, about 500 babies are born each year with herpes, and two-thirds of infected babies who are not treated die. Pregnant women who have had a prior genital herpes infection should tell their physicians in order to prevent transmission of HSV to their babies.

There is no cure for herpes, and individuals remain infected for life. Drugs such as acyclovir can only minimize the duration and severity of the symptoms of an initial infection or a recurrence.

Human Papillomavirus (HPV) and Genital Warts

Human papillomaviruses (HPV) are viruses that cause warts. Of the more than 100 types of HPV, about 25 produce warts on the genitals, anal region, and cervix. Warts on other parts of the body (hands, feet, lips, and tongue) are caused by different types of HPV.

Genital warts (*condylomata acuminata* or venereal warts) are among the most common STDs. Between 24 and 40 million Americans are infected with HPV, with 500,000 to 1 million more becoming infected each year (Saunders, 2000). A study of U.S. college women showed that nearly half experienced a case of genital warts during a three-year period. Approximately two-thirds of people who have sexual contact with a partner with genital warts will develop warts within three months of contact.

About two percent of sexually active people have visible genital warts, but many more are infected with HPV but have no signs or symptoms. Because the viral infection persists, individuals may not be aware of their infection or the potential risk of transmission to others and of developing complications.

In women, the warts occur on the outside and inside of the vagina, on the cervix (the opening to the uterus), or around the anus. In men, they occur on the tip and shaft of the penis, on the scrotum, or around the anus. Rarely, genital warts also can develop in the mouth or throat of a person who has had oral sexual contact with an infected person. Genital warts often occur in clusters and can be very tiny or can spread into large masses on genital tissues. Left untreated, genital warts often disappear. In other cases, they eventually may develop a fleshy, small raised growth with a cauliflower-like appearance. Because there is no way to predict whether the warts will grow or disappear, however, people who suspect that they have genital warts should be examined by a physician.

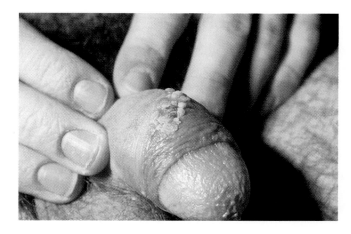

Genital warts on the penis are caused by infection of the skin by papilloma viruses. Genital warts can be removed by a variety of treatments but sometimes recur.

About 15 types of HPV are responsible for nearly all cases of cervical cancer, which number about 18,000 in the United States each year. Without early detection and treatment, cervical cancer can progress and become fatal. "Low-risk" types of HPV (types 6 and 11) cause warts but not cervical cancer. "High-risk" or "cancer-associated types" types of HPV (types 16, 18, 31, and 45) cause cervical cancer and also are associated with vulvar cancer, anal cancer, and cancer of the penis (a rare cancer). Even though they do not cause warts, types of HPV that cause cervical cancer can be transmitted sexually.

Genital warts are generally diagnosed by direct visual examination. Invisible infections may be identified by applying vinegar (acetic acid) to areas of suspected infection, which causes infected areas to whiten. Sometimes a colposcopy is performed, which is using a magnifying instrument to view the vagina and cervix. In some cases, a small sample of tissue is taken and examined under a microscope (biopsy) or submitted for HPV-DNA analysis. A Pap smear, a microscopic examination of cells scraped from the cervix, may indicate the presence of an HPV infection.

Genital warts are treated in different ways depending on their size and location. Self-treatments include covering the warts with 5 percent imiquimod cream, 20 percent podophyllin solution, or 0.5 percent podofilox solution. Pregnant women should not use podophyllin or podofilox because they are absorbed by the skin and may cause birth defects. Clinician-applied treatments include applying 10-25 percent podophyllin resin, trichloroacetic acid (TCA), bichloroacetic acid (BCA), physically excising the wart, cryosurgery (freezing), electrocautery (burning), or laser treatment. Treatments remove the warts, but they do not destroy HPV in cells, so warts can reappear after treatment.

Terms

herpes: sexually transmitted disease caused by *Herpes simplex virus, HSV*

genital warts: hard growths caused by an infection with human papillomavirus (HPV) that appears on the skin of the genitals or anus

human papillomavirus (HPV): a genus of viruses including those causing papillomas (small nipple-like protrusions of the skin or mucous membrane) and warts

As yet there are no vaccines against HPV, so the only way to prevent HPV infection is to avoid skin-to-skin contact with someone who has the virus. Avoid sexual contact if warts are visible in the genital area, and use a latex condom.

Hepatitis B

Hepatitis B is a disease of the liver caused by infection by hepatitis B virus (HBV), one of several types of hepatitis viruses (see chapter 12). Compared to other hepatitis viruses, which tend to be transmitted in fecally contaminated food, HBV is transmitted sexually and in blood, in a manner similar to HIV, the AIDS virus. About 150,000 sexually transmitted HBV infections occur in the U.S. each year; worldwide, the number of people infected with HBV is estimated at 300 million (Figure 11.2). Hepatitis B virus is sexually transmitted 100 times more effectively than HIV.

The symptoms of hepatitis B infection include low-grade fever, tiredness, headaches, loss of appetite, nausea, dark urine, and jaundice (i.e., yellowing of the white of the eyes and the skin). The first symptoms, which are flu-like, tend to occur 14 to 100 days after infection. Signs of liver disease (e.g., dark urine, jaundice) appear later. No specific therapy exists for HBV infection. Rest, proper nutrition, and avoidance of substances harmful to the liver (e.g., alcohol and drugs) are required for recovery, which may take many months. Long-term liver damage is possible, including liver cancer and death.

A vaccine against HBV exists and everyone is advised to be vaccinated, especially children, health workers, and others who are at high risk of exposure (see Chapter 12).

Molluscum Contagiosum

Molluscum contagiosum is caused by a virus of the same name. Fewer than 100,000 infections occur in the U.S. each year. The infection is characterized by the appearance of freckle-sized, smooth, rounded, shiny, whitish growths on the skin of the trunk and anogenital region. Generally, there are no associated symptoms. The lesions may resolve spontaneously, but it is best to have them removed by a health care provider, otherwise they may be transmitted to others or reoccur.

Pubic Lice

Pubic lice (*Phthirus pubis*), also known as "crabs," are barely visible insects that live on hair shafts primarily in the genital-rectal region and occasionally on hair in the armpits, beard, and eyelashes. The organisms' claws are specifically adapted for grasping hairs with the diameter of pubic and axillary hair, which differs in diameter from the shafts of scalp hair. Thus pubic lice are not usually found on the head. (Scalp hair is the ecological niche of the head louse, *Pediculus humanus capitis.*)

Lice feed on blood taken from tiny blood vessels in the skin, which they pierce with their mouth. Some people are sensitive to the bites and may experience itching, which is often the main symptom of infestation. The lice can also be seen; they look like small freckles. The eggs of lice are enclosed in small white pods (called "nits"), which attach to hair shafts. The presence of nits is also a sign of infestation.

Transfer of lice is via physical—usually sexual—contact. They can also be transmitted via contact with objects on which eggs might have been laid, such as towels, bed linens, and clothes. An infestation of pubic lice can be eliminated by washing the pubic hair with liquids or shampoos containing agents that specifically kill lice (e.g., pyrethrins, piperonyl butoxide, and gamma benzene hydrochloride). All of an infected person's clothes, towels, and bed linens should also be washed with cleaning agents made specifically for killing lice.

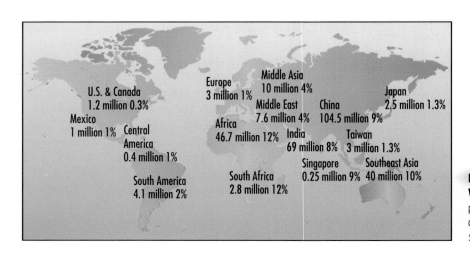

FIGURE 11.2   Hepatitis B Infection Worldwide   Number of people infected with hepatitis B virus in 1997 in the world and the percentage infected in each region.
Source: World Health Organization (1997).

Scabies

Scabies is an infestation of certain regions of the skin by extremely small (invisible to the naked eye) mites, *Sarcoptes scabiei.* The mites burrow into the skin where they live and lay eggs. The tiny lesions produced by the mites often cause intense itching, which is the major sign of a scabies infection. The mites produce tiny burrows across skin lines, which often go unnoticed. Occasionally, an infestation will produce small round nodules. The mites tend to live in the webs between the fingers, on the sides of fingers, and on the wrists, elbows, breasts, abdomen, penis, and buttocks. Rarely do mites live on the face, neck, upper back, palms and soles.

Scabies can be transmitted both sexually and nonsexually. All that is required is close personal contact. The itching and physical symptoms often take several weeks to appear. Scabies can be treated with topical agents that kill the mites and their eggs.

Acquired Immune Deficiency Syndrome (AIDS)

AIDS is caused by **human immunodeficiency virus,** or **HIV** (see Chapter 12). HIV infection causes disease by destroying immune system cells and weakening the body's immune system. Destruction of the body's immune system makes HIV-infected individuals susceptible to a variety of bacterial, viral, and fungal infections that a person with an intact immune system could readily ward off. HIV infection in the brain leads to loss of mental faculties (AIDS dementia).

HIV is mainly transmitted via blood, semen, or vaginal fluids of infected people. Sexual transmission is most common by having unprotected penis-anus sex with an infected person. Unprotected sex is exposure to sexual fluids and blood without consistent and correct use of a male or female condom.

When individuals become infected with HIV, within a few weeks they usually experience flu-like symptoms, from which they eventually recover. Their immune systems are still intact and they produce copious antibodies to HIV. The mounting of an immune response in the early phases of an HIV infection provides the basis for HIV testing. Nearly all of the tests for HIV infection detect antibodies to HIV. A positive result (seropositive) indicates that a person has been exposed to sufficient quantities of HIV particles to mount an immune response.

An HIV-infected individual may not manifest symptoms of AIDS for as many as 15 or 20 years after the initial infection. During this latency period, the infected person is contagious and can spread the infection to others, even though she or he is symptomless. The first signs of AIDS are usually mononucleosis-like symptoms (e.g., swollen lymph glands, fever, night sweats) and possibly headaches and impaired mental functioning caused by HIV infection of the brain. As the disease progresses, individuals most often suffer weight loss, infections on the skin (shingles) or in the throat (thrush), one or more opportunistic infections, and cancer.

Because there is no way to rid the body of HIV and hence cure AIDS, treatment of the disease relies on (a) medically managing the opportunistic infections that result from immune suppression and (b) attempting to suppress HIV infection within the affected person's body. Treating HIV infection involves administering combinations of different drugs, but unfortunately, the combination therapies are not a cure and not all HIV-infected individuals respond. Also, because the drugs only suppress HIV, even those who do respond must take the drugs for life lest the virus begin multiplying again. Because HIV mutates rapidly, in many cases drug resistance develops. Finally, combination drug treatments cost about $10,000 per person per year, so they are unavailable for the economically disadvantaged, who make up 90% of the more than 32 million HIV-infected people in the world.

Sex is like air . . .
It's not important unless
you aren't getting any.
ANONYMOUS

Because many viral diseases have been conquered by vaccination, much effort has gone into developing vaccines against HIV, but without success so far. The only effective way to control the spread of AIDS is to prevent the transfer of HIV from person to person. This is accomplished by using condoms and spermicides (which destroy the virus), reducing exposure to infected individuals, and avoiding casual sex.

Reducing the Risk of HIV/AIDS   Because the first reported cases of AIDS in the United States were among male homosexuals, and because many thousands of men in that group have died from AIDS, some people mistakenly believe that only homosexual men can get AIDS. This is not so. Anyone can get AIDS. The reasons that so many male homosexual males acquired AIDS include:

- Without knowledge of the infectious agent HIV, it was impossible to take precautions.

Terms

pubic lice: small insects that live primarily in hair in the genital and rectal regions

scabies: infestation of the skin by microscopic mites (insects)

human immunodeficiency virus (HIV): the virus that causes AIDS; it causes a defect in the body's immune system by invading and then multiplying within the white blood cells

Dollars and Health Sense

The Costs of AIDS Drugs

AIDS is still an incurable disease, but antiviral drugs have been developed over the last 20 years that can slow or halt the multiplication of the virus (HIV) and the progression of diseases associated with AIDS. A cocktail of three different antiviral drugs has proved to be effective in prolonging the lives of patients with AIDS; however, the costs of these drugs are usually at least $10,000 or more a year per patient. To date, this means that only wealthy AIDS patients and those with health insurance that covers the costs can afford such treatments.

The pharmaceutical companies that market the potent, antiviral drugs have spent millions of dollars to develop these drugs and want to reap the profits of their investment—thus, the high cost of the drugs. The companies argue that they simply cannot afford to sell the drugs cheaply. Moreover, they claim that poor countries in Africa, South America, and elsewhere do not have the means or medical structure to effectively treat AIDS patients. As a result, many millions of AIDS patients in underdeveloped countries (more than 30 million, according to estimates) receive no treatments of any

kind and die slowly with great suffering and pain. And before they become incapacitated, they spread the virus to others, largely through sexual intercourse. This has resulted in a staggering pandemic of AIDS in many underdeveloped areas of the world.

But some countries are fighting back. In 1998, Brazil decided to ignore the patents that the multinational pharmaceutical companies hold on the AIDS drugs and began to make the drugs in its own laboratories. (A drug patent usually gives a company the exclusive right to sell that drug for a period of about 20 years.) Brazil ignores the patents and produces the same drugs at a cost of about $3,000 per patient and expects to reduce the cost even more. (In 2001, a drug company in India agreed to make the same drugs and sell them to a humanitarian organization called Doctors Without Borders for $350 per year per patient. Doctors Without Borders will use the drugs to treat AIDS patients in Africa.) Brazil has AIDS clinics throughout the country and treats almost 100,000 AIDS patients with the effective drug cocktail. Even during

the financial crisis of 1999, Brazil refused to cut its AIDS program and eventually expects to treat its half-million HIV-infected persons, most of whom do not yet have symptoms and do not know they are infected.

In 2000, Brazil spent $444 million on AIDS drugs, but this money is regarded as well spent. Brazil is beginning to reduce the number of HIV-infected individuals in the country and also has reduced the incidence of tuberculosis. Brazil has become a role model for other poor countries who previously felt that they could not afford to treat AIDS patients and let the epidemic spread out of control, as it has in many countries in Africa. It has become clear to many countries that adherence to the rules of a global economy do not always benefit its citizens.

As the costs of drugs and health care continue to escalate in all countries, developed and underdeveloped, governments and citizens are beginning to realize that the right of people to appropriate medical care supersedes the right to profit.

- In the late 1970s and early 1980s, sexual mores among young people, including male homosexuals, permitted multiple sexual partners affording HIV rapid access to a large population.
- Anal intercourse provides HIV a highly efficient route of infection because microscopic tears in the rectum give the virus access to the recipient's blood. Microscopic tears in the penis also allow blood transmission and blood in semen provides a further avenue of infection.

After it was determined that HIV caused AIDS and once strategies were developed to stop its transmission, the frequency of new HIV infections among homosexual males declined dramatically. This decline demonstrated that educational efforts and motivation can prevent the transmission of HIV/AIDS and other STDs. Although AIDS is still a threat to male homosexuals, the majority of new cases of AIDS are among injection drug users who share their drug paraphernalia (needles and syringes) with others, and persons

who engage in sexual intercourse with these individuals. AIDS is increasing among heterosexuals around the world.

Testing for HIV Infection Health officials do not advocate that everyone be tested for HIV infection. But certainly those who suspect that they have been exposed to the virus are candidates for testing. These individuals include males who have had unprotected sex with other males and anyone who has:

- had unprotected sex with someone who is known or suspected to be infected with HIV.
- had a sexually transmitted disease.
- had unprotected sex with someone while drunk.
- had sex with someone whose AIDS-risky behaviors are unknown.
- had several sexual partners.
- shared needles or syringes to inject drugs of any kind.

Global Wellness

HIV Infections Worldwide

Of the millions of persons worldwide who are infected with HIV, about 90% live in the developing world and most of them are not aware of their infection. In the year 2000, 36 million people worldwide were infected with HIV. In 2000, more than 3 million people around the world died from AIDS; since the AIDS pandemic began, about 22 million people have died from AIDS. Of all the persons who have died from AIDS, about 600,000 have been children.

Sub-Saharan Africa is the region of the world with the most infections: 7.4% of all those aged 15 to 49 are infected with HIV. The region has 90% of the world's total of children born with HIV. Unprotected sex between men and women accounts for most of the adult infections. High fertility combined with poor access to information and services for the prevention of mother-to-child transmission of HIV accounts for infections among children.

East Africa was one of the first areas to suffer a massive regional epidemic, and one country in the region, Uganda, was among the first to respond with open and concerted efforts to prevent the spread of the virus. Today, Uganda's infection rate is about one-fifth of what it was in the early 1990s.

Infection rates in Asia are lower than Africa but the numbers are large. Indeed, with between 3 million and 5 million people living with HIV, India has the largest number of HIV-infected people in the world. In China, as many as 400,000 people may be infected.

In Thailand, the number of new infections has decreased, especially among prostitutes and their clients, which account for the majority of the

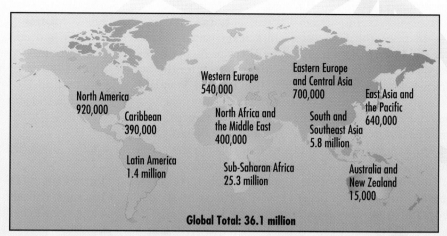

Source: World Health Organization, 2000.

750,000 persons currently infected (representing 2.3% of the adult population). The decrease in new infections is a result of prevention efforts aimed at increasing condom use, boosting respect for women, discouraging men from visiting prostitutes, and offering young women better educational and employment opportunities to discourage their entry into the commercial sex business.

In Latin America, the epidemic has taken its greatest toll on men who have sex with men and among injection drug users. In Latin America and the Caribbean as a whole, AIDS has already overtaken traffic accidents as a leading cause of death. HIV infection rates among pregnant women are 3% in some parts of Brazil, and 8% in Haiti and the Dominican Republic.

In Eastern Europe, drug injection is responsible for most HIV infections. The potential for sexual transmission also exists, since STDs are increasingly common. Increasing rates of non-HIV STDs indicate

that individuals are not practicing safe sex. Furthermore, an untreated STD makes HIV (when present) spread much more easily.

In Western Europe, North America, Australia, and New Zealand, the number of new AIDS cases has dropped considerably since 1995 because of better prevention and treatment. The fall is greatest in countries in which infection has been concentrated in homosexual men, in whom HIV infection rates began dropping in the late 1980s. Only in communities in which unsafe drug injection is the main mode of transmission do new AIDS cases show substantial rises.

Because the vast majority of people living with HIV are in the developing world, where access to prevention information, health care, and anti-AIDS medicines are often difficult or impossible to obtain, international public health officials are concerned that many of the millions of people currently infected with HIV will die within the next decade.

Testing begins with a counseling session. You will be given materials to read before the session with a counselor or doctor. In the session, you'll be asked why you want to be tested and about your behavior and that of your sex partner(s). This will help your counselor and you to determine whether testing is appropriate. If testing is appropriate, your counselor or doctor will describe the test and how it is done, provide basic AIDS education, explain confidentiality issues, discuss the meaning of possible test results and what impact you think the test result will have on you, and talk about whom you might tell about your result.

The most common HIV tests involve taking a small sample of blood from the arm. Less common are urine and oral-fluid tests. The blood, urine, or oral fluid is sent to a laboratory where it is analyzed for antibodies to HIV. Commonly, the results are returned in a week or two. A rapid HIV test, which produces results in 5 to 30 minutes, is also available. When your result is available, you will be asked to return to the counseling and testing center to receive the information. This is true for everyone tested regardless of the results.

Consumers should be wary of at-home HIV test kits. In 1999, the FDA tested kits advertised and sold over the Internet and found all of them to be faulty. In every case, the kits showed a negative test result on samples known to test positive for HIV by standard methods. Using one of these kits could give a person the false impression that he or she is not infected. At-home *collection* kits are less error-prone. The sample is collected in private at home and sent to a lab that does the analysis and returns the results. Reliable at-home HIV testing kits are in development. Check the FDA website (http://www.fda.gov/oashi/aids/test.html) for up-to-date information on at-home test kits.

HIV tests can be obtained from physicians and a variety of health agencies. There are two kinds of HIV-testing: anonymous and confidential. In the anonymous system, individuals are identified only by a self-selected number or alias, so the true identity is never recorded. In the confidential system, one's name is part of the medical record, which is supposed to be confidential. At-home HIV tests are also available. These require individuals to collect a drop or two of blood from a finger-stick and mail the sample to a laboratory for analysis and follow-up telephone counseling.

Before HIV tests became available, thousands of people were inadvertently infected with HIV as a result of receiving HIV-tainted products derived from blood or blood transfusions (for example, tennis star Arthur Ashe). In the 1980s thousands of people with **hemophilia** (a hereditary blood disease) received clotting factor derived from pooled blood that was contaminated with HIV, and many have since been stricken with AIDS. In France, a national scandal erupted when it was learned that French health officials knowingly

continued to allow hemophiliacs to receive contaminated blood products. All clotting factor products used today are manufactured by biotechnology companies and are free of viral contamination. In addition, all blood donations in the United States today are tested for HIV and other viral contamination. However, new strains of HIV continually arise, and tests are not available for all of them. For any elective surgery, patients often are advised to donate their own blood beforehand should a transfusion be required.

Preventing STDs

Preventing STDs requires that societies provide continuous, widespread public health programs and services for STD education and treatment. It is also crucial that infected individuals seek prompt treatment, take responsibility for not infecting other individuals, and practice safer sex to lower their risk of infection.

The stigma associated with STDs is a great hindrance to prevention efforts. Thinking about STDs in moral terms, i.e., associating them with dirtiness and immorality, makes people reluctant to think and talk about them. It also makes society want to ignore STD epidemics. During World Wars I and II, American society supported massive gonorrhea and syphilis control programs; as a result, the incidence of these infections dropped tremendously. When the threat of a postwar STD epidemic seemed to wane, moralistic concerns

Terms

hemophilia: a hereditary disease (primarily in men) caused by lack of an essential blood clotting factor; results in excessive bleeding in response to any scratch or injury

---

Managing Stress

Why It Is Vital to Stay HIV-free

It's hard for me to remember the seemingly carefree life that I led in Los Angeles, San Francisco, and New York City before my AIDS diagnosis. It's been so long that I can barely remember what it felt like. I don't wish for anyone to have to lose that feeling. I take 37 pills every day: 14 drugs with breakfast, 9 vitamins and herbs with lunch (to help counteract and balance the drugs), and 14 more drugs with

dinner. Doing this leads, of course, to the dreadful bouts of diarrhea, irritability, nausea, and fatigue that accompany these medications and take place at times, it seems, without any rhyme or reason. Yet I take them religiously because they appear to enhance the quality of my life, but not without paying a price: the constant anxiety and doubt that goes along with swallowing toxic chemicals that no

one really knows for sure what the long-term physical and mental effects may be. I don't wish this on anyone either.

Mark W. Baker
Provincetown Positive (newsletter)
Fall/Winter, 1997

Wellness Guide

Condom Sense

Always use latex condoms when using condoms to prevent the transmission of STDs. Natural, or skin, condoms, while effective as contraceptives, are too porous to block the transmission of microorganisms. Use fresh condoms to lessen the possibility of leakage or breakage. Condoms that have been in a wallet or a purse for several weeks may have small punctures or may have been weakened by exposure to heat. Store condoms in a cool, dry place, and do not expose them to sunlight. Condoms from damaged packages or condoms that are brittle,

sticky, or discolored should not be used.

Condoms should be taken carefully from their packages to avoid puncture. They should be used from the very beginning of a sexual episode and not put on just before the man ejaculates. This prevents contact with genital and rectal regions.

A condom is unrolled onto the erect penis. While unrolling, the tip of the condom is pinched to push out the air. This leaves space for the ejaculate and prevents breakage. If additional lubricant is desired, it should be a water-based one, not oil-based,

because oil-based lubricants weaken the latex.

After ejaculation, one of the partners should hold the condom on the penis as it is withdrawn. This prevents semen from spilling out of the condom. If the condom breaks before ejaculation, another condom should be put on immediately. If the condom breaks, leaks, or slips off after ejaculation, extra spermicide should be used. Discard the condom after use. Never reuse a condom.

---

thwarted the continuation of control efforts, and the incidence of STDs increased. Public health officials realize that ongoing efforts are the only way to control STDs.

Judgmental attitudes also make talking about STDs difficult. To have to tell a partner that you have an STD, or even to say that you once had an infection and are now perfectly okay, can bring feelings of guilt and shame, which can lead to the avoidance of discussion altogether. Similarly, to ask about a partner's previous STDs may be interpreted as an accusation that the person is "loose" or immoral. To avoid feeling embarrassed or risk offending a sexual partner, people are likely to avoid the topic of STDs. Prevention would be enhanced if sexually active individuals developed an open attitude about talking about STDs (and other aspects of sex) and acquired the necessary communication skills.

Practicing Safer Sex

The surest way to reduce the risk of acquiring a sexually transmitted disease is to abstain from sexual intercourse. This does not mean that one has to give up sexual interaction. There are many ways of giving and receiving sexual pleasure without engaging in sexual intercourse: touching, kissing, exchanging a massage, even sleeping together without intercourse.

Another way to reduce risk is to know a partner's sexual history, including all high-risk activities in which a partner may have engaged. Often this kind of information is difficult to gain early in a relationship, because exchanging information about sexual histories requires a certain level of trust, which takes some time to develop.

Until you have this knowledge, it is essential to protect yourself by using condoms together with spermicides when having sex. Women and men who are

sexually active should come to accept as standard practice with new partners the use of condoms together with spermicides, since birth control pills offer no protection against STDs. Sexually active women and men should carry condoms and spermicides whenever the possibility of sex exists and use them. This requires overcoming the gender role stereotypes that women who admit to being sexual are "sluts" and men who behave the same way are "studs." The female condom (see chapter 10), a polyurethane plastic sheath that a woman inserts into her vagina, has been shown to prevent the transmission of STDs.

Some barriers to safer sex include:

- **Denying that there is a risk.** Many people assume that STDs happen only to "dirty," "promiscuous," and "immoral" people, and since they themselves have sex only with people who are "clean" and "nice," getting an STD is impossible. Another form of denial is to tell oneself, "I eat right. I exercise. I can't get an STD."

- **Believing that the campus community is somehow insulated from STDs.** The truth is that about half of college students are sexually active before they enter college. As a result, students can arrive on campus with an infection. Also, on many campuses, students in the same living groups and student organizations have sex with one another. One infected person could lead to a whole chain of infections.

- **Feeling guilty and uncomfortable about being sexual.** This prevents individuals from planning sex and carrying condoms and spermicides, and talking about possible risks with new partners.

- **Succumbing to social and peer pressure to be sexual.** These pressures encourage people to be sexual in

Both partners need to be responsible for practicing safe sex.

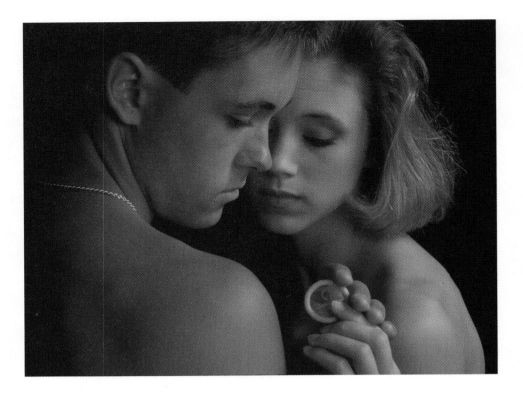

situations that are potentially risky, such as "one night stands" and brief relationships that are sexual virtually from the beginning. The risk of infection is lessened when individuals resist peer pressure to have sex with a relative stranger, and ask themselves instead, "Is this the right relationship?," "Is this the right partner?," "Am I going to feel OK about this afterwards?"

Effective Communication Skills

The pressure to be sexual early in a relationship, before the partners know each other well enough to talk about their past sexual experiences, may force partners to deny there may be a risk. A less risky strategy would be to postpone sexual interaction by saying, "I'd like to be close to you, but I'm not ready to have sex until we get to know each other better." "Not yet" and "maybe" are options when weighing an invitation to be sexual.

Even if a person is ready to talk about the sexual aspects of a new relationship, including birth control and possible exposure to STDs, it can be difficult because of fear of being rejected, offending the partner, or just spoiling the mood. Disclosing one's discomfort about talking about the subject is one way to relieve anxiety about it. A conversation could begin with one partner saying, "There's something I want us to talk about and I feel sort of uncomfortable about it, but I think it's important to both of us, so here goes."

After that introduction, the individual can offer information by saying something like, "We don't know each other very well; I'm concerned about sexual diseases. I want you to know this about me." That person should offer all of the information that he or she would like to be told. After hearing the disclosure, the other person is more likely to respond in kind. And if more information is desired, one could say something like, "Thanks for telling me all of that. I'd feel more comfortable if I knew a little more about . . ." whatever it is.

What if the other person gets offended or won't talk about this subject? Or what if the other person can't be trusted? If partners cannot discuss something as serious as STDs, it is prudent to postpone sexual interaction until the relationship has progressed to a greater level of trust. Potential sexual partners should remember that being under the influence of alcohol or other drugs can affect judgment in making decisions about what is and is not safe. Also, being drunk or stoned can impair using condoms effectively—or using them at all!

Safer sex does not mean no sex. It does not mean that sex is dangerous. It does not mean that sex cannot be fun. It does mean that sex is cooperative. It means that partners are making choices together.

Critical Thinking About Health

1. Research has consistently shown that a vast majority of college students know a lot about STDs and AIDS, and yet only 50% of students whose behavior puts them at risk for acquiring an STD or AIDS practice safer sex techniques. To many observers, such risk taking seems illogical, not to mention dangerous. One could postulate, however, that college students are behaving rationally (from their point of view) when they do not practice safer sex.

   a. Looking at your behavior and the attitudes of those of the people in your peer group, can you explain why some college students do not protect themselves from STDs and HIV?

   b. From your knowledge of your peer group's attitudes, how would you advise your college's administration to lessen the risk of STDs and HIV among its students?

2. From their first moments together it was obvious that Ilana and Jason were going to make a great couple. Every one of their friends said so. Yet Jason was troubled. Although they had agreed not to have sexual intercourse before marriage, as their intimacy deepened, Ilana felt obliged to tell him of the genital herpes infection she acquired when she was a wild 15-year-old. "I'm not that person anymore," she said, "and it's under control. Still, you never get rid of it."

   a. Do you think Jason should proceed in this relationship with Ilana?

   b. What factors should he consider in making his decision?

3. The monthly meeting of the Washington County School Board had never had so many attendees as the night of the vote on the new health curriculum for the county's middle schools. It seemed that everyone in the county had an opinion and was prepared to voice it to the seven board members. At issue was revising the module on sexual infections and HIV to include *how* such infections were actually transmitted. Some parents objected to including any discussion of STDs and HIV in the health curriculum, arguing that doing so only makes the students curious about sex and drugs and encourages experimentation. A second group of parents, while supporting a discussion of the diseases and the organisms that cause them, nevertheless objected to any discussion of behaviors involved in their transmission. They believed that the children ought to know about the biological aspects of the issue as a foundation for their own efforts at dissuading their children from any experimentation with unsafe sexual practices and experimentation with drugs. A third group of parents argued that the only way to ensure prevention was to discuss the behaviors involved. They claimed that the children would not take the discussion seriously unless all aspects of the issue were covered, and hence would be tempted either to disregard the information altogether or to become curious about what was not covered and put themselves at risk. If you were one of the school board members, how would you vote and how would you justify your vote to the parents in your district?

4. Because she had consistently voted to support research on HIV and AIDS, it shocked many people when Congresswoman Harmas refused to vote for the $7.8 billion appropriations bill to pay for protease inhibitor medicines for the medically indigent with AIDS in both the U.S. and around the world. "I have total compassion for these people," said Harmas, "but at $10,000 a year, we cannot afford to take care of everyone who is sick. Furthermore, in our country, most of the money will go to treating injection drug users, who ought to know better than to get the disease in the first place. And for all the poverty-stricken sick people, principally in Asia and Africa, all I can say is I'm sorry, complain to your own government. We're broke." Do you agree or disagree with the congresswoman's position?

Health in Review

- Sexually transmitted diseases (formerly called venereal disease, or VD) are infections passed from person to person, most frequently by sexual contact.
- Millions of sexually transmitted infections occur each year in the United States.
- STDs are epidemic in the United States because people are uninformed about them, because they engage in high-risk behaviors, and because vaccines and cures (for several) are unavailable.
- The most common STDs in the United States are: trichomonas and gardnerella vaginalis, chlamydia, gonorrhea, syphilis, herpes, genital warts, pubic lice, and AIDS.
- Preventing STDs involves supporting public health efforts to inform the populace about STDs and their prevention and treatment. It also requires individuals to practice "safer sex" and to comply with treatment when they are infected.
- PREVENTION is the key!

Health and Wellness Online

The World Wide Web contains a wealth of information about health and wellness. By accessing the Internet using Web browser software, such as Netscape Navigator or Microsoft's Internet Explorer, you can gain a new perspective on many topics presented in *Health and Wellness, Seventh Edition*. Access the Jones and Bartlett Publishers Web site at http://www.jbpub.com/hwonline.

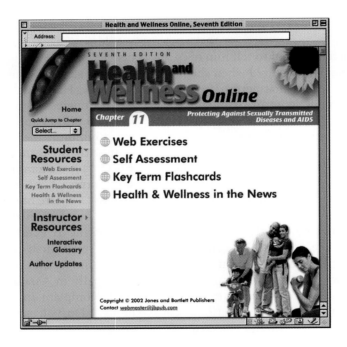

References

Graves, K. L., and Hines, A. M. (1997). Ethnic differences in the association between behavior with a new partner. *AIDS Education and Prevention, 3,* 219–237.

Santelli, J. B. et al. (1998). Multiple sexual partners among U.S. adolescents and young adults. *Family Planning Perspectives, 30,* 271–275.

Saunders, C. (2000, March 15). Monitoring HPV infection. *Patient Care,* 142–172.

World Health Organization/UN AIDS (2000). AIDS Surveillance Reports (http://www.unaids.org).

Suggested Readings

Handsfield, H. H. (1997). A look at sexually transmitted diseases. *Postgraduate Medicine, 101,* 268–277. A highly readable account of STDs in human history.

National Center for HIV, STD, and TB Prevention. Public health surveillance, prevention research, and programs to prevent and control human immunodeficiency virus (HIV) infection and acquired immunodeficiency syndrome (AIDS), other sexually transmitted diseases (STDs), and tuberculosis (TB) (http://www.cdc.gov/nchstp/od/nchstp.html).

National HIV Testing Resources. Information on HIV testing resources, from the U.S. Centers for Disease Control (http://hivtest.org/).

Royce, R. A. (1997). Sexual transmission of HIV. *New England Journal of Medicine, 336,* 1072–1078. Explains in detail how HIV is transmitted sexually and what contributes to the risk of infection. Surprising is the finding that HIV is transmitted in only about 1 per 1000 occasions of sexual intercourse in which one of the partners is HIV-positive.

U.S. Centers for Disease Control (2000). Tracking the hidden epidemics: Trends in STDs in the United States (http://www.cdc.gov).

Part ———— 4

Understanding and Preventing Disease

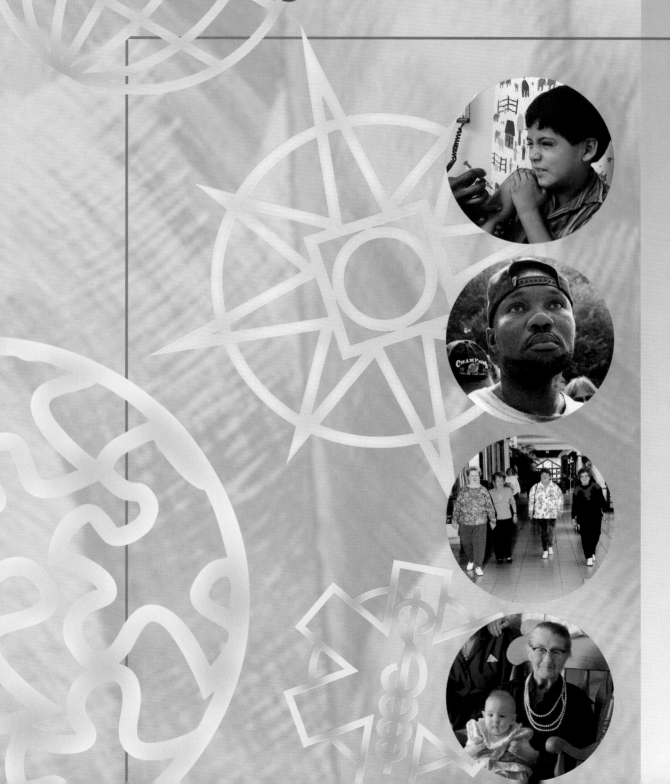

Learning Objectives

1. Define pathogen, communicable disease, vector, immunizations, opportunistic infections, nosocomial disease, immune system, antibodies, antigens, and autoimmune diseases.
2. Identify and explain how infectious diseases are prevented and treated.
3. Discuss the importance of antibiotics with regard to bacterial infections and the implications of antibiotic-resistant strains of bacteria.
4. Discuss how immunizations prevent infections.
5. Discuss the etiology, symptoms, and treatments for cold and flu, Lyme disease, mononucleosis, and ulcers.
6. Explain how antibodies battle infectious diseases.
7. Describe how unwanted activities of the immune system cause allergies.
8. Discuss organ transplants, blood transfusions, and the Rh factor.
9. Describe how HIV causes AIDS.

Study Guide and Self Assessment

Are You Current on All Your Vaccines?

Health and Wellness Online

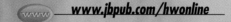 **www.jbpub.com/hwonline**

Chapter 12

Reducing Infections and Building Immunity: Knowledge Encourages Prevention

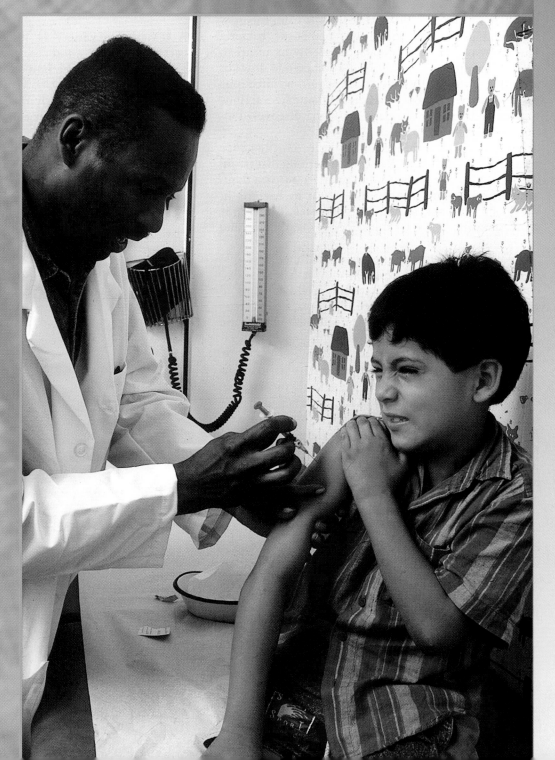

In past centuries, hundreds of millions of people died from infectious diseases caused by bacteria, viruses, protozoa, and other microorganisms. In this century, improvements in public sanitation, personal hygiene, nutrition, and immunizations have drastically reduced the amount of sickness and number of deaths from infectious diseases. However, infectious diseases such as malaria, tuberculosis, and cholera still cause millions of deaths each year, primarily in poor, underdeveloped countries. Poverty and undernutrition create conditions that foster the spread and lethality of infectious diseases. Globally, infectious disease is still the single most common cause of death.

After years of decline, many infectious diseases are again on the rise in the U.S. Deaths from tuberculosis and pneumonia and from food-borne bacteria have increased in recent years. People living in urban or rural poverty and those who are addicted to drugs or alcohol are especially at risk for acquiring infectious diseases. New viruses and bacteria that cause serious disease and death in humans are being discovered almost monthly.

Bacterial contamination of beef, chicken, ice cream, and other foods has caused serious disease in the U.S. in recent years. And in many countries, thousands of people are infected every year by bacteria in their food that makes them seriously sick. Concern is growing in the U.S. over the safety of meat, dairy, and other foods.

Bovine spongiform encephalitis ("mad cow disease") first emerged in Great Britain; it is a fatal disease caused by an unusual protein-like agent (prion) that infects cattle and, in rare instances, people who eat prion-contaminated beef. Considerable efforts are being made worldwide to prevent the spread of infected cattle to other countries.

A healthy body has a functionally active immune system that is able to cope with most infections. A nutritious diet, regular exercise, and low levels of stress are vital elements to maintaining a healthy immune system that can help ward off infections. However, even the healthiest person is exposed to microorganisms that may cause an infectious disease. We all have occasional colds, flu, or stomach upsets that are caused by viruses. Usually these infections are self-limiting, and we become well in a few days or weeks. Other infectious diseases such as pneumonia, tuberculosis, or "staph" infections are caused by bacteria that can be destroyed with antibiotics. However, there is growing concern over the upsurge in disease-causing bacteria that are resistant to many antibiotics.

Understanding how infectious microorganisms cause disease and how your immune system battles infections is essential for maintaining wellness and for recovering from an infectious disease.

Infectious Microorganisms

Not all microorganisms are harmful when they are present in or on the body. In fact, bacteria perform many essential functions in many parts of the body, but there are also areas of the body that must remain sterile (Table 12.1). If normally sterile areas of the body become infected by microorganisms, an infectious disease results. Any microorganism that infects the body and causes disease is called a **pathogen.**

Recognizing Agents of Infectious Disease

A remarkable variety of microorganisms, including bacteria, viruses, protozoa, yeast, and small worms, can infect cells in the human body and cause disease and sickness (Figure 12.1). Viruses are not alive in the same sense that a bacterium is; all microorganisms except viruses are cells that can grow and reproduce on their own. Viruses only grow and reproduce after they infect a cell and usurp the cellular machinery to make more viruses. Some common human diseases caused by viruses are colds, flu, polio, hepatitis, chicken pox, mumps, measles, herpes and AIDS. Each of the viruses

TABLE 12.1   Bacteria in the Body
Some areas of the body harbor millions of bacteria, most of which are beneficial; other areas of the body are sterile.

Sterile body areas
Respiratory tract (below the vocal chords)
Sinuses and *middle ear*
Liver and *gall bladder*
Urinary tract above the urethra
Bones, joints, muscles, and *blood*
Cerebrospinal fluid (the brain and spinal column)
The *linings around the lungs* (pleura) and *abdominal cavity* (peritoneum)
Body areas that are colonized with bacteria
Skin: Contains thousands of bacteria per square centimeter and some fungi. The microorganisms are beneficial or harmless unless the skin is damaged or a person is already sick.
Nasopharynx and oropharynx: May contain billions of bacteria per milliliter of fluid, including pathogenic bacteria that can cause pneumonia or influenza. These pathogens cause disease only in people whose immune systems are weak.
Esophagus and stomach: Thousands of bacteria are ingested with food. Most people have been infected with *Helicobacter pylori* but do not have any symptoms of ulcers.
Small intestine: Low concentration of bacteria; one of the more common ones is *Lactobacillus* species.
Large intestine: Billions of bacteria per milliliter of fluid are present; almost all anaerobic species (bacteria that only grow in the absence of oxygen). All fecal matter contains billions of bacteria.
Vagina: Contains millions of bacteria including *Lactobacillus* species and *Escherichia coli* as well as other anaerobic bacteria.

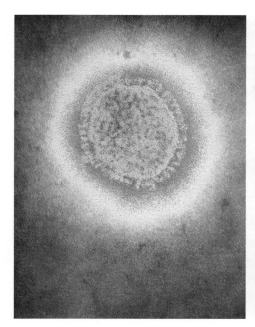
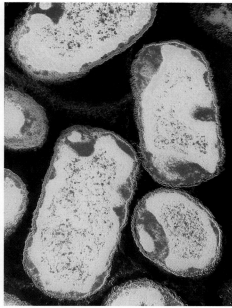

FIGURE 12.1   Infectious Organisms
Electron micrographs of (left) an influenza virus that causes flu and (right) *Salmonella* bacteria that cause food poisoning. Both the "flu" virus and the bacteria are easily passed from person to person and cause widespread epidemics.

that cause these diseases is different and infects a specific tissue or organ in the body.

Other infectious diseases, such as pneumonia, tuberculosis, cholera, plague, typhoid fever, and gonorrhea, are caused by specific pathogenic bacteria. Often pathogenic bacteria and viruses cause disease only if the individual is already in a weakened state, particularly if the immune system is not functioning optimally.

If an infectious disease is shown to be caused by a specific microorganism, that cause is called its **etiology.** For example, tuberculosis usually is caused by a specific bacterium called *Mycobacterium tuberculosis*; infectious mononucleosis is caused by the Epstein-Barr virus; and giardiasis (an infection of the small intestine) is caused by the protozoan *Giardia lambia*.

Infectious agents enter the body in a variety of ways. If the infectious organism is usually passed from person to person, the disease is called a **communicable disease.** Colds, measles, chicken pox, and gonorrhea are all communicable diseases. Infectious organisms also can be transferred to people from other animals, especially insects. In these instances the animal or insect is said to be the **vector,** or carrier, of the disease-causing

microorganism. For example, **malaria** is usually caused by a microscopic protozoan called *Plasmodium falciparum*. When a person with malaria is bitten by a mosquito, blood (and the parasite) is taken up by the mosquito and injected into another person by a bite from the same mosquito. Thus, mosquitoes are the vectors for malaria. (Only a few species of mosquitoes carry the malarial parasite.)

Rabies is a disease of the nervous system caused by the rabies virus present in infected dogs, cats, bats, skunks, and other animals. The infected animals are the vectors for rabies, and the virus is transmitted in the saliva of the rabid animal.

Whether or not a person gets an infectious disease depends on a wide range of factors, including the competence of the immune system, nutritional status, stress, the presence of other diseases, and environmental conditions (Figure 12.2). For example, many people are exposed to bacteria that can cause pneumonia. However, pneumonia usually develops in older people whose immune systems are weak or in younger people who are susceptible to infections for the reasons stated above. Some people are more resistant to infectious organisms than others because of genes that they inherited.

Tuberculosis (TB) is not simply caused by infection with the bacterium *Mycobacterium tuberculosis*. Robert Koch, a famous nineteenth-century microbiologist, called TB the "disease of poverty" because it was associated with squalor, overcrowding, poor

> *Life is still what it has always been, a battle of molecules, of our chemistry against the invaders.*
> RONALD J. GLASSER
> *THE BODY OF THE HERO*

Terms

pathogen: a disease-causing organism

etiology: specific cause of disease

communicable disease: an infectious disease that is usually transmitted from person to person

vector: the carrier of infectious organisms from animals to people or from person to person

malaria: a disease of red blood cells that produces fever, anemia, and death

Internal	External
Age	Infection in the community
Sex	Season of the year
Immunological competence	Hygiene and sanitation
Previous infections	Drugs and medications
Hormonal status	Environmental pollutants or toxins
Presence of other diseases	
Nutritional status	
Emotional stress level	
Heredity	

FIGURE 12.2   *Various internal and external factors determine if disease will result from infections by viruses, bacteria, and other kinds of infectious agents.*

nutrition, and poor sanitation. Today many people have small tubercular lesions in their lungs, but have no symptoms of disease because they enjoy good nutrition, good living conditions, and are in good general health. Today, in some urban areas where people live in squalor and poverty, TB is once again emerging as a communicable, infectious disease.

In many areas of the globe, millions of people still die from infectious diseases (Table 12.2). Various kinds of worms (roundworm, pinworm, hookworm, and tapeworm) infect at least a billion people worldwide. Another 200 million people are debilitated by the water-borne parasite that causes the disease schistosomiasis. Malarial parasites still infect as many as 300 million people each year and cause at least a million deaths annually in Africa. Surveys show that about a billion children in Asia, Africa, and Latin America contract severe diarrhea caused by infectious organisms, and about 4 million children die from diarrhea each year in these areas. Many countries lack the resources to ensure safe water supplies, public sanitation, safe waste disposal, and adequate health care—factors that can control the spread of most infectious diseases.

Fighting Infectious Diseases

Infectious diseases are fought in four ways: sanitation, treatment with antibiotics and other drugs, vaccinations, and healthful living. Stopping the spread of infectious organisms requires that they be destroyed in infected people, in the environment, or in both.

> *If you think nobody cares if you're alive, try missing a couple of car payments.*
> ANONYMOUS

Scientific understanding of the causes of infectious diseases first began in the late nineteenth century with the research of the French scientist Louis Pasteur, who established the "germ" theory of disease by showing that microscopic organisms could cause infections and disease. Pasteur discovered that these

TABLE 12.2   Estimated Deaths Worldwide from Infectious Diseases*

Cause of death	Estimated number
Acute respiratory infections	6,900,000
Diarrheal diseases	4,200,000
Tuberculosis	3,300,000
Malaria	1,000,000–2,000,000
Hepatitis	1,000,000–2,000,000
Measles	220,000
Meningitis, bacterial	200,000
Schistosomiasis (parasitic tropical disease)	200,000
Pertussis (whooping cough)	100,000
Amoebiasis (parasitic infection)	40,000–60,000
Hookworm (parasitic infection)	50,000–60,000
Rabies	35,000
Yellow fever (epidemic)	30,000
African trypanosomiasis (sleeping sickness)	20,000 or more

Source: World Health Organization.

microorganisms could be rendered harmless by heat or by treatment with antiseptic chemicals. Like many radically new scientific ideas, Pasteur's admonitions were ignored at first.

The use of antiseptic (sterile) techniques to reduce the number of infections and deaths after surgery was adopted slowly in the United States, despite the fact that a famous American physician, Joseph Lister, had successfully implemented Pasteur's advice in his hospital. (The antiseptic mouthwash Listerine is named in his honor.) Before antiseptic techniques were introduced in hospitals, surgery or giving childbirth in a hospital often led to death from subsequent infection.

Sanitation, sterile techniques, and public health programs were not actively implemented in the United States until the beginning of the twentieth century. Only then did the incidence of many infectious diseases, such as tuberculosis, plague, pneumonia, and diphtheria, begin to decline dramatically. Many medical historians argue that sanitation is the most significant medical advance of all time because it contributed to preventing millions of cases of infectious disease caused by contaminated water and food.

Understanding Antibiotics

In the late 1940s another highly effective tool was discovered for combatting infectious diseases caused by bacteria. The antibiotic **penicillin**, which is produced by a species of mold, was able to cure many kinds of bacterial infections. Today hundreds of antibiotic drugs are available for treating infectious diseases

Global Wellness

Urbanization and Emerging Health Problems

The global human population is still increasing and is expected to double in the next 25 to 30 years (see chapter 24). Asia, in particular, is expected to have a large number of megacities, in which the present populations will double or more than double in size (see figure). Many of the inhabitants of these potential megacities already live in abject poverty and have poor health. The explosion in size in these cities is likely to be accompanied by a corresponding explosion in the incidence of infectious disease, air and water pollution, toxic wastes from factories, psychological stress from overcrowding, and poverty. Inadequate food, shelter, and medical care will also be factors in potentially insurmountable problems in controlling infectious diseases.

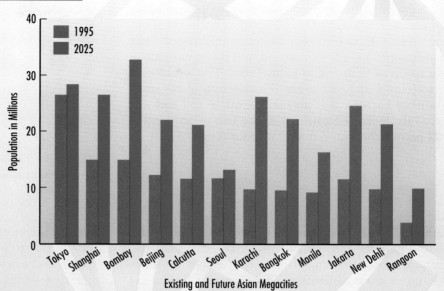

Existing (1995) and Predicted (2025) Populations of Asian Megacities in the Next Century.
Source: Asian Development Bank (1995).

caused by bacteria, yeast, worms, and other microorganisms, except for viruses.

Antibiotics block essential biochemical reactions of microorganisms that infect the body, thereby preventing them from growing. The most useful antibiotics selectively interfere with the growth of bacteria without affecting the functions of body cells. Antibiotics kill both harmful and helpful bacteria in the body; however, once the harmful bacteria have been killed, the helpful bacteria quickly repopulate their normal sites.

Antibiotics do not prevent the growth of viruses because viruses are not living cells. Viruses infect and take over the cellular functions of body cells, thus ensuring their own growth and propagation. Finding a drug that will specifically kill a virus but not also kill body cells is very difficult.

When antibiotics were first discovered they were greeted as wonder drugs capable of curing some of the most deadly infectious diseases, such as plague, tuberculosis, pneumonia, syphilis, and a slew of less serious diseases. Indeed, antibiotics have been exceptionally useful drugs over the past 50 years, but we are now witnessing a decline in their general effectiveness. One of the primary reasons is that many pathogenic bacteria have acquired new genes that make them resistant to one or several of the most common antibiotics.

Within a few years of the discovery of penicillin, penicillin-resistant bacteria began appearing in patients treated for bacterial infections. Bacteria also acquired resistance to later antibiotics, such as tetracycline, erythromycin, and chloramphenicol. Antibiotic resistance can be transferred among bacteria in nature in a small piece of **deoxyribonucleic acid (DNA)** that carries antibiotic-resistance genes. Harmless bacteria of one species can transfer antibiotic-resistance genes to many other species of bacteria, including ones that cause disease. In this way bacteria that cause gonorrhea, pneumonia, tuberculosis and "staph" infections have become resistant to many previously effective antibiotics.

For example, vancomycin is the only effective antibiotic for treating deadly bacterial infections of the circulatory system and surgical wounds. Since 1988, vancomycin-resistant bacteria have been increasing in patients with these infections; consequently, some patients die because the antibiotic is no longer effective.

Terms

penicillin: an antibiotic produced by mold and capable of curing many bacterial infections

DNA (deoxyribonucleic acid): a chemical substance in chromosomes that carries genetic information

The antibiotics rifampin and isoniazid had been very effective in treating TB, but now these drugs are sometimes ineffective because the TB bacteria have acquired multiple antibiotic resistance.

New antibiotics are constantly being developed, but nature is never far behind in the selection of resistant strains of bacteria. For example, millions of tons of antibiotics have been released into the environment as a result of their use in animal feed. The antibiotics in soil and water encourage the selection of resistant strains of bacteria that normally grow in soil and water. Only increased caution in the use of antibiotics will permit them to remain "wonder drugs."

How the Body Protects Itself

The best way to avoid infectious diseases caused by pathogenic microorganisms is to keep them out of the body. The skin and mucous membranes prevent the entry of most microorganisms into the body by functioning as physical barriers. That is why a wound often exposes the body to infection (Figure 12.3). The skin is mildly acidic and provides a poor habitat for most harmful microorganisms, although the skin is covered with beneficial bacteria.

The eyes, nose, throat, and breathing passages are protected by mucous membranes that continuously

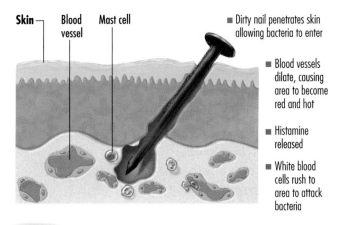

FIGURE 12.3   Inflammation Response   Penetration of the skin by any unsterile sharp object often produces an inflammation response, the normal response of the body to injury or infection.

- Dirty nail penetrates skin allowing bacteria to enter
- Blood vessels dilate, causing area to become red and hot
- Histamine released
- White blood cells rush to area to attack bacteria

Skin — Blood vessel — Mast cell

produce secretions that flush away harmful organisms and particles. Mucous membranes also secrete enzymes that can destroy toxic substances. The mouth, digestive system, and excretory organs also are protected by membranes that guard the internal organs.

Tears keep the surface of the eyes moist and serve to wash away foreign particles. Wax secreted from the ears protects the delicate hearing apparatus. The mucus coating of the respiratory tract is sticky and provides a trap for irritating particles and microorganisms

Dollars and Health Sense

Industry Pressures Block Government Health Regulations

Bacterial infections are responsible for a wide range of diseases—cholera, pneumonia, typhoid fever, plague, tuberculosis—and food poisoning. Since penicillin was discovered in the mid 1940s, antibiotics have been invaluable in treating bacterial infections. However, bacteria can evolve to become resistant to antibiotics, especially ones used in large quantities. Since animals also suffer from bacterial diseases similar to humans, antibiotics are added to animal feed or given to animals directly to control infections in chicken flocks and animal herds. For more than 30 years scientists have been urging the government to ban the use of antibiotics in animal feed or at least not use the same antibiotics that are used to treat people with serious infections. Despite years of warnings, the drug companies and animal husbandry industries have prevented government

regulatory agencies from banning the routine use of antibiotics in animal feed. Now the situation has become critical.

Fluoroquinolones are an especially important class of antibiotics used to treat people infected by *Campylobacter*, a bacterium that is the most common cause of diarrheal illness in the United States. More than 2 million people are infected by this bacterium every year, mostly from eating undercooked chicken or turkey (Bren, 2001). Fluoroquinolones are the most important antibiotics available for treating *Campylobacter* and other hard-to-treat bacterial infections. But fluoroquinolones are also used to treat chickens and turkeys to prevent bacterial diseases in crowded poultry farms. As a result of the widespread use of fluoroquinolone antibiotics in

poultry, many of the *Campylobacter* strains that infect people are now resistant to fluoroquinolones.

In 2001 the FDA finally decided to take action to ban the use of fluoroquinolones to treat infections in poultry, but not without a battle. Abbott Laboratories, one of the manufacturers of fluoroquinolones, volunteered to stop selling the antibiotic to treat poultry. However, Bayer Corporation, another manufacturer, decided to fight the ruling and wants to continue to market fluoroquinolones to poultry growers.

The losers in the indiscriminate use of antibiotics are the millions of patients who become infected with disease-causing bacteria that are resistant to one or more antibiotics. These patients often cannot be treated effectively, and some with weakened immune systems may die.

in the air; microscopic hairs called **cilia** keep the mucus moving out of the bronchial tubes. Coughing and spitting are mechanisms that remove foreign material from the breathing passages. Sneezing and blowing the nose eliminate irritating particles that are inhaled.

Cells and enzymes in the blood quickly form clots that seal off any break in the skin, thereby preventing the entry of harmful substances and infectious organisms. If some bacteria do enter the wound before it is sealed off, other special cells that are part of the immune system attack and destroy the invaders.

If microorganisms or foreign particles penetrate the skin and enter the blood, they soon encounter specialized cells called **leukocytes,** the colorless white blood cells that can be distinguished from the red blood cells that transport oxygen. Only about 1 in 700 cells in the blood is a leukocyte, but their number can increase dramatically if an acute infection occurs. That is why blood is tested for the number of white blood cells when an infection is suspected.

Specialized white blood cells called **macrophages** are associated with specific organs and are vital to the body's internal defense mechanisms. Macrophages are able to engulf and digest foreign cells and particles that invade the body. Organ-specific macrophages protect the lungs, stomach, and other organs from damage by foreign substances (Figure 12.4).

Common Infectious Diseases

Some infectious diseases, such as AIDS and Lyme disease, have received more-than-average public attention and press coverage. Colds and flu are so common that almost everyone gets one or more infections each year. Infectious diseases, depending on their cause and consequences, present special public health problems and personal concerns for many people. To better understand how to cope with infectious disease, we'll review colds and flu, Lyme disease, mononucleosis, hepatitis, prion diseases, and ulcers. AIDS is discussed later in this chapter and also in chapter 11.

Colds and Flu

Most people especially children, contract several colds and flu every year. Both diseases are caused by viruses

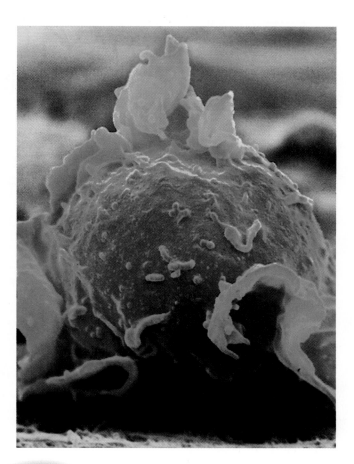

FIGURE 12.4   Macrophage   A lung macrophage as seen in the electron microscope. These cells "eat and destroy" foreign particles and microorganisms that are breathed into the lungs.

that infect cells of the respiratory tract. Colds are caused by more than 200 different species and strains of viruses. A cold caused by one virus does not protect a person from catching a cold caused by a different one, which explains why colds can occur one after another or several times a year.

While cold symptoms may be quite discomfiting, colds generally do not result in long-term illness or death. Billions of dollars are spent by Americans every year on medications that are supposed to alleviate cold symptoms, such as sore throat, cough, congestion, runny nose, and pain. Physicians joke that a cold will go away in about a week with rest and medications or in about 7 days if nothing is done. It takes the immune system of the body about a week to produce the specific proteins that inactivate the viruses and for all the tissues to heal.

High-tech modern medicine has nothing to offer that can prevent a cold, although enormous research efforts have been expended to find a drug that would reduce the risk of catching a cold. While many of the "discoveries" of cold research were announced with great fanfare, none have worked.

Terms

cilia: microscopic hairs in the lining of the bronchial tubes

leukocytes: white blood cells that fight infections

macrophages: specialized cells that destroy and eliminate foreign particles and microorganisms from the body

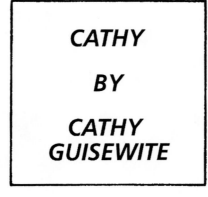
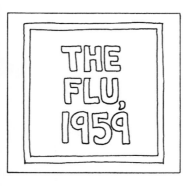
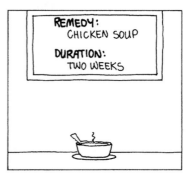
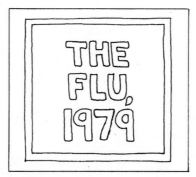
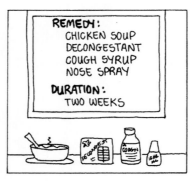
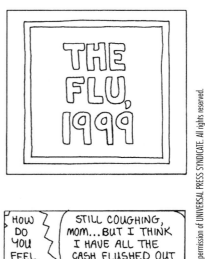
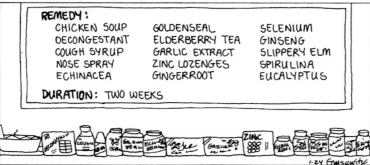
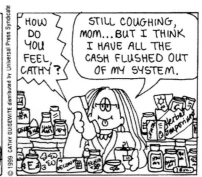

Influenza, or flu, is caused by a different kind of virus than the ones that cause colds. Flu is a much more serious disease. The symptoms of flu are body aches, high fever, loss of appetite, and other complications that may result from the infection. Infections of the respiratory system by a flu virus can so weaken people that they contract pneumonia, a bacterial infection, and die.

There are many different strains of flu virus and new strains arise continually. Because flu is so debilitating and serious, vaccines are prepared each year that are supposed to be specific to the expected yearly epidemic. The problem is that scientists have to guess which flu strain will be the cause of the next epidemic, because it takes about a year to prepare and distribute the vaccine.

In some years, flu vaccine is quite effective, but in others, it is not effective at all because it was prepared with the wrong strains of the virus. People with respiratory problems such as asthma, people with immune system deficiencies, or the elderly, who are most susceptible to pneumonia, are advised to get a flu shot each year to help prevent infection.

Never catching a cold or flu is probably impossible in modern society. However, certain precautions can help reduce the risk. During seasons when colds and flu are present, try to stay away from crowds as much as possible. The viruses are easily transmitted in droplets from people who are coughing or sneezing. Being in a classroom, theater, bus, or any crowded place increases the risk of being infected. The viruses also are easily transmitted by bodily contact, such as shaking hands with someone with a cold who has recently wiped his or her nose or mouth. So it's a good idea to wash your hands frequently during cold and flu season.

Lyme Disease

Lyme disease first received public attention when numerous cases were diagnosed in Old Lyme, Connecticut in the 1970s. Since 1991 it has been mandatory to report all cases of Lyme disease; 10 to 20 thousand cases occur each year in the United States. Most cases occur in eight states—Connecticut, Rhode Island, New York, New Jersey, Delaware, Pennsylvania, Maryland, and Wisconsin—but cases have been reported from almost all states except Alaska and Hawaii. Most infections occur in the summer when people are hiking and walking in the woods.

Lyme disease is a tick-borne disease. The ticks are normal inhabitants of deer and other small mammals that roam the woods. When dogs run in the woods, they also pick up ticks that may eventually become attached to a person. A specific bacterium called *Borrelia burgdorferi* is carried by a few species of tick (mainly, *Ixodes scapularis*). When this tick attaches to the skin and bites, the bacterium is injected into the blood and causes the disease.

The first sign of Lyme disease is a red rash at the site of the tick bite. Over several days, a person may experience fever, headache, tiredness, muscle pains, and joint inflammation. Because these symptoms can occur with many diseases and infections, Lyme disease is often difficult to diagnose. However, an antibody test for the specific bacterium that causes Lyme disease can rule out other possible causes.

In 1998, the FDA approved a vaccine that was 75% effective in protecting against Lyme disease (Rusk and Gluckman, 1999). However, the vaccine is not generally recommended for several reasons. Three injections are needed, and protection lasts less than a year. The effectiveness of booster injections is not known. The vaccine is effective only against Lyme disease, does not protect against other tick-borne diseases, and is effective only against U.S. strains of *Borelia burgdorferi*; it does not protect against strains found in Europe or other parts of the world. Finally, the cost is high (about $200) and the vaccine is approved only for those 15 to 70 years of age, so children cannot be vaccinated.

It is important to detect Lyme disease in its early stages when antibiotics can be taken that will cure the bacterial infection. If left untreated, more serious complications can occur later that may affect the joints, heart, or nervous system. To avoid contracting Lyme disease, it is important to be completely covered with clothing—especially when hiking—in tick-infested areas. Pants should be tucked into boots. Use light-colored clothing so that ticks can be seen more easily. If pets hike with you, examine them carefully afterwards for ticks. Ticks embedded in the skin can be removed by pulling on them carefully with a tweezer, making sure that the head is removed, also.

Mononucleosis

Mononucleosis (commonly called "mono") is an infectious disease caused by the Epstein-Barr virus (EBV) that is ubiquitous in all human populations (Cohen, 2000). It is spread easily from person to person, especially in crowded conditions. It sometimes is called the "kissing disease" because the virus is present in saliva and readily transferred by mouth-to-mouth contact. About half of all children in the United States are infected by EBV by age 5, but, in most children, the infection goes unnoticed because there are no symptoms. Once someone has been infected by EBV, he or she usually carries the virus for life without having symptoms or signs of disease. A number of other viruses also can become permanently established in the body (Table 12.3).

If a teenager or young adult becomes infected by EBV, symptoms develop but usually clear up in several weeks without further illness. Symptoms of mononucleosis include swollen glands, sore throat, fever, chills, and, above all, complete exhaustion and loss of energy. About half of those infected develop an enlarged spleen and a small percentage develop jaundice (yellow coloration of the skin and eyes). Fortunately, these symptoms resolve in two to four weeks in a healthy young adult.

A diagnosis of mononucleosis can be confirmed by a blood test for EBV. There is no specific treatment for mononucleosis, but there are precautions that can facilitate recovery. The primary focus is rest and more rest. For the first two weeks you may hardly be able to drag yourself out of bed. When you start to feel stronger, however, it is important to continue to rest. Trying to resume normal activities too soon can cause a relapse and extend the illness. Fluid intake is also important; drink as much water, juice, soup, or tea as you can. Some people find that taking herbs that act as immune system boosters (echinacea and astragalus) can speed recovery.

Terms

Lyme disease: a serious, difficult-to-diagnose infectious disease caused by bacteria deposited by ticks when they bite

mononucleosis: an infectious disease caused by the Epstein-Barr virus, common among college-age adults

The primary reason to avoid strenuous activities, especially contact sports, for a month or more after a diagnosis of mononucleosis is to protect the spleen. If the spleen is enlarged, an injury could rupture it and create a serious medical problem that may necessitate surgery and removal of the spleen. Because mono affects young people who may be involved in competitive athletics, it is important that they understand why they must continue to be relatively inactive even when they no longer feel sick. Also, because EBV infection affects the liver, it is important not to drink alcohol or take other drugs that may further injure the liver.

The incubation time for EBV is quite long. Children may show symptoms in one to two weeks after infection; however, adults may not develop symptoms for one to two months. Thus, it is often difficult to know from whom you received the virus. Once you know that you have mononucleosis, it is important to try not to spread it among family and friends. Do not kiss anyone, and avoid sharing drinks or food. Try not to sneeze or cough when others are close by, and carry tissues to cover your mouth and nose. Even after all symptoms of mono have disappeared, active virus particles remain in the saliva for many months—up to six months in some studies—so you still need to exert caution so as not to spread EBV to close associates and loved ones.

Ulcers

For most of the last century, it was thought that stomach **ulcers** (sores or holes in the lining of the stomach or duodenum, the first part of the small intestine) were due to stress, anxiety, smoking, and alcohol consumption. However, in 1983, two medical researchers in Australia shocked the medical world by announcing that most stomach ulcers were caused by a bacterial infection in the lining of the stomach of susceptible persons. For several years this view was treated with skepticism but now it has been established unequivocally that as many as 90% of ulcers are caused by particular stomach bacteria (*Helicobacter pylori*). Without the presence of these bacteria in the stomach, ulcers hardly ever occur.

Approximately 30% of the U.S. population is infected with *H. pylori* and in developing nations the incidence of infections is estimated at 70% or higher. Most people become infected as children and do not experience any symptoms at the time. However, later in life some of those carrying the bacteria will develop ulcers. People get ulcers at any age, and men and women are affected equally. In addition to causing ulcers, *H. pylori* is associated with an increased risk of stomach cancer. About 1% to 3% of infected persons eventually will develop stomach cancer. That rate is six times greater than the rate for uninfected persons.

The most common ulcer symptom is a gnawing or burning pain in the abdomen between the breastbone and the belly button. The pain often occurs when the stomach is empty, between meals, and in the early morning hours, but it can occur at any other time. It may last from minutes to hours and may be relieved by eating food or taking antacids. Less common symptoms include nausea, vomiting, or loss of appetite. Sometimes ulcers bleed. If bleeding continues for a long time, it may lead to anemia with weakness and fatigue.

A physician can determine if an ulcer is caused by *H. pylori* infection by the following tests:

- Blood: A blood test can confirm if you have *H. pylori*.
- Breath: A breath test can determine if you are infected with *H. pylori*. In this test, you drink a harmless liquid and, in less than one hour, a sample of your breath is tested for *H. pylori*.
- Endoscopy: Your health care provider may decide to perform an endoscopy. This is a test in which a

TABLE 12.3   **Viruses That Remain in the Body for Life After Infection**

Virus	Symptoms	Spread by	Remains in
Herpes simplex I	Cold sores on lips or in mouth	Direct contact; most infectious when lesions are present	Nerve cells
Herpes simplex II	Painful blisters on genital organs	Direct contact; oral-genital sex can transmit type I or II to mouth or genital area	Nerve cells
Cytomegalovirus (CMV)	No symptoms in most children and adults; CMV can cause stillbirth and mental retardation in fetuses	Body fluids: blood, urine, saliva	White blood cells
Varicella zoster virus	Chicken pox in children; shingles in adults	Person to person	Nerve cells
Epstein-Barr virus (EBV)	Mononucleosis	Saliva (kissing)	Lymph glands
Human immunodeficiency virus (HIV)	From none to full symptoms of AIDS	Sexual intercourse (homosexual or heterosexual), blood transfusions, contaminated needles of injection drug users, mother-to-child transmission before or after birth	T-cells of the immune system and other body cells

small tube containing a camera is inserted through the mouth and into the stomach to look for ulcers. During the endoscopy, small samples of the stomach lining can be obtained by biopsy and tested for *H. pylori.*

Antibiotics are the new cure for ulcers; therapy is one week to two weeks of one or two antibiotics and a medicine that will reduce the acid in the stomach. This treatment is a dramatic medical advance, because eliminating *H. pylori* with antibiotics means that there is a greater than 90% chance that the ulcer can be cured for good. It is very important to continue taking all of the antibiotics until they are gone, even when you begin to feel better.

Hepatitis

Serious liver disease is known as **hepatitis.** It can be caused by environmental agents such as excess alcohol consumption, exposure to pesticides, and drugs. Hepatitis also is caused by infection by any one of several different viruses that infect liver cells; the most common infections are due to hepatitis A, hepatitis B, and hepatitis C viruses. The sources of infection and their severity vary for each of these viruses.

Hepatitis A This virus (HAV) causes liver disease in approximately 200,000 Americans each year but is fatal in less than 100 persons. At least one-third of Americans have been infected with hepatitis A at some time in their lives, and most suffer only mild symptoms and recover completely. The primary source of HAV infection is fecal-oral transmission; one can become infected from contaminated water or from eating food that has been handled by an infected person. Not washing hands after going to the toilet and subsequently handling food is the primary means of transmitting HAV. The symptoms of being infected include jaundice, fatigue, loss of appetite, abdominal pain, and intermittent diarrhea. The symptoms usually clear up within a few weeks, and there is no persistent liver infection. A very effective vaccine is available for those individuals who are at high risk of exposure to HAV or who travel to areas of the world where hepatitis A disease is widespread.

Hepatitis B Infection of the liver by hepatitis B virus (HBV) causes much more serious liver disease; it persists as a chronic infection and may eventually cause liver failure or liver cancer and death. More than one million Americans have a chronic HBV liver infection, and approximately 300,000 new cases are diagnosed yearly. Not all infections by HBV produce symptoms but when they do the symptoms include jaundice, fatigue, abdominal pain, loss of appetite, nausea, and vomiting. Hepatitis B disease causes about 6,000 deaths each year from liver failure and liver cancer.

HBV is transmitted via blood; infection can result from blood transfusions, use of contaminated needles by injection drug users, sexual intercourse (heterosexual or homosexual) in which minute amounts of blood are exchanged, and by perinatal transmission, in which an infected pregnant woman passes the virus to her fetus. The incidence of hepatitis B disease has been decreasing due to the availability of a highly effective vaccine and prevention programs aimed at high-risk groups of people such as injection drug users and sexually active individuals. The blood used for transfusions now is screened routinely for the presence of HBV, and infection by this means is no longer a danger.

A vaccine is available, and it is recommended that all children be vaccinated for hepatitis B. In addition, all persons who are at high risk of exposure to hepatitis B—health care workers, hemodialysis patients, sexually active individuals, and injection drug users—are advised to obtain the HBV vaccination.

Hepatitis C Liver disease caused by hepatitis C (HCV) is sometimes called the silent epidemic because, until recently, relatively little was known or publicized regarding this infection. However, HCV infection is now the most common reason for liver transplantation. It is estimated that 4 million people in the United States are chronically infected by HCV and that many eventually will develop serious liver disease (Thomas et al., 2000). Hepatitis C is found worldwide, and about 170 million of the world's population is thought to be infected. The development of liver disease after HCV infection depends on environmental factors and the health of each individual.

Hepatitis C virus has been well characterized only since 1989, and prior to that time millions of people became infected from contaminated blood without knowing it. HCV is not a single viral strain but consists of many related viruses. Like the flu virus, HCV can change its genetic information easily, which is one of the reasons that it is difficult to treat and why no vaccine has been developed. HCV is transmitted exclusively in blood and blood products; it is not transmitted by casual contact. People who are at risk for HCV infection are the same groups that are at risk for HBV infection.

Because HCV is so widespread in this country and the rest of the world, preventing infection is vital to

T e r m s

ulcers: open sores that occur in the stomach or small intestine for reasons largely unknown

hepatitis: serious disease of the liver caused by hepatitis viruses B, C, or D; also caused by chemicals and alcohol

avoid long-term liver disease and liver cancer. No vaccine is available, and it is unlikely that one will be developed in the foreseeable future. The only treatments for HCV infection involve the use of antiviral drugs (also used to treat AIDS), which can suppress replication of the virus. However, these drugs have serious side effects and are only marginally effective (Koff, 1998).

Hepatitis D This virus (HDV) is defective, is unable to grow by itself, and is only detected in the presence of HBV infection.

Hepatitis E This virus (HBE) is similar to HAV in that it is transmitted by a fecal-oral route in contaminated food and water. It causes the same symptoms as hepatitis A and does not result in chronic infection. Hepatitis E occurs primarily in underdeveloped countries where sanitation is poor. Travelers to such areas should avoid drinking unbottled water, using ice, or eating fresh fruits and vegetables that may be contaminated. No vaccine currently is available for hepatitis E.

Although viruses are the primary cause of hepatitis, remember the golfer in Ireland who suffered from nonviral hepatitis. It turned out that at each hole he licked his golf balls to clean them before teeing off. The herbicide residue on the balls eventually damaged his liver and caused hepatitis. The herbicide was used heavily on the golf course to control weeds, and the chemicals were picked up by the golf balls as they rolled in the grass.

Prion Diseases

All bacteria and viruses carry genetic information in a chemical substance called DNA (or occasionally in a related chemical called RNA). All cells in plants and animals also carry their genetic information in DNA. When the idea was proposed many years ago that some infectious agents did not contain any genetic information (DNA or RNA) but could still cause disease, the idea was met with skepticism. However, in the last few years the evidence for such disease-causing agents has grown stronger. The term given to such unusual infectious agents is **prions** (proteinaceous infectious particles), and they now are thought to be the cause of several rare human brain diseases called spongiform encephalopathies. This hard-to-pronounce disease simply means that people who die from a prion infection have a "spongy" appearing brain that is full of holes when it is examined at autopsy.

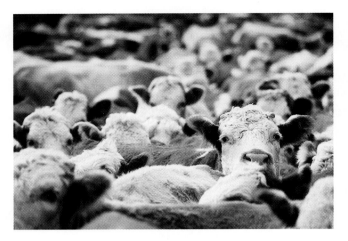

So far, U.S. herds seem to be free of prions; however, concern and surveillance of the herds continue.

For some time it has been known that prion diseases occur in sheep, cattle, and other animals, but it was not thought that these diseases could be transmitted to people. That all changed a few years ago when a small number of people in England died from what appeared to be a prion-like brain disease (a variant of Creutzfeldt-Jacob disease, one form of spongiform encephalopathy). It was shown that the type of prion that infected these individuals was the same as the one found in the brains of cattle that also had died from a prion brain disease. This gave rise to the term "mad cow disease" and focused worldwide attention on prion diseases and the possibility that they could be transmitted from contaminated animal meat and meat by-products to humans who consumed them. (By the end of year 2000, almost 100 people in Europe had died from mad cow disease.)

Millions of cattle in England were slaughtered to eliminate mad cow disease from all remaining herds. English beef and feed made from cattle were banned in Europe and other countries for several years. However, in recent years, infected cattle also have appeared in other European countries, and a few people have died from the variant Creutzfeldt-Jacob disease. Cattle in other countries may have become infected because their feed was derived partly from infected sheep or cattle remains that were used to make animal feed. Fortunately, no case of mad cow disease has appeared in the United States, and the beef supply in America is safe. However, there is ongoing concern in the United States because many animal-derived products that may have been untested and unlabeled have entered this country (Blakeslee, 2001). As an indication of the concern over this disease, the American Red Cross announced in early 2001 that it no longer would accept blood from any American who had traveled to Europe since 1980! Prions and their ability to cause disease still are controversial. It may be that prion diseases occur only in susceptible individuals and that most people are not affected by them. If the prions could readily be transmitted in meat that people eat, it is likely that many more people would have died in England, where the meat probably had been contaminated for years. However, because symptoms take decades to manifest, the possibility of an epidemic originating from prion-infected meat still is a concern.

While prion diseases in humans are extremely rare and are not considered a public health problem, many people have stopped eating meat because of concern about prion contamination. Tests are now available that can detect the presence of prions in meat and are being used to assure the safety of American beef. So (presumably) one need not worry about catching a prion disease from the next hamburger, although bacterial contamination of meat is still a problem.

An Emerging Infectious Disease

West Nile Virus (WNV) is found throughout much of the world—Africa, the Mideast, India, Indonesia, and some areas of Europe. However, until the summer of 1999, WNV had never been reported in the United States (Enserink, 2000). The first clue to its presence here occurred at the Bronx Zoo in New York. A large number of crows were found dead on the zoo grounds; this was followed by the death of a number of other birds in the zoo's collection. Soon afterward, several people in the New York area were hospitalized with symptoms of encephalitis. Blood samples were analyzed, and it was found that the DNA of the virus matched that of a West Nile virus strain isolated in Israel several years ago.

Mosquitoes that bite infected birds can transmit WNV to people. After about two weeks of incubation in a person, WNV may cross the blood-brain barrier (which restricts many infectious agents from reaching the brain) and infect the nervous system. In a few people, once the virus has infected the brain and nervous system, symptoms such as tremors, convulsions, paralysis, coma, and death may follow. The good news is that most people who are bitten by a WNV-infected mosquito will *not* develop serious symptoms and will recover completely without any lasting effects.

Although no one can be certain, the virus may have arrived with an infected bird that was imported. If a mosquito bit this bird, it could have started the cycle of infections. Or a WNV-infected individual may have come to the United States and been bitten by a mosquito that subsequently bit other people or birds. Although the virus infects people and other mammals, the primary reservoirs for the virus are bird populations. The outbreak of West Nile encephalitis in New York killed many birds and several horses and cats. It also caused severe illness in 62 people, seven of whom died.

With the onset of winter 1999 in the eastern part of the United States, the mosquitoes vanished along with the virus. But the worry was that infected birds may have migrated south for the winter and would return in the spring, bringing the virus back with them.

Wellness Guide

Are the Hamburgers Safe? Maybe Yes, Maybe No

The United States has an enviable record for the safety of its meat products, but bacteria are gaining ground. A particular strain of *Escherichia coli* bacteria (0157:H7), now found worldwide, causes serious outbreaks of disease when people eat food contaminated with it. In 1997, 25 million pounds of frozen hamburger were destroyed in the U.S. when a large meat processing plant was found to be contaminated with *E. coli* 0157:H7.

The symptoms of infection by this pathogen include acute diarrhea and blood infections. The bacteria release a toxin that causes the symptoms; killing the bacteria with antibiotics does not destroy the toxin which, once released, circulates in the blood. (Thoroughly cooking meat destroys both bacteria and toxins.)

The public health problem associated with *E. coli* 0157:H7 infection was recognized in the 1980s and has increased in magnitude ever since. The bacteria are usually found in beef products but occur in poultry, pork, lamb, and other meat and dairy products as well. The bacteria can also be passed from person to person. Some people have stopped eating meat, especially hamburgers, because of fear of infection. In 1998, TV talk-show personality Oprah Winfrey was acquitted by a jury in Texas on the charge of libeling the Texas meat industry. She had said on her TV show that she would not eat hamburgers again because of the risk of "mad cow" disease. The Texas meat industry claimed that they lost millions of dollars in beef sales because of her comment.

Sensitive tests for detecting bacterial contaminants in foods are being developed. Also, meat products have been approved by the FDA for sterilization by gamma irradiation to ensure that the meat is absolutely free of microbial contamination. However, most meats are not being irradiated due to consumer resistance.

When spring arrived, the virus did return. By winter of 2001, it became clear that WNV infections pose a serious threat to human and animal health. A new, aggressive mosquito from Asia, presumed to have arrived in a shipment of tires, is particularly effective as a vector for the virus. More than 60 species of birds already have been infected by WNV and some, like the bald eagle, are in danger of extinction. Other bird populations will be seriously depleted. Horses and other animals also will be infected and some may die. The virus already is moving into other parts of the country, and it is estimated that within three to five years WNV will be present throughout the continent. Scientists hope to develop a vaccine or other treatments to help contain the expected epidemic.

Steps to prevent infection in areas where the virus is found include:

- Reducing outdoor activities in early evening when mosquitoes are active.
- Wearing clothing that covers the arms and legs when going into mosquito-infested areas such as woods and wetlands.
- Spraying clothing with insect repellent.
- Applying insect repellent sparingly to exposed areas of the body. (Read all precautions for using insect repellent.)
- If there are many mosquitoes in the house, putting up mosquito nets around beds, especially those where children sleep.

As the world becomes a single global community in which people and other animals move rapidly from one part of the world to another, it is likely that more infectious diseases will appear. In fact, emerging infectious diseases have become one of the serious health problems in the United States (Holloway, 2000).

Hospital-Acquired Infections

We usually regard the hospital as a safe, sterile environment. Unfortunately, the modern hospital has become a place that sometimes endangers the health of patients, because it is a source of serious infectious diseases. About 5% of hospital patients in this country contract an infectious disease while hospitalized for an unrelated problem. These infections are called **nosocomial diseases.** Each year, approximately 7.5 million Americans undergo bladder catheterization in hospitals because they are immobilized. About a half million of these patients develop serious bacterial urinary tract infections, and some patients die from the hospital-acquired infections.

The two bacteria mainly responsible for nosocomial diseases are *Escherichia coli* and *Staphylococcus aureus.* These bacteria normally are present in healthy individuals and usually do not cause disease. In hospital patients, however, antibiotic resistant strains of these bacteria may invade other tissues and cause an infectious disease. Because hospitals use large quantities of antibiotics, bacteria that grow in hospitals are often resistant to the antibiotics. Thus, nosocomial diseases are difficult to treat and prolong patients' stay in the hospital.

Because of the problem of nosocomial diseases, the U.S. Centers for Disease Control and Prevention established a program that monitors frequency of nosocomial infection in hospitals across the country. Hospitals are supposed to keep records of nosocomial diseases. Rates have been found to vary considerably among hospitals. If you need to be hospitalized, you might want to find out the hospital's rate of nosocomial diseases and how the rate compares to other hospitals in your area.

The Immune System Battles Infections

The world teems with infectious viruses, bacteria, and other microorganisms that can cause disease if they invade the body. Most people stay well most of the time because the body contains a remarkable array of defense mechanisms that help keep disease-causing microorganisms out or that can destroy them if they invade the body. We only occasionally have an infectious disease because the **immune system** acts to protect the body from infectious organisms and foreign substances.

The immune system takes time to develop. At birth, a baby is protected from infectious diseases by antibodies that were present in the mother's blood and passed on to the newborn. **Antibodies** are proteins that recognize and inactivate viruses, bacteria, and harmful substances that can cause disease. Babies also receive antibodies in breast milk, which helps to protect them while their own immune systems mature during the first year or so of life.

Many factors can adversely affect the development and functioning of the immune system. Perhaps the most important factor is poor nutrition, especially early in life. Without a healthy diet, a child is extremely susceptible to infections that a weak immune system cannot fight. Inadequate nutrition and starvation are the principal reasons that children die in many undeveloped and impoverished countries of the world. Other factors that affect the development or functions of the immune system are hereditary disorders, viral infections, stress, and many drugs and chemicals, including alcohol and tobacco.

FIGURE 12.5 **The Lymphatic and Immune Systems** Bone marrow, lymph nodes, and other organs of the immune system are shown. The lymphatic system performs many functions in protecting the body from infectious diseases.

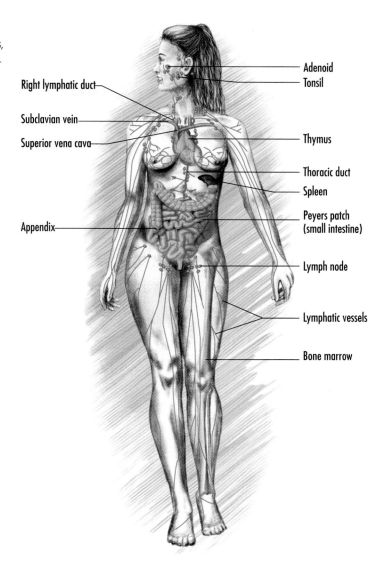

Right lymphatic duct

Subclavian vein

Superior vena cava

Appendix

Adenoid

Tonsil

Thymus

Thoracic duct

Spleen

Peyers patch
(small intestine)

Lymph node

Lymphatic vessels

Bone marrow

The Lymphatic System

The immune system, which is part of a larger and more complex system called the **lymphatic system,** has many organs and cells that must act in concert to protect people from infectious diseases (Figure 12.5). The lymphatic vessels contain fluid called lymph. At various intervals along the lymphatic vessels are nodules called **lymph nodes.** The "swollen glands" that people experience in the neck, under the arms, in the groin, or in other areas of the body are due to enlarged lymph nodes that are engaged in filtering out infectious organisms or foreign particles capable of causing disease. Thus, swollen and sore lymph nodes are a sign that the body is fighting an infection.

Bone marrow, tonsils, adenoids, spleen, and thymus all produce cells that allow the body to mount an immune response against infectious microorganisms. When bacteria or viruses infect the body, the immune system produces diverse kinds of white blood cells that function in different ways to destroy infectious organisms (Figure 12.6).

Terms

nosocomial diseases: an infectious disease contracted while in the hospital for an unrelated disease or problem

immune system: an interacting system of organs and cells that protect the body from infectious organisms and harmful substances

antibodies: proteins that recognize and inactivate viruses, bacteria, and other organisms and toxic substances that enter the body

lymphatic system: a system of vessels in the body that trap foreign organisms and particles; the immune system is part of the lymphatic system

lymph nodes: nodules spaced along the lymphatic vessels that trap infectious organisms or foreign particles

WHITE BLOOD CELL TYPE	DESCRIPTION	FUNCTION	LIFE SPAN
Neutrophil 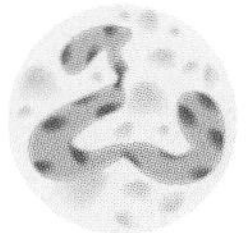	Spherical; with many lobed nucleus, no hemoglobin, pink-purple **cytoplasmic granules**.	Cellular defense-phagocytosis of small microorganisms.	Hours to 3 days.
Eosinophil 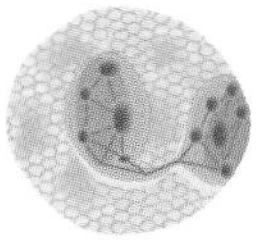	Spherical; two-lobed nucleus, no hemoglobin, orange-red staining **cytoplasmic granules**.	Cellular defense- phagocytosis of large microorganisms such as parasitic worms, releases anti-inflammatory substances in allergic reactions.	8 to 12 days.
Basophil 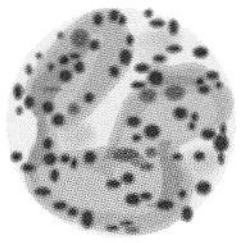	Spherical; generally two-lobed nucleus, no hemoglobin, large purple staining **cytoplasmic granules**.	Inflammatory response - contain granules that rupture and release chemicals enhancing inflammatory response.	Hours to 3 days.
Monocyte 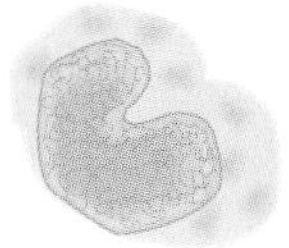	Spherical; **single nucleus** shaped like kidney bean, no cytoplasmic granules, cytoplasm often blue in color.	Converted to macrophage which are large cells that entrap microorganisms and other foreign matter.	Days to months.
B-lymphocyte 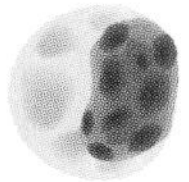	Spherical; round **singular nucleus**, no cytoplasmic granules.	Immune system response and regulation, antibody production sometimes cause allergic response.	Days to years.
T-lymphocyte 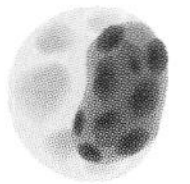	Spherical; round **singular nucleus**, no cytoplasmic granules.	Immune system response and regulation; cellular immune response.	Days to years.

FIGURE 12.6   Specialized White Blood Cells   All white blood cells originate in bone marrow and become specialized as they mature in different organs. Specialized cells carry out different functions of the immune system. The B-cells and T-cells recognize foreign proteins on infectious bacteria, viruses, and other organisms and substances. B-cells are converted to plasma cells that manufacture antibodies.

The **T-cells** (also called T-lymphocytes) circulating in the blood are ready to attack infectious organisms immediately, because T-cells recognize the "foreignness" of specific proteins on the surface of bacteria, viruses, and other pathogens. The response of the T-cells is called **cell-mediated immunity** because the T-cells attach directly to the infectious organisms and inactivate them. Once cells have been identified as foreign by the T-cells, the macrophages and other immune system cells complete the process of their destruction and elimination from the body.

The **B-cells** (also called B-lymphocytes) comprise the final and most effective immune system defense; the response of the B-cells is called **humoral immunity.** The B-cells function by producing antibodies, which recognize all proteins that are foreign and potentially harmful to the human body.

All mammals have similar immune systems and manufacture antibodies; these immune systems evolved with the earliest animals on earth. Without a functional immune system, people and animals would quickly succumb to the countless infectious microorganisms in the environment. Because the immune systems of all mammals are quite similar, researchers use rats, mice, and other small animals to study how cells of the immune system are synthesized and how they function.

The foreign proteins on viruses, bacteria, and other infectious organisms are called **antigens** (*anti*body *gen*erators). Every person has a collection of B-cells circulating in the blood that can recognize any foreign protein on any infectious organism in the world that may be encountered during a person's lifetime. How this collection of many millions of different B-cells develops in the human body is a fascinating but complex story, much of which is now well understood.

A particular B-cell can recognize a particular foreign antigen on a virus or bacterium and begin to make more B-cells just like itself. Eventually these B-cells (at this stage called plasma cells) synthesize vast amounts of one specific kind of antibody that attaches to all of the infectious bacteria or viruses in the body. Once the antibodies have recognized and inactivated an invader, other white blood cells finish the job of destruction. To produce the correct antibodies in large amounts takes about a week after an infection, which is why other quicker-acting immune system defense mechanisms are also needed.

The B-cells and T-cells interact among themselves in complex ways to produce a full-fledged immune response. Small molecules called **cytokines** coordinate the activities of the B-cells and T-cells. Many of the natural cytokines, such as interferons and interleukins, that regulate functions of the immune system are now also manufactured by biotechnology companies. Some of these products are being tested as potential drugs in the treatment of cancer and other diseases in which the functions of the immune system are impaired.

T-cells are also divided into different classes according to their specific functions. Helper T-cells increase the proliferation of B-cells; killer T-cells destroy cancer cells and other pathogenic organisms; and suppressor T-cells retard the growth of other immune system cells. A special class of T-cells called CD4 cells are important indicators in the diagnosis and development of AIDS. When the level of CD4 cells in the blood falls, a person becomes extremely susceptible to infection by many different microorganisms, causing one of the more than two dozen infectious diseases that characterize AIDS.

Immunizations

One of the great achievements of modern medicine has been the development of **immunizations** (vaccinations) to prevent many serious infectious diseases caused by bacteria and, more importantly, by viruses (Beardsley, 1995). Viral diseases (whooping cough, measles, mumps, and hepatitis) have been eliminated in the U.S. (smallpox, polio) or markedly reduced.

Vaccination is the administration, usually by injection (hence, the name "shot"), of substances called **vaccines.** When you are vaccinated, specific proteins from inactivated viruses, bacteria, or toxins are injected into the body. The body's immune system responds by producing antibodies (proteins) that can inactivate the infectious organisms. If you later encounter the active, disease-causing viruses, you are protected by the vaccination and the antibodies.

For example, the crippling disease poliomyelitis has been virtually eradicated in the United States as a result of the widespread use of the polio virus vaccine. The first polio vaccine was developed in 1954 by Jonas Salk, using chemically inactivated viruses. The polio vaccine now used is derived from a genetically inactivated virus developed in 1957 by Albert Sabin. Both methods of viral inactivation prevent the dead virus from causing disease and confer long-lasting immunity. However, a handful of polio cases occur each year as a result of the polio vaccine now in use. A change from the Sabin vaccine (live, weakened virus) to the Salk vaccine (killed virus) is being considered.

In general, vaccination is safe and effective in preventing a number of infectious diseases. Vaccinations are recommended for both children and adults, but vaccinations are crucial for young children (Figure 12.7). Other vaccinations are recommended only for people at particular risk of exposure to a certain disease. For example, travelers to a country where cholera, typhoid fever, or polio is prevalent should be vaccinated for these diseases (Ryan and Kain, 2000).

Workers who handle food may be exposed to the hepatitis A virus and should be vaccinated for that particular virus. Vaccination for a disease such as influenza usually is recommended for people susceptible to lung infections, such as those who are elderly or have asthma. Since the flu shot is only partially effective, and in some years not effective at all, it is not recommended for healthy persons.

A recent addition to the list of effective vaccines is one for the hepatitis B virus. About 300,000 cases of hepatitis B (HB) are diagnosed in the United States

Terms

T-cells: cells of the immune system that attack foreign organisms that infect the body

cell-mediated immunity: the response of T-cells to infections

B-cells: cells of the immune system that produce antibodies

humoral immunity: the response of B-cells to infections

antigens: foreign proteins on infectious organisms that stimulate an antibody response

cytokines: small molecules that coordinate the activities of B-cells and T-cells

immunizations: vaccinations to prevent a variety of serious diseases caused by both bacteria and viruses

vaccines: inactivated bacteria or viruses that are injected or taken orally; the body responds by producing antibodies and cells that provide lasting immunity

Wellness Guide

Boosting Immunity with Herbs

Several herbal remedies have been shown to safely and effectively stimulate the immune system. The herb echinacea, commonly known as cornflower, is an "immune booster"; that is, it stimulates certain cells of the body so that the immune system is better able to ward off disease and fight infection. Laboratory studies of echinacea have shown that it stimulates phagocyte cells that help destroy cancer cells and infectious microorganisms. Echinacea also has been shown to stimulate the formation of interferon and tumor necrosis factor, substances in

the body that fight infectious microorganisms and cancer cells. Other studies have shown that echinacea is about half as effective as steroid therapy in controlling the symptoms of arthritis. Some people who use echinacea take it at the first sign of a cold and report that symptoms disappear within a day. Because some studies show that echinacea loses its ability to stimulate the immune system if taken on a daily basis, it is suggested that echinacea be taken for a few days, then stopped for a few days, to maintain its stimulatory effects.

Another herb used to stimulate the immune system is *Astragalus membranaceus,* which has been used in China and other parts of Asia for thousands of years. The root is used in a dried form or boiled to make a broth or tea. Scientific studies of this herb show that it stimulates all functions of the immune system—in particular, the production of stem cells in bone marrow that are precursors to other immune system cells. Goldenseal is another herb purported to have immune boosting properties.

annually. HB is a serious viral disease that can lead to death from liver disease or liver cancer. Some people experience only mild symptoms after being infected, but others develop a chronic infection that gradually destroys the liver. Because HB causes such a serious disease, vaccination of infants with hepatitis B vaccine is strongly advised.

Understanding Allergies

Allergies are the immune system's response to foreign substances called **allergens** that the body thinks are harmful, but which usually are not. Pollens, molds, house dust, animal hair, foods, drugs, chemicals, and many other substances can act as allergens. The body responds by synthesizing a particular class of antibodies (immunoglobulin E, or IgE) that triggers the allergic re-

action (Figure 12.8). No one knows why allergic responses evolved or what benefit they might have provided, but millions of people today can attest to the misery caused by allergic responses.

The allergic reaction is usually accompanied by the secretion of mucus and the release of **histamine,** an inflammatory chemical that is abundant in cells of the skin, respiratory passages, and digestive tract. That is why most allergic reactions are associated with the skin (eczema, hives, contact dermatitis), the respiratory passages (asthma, hay fever), and the digestive tract (swelling, vomiting, diarrhea).

Contact Dermatitis

Contact dermatitis affects millions of people because many of the things we touch or put on our skin can cause allergic reactions that manifest as rashes. Walking in the woods where poison ivy or poison oak

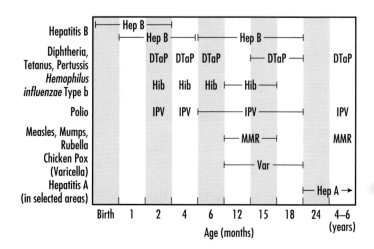

FIGURE 12.7   **Recommended Immunizations for Children**   Chickenpox immunization is recommended but optional. The brackets indicated the accepted time interval for the vaccination.

Wellness Guide

A Cure for Asthma

One of the first successful treatments for an allergy dates from the sixteenth century. An Italian physician, Girolamo Gardano, was asked to come to Scotland to treat John Hamilton, Archbishop of St. Andrews, who suffered from asthma. After watching his patient for several days, Gardano asked the archbishop to give up his swan-feather pillows. This was almost heresy because only the upper classes were allowed to use such pillows. However, the archbishop did give them up and was cured.

Today avoidance of allergy-causing foods and environmental substances that cause allergic reactions is still the best therapy. In many patients with allergies, mental imagery, hypnosis, or suggestion are also effective in reducing or eliminating allergic reactions.

---

grows can produce serious rashes in susceptible persons. Peeling a mango can cause people who are allergic to the skin of this fruit to break out in a rash; however, they usually can eat the flesh of the fruit without experiencing a reaction.

One increasingly common form of contact dermatitis is latex allergy. It is estimated that latex allergies range from 1% to 6% in the general population, and among people who work in hospitals, such as nurses, the frequency is as high as 8%.

Latex is a form of sap extracted from rubber trees and is used in tires and rubber products of all kinds, especially protective gloves, which are used throughout the health care industry and other industries where materials must not be contaminated by touch. In the 1980s, the epidemics of AIDS and hepatitis B, both of which are caused by viruses transmitted in blood, created an unprecedented increase in the use of protective latex gloves. In 1987, the use of latex gloves in the United States jumped from 1 billion to 8 billion pairs, and it has been increasing ever since.

The milky latex sap extracted from rubber trees contains hundreds of different proteins; more than fifty have been purified and have been found to be allergenic. (Most allergies are caused by some kind of protein.) When these latex proteins interact with the skin, they can cause blisters and rashes. When they interact with sensitive mucus membranes in the vagina, rectum, or urethra from using condoms or other contraceptive devices, or during medical exams, the latex proteins can cause **anaphylactic shock** and death. Surgical instruments containing latex coverings or surgical gloves can cause severe reactions in sensitive patients.

The proteins in latex are similar to many proteins found in such fruits as banana, mango, papaya, cherry, peach, and avocado. Latex-related proteins also are found in milk, potatoes, and tomatoes. People who notice that they have become allergic to certain foods may, in fact, have become sensitive to latex. Physicians can test for latex allergies and can advise sensitive people on what foods to avoid.

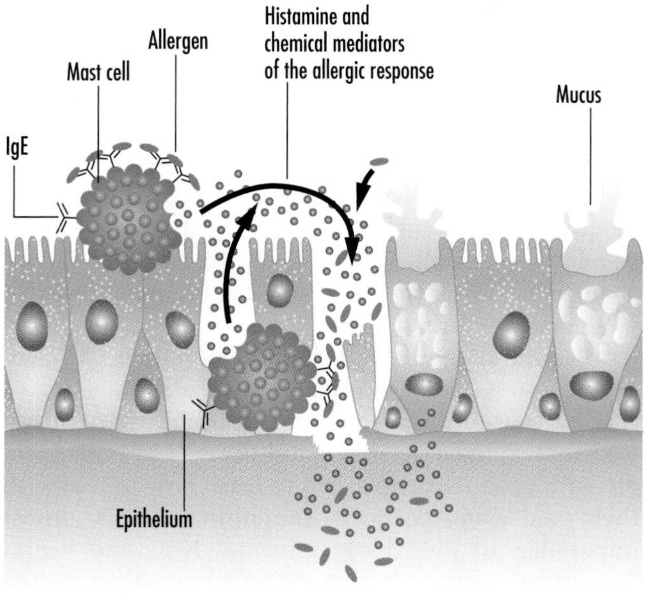

FIGURE 12.8   Chemistry of an Allergic Response   An allergen (a substance from a plant, insect, or other organism) binds to antibody proteins (IgE) on mast cells. This triggers the release of histamines and other inflammatory substances that characterize the allergic response. These reactions occur mainly in the nose, lungs, skin, and digestive tract.

Terms

allergens: foreign substances that trigger an allergic response by the immune system

histamine: a chemical released by cells in an allergic response; causes inflammation

contact dermatitis: an allergic reaction of the skin to something that is touched

anaphylactic shock: a severe allergic reaction involving the whole body that can cause death

Asthma

Although allergies are caused by physiological and immunological responses in the body, they can also arise or be made worse by a person's emotional and psychic state. Some asthmatic children often improve dramatically when separated from family situations that are stressful and emotionally upsetting. Adult asthmatics often notice that their attacks occur more frequently or become worse when they are upset or under stress that cannot be managed. Thus, asthmatics have an immunological make-up that makes them sensitive to allergens, but also respond to emotions and stress in ways that other people do not.

For example, an asthmatic who gets into a violent argument with a husband, wife, or parent may begin to experience breathing difficulties, whereas an equally angry, nonasthmatic person would not. For these reasons asthma is classified as a psychosomatic disease, meaning that both the body and the mind contribute to the symptoms (see chapter 2).

The incidence of asthma has been increasing in both adults and children in developed countries and has more than doubled in the U.S. in the past 20 years (Alpert, 1999). The increase does not appear to be caused by air pollution (although that certainly exacerbates symptoms), and the reasons for the upsurge are still not clear.

Although the biological basis for allergies and asthma has been well documented by research, environmental factors also play a crucial role. Black American children living in urban areas suffer from asthma much more frequently than other children, especially children living in the suburbs. Exposure to dust mites, cockroach feces, and other allergens may account for their higher rates of asthma. However, in the view of some physicians, asthma is a lifestyle disease like hypertension (Platts-Mills and Carter, 1997).

While the symptoms of asthma vary from mild to very severe, deaths due to asthma are rare, although increasing. People no longer need to suffer from asthma and endure the fear of not being able to breathe. A range of effective medicines are now available that can control any asthmatic's symptoms, even the most serious. Short-acting bronchodilators that are inhaled at the onset of symptoms can provide immediate relief. For persistent asthma, short-term and long-term corticosteroid inhalers are available. With daily use, these can effectively suppress wheezing symptoms and breathing difficulties. Cromolyn inhalers also suppress symptoms in many people, and oral corticosteroids prevent asthma in the most severe cases.

Recently, a new class of drugs became available that blocks the actions of leukotrienes, chemicals produced in the body that cause muscles in the air passages to constrict. The goal of asthma treatment is to find the right medication at the lowest dose that leaves an asthmatic free of symptoms. And, of course, it is still important to eliminate from an asthmatic's environment as many allergens as possible to which the individual is sensitive.

Many people with asthma receive allergy shots that are supposed to desensitize them to the substances (such as pollens or house dust) to which their bodies react. Some people do believe they benefit from the shots and that their asthma symptoms are reduced. However, scientific studies indicate that immunotherapy for asthma is of marginal benefit (Barnes, 1996). It is likely that getting a weekly shot acts as a powerful placebo in many asthmatics who believe in the efficacy of the injection.

Food Allergies

Food allergies, also called food intolerance, are allergic responses to a particular food. The reaction can be local (such as a stomach upset or swelling in the mouth) or it can involve the whole body. For example, an allergic reaction to a food or to an insect bite can cause hives to break out all over the body. Food allergies are most common in children but can occur in anyone at any age.

When people are tested for food allergies, six substances account for 90 percent of the allergic reactions—eggs, peanuts, milk, fish, soy, and wheat. Severe allergic reactions produce anaphylactic shock, a systemic reaction that can quickly cause death. Anaphylactic shock can be brought on by an immediate, strong allergic reaction to food, a bee sting, or a drug.

Children are at particular risk of developing allergies to nuts, particularly peanuts. (Strictly speaking, the peanut is a legume, not a nut). Children tend to outgrow most of their childhood allergies, but this is not true for nut allergies. In addition to peanuts, many persons are allergic to Brazil nuts, almonds, hazelnuts, and walnuts. Because the reactions in nut allergies can be quite serious, including anaphylactic shock, most people with nut allergies have to be extremely careful about what foods they eat, since many manufactured products contain nuts.

Peanut allergies are especially common and dangerous—some people suffer to such a serious degree that even a minuscule amount of peanut protein can lead to anaphylactic shock and death. For years, people with peanut allergies had to learn how to live with them and avoid peanuts—something that is almost impossible to do all of the time. Now the health dangers of peanut allergies are widely recognized, and a number of steps have been taken to reduce potential exposure. Many airlines no longer serve peanuts. And many school lunch programs have eliminated peanuts or post warnings when they are served.

Eating in restaurants is always hazardous for those with peanut allergies, especially in Thai, Indonesian, or Vietnamese restaurants. If a pan has had peanut oil in it, enough remains to cause a reaction, even if it is cleaned before being used again. A 50-pound bag of dried molé from which the sauce is made has a handful of peanuts in it, more than enough to cause a reaction for someone eating in a Mexican restaurant.

A cutting board that has been used to cut peanuts a week ago still has enough peanut protein and oil on it to produce a reaction if it is used to cut something that goes into your dinner. A jelly jar also is very dangerous. If a spoon or knife that touched peanut butter is used to scoop out jelly, that jar is potentially harmful to someone with severe peanut allergies.

Shopping in a health food store is risky, although it is much better than it used to be when there were only a few scoops for all of the bins. Suppose someone uses a scoop to get some trail mix that has peanuts in it. That scoop is now contaminated. If it is used to scoop food out of other bins, they all become contaminated with enough peanut protein to cause a reaction. Today, most health food stores have a separate scoop for each bin, and the scoop is wired down so it cannot be moved.

About 20% of people report food intolerance of one sort or another at some time in their lives, yet studies show that the actual number of people who are physiologically sensitive to foods actually is less (Sampson, 2000). The discrepancy between what people report as an allergic reaction and what is demonstrated by allergy tests probably results from the power of suggestion. If someone reads or is told that many people are allergic to eggs, he or she may begin to experience a reaction when eggs are eaten. Also, vomiting after eating a particular food can produce a subsequent aversion or apparent allergic reaction to that food.

The power of suggestion in causing food allergies has been demonstrated by experiment (Jewitt, 1990). In this study, patients who reported that they had a food allergy were given a series of injections to desensitize them to the food causing the allergy. One group was desensitized with a placebo (saline) injection; another group was desensitized with an injection of the allergen. Neither the patients nor the doctors knew which injections contained saline and which contained the allergen. Seven of eighteen patients reported that their food allergies were prevented by the placebo shots. Others reported that their symptoms worsened when they received the saline placebo. Thus, placebo effects can cure food allergies or they can make them worse as in this experiment. How we view food in our minds has a powerful effect on how it is received by the body (see chapter 2).

However, food allergies should not be regarded as the result of imagination and, therefore, in some sense, "unreal." Whether the allergic reaction is brought on specifically by the interaction of an allergen with IgE antibodies or by a state of mind is largely irrelevant. In both instances, the physiological responses are real and need to be treated. For centuries, allergies have been successfully treated by eliminating the cause of the allergic reaction, by the power of suggestion, or both.

Recognition of "Self"

The immune system is able to recognize and destroy virtually any foreign cell, which is how it protects the body from infectious diseases. What prevents the immune system from recognizing and attacking the body's own cells and organs? By mechanisms that are not yet completely understood, the immune system can distinguish cells of the body that are recognized as "self" from all other cells (even those of another person) that are "nonself."

During fetal development, as the body's tissues are being formed, all of the antibody-producing cells that could attack the body's own cells are destroyed. It is not yet known how these particular antibody-producing cells are selected out of the millions of different cells and destroyed, but such a mechanism is vital to protect the organs and tissues of the body from destruction.

Autoimmune Diseases

The immune system must function without mistakes to distinguish "self" from "nonself" because any mistake that caused antibodies to attack the body's own cells could result in serious disease or death. Unfortunately, mistakes in the functioning of the immune system do occur and produce **autoimmune diseases** (Figure 12.9). Some inherited disorders, fortunately quite rare, can result in the loss of the immune system's ability to distinguish "self" from "nonself." Environmental factors, such as viral infections, nutritional problems, and other unknown agents may also cause the immune system to make mistakes that lead to autoimmune diseases.

Lupus erythematosus is an autoimmune disease that most frequently affects women between the ages of 18 to 35. In this disease, for reasons still unknown, antibodies are synthesized that attack the genetic

Terms

food allergies: allergic responses to something that is eaten

autoimmune diseases: mistakes in the functioning of the immune system that cause it to attack tissues in the body

lupus erythematosus: an autoimmune disease that mostly affects women

Various autoimmune diseases

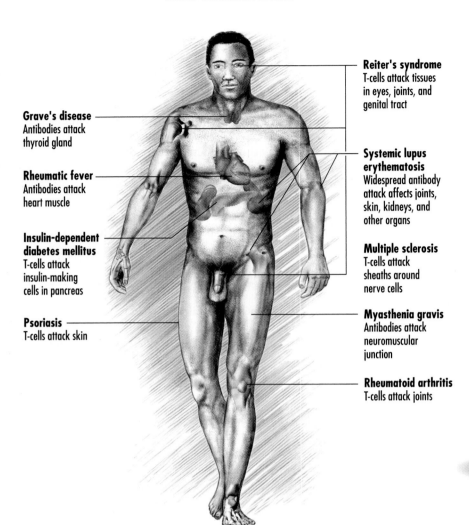

Grave's disease
Antibodies attack
thyroid gland

Rheumatic fever
Antibodies attack
heart muscle

**Insulin-dependent
diabetes mellitus**
T-cells attack
insulin-making
cells in pancreas

Psoriasis
T-cells attack skin

Reiter's syndrome
T-cells attack tissues
in eyes, joints, and
genital tract

**Systemic lupus
erythematosis**
Widespread antibody
attack affects joints,
skin, kidneys, and
other organs

Multiple sclerosis
T-cells attack
sheaths around
nerve cells

Myasthenia gravis
Antibodies attack
neuromuscular
junction

Rheumatoid arthritis
T-cells attack joints

FIGURE 12.9   **Autoimmune Diseases**
These occur when the body's immune system goes
awry and cells of the immune system begin attacking the body's own cells because they are mistakenly
recognized as foreign.

information in cells (DNA), especially in cells of the blood vessels, skin, and kidneys. Many organs of the body are affected, and the symptoms—rashes, pain, and anemia—flare up and wane throughout life, which usually is shortened.

Arthritis is one of the most common chronic diseases; approximately 1 in 7 Americans has some form of arthritis. There are about 100 forms of arthritis and arthritis-related conditions, but the common denominator is pain and stiffness in joints throughout the body (Figure 12.10). The causes of arthritis vary widely, but many forms are the result of autoimmune disease in which the body's immune system mistakenly attacks cartilage and bone. Drugs can relieve many of the symptoms of arthritis, such as pain and inflammation, but the diseases themselves have no cure.

As with most chronic diseases of unknown etiology, the mind can exert a powerful role in controlling the symptoms of arthritis or in aggravating them. Relaxation and visualization exercises that emphasize mobility and comfort can be of great benefit in relieving the pain, stiffness, and inflammation associated with arthritis.

An autoimmune disease that affects the central nervous system is **multiple sclerosis (MS)**. Recent research suggests that MS may be initiated by a viral infection that somehow causes the immune system to produce antibodies that attack **myelin,** a substance that sheaths and insulates nerve fibers in the brain and spinal cord.

Although drugs can help reduce the symptoms of autoimmune diseases, these diseases are caused by complex malfunctions of the immune system. Because the mind also affects the functions of the immune system, many people who suffer from autoimmune diseases find relief in alternative therapies, mental relaxation techniques, and nutritional changes.

Common forms of arthritis and arthritis-related diseases and their symptoms

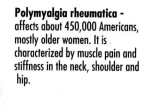

Ankylosing spondylitis - affects about 300,000 Americans, usually younger men. It is due to a spinal inflammation that spreads to other areas of the body.

Fibromyalgia - affects about 4 million Americans, the majority of them women. The symptoms include fatigue, pain, insomnia, and stiffness but usually no inflammation of the joints.

Osteoarthritis - affects an estimated 15 million older Americans. It is caused by the erosion of cartilage which acts as a shock absorber at the tips of bones.

Gout - affects about 1 million Americans, the majority of them men. It is caused by the build up of uric acid in the blood, crystals of which accumulate in joints, especially the big toe for unknown reasons. Overeating and alcohol are linked to the condition.

Polymyalgia rheumatica - affects about 450,000 Americans, mostly older women. It is characterized by muscle pain and stiffness in the neck, shoulder and hip.

Rheumatoid arthritis - affects about 2 million Americans, the majority of them women. It strikes at any age and can eventually be crippling due to destruction of joints.

Scleroderma - affects about 100,000 Americans. It is characterized by a thickening of the skin and inflammation of joints and internal organs.

FIGURE 12.10   Common Forms of Arthritis and Arthritis-Related Diseases and Their Symptoms

Organ Transplants

Like blood cells, all body cells have antigens on their surfaces that are different for everyone except identical twins. If tissue or organs from one person are grafted onto another, the immune system produces antibodies to the foreign cell antigens, causing destruction of the cells and rejection of the transplanted organ.

The more alike two persons are genetically, the more likely it is that the transplanted tissue will be accepted by the body. Identical twins are genetically identical; this is why tissue transplants between identical twins have the greatest chance of success. To minimize the rejection of transplanted organs, the **histocompatibility** (similarity of cell surface antigens) between the donor and recipient is determined by immunological tests. Just as red blood cells have particular groups of strongly antigenic proteins on their cell surfaces, other cells in the body have antigenic proteins called **HLA**

(human leukocyte antigens) that are crucial in determining whether a transplanted organ is accepted or rejected (Figure 12.11). The greater the similarity in HLA antigens between donor and recipient, the greater the chance that the tissue will be accepted and function normally in its new host. From the number of HLA

Terms

multiple sclerosis (MS): an autoimmune disease that affects the central nervous system

myelin: a substance that sheaths and insulates nerve fibers in the brain and spinal cord

histocompatibility: the degree to which the antigens on cells of different persons are similar

HLA (human leukocyte antigens): antigens that are measured to determine the suitability of an organ for transplantation from donor to recipient

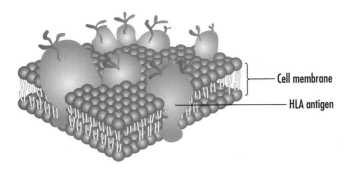

Cell membrane

HLA antigen

FIGURE 12.11   Antigens and the Immune System   A vast array of different HLA antigens are embedded in the outer membranes of cells, projecting beyond their surfaces. These antigens can be recognized by the body's immune cells and antibodies. Since every person's antigens are different, tissue transplanted from one person to another is usually rejected because the donor's HLA antigens are recognized as foreign and destroyed by the immune response of the recipient.

antigens already determined, calculations show that there are so many different HLA combinations that each unrelated person is immunologically unique.

Today, the transplantation of hearts, kidneys, livers, and other organs has become a relatively common procedure in many hospitals. However, organ transplants are extremely costly, complicated procedures and are not always successful. Many more people are waiting for suitable organs than can be supplied from living donors or accident victims. Patients whose survival depends on the availability of a suitably matched organ often wait months to receive one. And often no organ becomes available before the patient dies.

The organ transplanted most often is the kidney. Since people have two kidneys, relatives sometimes donate one of their healthy kidneys to another close relative if their HLA genes are well matched. If the match is perfect for HLA antigens and ABO blood type, the success rate is 90% survival at 1 year. Brothers and sisters have one chance in four of inheriting the same HLA genes from their parents, which is why close relatives are examined first as possible donors. Bone marrow transplants also are used as a last resort in cases of aplastic anemia, acute leukemia, and radiation sickness.

The rejection of transplanted organs can be controlled to some degree with **immunosuppressive drugs** (corticosteroids, cyclosporine); however, treatment with these drugs lessens resistance to infections and sometimes enhances development of other diseases. Long-term immunosuppressive drug therapy itself results in increased susceptibility to cancer. It makes more sense to seek ways to prevent kidney and heart diseases, so that surgical transplants are not necessary.

Blood Transfusions and Rh Factors

In the early part of the twentieth century, a blood transfusion often led to the patient's death. Because the patient's immune system recognized the donor's blood cells as being "foreign," it attacked them with both T-cells and antibodies. The antibodies caused clumps of blood cells to form in the veins and arteries, impeding the flow of blood and oxygen and causing death.

The two most important human red blood cell surface antigens are the ABO and Rh-positive/Rh-negative proteins. There are actually many other groups of antigens on red blood cells, but these two are by far the most important ones in evoking an immune response that can endanger health. Table 12.4 shows the pattern of donor-recipient ABO blood types that must be matched for a successful transfusion.

People with type O blood have neither A nor B antigens on their red blood cells and are **universal donors;** their blood cells will not stimulate an antibody response in the recipient, no matter what the blood type. People with type AB blood have both antigens present on their red blood cells and do not synthesize A or B antibodies, because these antigens were recognized as "self" and those antibody-producing cells were destroyed. People with type AB blood are **universal recipients** and accept blood from any of the four groups.

The Rh-positive antigen and the antibody that reacts against it cause problems primarily in pregnancy. A woman is Rh-negative if her red blood cells do not contain any of this antigen. If the red blood cells of a developing fetus have the Rh-positive antigen (inherited from the father) and if some of the fetus' red blood cells enter the mother's blood supply, production of anti-Rh antibodies can be stimulated by her immune system, which

TABLE 12.4   Blood for Transfusions Is Chosen by ABO Blood Group

Blood group	Genotype	Antigens on red blood cells	Transfusions cannot be accepted from	Transfusions are accepted from
O (universal donor)	OO	None	A, B, AB	O
A	AA, AO	A	B, AB	A, O
B	BB, BO	B	A, AB	B, O
AB (universal recipient)	AB	A, B	None	A, B, AB, O

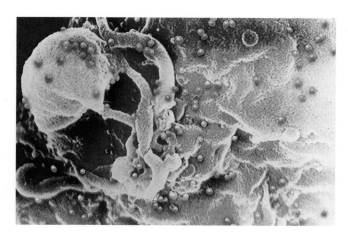

The AIDS virus as seen under the electron microscope. The red dots are presumed to be human immunodeficiency viruses being released from infected cells.

AIDS and HIV

AIDS (Acquired Immune Deficiency Syndrome) was first recognized as a distinct disease in the early 1980s in the United States. It has progressively spread worldwide and now is a major threat to global health. More than 50 million people are infected worldwide and approximately 6 million new infections occur each year. More than half of the world's AIDS victims live in Africa, and most have no access to drugs that can provide relief and retard the spread of **HIV (human immunodeficiency virus)**, which is the cause of AIDS (Figure 12.12).

Although diseases such as smallpox and polio can be traced back in human history for thousands of years,

recognizes the fetal cells as foreign. This usually does not cause any difficulty during the first pregnancy and might even go unnoticed until the woman becomes pregnant again.

Now, if the second fetus is also Rh-positive, the Rh-positive antibodies (synthesized during the first pregnancy) in the mother's blood attack the developing infant's red blood cells, resulting in anemia, brain damage, or even death. Fortunately, doctors can manage this problem safely and effectively. At the time the first child is delivered, the mother is given an injection of anti-Rh antibodies that destroys any Rh-positive antibodies in her blood. In this way, any danger to the fetus during a subsequent pregnancy is avoided.

Terms

immunosuppressive drugs: drugs to suppress the functions of the immune system (e.g., after organ transplants)

universal donor: a person whose blood is accepted by everyone during transfusion

universal recipient: a person whose blood type is compatible with anyone else's blood

AIDS (acquired immune deficiency syndrome): a syndrome of more than two dozen diseases caused by HIV

HIV (human immunodeficiency virus): the virus defined as the cause of AIDS

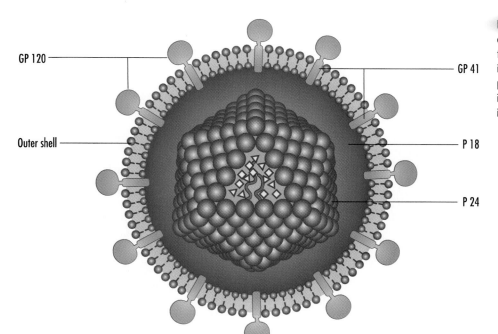

GP 120
GP 41
Outer shell
P 18
P 24

FIGURE 12.12   Human Immunodeficiency Virus (HIV) Protein spikes extrude from the outer shell of the virus. The genetic information is carried in two RNA molecules in the core. Other proteins form protective layers. Reverse transcriptase is the enzyme that the virus uses to copy its genetic information and make new viruses.

it is thought that AIDS is a disease of very recent origin; the first cases emerged less than 50 years ago. Considerable evidence now indicates that the virus originally infected chimpanzees and probably infected humans who butchered and/or ate chimpanzee meat, or who received bites or scratches while handling chimpanzees. After infecting people, the virus gradually changed its genetic makeup, evolving into a virus that could infect human immune system cells and destroy them. At least two distinct strains of HIV have been isolated from patients with AIDS, and it is likely that other strains will emerge as the virus spreads around the world.

AIDS is called a syndrome because it is defined by the appearance of any one or several different infectious diseases. It also is characterized by a very low level of a particular immune system cell called the CD4 T-cell. In an uninfected person the CD4 T-cell level is 800–1200 cells/milliliters; in an AIDS patient the level can be 100 cells/milliliters or less. Once HIV infects CD4 T-cells, it replicates and releases viruses that infect additional cells.

AIDS and the Immune System

Infection with HIV gradually weakens the body's immune system, exposing it to **opportunistic infections,** caused by any of a wide variety of microorganisms. AIDS patients become progressively weaker with each infection and eventually die. The course of HIV infection is unpredictable; some individuals progress to full-blown AIDS and die within months. Oth-

> *Nothing in life is to be feared, it is only to be understood.*
> MARIE CURIE

ers have no symptoms even after 10 years or more of HIV infection (Figure 12.13).

About 1% of HIV-infected persons have remained healthy for as long as 15 years after they were infected, demonstrating that HIV infection does not inevitably lead to AIDS (at least within a certain timeframe) in everyone. Studies of these long-term survivors revealed that these lucky persons carry two copies of a rare gene (CCR5) that makes them resistant to HIV infection. People who carry one copy of the rare gene along with a copy of the more common gene also survive longer than average with HIV infection (O'Brien and Dean, 1997). This important finding paves the way for scientists to devise drugs that can mimic the effect of the desirable gene in people who are not genetically resistant to HIV infection.

For the majority of HIV-infected patients, powerful drugs must be taken (more than 50 pills a day) to keep HIV in check and prevent progression to AIDS. Three classes of drugs that block HIV multiplication in infected individuals are available: reverse transcriptase inhibitors (AZT and 3TC), nonnucleoside reverse transcriptase inhibitors (Nevirapine, Delavirdine, and Loviride), and protease inhibitors (Saquinavir, Rotonavir, and Indinavir). These or other drugs must be taken daily to prevent HIV proliferation. Since all of these drugs are toxic, there is a time limit as to how long they can be taken. Also, because of cost and other considerations, not all AIDS patients are receiving the most effective drug regimens (Binswanger, 2001).

Although optimism for treating HIV infections has increased, a cure for AIDS is still a remote hope. Eventually, scientists hope to develop a vaccine for HIV infection; although many potential vaccines have

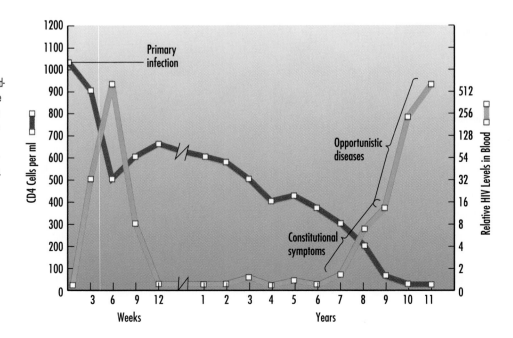

FIGURE 12.13   HIV and the Immune System   After infection, the virus level rises sharply in the blood, but within 3 months is undetectable. However, the virus is usually multiplying slowly in lymph nodes. The infected CD4 T-cells gradually decrease in number over many years. At some point, the immune system is weakened so that the person becomes susceptible to any of dozens of infectious diseases. Although this figure shows a disease latency of 8 years, some HIV-positive individuals have had no symptoms for as long as 15 years.

been tested, none have proved effective as yet. In Asia and Africa, millions of people are still becoming infected with HIV; however, they have little hope of receiving the expensive and complicated treatments being developed in the U.S. In 16 countries in Africa, HIV infection rates exceed 10 percent. In South Africa and Zimbabwe as many as one fourth of the population is infected. Average life expectancy in these countries is falling rapidly. For poor countries, prevention is the best way to reduce HIV infections and AIDS.

The AIDS Antibody Test

Upon infecting a person, HIV acts like all other viral infections by stimulating synthesis of antibodies capable of inactivating the virus. Detection of these antibodies is the basis of the **AIDS antibody test.** In reality, the test is an indirect measure of HIV infection; it does not measure whether a person has AIDS or will get AIDS.

The test is positive only after antibodies have reached a detectable level, which can take several weeks or even months after infection. In the interim, a person is highly infectious, but will show negative results on the AIDS antibody test. Thus, even a recent negative AIDS antibody test may not mean that a person is uninfected if they have been sexually active or use injected drugs.

Another problem with AIDS antibody tests is false-positive results that create unnecessary anxiety. A false-positive means that the test shows that the person has antibodies in his or her blood that resemble ones produced in response to HIV. In reality, the person is not infected and the test is in error. Infection by other viruses or bacteria whose antigens resemble those of HIV can lead to a false-positive result on the HIV antibody test. Any positive AIDS test result should be rechecked. The most accurate test for HIV infection is the **Western blot,** which tests for the presence of specific HIV proteins.

Preventing HIV Infection

Compared to other viral infections, such as ones that cause colds, flu, or hepatitis, HIV is not very infectious. The virus is *never* transmitted by casual contact between an infected person and uninfected persons. Never, in this context, means that no well-documented cases of HIV infection have been reported except as a result of sexual intercourse or the receipt of HIV-contaminated blood (see chapter 11 for a discussion of the sexual transmission of HIV). HIV is not transmitted in saliva, spit, sweat, air, water, or other objects that have been used by an HIV-infected person. You can protect yourself from HIV infection by understanding the facts about HIV and AIDS.

Preventing Infections

Infections to some degree are unavoidable. However, the elements of healthy living that we have been emphasizing can both reduce the risk of contracting an infectious disease and also hasten recovery. Foremost is maintaining health by proper nutrition and a reasonable amount of exercise. These factors, as well as sufficient rest and sleep, increase the ability of the immune system to fight infectious organisms.

Vaccinations against certain infections can provide almost complete protection in most cases. Check your record of immunizations with your family physician and update any that have not been received on schedule or that you are not sure that you received as a child. Many infections, such as mumps or measles, that are usually mild in childhood, can be serious if acquired as an adult.

Never forget that the mind interacts with the immune system and also contributes to the body's propensity to ward off or to succumb to infections. Stressful situations and emotional disturbances lower the body's defenses and make it more vulnerable to infectious microorganisms. Finally, use common sense and stay away from people and situations that are known to carry a high risk of infection. For example, do not travel to an area that is having a cholera epidemic. Do not expose yourself unnecessarily to people with colds, flu, hepatitis or other highly contagious diseases. With reasonable precautions many infectious diseases are preventable. And by maintaining good health, the body will quickly and completely recover from most infections when they do occur.

Terms

AIDS antibody test: detects antibodies in blood that are produced in response to infection by HIV

Western blot test: a test to determine the presence of specific HIV proteins; very accurate

Critical Thinking About Health

1. Describe one infectious disease you have had in the past few years (other than a cold). Discuss the following: (a) how you think you caught the disease, (b) what kind of microorganism caused it, (c) what the symptoms were, (d) how the disease was treated, and (e) any advice you were given on how to avoid contracting the disease in the future. Have you made any changes in your lifestyle to reduce the risk of contracting an infectious disease as a result of this experience?

2. What kind of infectious disease worries you the most: Lyme disease, AIDS, hepatitis, tuberculosis, sexually transmitted diseases in general, or others? Explain your concerns over contracting this disease, including any circumstances in your life that might have given rise to your concerns. Describe all that you know about this particular disease and how your concerns have altered your lifestyle or behaviors.

3. Find out all that you can on food-borne infectious diseases. Describe the kinds of microorganisms in foods that cause disease and ways that people can protect themselves from becoming infected. Do you have any concerns about the foods that you eat? Can you reduce or eliminate these concerns by making changes in your diet?

4. A variety of mind-body exercises are effective in controlling the symptoms of allergies, asthma, arthritis, and other immune system diseases. Learn as much as you can about how the immune system works. Discuss how you think the mind affects the immune system and how it can affect symptoms of the diseases mentioned above. Have you had any personal experience in using your mind to change the symptoms of a disease that has its roots in some form of immune system malfunction?

Health in Review

- Infectious diseases are caused by a myriad of pathogenic organisms: viruses, bacteria, fungi, protozoa, and worms. Growth of certain microorganisms in the body can cause a wide range of diseases and sickness; some produce only mild symptoms, but others produce serious disease and death.
- Some pathogenic microorganisms are easily passed from one person to another and cause communicable diseases.
- Some infectious diseases are caused by a vector such as an insect or other animal that transmits the pathogenic microorganism to an uninfected person.
- Hepatitis B and C infections affect millions of people worldwide.
- Prion diseases (mad cow disease) are of growing concern worldwide.
- In the United States emerging infectious diseases are of concern: West Nile virus that causes encephalitis is one.
- Many pathogenic bacteria are becoming resistant to common antibiotics, making treatment of serious infectious diseases difficult.
- Antibiotics kill microorganisms but do not kill viruses, which are not alive in the sense that cells are.

- Nosocomial infections can be acquired in hospitals and are difficult to treat because the pathogenic bacteria are often antibiotic-resistant.
- Infectious disease is fought in four ways: sanitation, antibiotics, vaccination, and healthful living.
- The skin and mucous membranes keep harmful substances from entering the body.
- Specialized white blood cells circulate in the body, attacking and destroying invading foreign organisms.
- The immune system produces cells that make antibodies, which are proteins that recognize any foreign substance or organism.
- Malfunctioning of the immune system causes autoimmune diseases and allergies.
- Each person carries a unique set of antigens on cells of the body that make tissues and organs unique to each individual.
- Transplantation of organs or blood requires that the donor and recipient be matched with respect to histocompatibility, which is the matching of HLA or ABO antigens.
- Foods contaminated by bacteria and prions, especially meats, can cause serious infectious diseases.

- AIDS results from infection by HIV, which destroys CD4 cells of the immune system. Immunodeficiency leads to opportunistic infections that eventually cause death.
- Long-term survivors of HIV infection have genes that make them resistant to infection by HIV and to development of AIDS.
- New drugs help to keep the virus in check in persons infected with HIV.

Health and Wellness Online

The World Wide Web contains a wealth of information about health and wellness. By accessing the Internet using Web browser software, such as Netscape Navigator or Microsoft's Internet Explorer, you can gain a new perspective on many topics presented in *Health and Wellness, Seventh Edition.* Access the Jones and Bartlett Publishers Web site at http://www.jbpub.com/hwonline.

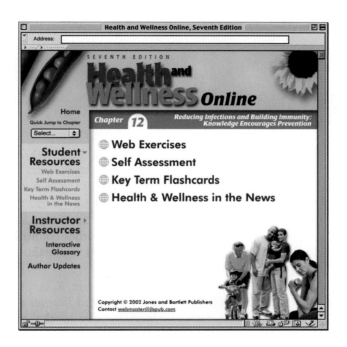

References

Alpert, M. (1999, November). The invisible epidemic. *Scientific American*, 19–20.

Barnes, P. J. (1996). Is immunotherapy for asthma worthwhile? *New England Journal of Medicine, 334*, 530–531.

Beardsley, T. (1995, January). Better than a cure. *Scientific American*, 88–93.

Binswanger, H. P. (2001). HIV/AIDS treatment for millions. *Science, 292*, 221–223.

Blakeslee, S. (2001, January 14). Stringent steps taken by U.S. on cow illness. *New York Times*, 1,25.

Bren, L. (2001, January/February). Antibiotic resistance. *FDA Consumer*, 10–11.

Brunton, S. A., and Saphir, R. L. (1999, September 15). Dust mites and asthma. *Hospital Practice*, 67–76.

Cohen, J. I. (2000). Epstein-Barr virus infection. *New England Journal of Medicine, 343*, 481–490.

Enserink, M. (2000). The enigma of west nile. *Science, 290*, 1482–1484.

Holloway, M. (2000, April). Outbreak not contained. *Scientific American*, 20–22.

Jewett, D. L. et al. (1990). A double blind study of the symptom provocation to determine food sensitivity. *New England Journal of Medicine, 323*, 429–433.

Koff, R. S. (1998, June 15). Chronic hepatitis C: Early intervention. *Hospital Practice*, 101–114.

Lanchester, J. (1996, December 2). A new kind of contagion. *The New Yorker*, 70–81.

Lederberg, J. (1996). Infectious diseases—A threat to global health and security. *Journal of the American Medical Association, 276*, 417–419.

Morse, S. S. (1996, April 15). Patterns and predictability in emerging infections. *Hospital Practice*, 85–91.

Platts-Mills, T. A. E., and Carter, M. C. (1997). Asthma and indoor exposure to allergens. *New England Journal of Medicine, 336*, 1382–1384.

Raloff, J. (1996). Family allergies? Keep the nuts away from baby. *Science News, 149*, 279.

Rusk, M., and Gluckman, S. (1999, August 15). The new vaccine for Lyme disease. *Hospital Practice*, 37–40.

Ryan, E. T., and Kain, K. C. (2000). Health advice and immunizations for travelers. *New England Journal of Medicine*, 1716–1724.

Sampson, H. A. (2000, May 15). Food allergy: from biology toward therapy. *Hospital Practice*, 67–79.

Sands, K. E. et al. (1997). Epidemiology of sepsis syndrome in 8 academic medical centers. *Journal of the American Medical Association, 278*, 234–240.

Thomas, D. I. et al. (2000). The natural history of hepatitis C virus infection. *Journal of the American Medical Association*, 450–454.

Walsh, J. H., and Peterson, W. L. (1995). The treatment of *Heliobacter pylori* infection in the management of peptic ulcer disease. *New England Journal of Medicine, 333*, 984–991.

Suggested Readings

Blaser, M. J. (1996, February). The bacteria behind ulcers. *Scientific American*, 104–107. The story of how the ulcer bacterium was discovered; one of the great medical stories of the century.

Defeating AIDS: What will it take? (1998, July). *Scientific American*, 81–105. A series of articles discussing all aspects of AIDS including preventing infection in children and adults and possibilities for a vaccine.

Guenno, B. L. (1995, October). Emerging viruses. *Scientific American*, 56–64. Explains the health danger of the many new viruses that are causing disease.

Lederberg, J. (2000, April 14). Infectious history. *Science*, 287–293. A Nobel Prize winner discusses the history of the human battle with infectious diseases.

Morganthau, T. (1997, September 1). *E. coli* alert. *Newsweek*, 26–32. Discusses the bacteria that contaminate meat and other foods and how to protect yourself from infection.

Nemecek, S. (2000, March). Granting immunity. *Scientific American*, 15–16. A brief explanation of the importance of vaccinations in children.

Rosenberg, T. (2001, January 28). Look at Brazil. *The New York Times Magazine*. 26–63. Describes how Brazil and other countries are defying the drug companies' patents and making their own drugs to treat AIDS patients.

Sepkowitz, K. A. (2001). AIDS—The first 20 years. *New England Journal of Medicine, 344*, 1764–1772. A brief history of the AIDS epidemic and the global problems that lie ahead.

Smaglik, P. (1997). Proliferation of pills. *Science News, 151*, 310–311. Discusses the overuse of antibiotics by physicians and how this contributes to the development of antibiotic-resistant bacteria.

1. Identify and describe the most important ways to prevent cancer.
2. Briefly discuss the incidence of cancer today and why mortality has not fallen.
3. Define the following terms: cancer, tumor, benign tumor, malignant tumor, metastasis, and xenoestrogen.
4. Explain the difference between inherited diseases and genetic diseases.
5. Describe the kinds of environmental agents that cause cancer.
6. Explain ways to prevent skin cancer.
7. Discuss some risk factors associated with breast cancer.
8. Describe how to do a breast self-exam (BSE).
9. Discuss how cigarette smoke contributes to cancer.
10. Discuss the association between diet and cancer.
11. Briefly describe the three medical treatments for cancer.
12. Describe several coping mechanisms for someone with cancer.
13. Explain the risks and benefits of being tested for a cancer susceptibility gene.

Study Guide
and
Self Assessment

Reduce Environmental Cancer Risks

Health
and Wellness
Online

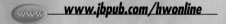 **www.jbpub.com/hwonline**

Chapter 13

Cancer: Understanding Risks and Means of Prevention

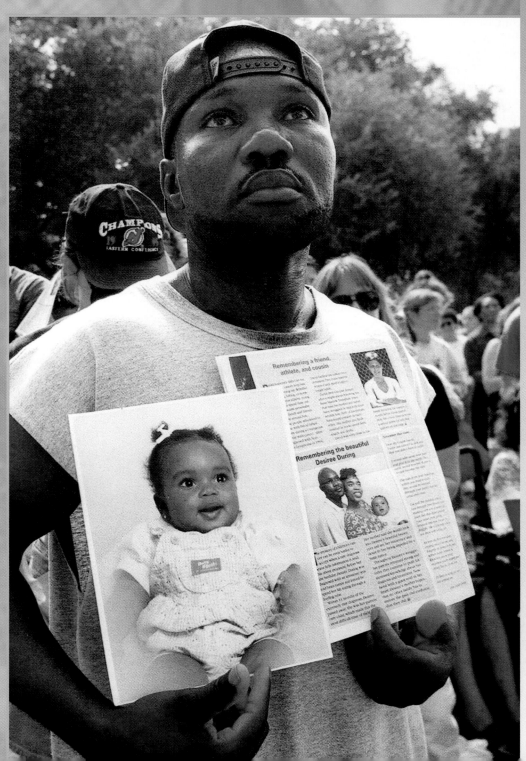

On the basis of recent statistics, one out of two men and one out of three women in the United States will develop some type of cancer during their lifetime; in 2000, approximately 552,000 Americans died from cancer. Despite the dismal statistics, the news about cancer is not all bad. Most cancers *are* preventable if people adopt healthy lifestyles. Avoiding cigarette smoke and tobacco in *any* form is the most important action anyone can take to avoid cancer, especially lung and pancreatic cancers, which are most often incurable. Cigarette smoke is estimated to be the primary cause in the development of at least 30% of all cancers (see chapter 17).

> *Pain has an element of blank;*
> *it cannot recollect*
> *when it began, or if there were*
> *a day when it was not.*
> EMILY DICKINSON

A healthy diet that includes low levels of animal fat and high levels of fresh fruits, vegetables, and fiber from grains will also markedly reduce the risk of cancer. Avoiding as much as possible ultraviolet (UV) radiation in sunshine is essential to prevent skin cancer later in life. Finally, knowing what chemicals in the environment are cancer-causing can help you avoid dangerous substances. Overall, if everything known about cancer prevention were practiced by everyone, up to two-thirds of *all* cancers could be prevented. About one third are caused by cigarette smoking.

Another positive note is that about half of all cancer patients can be cured if their cancer is detected at an early stage before cancer cells have spread. Being "cured" of cancer means that a person's life expectancy is the same as for a person who never had cancer. It is important to have cancer screening tests as indicated for your age and risk group; tests for the early detection of breast, colon, prostate, and cervical cancers are recommended by the American Cancer Society (Table 13.1). You should also watch for early warning signs in functions of the body that may indicate that a cancer is developing (Figure 13.1).

Understanding Cancer

Incidence of Various Cancers

Cancers of certain organs have declined significantly in recent years (Figure 13.2). However, cancers of the lung, skin, liver, prostate, and kidney and non-Hodgkin's lymphoma have all increased in frequency. Overall, the mortality from cancer has remained virtually unchanged over the last generation, despite intensive research and improved medical treatments.

The most serious increase has been the continuing rise in lung cancer in both men and women. Increases in lung cancer in men began to be noticed in the 1940s; in women, the increase did not become apparent until the 1960s. As everyone knows, the reason for the increase in lung cancer among both men and women is cigarette smoking. Women now die from lung cancer about half as often as men, and their rate of death is still increasing.

Addiction to nicotine and to cigarette smoking begins for both sexes as soon as smoking begins, during teenage years or even earlier. For this reason, government agencies and health organizations are now making a concerted effort to stop teenagers from smoking and thereby reverse the upward trend in cancer mortality.

What Is Cancer?

The term *cancer* comes from the Latin word meaning crab. Cancer was characterized as a crablike disease by the Greek physician Hippocrates, who observed that cancers spread throughout the body, eventually cutting off life. Now **cancer** generally is defined as the unregulated growth of specific cells in the body. The word cancer actually refers to over 100 different diseases, but in all cases, certain body cells multiply in an abnormal, unregulated manner.

Normally, the growth and reproduction of every cell in the body are regulated; this regulation, in turn, determines the size and functions of tissues and organs. If a normal body cell begins to grow abnormally and reproduces too rapidly, a mass of abnormal cells eventually develops that is called a **tumor.** A tumor generally contains millions of genetically identical abnormal cells before it can be detected or felt.

If the cells of the tumor remain localized at the site of origin in the body and if they multiply relatively slowly, the tumor is said to be benign. **Benign tumors,** such as cysts, warts, moles, and polyps, do

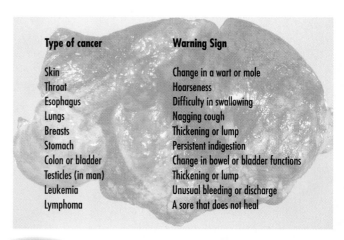

Type of cancer	Warning Sign
Skin	Change in a wart or mole
Throat	Hoarseness
Esophagus	Difficulty in swallowing
Lungs	Nagging cough
Breasts	Thickening or lump
Stomach	Persistent indigestion
Colon or bladder	Change in bowel or bladder functions
Testicles (in man)	Thickening or lump
Leukemia	Unusual bleeding or discharge
Lymphoma	A sore that does not heal

FIGURE 13.1   Some Warning Signs of Cancer   If any of these symptoms occur, see a physician promptly.

TABLE 13.1   American Cancer Society Recommendations for the Early Detection of Cancer

Test	Population		Frequency of testing
	Sex	Age	
Sigmoidoscopy, preferably flexible	M & F	50 and over	Every 3–5 years
Fecal occult blood test	M & F	50 and over	Every year
Digital rectal exam	M & F	40 and over	Every year
Prostate exam*	M	50 and over	Every year
Pap test	F		All women who are, or who have been, sexually active, or have reached age 18, should have an annual Pap test and pelvic examination. After a woman has had three or more consecutive satisfactory normal annual examinations, the Pap test may be performed less frequently at the discretion of her physician.
Breast self-examination	F	20 and over	Every month
Breast clinical examination	F	20–40 Over 40	Every 3 years Every year
Mammography†	F	40–49 50 and over	Every 1–2 years Every year

*Annual digital rectal examination and prostate-specific antigen test should be performed on men 50 years and older. If either result is abnormal, further evaluation should be considered.

†Screening mammography should begin by age 40.

Source: Reprinted by the permission of the American Cancer Society.

not spread to other parts of the body. Benign tumors usually can be removed surgically and generally are not a threat to life. In fact, benign tumors weighing several hundred pounds have been surgically removed from persons who then recovered fully. Benign tumors cannot regrow if all of the abnormal cells are removed by surgical excision of the tumor.

Malignant tumors are composed of cells that grow rapidly, have other abnormal properties that distinguish them from normal cells, and invade other normal tissues. In particular, malignant cells may have altered shapes and cell-surface characteristics that contribute to their rapid proliferation. Many malignant cells also have abnormal chromosomes or altered genes, and they manufacture abnormal proteins. The numerous altered properties of malignant cells enable a **pathologist,** a physician who specializes in the causes of diseases, to determine whether the cells removed from a tumor are abnormal and to what degree.

The cells of most malignant tumors also undergo **metastasis,** a process in which cells detach from the original tumor, enter the lymphatic system and bloodstream, and are carried to other organs. Once the malignant cells spread to other organs, they develop into new tumors that often grow more rapidly than cells in the original tumor. Metastases and the growth of new tumors in many organs of the body eventually disrupt a vital body function, which is the cause of death.

Cancers are medically classified according to the organ or kind of tissue in which the tumor originates. The four major categories of cancers are *carcinomas, sarcomas, leukemias,* and *lymphomas* (Figure 13.3). Within these major categories are numerous subgroups that generally describe the organ in which the cancer originates, such as adenocarcinoma of the stomach or oat cell carcinoma of the lung. About half of all human cancers originate in one of four organs: the lung, breast, prostate, or colon, which is why so much research is devoted to these particular forms.

Cancer does not develop all at once in a cell. Several changes must occur in the genetic information (i.e., DNA) carried in a single cell before it can become a cancer cell and multiply into a tumor. Cells change their abnormal growth properties one step at a time; each genetic change pushes the cell further along the spectrum of abnormal growth. Not all cells acquire the same genetic changes nor can anyone predict when the changes will occur. That explains why some cancers develop and grow rapidly and cause death in months while other cancers grow so slowly that the person eventually dies from a cause other than cancer.

Terms

cancer: unregulated growth of cells in the body

tumor: a mass of abnormal cells

benign tumor: a tumor whose cells do not spread to other parts of the body

malignant tumor: a tumor whose cells spread throughout the body

pathologist: a physician who specializes in the causes of diseases

metastasis: the process by which cancer cells spread throughout the body

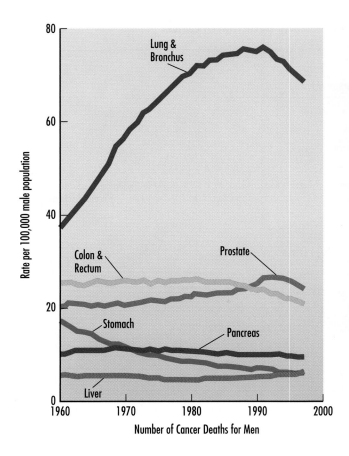

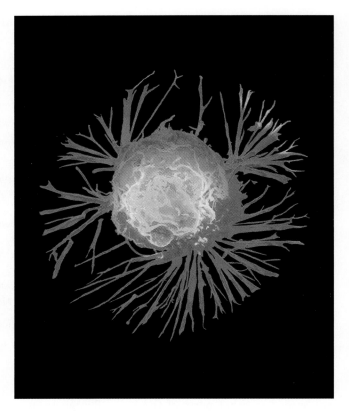

Electron micrograph of a breast cancer cell.

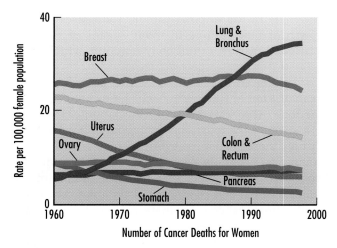

FIGURE 13.2 **Age-adjusted Cancer Death Rates for Men and Women in the United States from 1960 to 1999** Deaths from cigarette smoking have caused a dramatic rise in lung and bronchus cancers. The only cancers to have declined significantly in this period are of the uterus and stomach.

Source: Reprinted by permission of the American Cancer Society.

Once a tumor has been detected, cells can be removed from it in a procedure called a **biopsy;** the cells are then examined under the microscope by a pathologist. In stage I, cancer cells can be distinguished from normal cells. The cancer cells are still localized (usually referred to as cancer *in situ*) and surgical removal

of the tumor usually results in a cure. In stage II, the cancer cells have begun to metastasize and may have migrated to nearby lymph nodes. That is why lymph nodes near the tumor are removed and examined during surgery to determine if cancer cells have spread. By stage III, the cancer cells have spread throughout the body, and tumors may have begun to grow in other organs. In stage IV, often a terminal stage, tumors are found throughout the body and usually are resistant to treatment.

The number of deaths from cancer by organ and by sex are shown in Figure 13.4. In 2000, prostate cancer was exceeded only by lung cancer as a cause of death in men. And among women, lung cancer now exceeds breast cancer as the leading cause of death. Cancer of the colon and rectum, the third leading cause of death for both men and women, is believed to be strongly associated with fat-rich diets that are low in fiber.

Causes of Cancer

Most Cancers Are Not Inherited

Many people live in fear of cancer, often because one or more closely related family members have died from some type of cancer. They believe that cancer is passed on in the genes or that, at least, the suscepti-

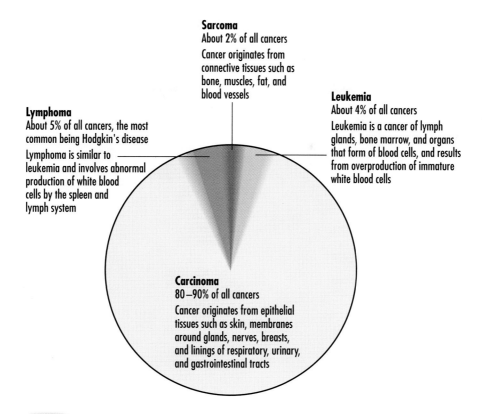

Sarcoma
About 2% of all cancers
Cancer originates from connective tissues such as bone, muscles, fat, and blood vessels

Lymphoma
About 5% of all cancers, the most common being Hodgkin's disease
Lymphoma is similar to leukemia and involves abnormal production of white blood cells by the spleen and lymph system

Leukemia
About 4% of all cancers
Leukemia is a cancer of lymph glands, bone marrow, and organs that form of blood cells, and results from overproduction of immature white blood cells

Carcinoma
80–90% of all cancers
Cancer originates from epithelial tissues such as skin, membranes around glands, nerves, breasts, and linings of respiratory, urinary, and gastrointestinal tracts

FIGURE 13.3   **Four Major Categories of Cancers and Approximate Frequencies of Occurrence**

bility to cancer is inherited. Neither of these beliefs is correct for the vast majority of people. However, a constant fear of developing cancer can generate stress that may weaken the immune system and contribute to the development of disease, including cancer.

Scientific studies indicate that 90% to 95% of all cancers, including breast, lung, stomach, colon, skin, or prostate, are *not* inherited from parents except in a few rare families in which members do inherit one or more cancer susceptibility genes (Lichtenstein, 2000).

Confusion about genes often stems from misunderstanding the meanings of the words "genetic" and "inherited." The two are not synonymous. All of your cells (except for red blood cells) contain exact copies of the chromosomes and genes that were in the fertilized egg from which you developed. The genes in the chromosomes of any cell of your body, such as skin, lung, or stomach cells, can be chemically changed by environmental agents. These genetic changes in skin, lung, or stomach cells may transform them into cancer cells. Thus, cancer is a genetic disease in that genes are changed in a person's body cells; however, it is *not* an inherited disease because defective genes

were not passed on from parents. Thus, a parent who acquires cancer cannot pass it on to his/her child

Even if several close family members have died of cancer, it does not mean that cancer "runs in the family" and is an inherited disease. Currently, one out of every five deaths each year in the United States is due to cancer (American Cancer Society, 2000). If your parents and eight aunts or uncles have died, probably two or three of them died of cancer simply by chance. If they all smoked cigarettes, it would not be surprising if more than three close relatives out of ten died of cancer.

One of the best pieces of evidence showing that most cancers are *not* inherited comes from a study of World War II veterans. The health of 15,000 pairs of identical or nonidentical (fraternal) twin brothers was followed for many years after WWII. No difference was observed in the different twin pairs in the development of cancer. That is, if one identical twin contracted cancer, his identical twin was no more likely to get cancer than the average person.

Because identical twins share identical genes (i.e., they are natural clones that developed from the same fertilized egg that split into separate embryos), they should carry identical cancer-causing genes. The fact that identical twins do not *both* have cancer at significantly higher rates than the average person means that most cancers are *not* caused by inherited genes. For most people, lifestyle (e.g., diet, smoking, drinking

Terms

biopsy: removal of cells from a tumor for examination under a microscope

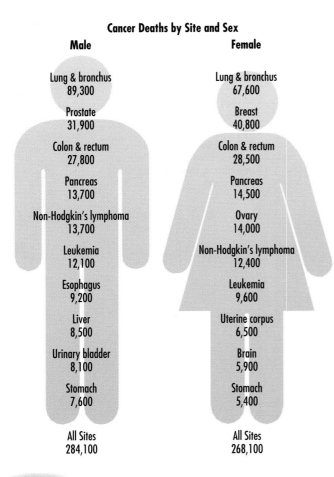

Cancer Deaths by Site and Sex

Male	Female
Lung & bronchus 89,300	Lung & bronchus 67,600
Prostate 31,900	Breast 40,800
Colon & rectum 27,800	Colon & rectum 28,500
Pancreas 13,700	Pancreas 14,500
Non-Hodgkin's lymphoma 13,700	Ovary 14,000
Leukemia 12,100	Non-Hodgkin's lymphoma 12,400
Esophagus 9,200	Leukemia 9,600
Liver 8,500	Uterine corpus 6,500
Urinary bladder 8,100	Brain 5,900
Stomach 7,600	Stomach 5,400
All Sites 284,100	All Sites 268,100

FIGURE 13.4 Estimated Cancer Deaths by Site and Sex for 2000

Source: Reprinted by the permission of the American Cancer Society.

alcohol) plays a far greater role in causing cancer than any genes that are passed on from parents.

Cancer Susceptibility Genes

Although only a small fraction (estimates range between 5% to 10%) of all cancers are strongly influenced by heredity, some families do transmit **cancer susceptibility genes** to children. A cancer susceptibility gene does not cause cancer directly; however, it makes a person carrying such a gene more vulnerable to environmental factors that contribute to the risk of developing cancer.

Quite a few cancer susceptibility genes have been identified in recent years (Table 13.2). Most of these genes appear to contribute to the development of cancer in a particular organ: BRCA1 and BRCA2 genes are susceptibility genes for breast or ovarian cancer; APC, MSH2, and MLH1, for colon cancer. People who carry mutant (abnormal) copies of these genes are at higher risk for certain cancers than are people who carry normal copies (O'Leary, 1999).

Many genes that increase the risk of colon cancer have been identified and some of their biological

TABLE 13.2 **Cancer Susceptibility Genes**
Abnormalities (mutations) in these genes can be inherited or acquired. Each abnormal gene contributes to the development of cancer in a specific organ.

Gene	Organ affected
Breast cancer	
BRCA1	Breast, ovary
BRCA2	Breast
p53	Breast, brain
Colon cancer	
MSH2	Colon, uterus
MLH1	Colon, uterus
PMS1, PMS2	Colon, other
APC	Colon
Melanoma	
MTS1 (CDKN2)	Skin, pancreas
CDK4	Skin
Prostate cancer	
HPC1	Prostate

functions in cells also are understood (Figure 13.5). If a person inherits an abnormal form of any one of three genes, APC, MSH2, or MLH1, the risk of colon cancer is increased. However, fewer than 5% of all colon cancer patients inherit any of these colon cancer susceptibility genes, so colon cancer is *not* inherited in over 95% of patients.

During a person's lifetime, mutations continue to arise and accumulate in cells lining the colon. For example, suppose a person inherited a MSH2 mutation and 20 years later a colon cell acquired an APC mutation. Those two mutations make that colon cell begin to reproduce itself at a faster rate; at some point, one cell among the faster growing ones acquires a third mutation in either a K-*ras*, DDC, or p53 gene. That cell now has three mutations and may develop into cancer of the colon. Along the way to tumor formation, other mutations also may occur. On average, when colon cancer cells are examined, they have at least three of the mutations described in Figure 13.5.

Terms

cancer susceptibility gene: gene responsible for familial breast cancer and genes that cause susceptibility to colon cancer; increases the risk of a person developing cancer in his or her lifetime

epidemiology: a branch of science that studies the causes and frequencies of diseases in human populations

mutation: a permanent change in the genetic information in a cell; only mutations in sperm and eggs are inherited

ionizing radiation: radiation, such as x-rays, that can damage cells and cause cancer; also used to treat cancer

Now you can understand why chance genetic changes and exposure to environmental agents that cause mutations play such important roles in the development of cancer (Byers, 2000).

Environmental Factors

The causes of cancer or, more correctly, the risk factors associated with the development of cancer are numerous and complex (Shields and Harris, 1991). It often is difficult to point to a single cause of a cancer, but certain environmental factors are strongly correlated with the occurrence of particular cancers. Two examples are the strong correlation between cigarette smoking and lung cancer and exposure to ultraviolet (UV) light and skin cancer. Even in these examples, not everyone who smokes heavily or stays in the sun day after day will get lung or skin cancer.

Epidemiology is the branch of science that investigates the causes and frequencies of diseases in human populations. Many epidemiological studies show that as many as 80% to 90% of cancers are caused by exposure to environmental factors that are known to increase the risk of cancer (Table 13.3). For example, smoking cigarettes while young puts a person at 10 to 20 times higher risk of developing cancer later in life than persons who do not smoke. Eating fat-laden fast food frequently may be convenient, but it is ultimately unhealthy and may contribute to the development of certain cancers (Raloff, 1999). Because each of us can change our diets, stop smoking, and avoid other cancer-causing risks in the environment, pre-

venting cancer is a realistic and attainable goal for most people.

Three classes of environmental agents—ionizing radiation, tumor viruses (viruses that cause cancer in animals), and chemical carcinogens (cancer-causing chemicals)—have been shown to increase the risk of cancer in both laboratory animals and people. Each of these agents increases the risk of cancer by producing chemical changes in genes, called **mutations,** that can occur in any cell in the body and cause it to grow abnormally. If a cell undergoes one or more mutations in genes that regulate its growth, it may begin to multiply rapidly and develop into a tumor. Environmental factors cause mutations and also affect the rate of abnormal cell growth (Figure 13.6).

Ionizing Radiation

Ionizing radiation consists of x-rays, UV light, and radioactivity whose energy can damage cells and chromosomes. The high rate of leukemia among survivors of the Hiroshima and Nagasaki atomic bomb blasts in 1945 leaves no doubt that radioactivity increases the risk of cancer.

In the United States, among children born in southern Utah in the 1950s who were exposed to radioactive fallout from nearby atomic tests, leukemia deaths were two to three times greater than among children born in southern Utah before and after the atomic tests. In a landmark legal decision in 1984, a federal court ruled that the U.S. government was negligent in conducting atomic bomb tests in southern Utah in the 1950s because they released radioactive material into the

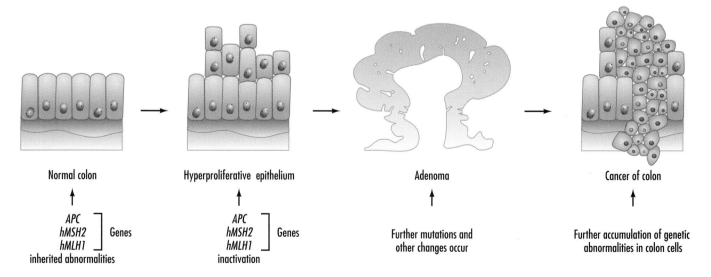

Normal colon	Hyperproliferative epithelium	Adenoma	Cancer of colon
↑	↑	↑	↑
APC *hMSH2* *hMLH1*] Genes inherited abnormalities	*APC* *hMSH2* *hMLH1*] Genes inactivation	Further mutations and other changes occur	Further accumulation of genetic abnormalities in colon cells

FIGURE 13.5   Mutant Genes Contribute to Development of Cancer Cells   Genetic changes in several genes can lead to increased risk of colon cancer. Abnormalities in APC, hMSH2, or hMLH1 genes can be inherited from parents. Other genetic changes may occur in colon cells during the course of a person's life before development of a cancer. Examination of colon cancer cells indicates that most of them have accumulated several genetic changes, either inherited or acquired.

TABLE 13.3   Environmental and Lifestyle Risk Factors that Contribute to Cancer

Factor	Amount of risk	Types of cancer
Nutrition	About *half* of cancer deaths are caused by nutritional problems: Excess calories Excess fat consumption Obesity Nutritional deficiencies, especially fiber and vitamin A	Cancers of the colon, rectum, stomach, breast, and ovaries
Cigarettes and alcohol	About *one-third* of cancer deaths are caused by smoking cigarettes and excessive alcohol consumption	Cancers of the lung, pancreas, mouth, larynx, liver, esophagus, and bladder
Occupation	About 5% of cancer deaths are caused by substances in the workplace such as asbestos, benzene, and vinyl chloride	Cancers of the bladder, lung, stomach, blood, liver, bones, and skin
Radiation	About 3% of cancer deaths are caused by ionizing radiation, such as x-rays and ultraviolet light	Blood, skin
Other	Other cancer deaths result from heredity, chronic disease, drugs, and chemotherapy	Various cancers

atmosphere. The court ruled that the families who were exposed to radioactivity as a result of these tests, and whose members died as a result of exposure to the radioactivity, were entitled to compensation.

The nuclear reactor accident at Chernobyl in the Ukraine in 1986 also released large amounts of radioactivity, particularly radioactive iodine, strontium, and cesium, into the atmosphere. Not only was the region around the reactor affected, but radioactive fallout occurred over much of Europe. In some countries, milk and crops were so contaminated that they had to be destroyed. Some of the radioactivity was detected in countries as distant as the United States and Japan.

The toll in human sickness and deaths from this nuclear accident continues to mount even today. Approximately 32,000 persons died directly or indirectly as a result of the reactor explosion; another 30,000 suffered some degree of radiation sickness. Children are especially at risk from radioactive iodine, which causes thyroid cancer; in the Ukraine, thyroid cancer among children is currently 10 times higher than it was before the accident occurred.

Because any amount of ionizing radiation, however small, has the potential for causing damage to chromosomes and genes, one should minimize exposure to x-rays. For example, if you are healthy, periodic chest x-rays are unnecessary. Dental x-rays with each 6-month checkup also pose a cumulative risk. Some homes release radon, a radioactive gas present in some building materials. Long-term exposure to the invisible radon gas contributes to the risk of cancer (see chapter 24).

The most common source of ionizing radiation in nature is UV radiation in sunlight. Because children and young people spend long hours in the sun, people acquire as much as 80% of their lifetime UV exposure by age 20.

Ultraviolet radiation in sunlight is characterized by two different wavelengths, called UVA and UVB. Until recently, it was thought that only UVB was dangerous, but now it appears that both forms of UV radiation are harmful. Reducing the time of exposure to intense sunlight and using sunscreen creams to protect exposed areas of the body reduce the risk of skin cancer.

Tumor Viruses

In 1911, Peyton Rous, a scientist working at the Rockefeller Institute in New York, showed that cancer could be produced in chickens by injecting them with a virus isolated from chicken tumors. Since then, other viruses, called **tumor viruses,** have been found in animals such as mice, cats, and monkeys.

Finding tumor viruses that infect people has been generally unsuccessful despite considerable research. Only four viruses have been associated with specific human cancers; in the vast majority of people, infection by these viruses will not cause cancer,

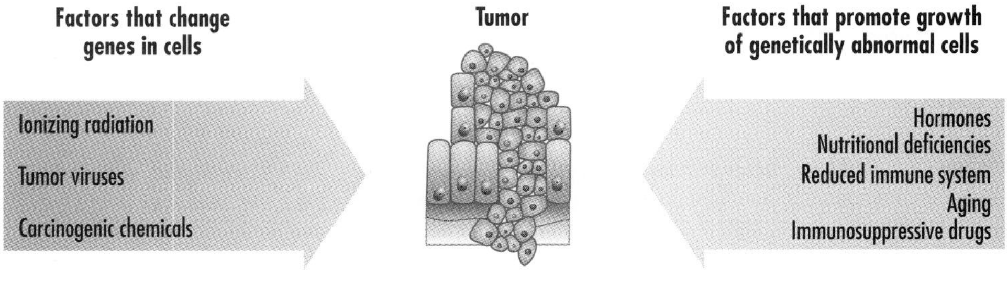

Factors that change genes in cells	Tumor	Factors that promote growth of genetically abnormal cells
Ionizing radiation Tumor viruses Carcinogenic chemicals		Hormones Nutritional deficiencies Reduced immune system Aging Immunosuppressive drugs

FIGURE 13.6   Environmental factors change both genes and the growth properties of cells that may lead to the development of cancer.

TABLE 13.4   Examples of Occupational Cancers

Chemical/physical agent	Cancer type	Exposure of general population	Examples of workers frequently exposed or exposure sources
Arsenic	Lung, skin	Rare	Insecticide and herbicide sprayers; tanners; oil refinery workers
Asbestos	Mesothelioma, lung	Uncommon	Brake-lining, shipyard, insulation, and demolition workers
Benzene	Myelogenous leukemia	Common	Painters; distillers and petrochemical workers; dye users; furniture finishers; rubber workers
Diesel exhaust	Lung	Common	Railroad and bus-garage workers; truck operators; miners
Formaldehyde	Nose, nasopharynx	Rare	Hospital and laboratory workers; manufacture of wood products, paper, textiles, garments, and metal products
Man-made mineral fibers	Lung	Uncommon	Wall and pipe insulation; duct wrapping
Hair dyes	Bladder	Uncommon	Hairdressers and barbers (inadequate evidence for customers)
Ionizing radiation	Bone marrow, several others	Common	Nuclear materials; medicinal products and procedures
Mineral oils	Skin	Common	Metal machining
Nonarsenical pesticides	Lung	Common	Sprayers; agricultural workers
Painting materials	Lung	Uncommon	Professional painters
Polychlorinated biphenyls	Liver, skin	Uncommon	Heat-transfer and hydraulic fluids and lubricants; inks; adhesives; insecticides
Radon (alpha particles)	Lung	Uncommon	Mines; underground structures; homes
Soot	Skin	Uncommon	Chimney sweeps and cleaners; bricklayers; insulators; firefighters; heating-unit service workers

although it will increase its risk. Increased cancer risk is associated with infection by hepatitis B virus (liver cancer), papillomavirus (genital cancer), human T-cell leukemia-lymphoma virus (leukemia and lymphoma), and Epstein-Barr virus (cancer of the nose or pharynx).

Chemical Carcinogens

A **chemical carcinogen** is an environmental substance that can interact with cells to initiate cancer, usually by chemically altering the chromosomes or genes in cells. Genes are responsible for manufacturing the enzymes and other proteins a cell needs to function properly. An altered gene usually makes an abnormal protein that may change the growth properties of a cell and cause it to become a cancer cell.

Many chemicals that are developed are now tested to determine their cancer-causing potential. Unfortunately, many thousands of chemical substances already in use have not been adequately tested. Of the thousands of chemical substances that have been tested, many have been found to be carcinogenic and should be avoided if at all possible. Carcinogens include cigarette smoke, pesticides, asbestos, heavy metals (lead, mercury, cadmium), benzene, and nitrosamines (Table 13.4).

Despite the long list of carcinogenic substances, some scientists and public health officials argue that tobacco is the only substance of consequence with respect to the numbers of cancers caused. While the argument has some basis, it is of small consolation to persons who acquire cancer from exposure, often without their knowledge, to carcinogenic substances in the environment or workplace.

In some industries, workers have cancers that almost never arise in the general population. For example, **mesothelioma** is a rare form of lung cancer that only occurs among persons exposed to asbestos fibers. Long-term exposure to the heavy metals beryllium and cadmium increases workers' risk of prostate cancer. Workers exposed to vinyl chloride, the starting material for polyvinyl chloride (PVC) pipes and other products, develop a rare form of liver cancer not found in the general public. Fortunately, with current occupational and safety regulations, these types of cancer occur infrequently.

The total number of cancers attributable to industrial chemicals is small compared to those caused by tobacco and diet; however, cancers caused by industrial chemicals are preventable or avoidable. Before you accept a job it might be wise to determine what chemicals you will be exposed to for long periods.

Do Xenoestrogens Cause Cancer?

Estrogens are hormones that regulate a variety of biological functions in women, including the growth and

Terms

tumor viruses: viruses that infect cells, change their growth properties, and cause cancer

chemical carcinogen: a chemical that damages cells and causes cancer

mesothelioma: a form of lung cancer caused by asbestos

development of breast tissue. Many chemicals that we are exposed to in the environment mimic the action of normal estrogen to some degree; such chemicals are called **xenoestrogens** (literally, foreign estrogen). Exposure to xenoestrogens in the environment may increase the risk of breast cancer (Davis and Bradlow, 1995).

Substances that contain xenoestrogens include the pesticides DDT (now banned in the U.S., but still used elsewhere), methoxyclor, kepone, chlordane, atrazine, and endosulfan. Polychlorinated biphenyls (PCBs), which were used in electrical transformers for many years, also are xenoestrogens. Bisphenol-A, a component of polycarbonate plastics that are widely used, can leach into liquids when the plastic bottles are heated. Even the gasoline vapor inhaled at the pump can act as a xenoestrogen.

A variety of evidence points to environmental xenoestrogens as possible agents in the formation of cancer. Clues came from wildlife that suffered reproductive abnormalities after being exposed to xenoestrogens. Male fish collected near the outflow from sewers showed production of vitellogin, a female protein. Alligators hatched in a lake in Florida contaminated with a pesticide grew abnormally small penises and had altered hormone levels. And military dogs that served in Vietnam (where Agent Orange, a xenoestrogen, was widely dispersed) have twice the rate of testicular cancer and reproductive defects compared with dogs that did not serve in Vietnam. So xenoestrogens may not only be involved in breast cancer, but may also play a role in reproductive problems and testicular cancer.

The effects of xenoestrogens can be tested on human cells grown in the laboratory. Normal estrogen binds to many cells and affects their growth. Xenoestrogens bind to the same cellular receptors as normal estrogen and exert some of the same effects on the growth of cells. The evidence that xenoestrogens can affect cell proliferation and reproductive organs is now well established.

Since 1976, when chlorinated pesticides were banned in Israel, and all pesticide residues eliminated from milk products, the incidence of breast cancer among Israeli women has been declining. Israel is the only industrialized country that has not experienced an increase in breast cancer in the past 20 years. These observations also lend support to the idea that xenoestrogens contribute to development of breast cancer.

However, a large study that included more than 100,000 nurses in the U.S. concluded that breast cancer is not associated with any differences in the level of PCBs (polychlorinated biphenyls) or DDE (dichloro-bischlorophenyl-ethylene), which are xenoestrogens. There was no significant difference in the levels of these chemicals in the blood of women with breast cancer compared with women who are healthy.

Therefore, some medical experts now believe that the breast cancer risk resulting from xenoestrogens is very small (Safe, 1997).

It is impossible to avoid all exposure to xenoestrogens since they are everywhere in the environment. Also, eating broccoli, cabbage, and soy products may help counteract the effects of xenoestrogens. This advice comes from the observation that Asian women have much lower rates of breast cancer in comparison to white or black American women. Asian diets are richer in these vegetables, which may contain chemicals that block the biological activities of the xenoestrogens.

Facts About Common Cancers

Lung Cancer

Lung cancer causes more deaths among men and women than any other form of cancer. In the U.S. in 2000, lung cancer was the cause of about 157,000 deaths. Smoking cigarettes is the primary cause of 80% to 90% of lung cancers; thus, it is almost completely preventable if people would stop smoking (see chapter 17). Most cases of lung cancer are detected only after considerable development and only after cancer cells have already spread to other parts of the body. And most lung cancers are resistant to chemotherapy, except for one form called small-cell carcinoma. Overall, the 5-year survival rate for people with a diagnosis of lung cancer is between 10% and 15%—not very good odds.

The rate of lung cancer in other nations is rising rapidly as more and more people take up cigarette smoking. China and other developing nations will have to cope with epidemics of lung cancer soon. The concerted effort in the U.S. to get people to stop smoking and to prevent access of young people to cigarettes is an attempt to reverse the epidemic of lung cancer in this country.

Breast Cancer

Both men and women can develop breast cancer, but it occurs very rarely among men. Although more women die from lung cancer than breast cancer, more than twice as many women had breast cancer as had lung cancer in 1997 in the U.S. Since 1940, the incidence of breast cancer among American women has more than doubled (Hortobagyi, 1998).

Increased weight, less exercise, and increased dietary fat have all been proposed as factors contributing to the increased rate of breast cancer (Figure 13.7). However, other research does not substantiate the view that the amount of fat in the diet increases the

Wellness Guide

How to Examine Your Breasts

1. Lie down and put a pillow under your right shoulder. Place your right arm behind your head.

2. Use the finger pads of your three middle fingers on your left hand to feel for lumps or thickening. Your finger pads are the top third of each finger.

3. Press firmly enough to know how your breast feels. If you're not sure how hard to press, ask your health care provider. Or try to copy the way

your health care provider uses the finger pads during a breast exam. Learn what your breast feels like most of the time. A firm ridge in the lower curve of each breast is normal.

4. Move around the breast in a set way. You can choose either the circle (a), the up and down line (b), or the wedge (c). Do it the same way every time. It will help you to make sure that

you've gone over the entire breast area, and to remember how your breast feels.

5. Now examine your left breast using right hand finger pads.

6. If you find any changes, see your doctor right away.

Source: The American Cancer Society.

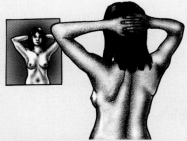

1. Under bright light, examine your breasts for any dimpling, puckering or change from the previous month.

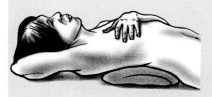

2. Lie down and put a pillow under your right shoulder. Place your right arm behind your head.

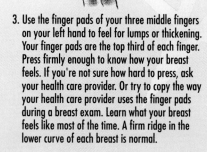

3. Use the finger pads of your three middle fingers on your left hand to feel for lumps or thickening. Your finger pads are the top third of each finger. Press firmly enough to know how your breast feels. If you're not sure how hard to press, ask your health care provider. Or try to copy the way your health care provider uses the finger pads during a breast exam. Learn what your breast feels like most of the time. A firm ridge in the lower curve of each breast is normal.

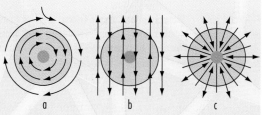

4. Move around the breast in a set way. You can choose either the circle(a), the up and down line (b), or the wedge (c). Do it the same way every time. It will help you to make sure that you've gone over the entire breast area, and to remember how your breast feels.

5. Now examine your left breast using right hand finger pads

6. If you find any changes, see your doctor right away.

risk of breast cancer (Holmes et al., 1999). Other factors that increase the risk of breast cancer among women to varying degrees are:

- Mother who had breast cancer before age 60
- Onset of menarche before age 14
- First child born after age 30
- No biological children
- Menopause after age 55

Terms

xenoestrogens: environmental chemicals that mimic the effects of natural estrogen

- Benign breast disease
- Estrogen replacement therapy after age 55
- Consuming more than 3 ounces of alcohol a day
- Inheritance of BRCA1 or BRCA2 genes

However, all of the risk factors described above still account for only a small fraction of breast cancer cases.

Some recent evidence suggests that the risk of breast cancer may begin in the uterine environment in which the female fetus develops (Fackelmann, 1997). Elevated levels of estrogen in the circulation during pregnancy and heavier birth weights (newborn in excess of eight pounds) are associated with a higher-than-average risk for breast cancer. If uterine estrogen (and possible xenoestrogen) levels during pregnancy do

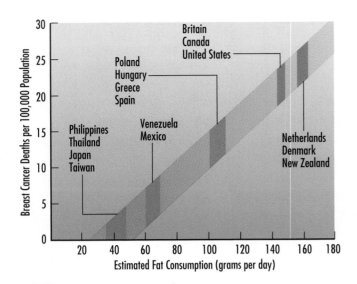

FIGURE 13.7   **Dietary Fat and Breast Cancer**   A strong association is observed between consumption of fat in the diet and the number of breast cancer deaths in various countries. Asian and Central and South American countries have the lowest number of breast cancer deaths. European and North American countries have the highest.

indeed predispose to breast cancer later in life, it may be possible to develop preventive strategies.

In 1997, a blue ribbon panel at the National Institutes of Health (NIH) created a furor when it recommended that routine mammogram screening for breast cancer need not begin until women reached age 50; the panel concluded that women in their 40s would not benefit from **mammograms.** The American Cancer Society still recommends mammograms every 1 to 2 years for women in their 40s and monthly breast self-exams beginning at age 20.

However, even breast self-exams are controversial and may not help in early detection or reduced mortality from breast cancer. Preliminary results from 265,000 women participating in a breast self-exam study showed no benefits; equal numbers of women died of breast cancer irrespective of whether they performed a regular breast self-exam or not (Moon, 1997).

The drug tamoxifen has been used both as a treatment for breast cancer and as a means of protection for women at high risk of developing breast cancer. Tamoxifen (and a related drug, raloxifene) blocks certain estrogen receptors on cells, which appears to reduce the risk of breast cancer. Some trials have shown a benefit; others have not. In any case, women are advised to take tamoxifen for no longer than five years, as further use does not appear to offer any additional protection (Chlebowski, 2000).

Testicular Cancer

The rate of testicular cancer among young men has been increasing but, as with breast cancer, the causes for the increase are unknown. It may be that expo-

Wellness Guide

Inherited Genes for Breast Cancer: What to Do?

The genes BRCA1 and BRCA2 confer an inherited predisposition to development of breast and ovarian cancer. About 5% to 10% of all breast cancer cases is thought to be influenced by inheritance of these cancer susceptibility genes. These genes do not cause breast cancer but they increase a woman's lifetime risk. However, any estimated risks are really only educated guesses from studies of a few families whose female members have an exceptionally high rate of breast or ovarian cancer. Whether the risks calculated for these families can be extrapolated to other families is speculative. The increased risk, however great, is vitally important to each woman who has to make crucial health decisions.

Knowing that one is carrying a BRCA1 or BRCA2 gene (or other cancer susceptibility genes) creates stress and problems for any woman (or couple) who choose to use the available tests for screening for these genes. Insurance coverage may be lost, job security may disappear, personal relations (including decisions on childbearing) are bound to be affected. And for the rest of her life, a woman will worry about the appearance of breast or some other cancer; such ongoing stress is bound to have a negative effect on health and on relationships.

For some women, knowing that they are at very high risk of developing breast cancer is sufficient cause for them to opt for prophylactic mastectomy; that is, they have their breasts removed while young to avoid the chance of breast cancer later in life. Prophylactic oophorectomy is an option for women who are at high risk for ovarian cancer. Whether these procedures prolong life or whether the potential benefits offset the damage to the quality of life are still very controversial (Eisen and Weber, 1999).

Medical technology already can detect cancer susceptibility genes for breast cancer, ovarian cancer, and colon cancer. Tests for many more will become available in the near future. The only measure that people who have cancer susceptibility genes can take is to wait, worry, and watch for signs of a tumor. That is why many counselors and individuals believe that testing for these genes is a poor substitute for healthy living.

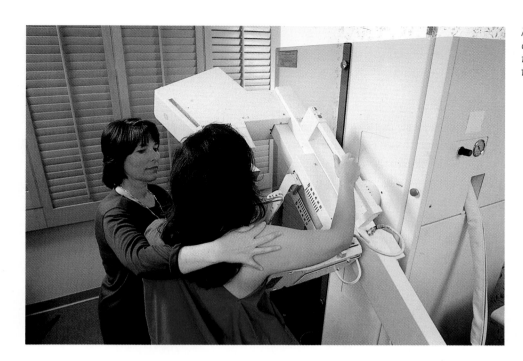

Mammograms can detect breast cancer at an early stage and improve chances for successful treatment.

sure to xenoestrogens plays a role, but that has not been confirmed. Testicular cancer is still quite rare but usually can be cured if detected early. That is why it is recommended that young men perform a testicular self-exam regularly. The most public example of a testicular cancer cure is that of bicyclist Lance Armstrong, who won the grueling Tour de France two years in a row after recovering from testicular cancer.

Prostate Cancer

Prostate cancer occurs primarily in men over age 65, although abnormal prostate cells can be detected at autopsy in young men who die from other causes. Generally, prostate cancers are very slow-growing and may never become life-threatening.

Early diagnosis of prostate cancer is facilitated by two tests. One is the finger rectal exam, in which a trained person can detect if the prostate is enlarged or otherwise feels abnormal. The **prostate-specific antigen (PSA)** test detects a protein in blood that is associated with abnormal growth of the prostate gland. A high PSA level may indicate prostate cancer, but also occurs with many other noncancerous conditions. Only additional tests can confirm the meaning of a high PSA level in blood.

An estimated 25 million men over age 50 have some detectible abnormal prostate cells; however, the majority never develop prostate cancer. And even among those who do, most eventually die from causes other than prostate cancer. Thus, the first question is whether it is worth screening for prostate cancer, and second, whether slow-growing prostate cancers should even be treated (Albertsen, 1997).

In 1996, a U.S. Preventive Services Task Force recommended *against* any routine screening for prostate cancer, including the digital exam, the PSA test, and ultrasound scan (Kuritzky, 1996). These medical experts concluded that screening would not reduce mortality from prostate cancer and would lead to treatments that would adversely affect the health and lives of many men. One form of treatment for prostate cancer, radical prostatectomy, usually causes urinary, sexual, and bowel dysfunction and makes life generally miserable. As one critic observed:

> The rates at which radical prostatectomy was performed increased almost sixfold from 1984 to 1990. . . . The increase in surgical rates has continued despite substantial mortality and morbidity after prostatectomy. . . . Physicians (and not only urologists) appear to find it difficult not to intervene when cancer is present. Yet a careful review of the available literature reveals no studies definitely supporting benefit from aggressive treatment (Eisenberg, 1995).

As with breast cancer and colon cancer, a susceptibility gene for prostate cancer (HPC1) has been identified. When screening tests for this gene become available, men will have to decide whether or not they want to know if they carry a gene that puts them at higher-than-average risk for prostate cancer.

Terms

mammogram: x-ray picture used to detect tumors in the breast

prostate-specific antigen: a blood test that detects a protein associated with abnormal growth of the prostate gland

Wellness Guide

Ways to Prevent Skin Cancer

The number of people in the U.S. with various types of skin cancer, especially melanoma, has been increasing yearly. This need not be so, because skin cancers are among the most preventable of all cancers. The primary cause of most skin cancers is overexposure to sunlight, particularly its ultraviolet (UV) rays, which have enough energy to damage the DNA in skin cells and cause mutations. The best way to prevent skin cancer is to follow the **WAR** rule:

- **W**ear protective clothing.
- **A**void the sun between 10 AM to 3 PM.
- **R**egularly apply sunscreen with an SPF greater than 15 when outdoors, even on cloudy days. Sunscreen should be reapplied every 2 hours, and more often to replace what is washed from the body if swimming or exercising.

Protecting children from sunburn and overexposure is especially important since it is the lifetime exposure to UV that is associated with skin cancers in later life. By age 65, about one American in two has had some form of skin cancer. The ozone layer in earth's upper atmosphere filters out much of the sun's UV light; thinning of the ozone layer in recent years markedly increases the danger of overexposure to sunlight. Unless more people follow the **WAR** rule, the incidence of skin cancers is expected to continue to rise in the years ahead.

Wearing sunglasses that block at least 99% of all UV light is important for protecting eyes. Polarized lenses block glare but do not necessarily block UV unless the label says so. "Photochromic" lenses that darken in bright light also may not block UV light; always read the label. Over time, eye exposure to UV can cause cataracts.

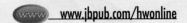 **www.jbpub.com/hwonline**

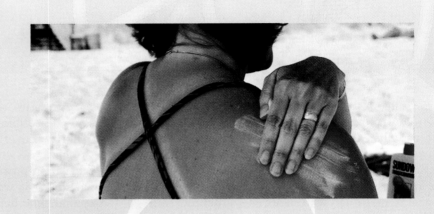

Skin Cancer

Skin cancers are on the rise everywhere, but they are especially prevalent in regions of the world exposed to intense sunlight. **Melanoma,** a malignant form of skin cancer, has increased almost 20-fold since 1930. Melanoma is now the most common cancer in women aged 25 to 29 and the second most common in women aged 30 to 34. Overall, melanoma is the fifth most frequent cancer diagnosed among Americans.

The skin (epidermis) consists of several layers and kinds of cells. The upper layer consists of flat squamous cells and the bottom layer contains basal cells. Interspersed among the squamous and basal cells are melanocytes, cells that give skin its characteristic pigmentation. People with more melanocytes, i.e., dark-skinned people, are less susceptible to skin cancer than light-skinned people.

Exposure to sunlight is the primary cause of all forms of skin cancer. The exposure to sunlight that most of us receive as children largely determines the risk of skin cancer later in life. Two factors contribute to the dramatic rise in the rate of skin cancers. First, in the last generation or two we have become a nation of sun bathers and sun worshipers. Tans are associated with health, vigor, and beauty. Second, the continuing depletion of the ozone layer (see chapter 24) has resulted in more UV radiation reaching the earth's surface; it is the UV radiation in sunlight that causes mutations in skin cells that may lead to cancer. To reduce the risk of skin cancer, you must reduce your exposure to sunlight.

About a million cases of skin cancer are diagnosed every year in the U.S. **Basal cell carcinoma** and **squamous cell carcinoma** are usually not life-threatening, and the abnormal cells can be removed surgically or by scraping, freezing, or burning. Even melanomas, if discovered and removed while the tumor is less than 1 millimeter thick, can be treated successfully. However, melanomas grow rapidly and once the cells have metastasized, malignant melanoma often leads to death.

To protect yourself from melanoma remember these "ABCD" rules when examining moles on your body for any changes. If you suspect anything, consult a physician immediately.

- **A**ssymetry—one half of a mole looks different from the other half.

- **B**order irregular—the edges of a mole are ragged or indistinct.
- **C**olor—the pigmentation in the mole is uneven.
- **D**iameter—any mole that is larger than the diameter of a pencil or that has increased in size.

Colon Cancer

Mortality from colon cancer is exceeded in the U.S. only by that from lung cancer. Colon cancer affects men and women equally and causes about 60,000 deaths annually in the U.S. As with many cancers, if discovered in its earliest stages, many cases of colon cancer can be cured surgically.

Colon cancer is rarely diagnosed in persons under age 40 but begins to appear more frequently in persons over age 50. The primary screening tests for colon cancer are occult blood tests and flexible sigmoidoscopy. In the occult blood test, stool samples are analyzed for the presence of blood, which may be a sign of colon cancer. In sigmoidoscopy, a flexible instrument is inserted via the rectum into the lower part of the colon to allow the physician to visually examine the lining of the colon. If any abnormal tissue is observed, a complete examination of the colon (colonoscopy) is recommended.

No screening test for colon cancer is completely accurate, and risk is often involved because accurate diagnostic procedures are invasive. A positive sign from an occult blood test in a stool is usually cause for invasive tests for colon cancer. In a colonoscopy, for example, death occurs in approximately one out of 10,000 procedures. However, the rate of death from colon cancer in persons age 50 to 54 is only about 1.8 per 10,000, so deciding to have a colonoscopy is not a simple decision. Each person needs to weigh the risks and benefits for his or her particular situation.

Certain inherited genes (Figure 13.5) are known to increase a person's risk for colon cancer. Persons from families known to be at high risk can be genetically tested to see if they have inherited a colon cancer susceptibility gene. They may benefit from the genetic information by more frequent examination of their colon, but they also must be willing to accept the lifelong stress that comes with knowing that they are at high risk for colon cancer.

Diet and Cancer Risk

Many epidemiological studies show that the risk of certain cancers is influenced by diet. For example, stomach cancer is very common in Japan but uncommon among white Americans in Hawaii. Japanese-Americans in Hawaii have stomach cancer rates that are almost as low as the white American population. Excessive consumption of smoked and pickled foods may contribute to the higher rates of stomach cancer in Japan. However, as with the association of dietary fat and breast cancer, it is not known what foods increase the risk of most cancers.

Despite the scientific uncertainty over what specific foods increase the risk of cancer, certain dietary choices may help in preventing cancer (Table 13.5). Most of these dietary recommendations also help boost the immune system, which is the body's main defense against foreign cells (see chapter 12). B vitamins, vitamin C, vitamin E, folic acid, and carotenoids have been shown to boost the immune system and, as a consequence, may also help destroy cancer cells. These substances can be taken as supplements, but also are readily available in fresh fruits and vegetables (Table 13.6).

Over the years, vitamin C has received much attention both as a preventive agent and as a cure for cancer when taken in extremely high doses. Some cancer patients who received megadoses of vitamin C have survived longer than expected, but other studies involving vitamin C and cancer have shown no positive therapeutic effect. However, keep in mind that the effects of any cancer treatment vary from person to person and vitamin C may help some people even if it acts only as a placebo.

Scientists continue to speculate over why certain kinds of cancer are so dependent on diet. One possibility is that we are asking the body to do things chemically for which it is unprepared by the course of human evolution. That is, cancer may be thought of as a disease of maladaptation.

Our ancestors foraged for their food. They collected and ate seeds, roots, fruits, vegetables, and rarely ate meat. Thus, the diet we consume today, filled with excess sugar, salt, fat, and meat, may be incompatible with the body chemistry we have inherited from our ancestors. The modern diet, heavy with processed foods, may result in the accumulation of

> *Life is not a matter of holding good cards but of playing a poor hand well.*
> ROBERT LOUIS STEVENSON

Terms

melanoma: a particularly dangerous form of skin cancer

basal cell carcinoma: a form of skin cancer which usually can be removed surgically

squamous cell carcinoma: cancer of the bottom layer of skin; most are curable if removed early

TABLE 13.5   Dietary Recommendations to Help Prevent Cancer
About 50% of all cancers are thought to derive from nutritional deficiencies.

Substance or food	Effect on cancer risk	Advice
Fiber	Helps decrease colon and rectal cancer	Obtain fiber from vegetables, fruits, whole grains
Cruciferous vegetables (broccoli, cauliflower, brussels sprouts)	Phytochemicals in these vegetables may detoxify cancer-causing chemicals	Eat more; raw or undercooked is best
Allium vegetables (onion, garlic, chives)	Sulfur-containing chemicals in allium vegetables may help prevent cancer	Eat more
Beta-carotene (15 mg), vitamin E (400 IU), and selenium (50 mcg)	A daily supplement reduced cancer (mainly stomach and esophagus) in a large Chinese population	Use supplements in moderation; selenium in high doses is toxic
Folic acid	Deficiency in this vitamin increases genetic damage that may contribute to cancer	Supplement if diet is deficient
Green tea	Reduced esophageal cancer in Chinese population	Most tea drunk in U.S. is black tea; try green tea
Shiitake mushrooms	Extracts of shiitake mushrooms reduced tumors in laboratory animals; also reduces blood cholesterol	Add to diet
Vitamins C and E	Boost immune system and may help prevent cancer	Supplement diet if desired

toxic chemicals or an insufficient amount of some essential nutrients found in fresh fruits and vegetables, nuts, and grains.

 Cancer Treatments

The three medical treatments for cancer are surgery, **radiation therapy,** and **chemotherapy.** Surgical removal of all or as much of a tumor as possible is considered

TABLE 13.6   Foods That Contain Cancer-Preventing Substances
Chemical compounds such as carotenoids, flavonoids, saponins, indoles, and phytochemicals inhibit the growth of cancer cells in laboratory experiments. Eat at least three different colors of fruits and vegetables daily.

Vegetables			
Cruciferous	Pigmented	Green, leafy	Fruits
Broccoli	Acorn squash	Chard	Apricot
Bok choy	Beets	Collard greens	Cantaloupe
Brussels sprouts	Carrot	Green tea	Grapefruit
Cabbage	Pumpkin	Kale	Grapes
Cauliflower	Red pepper	Kohlrabi	Guava
Turnips	Sweet potato	Lettuce	Mango
	Tomato	Okra	Orange
		Spinach	Papaya
			Peach
			Plum
			Watermelon

the best treatment for cancer, particularly if the tumor is small and cells have not spread throughout the body. If even a few cancer cells remain, however, they may grow into new tumors, which is the reason that surgery, such as mastectomy, often removes a great deal of tissue in addition to the tumor.

If there is evidence that tumor cells have spread, or if some of the tumor could not be removed surgically, then radiation or chemotherapy, or both, are used to kill the remaining cancer cells. X-rays or other forms of high-energy radiation can destroy cancer cells as can the powerful drugs used in chemotherapy. Because radiation therapy and chemotherapy destroy normal cells as well as cancer cells, only limited amounts of each treatment can be administered.

Despite improvements in surgical techniques and development of new chemotherapeutic drugs, cancer treatments today are not noticeably more successful than they were in the past, a fact that is reflected in the more or less unchanged death rates for most cancers. Because of the limited success of current cancer therapies, new approaches are being tested.

An analysis of cancer mortality over the past 40 years in the U.S. led to the following conclusion:

The best of modern medicine has much to offer to virtually every patient with cancer, for palliation if

T e r m s

radiation therapy: use of high-energy radiation, such as x-rays, to kill cancer cells and treat some forms of cancer

chemotherapy: use of toxic chemicals to kill cancer cells and treat some forms of cancer

not always for cure, and every patient should have access to the earliest possible diagnosis and the best possible treatment. The problem is the lack of substantial improvement over what treatment could already accomplish some decades ago. A national commitment to the prevention of cancer, largely replacing reliance on hopes for universal cures, is now the way to go (Bailar and Gornik, 1997).

As might be expected from such a radical suggestion, the restructuring of the nation's priorities toward cancer prevention rather than cures of advanced cancers was vigorously opposed by the head of the National Cancer Institute and other medical researchers (Kramer and Klausner, 1997). Scientists seeking cancer cures will continue to do battle with scientists hoping to prevent cancer in the future as they have in the past.

Cancer patients often become desperate and depressed about their condition, the pain of treatments, and the prospect of death. In this state, some patients turn to unconventional therapies and promises of "miracle" cures (Table 13.7). Many cancer patients turn to alternative therapies in hope of a cure when conventional medicine has nothing to offer. Although unconventional therapies may be helpful or at least produce more peace of mind, patients and their families need to be wary of practitioners who make unfounded claims for unlicensed drugs and unproven therapies. Things that are "too good to be true" usually are.

Experimental Cancer Therapies

When abnormal cells arise in the body, in most instances they are recognized and destroyed by the body's immune system. Only when abnormal cells fail to be eliminated and continue to grow and reproduce does a cancer develop. Medical researchers are currently looking for ways to boost the body's immune system so that it is better able to fend off cancer, and they also are working to develop novel immune therapies. For example, it may be possible to develop vaccines that would immunize people against development of specific cancers such as melanoma or prostate cancer. Another approach involves immune therapies that would target proteins that appear only on the surface of cancer cells, and not on normal ones. Once the cancer cells were recognized by the immune system, they would be destroyed.

For a tumor to grow rapidly it must be well supplied with nutrients. To accomplish this, the tumor develops a network of new blood vessels that can supply the necessary nutrients, a process called angiogenesis. More than thirty years ago, physician Judah Folkman proposed that finding ways to destroy the new blood vessels in tumors might be a powerful way to

arrest cancer growth and destroy tumors. Today, drugs that inhibit angiogenesis in tumors are being developed and tested in clinical trials (Eckhardt, 1999). While the results of angiogenesis inhibitors in treating cancers are promising, it will probably be years before truly effective drugs are available. However, if and when such angiogenesis inhibitors are shown to be effective, they will provide powerful new therapies for treating cancer.

> More harm is done by fools through foolishness than is done by evildoers through wickedness.
> SUFI PROVERB

Coping with a Diagnosis of Cancer

A diagnosis of cancer raises serious problems for the patient and for family and friends. Often the patient enters a state of disbelief or shock. The family has to cope with new problems. The patient must face surgery or other treatment. Along with treatment, the patient usually must deal with fear of death, anger at the disease, loss of income, changes in living habits, and, above all, the uncertainty of the outcome, which may last for months or years. These are some of the reasons why coping with cancer can be difficult. Stress and emotional upset can depress the normal functions of the immune system. There also is evidence that hostile feelings, resentment, deeply felt personal loss, and feelings of hopelessness may be important factors in cancer development and lowering of disease resistance.

Pain also contributes to a cancer patient's stress and depression. Some cancers cause intense, unremitting pain that can be relieved only by opioid

TABLE 13.7   Unproven Cancer Therapies
Many cancer patients who are desperate or who have exhausted all medical treatments turn to unconventional therapies for which benefits are scientifically unproven.

Therapy	Rationale
Metabolic therapy	Toxins and wastes in the body cause cancer. Treatments remove cellular poisons and detoxify the body.
Herbal remedies	Herbs have natural, sacred, curative properties not known to science.
Megavitamins	High doses of vitamins kill cancer cells and rejuvenate the body.
Diet therapy	Special diets (grape, macrobiotic, shark cartilage) restore balance to the body and cure the cancer.
Electronic devices	Electrical or magnetic energy harmonizes the life forces and kills the cancer cells.
Immunotherapy	Treatments stimulate or restore immune system functions, which will then be able to destroy cancer cells. (Immunotherapies are being tested by scientists but are a long way from clinical use.)

Managing Stress

The Art of Visualization

The new field of psychoneuroimmunology has provided some amazing insights into the mind-body-spirit connection. For example, several people with terminal cancer so severe that no medical treatment was suggested began to work with alternative methods of healing. To the surprise of many, their tumors went into remission. What was their secret? When these people were studied to find what they did to initiate their own healing process, one common theme emerged: a change in attitude. As director of Biofeedback Research at the Menninger Clinic in Topeka, Kansas, Dr. Patricia Norris has documented several cases where mental imagery and visualization were used successfully to complement traditional medical treatment. Dr. Norris cites eight specific characteristics which help to make mental imagery and visualization effective as a healing tool, specifically with regard to cancer:

1. **Make the visualization personal.** The images must be self-generated. Images that are created by the practitioner and not the patient appear to be ineffective.

2. **Make the imagery "egosyntonic."** Egosyntonic means that the image must fit the values and ideals of that person. If, for example, the individual is pacifistic, then combative or warlike imagery will undermine the effectiveness of this type of treatment.

3. **Make the imagery positive.** Negative imagery reinforces negative thoughts, which are not conductive to healing. As an example, Norris notes that sharks, as a healing image, are not a good idea.

4. **Take an active role in the imagery.** Rather than imagining watching the imagery on a movie screen, you must feel the sensations of your images in the first person. You must have a sense that what you are seeing is happening inside your body, not "out there somewhere."

5. **Make the image anatomically correct and accurate.** Knowing exactly what body region and physiological system is in a disease state will dictate the type of imagery used. Consequently, you need to know whether to access the central nervous system or the immune system. Norris states that more than one image can be used in the healing process.

6. **Be constant, use dialogue.** Constancy means to be regular in generating your imagery. Norris suggests three 15-minute sessions per day, with intermittent shorter sessions throughout the day. When you feel pain, your body is communicating to you. She suggests making pain your friend. In the dialogue style of self-talk, she suggests thanking the pain for making you aware of the problem so that you may be able to fix it. Finally, she suggests "destroying" a tumor with its permission. Respond with love. Make peace with your body.

7. **Create a blueprint.** The concept of the blueprint is a strategy. A blueprint visualization is like time lapse photography where a flower (symbolizing a tumor) is shown to bloom within seconds, and then closes up again and fades away. An example would be to see the construction of a building, starting from the hole in the earth to opening day, where you are cutting the ribbon at the front entrance.

8. **Include the treatment in the imagery.** Norris has found that patients who use mental imagery with chemotherapy treatment and radiation do better than those who "fight" these medical procedures. She notes that it helps to have benevolent feelings versus ambivalent feelings toward the treatment. She suggests one mentally "welcome the treatment into the body." Consider the treatment as a guest in your house. Based on her patient research, she offers these examples:

(a) *Chemotherapy*—a gold-colored fluid that healthy cells, acting as a bucket brigade, pass along to the cancer cells, who in turn drink up the chemotherapy

(b) *Radiation treatment*—a stream of silver energy aimed at the cancerous tumor(s). Ask the white blood cells to move away or to shield themselves and act like mirrors to reflect the radiation toward the cancer cells, then watch the cancer cells die.

therapy. Yet many physicians still are reluctant to prescribe adequate doses of appropriate drugs to alleviate the pain of cancer patients, even among those who clearly are dying (Foley, 2000). Some physicians worry more about creating addiction in their patients than about relieving their pain and suffering. Attitudes are changing slowly, but many—probably a majority—of cancer patients undergoing therapy do not receive adequate relief for their pain. In June 2001, a physician in Berkeley, California was convicted of not providing adequate pain relief to a patient dying from cancer. The family of the deceased sued the physician; a jury agreed and awarded significant monetary damages.

The coping strategies for dealing with the emotional distress resulting from cancer, AIDS, and other serious diseases are similar. They all depend on using the mind in positive ways. The effectiveness of any therapy and the ability to cope with a life-threatening illness depend on focusing the mind on ways to enhance the healing process. Meditation and relaxation techniques are important in reducing stress. Learning how to use visual imagery can help with the effectiveness of treatments. Along with mental relaxation techniques, the mind can focus on images and suggestions that may help the immune system fight and destroy cancer cells.

A dramatic illustration of the power of belief in altering the course of cancer is the case of Mr. Wright, a patient in the 1950s. At that time, a drug called krebiozen was touted by some as a "miracle drug" that could cure cancer. Mr. Wright, who had terminal lymphosarcoma, was given a life expectancy of two weeks by his physician. However, Mr. Wright had enormous faith in the miracle drug and insisted that he be treated with it. After a single injection, his doctor noted that "the tumor masses had melted like snowballs on a hot stove, and in only these few days, they were half their original size" (Klopfer, 1957).

Mr. Wright was symptom-free for 2 months until he read in the newspaper that krebiozen was worthless in treating cancer, whereupon he relapsed and was readmitted to the hospital. With nothing to lose, his doctor assured him that a fresh, double-strength injection of krebiozen would cure him. In actuality, Mr. Wright received an injection of salt water. Once again he was symptom-free for 2 months. Then headlines again proclaimed "nationwide tests show krebiozen to be a worthless drug in treatment of cancer." Mr. Wright relapsed and died in 2 days.

Coping with cancer requires courage and conviction. A cancer patient must not give up hope, despite what the statistics predict or what physicians say about the prognosis. The patient must believe that a cure is possible and work toward that end. For many people, coping with cancer is a transforming experience and gives renewed meaning to life.

The most important thing to remember about cancer is that most cancers *are* preventable. Abstain from smoking or using tobacco and follow a diet rich in fresh fruits and vegetables. Also avoid excess exposure to sunlight and to chemicals that are known to be carcinogenic.

Critical Thinking About Health

1. Consider this hypothetical case of a female college student. Several women in her family, including her grandmother and an aunt, died of breast cancer before they reached 65 years of age. She is only 21 years old but is very concerned about her own risk of developing breast cancer. She decides to be tested for the breast cancer susceptibility genes BRCA1 and BRCA2, even though her physician explains that no medical treatment short of prophylactic mastectomy is available. The genetic test is positive for gene BRCA1, and her risk of breast cancer is significantly higher than for other women who do not have this gene. Discuss, from your own perspective, what this woman should now do to preserve her health. Gather as many facts as you can on breast cancer and the effects of these susceptibility genes.

2. Make a list of all the factors you can think of that increase the risk of developing cancer. Order the items in your list from highest risk to lowest in your judgment. Are any of the risk factors relevant to your life? If so, describe how you could modify your lifestyle or behaviors to reduce the risk of developing cancer.

3. Table 13.6 (on page 292) lists fruits and vegetables that contain compounds that inhibit the growth of cancer cells in the laboratory and, hence, are thought to be cancer-preventing foods. Using this list, indicate how many of the fruits and vegetables are currently in your diet on a daily and weekly basis. Describe what other items in Table 13.6 could be added to your diet and whether you also could increase consumption of ones you already eat. Indicate what efforts you intend to make to add more of these foods to your diet in the future.

4. The "war against cancer" is fought by physicians and scientists in two fundamentally different ways. On the one hand, medical research tries to discover better treatments for all forms of cancer. On the other hand, epidemiologists and other researchers believe that we need to shift the scientific emphasis from seeking cures to prevention, since we understand many of the environmental factors that cause cancer. Reducing exposure to risk factors could prevent as many as half of all human cancers. In your judgment, which of these positions is correct; or do you believe both positions are equally valid? Develop facts and arguments that substantiate your views and write a report of your conclusions.

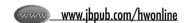 **www.jbpub.com/hwonline**

Health in Review

- Cancer refers to a number of different diseases, all of which share the common property of abnormal, unregulated cell growth in the body.
- Dietary factors and environmental agents, such as smoking and sunlight, act on the genetic material in cells to cause chemical changes that may initiate a tumor, which is a mass of abnormal cells.
- Both breast and testicular self-examinations are positive means of early cancer detection.
- The principal environmental agents that cause cancer are ionizing radiation, tumor viruses, carcinogenic chemicals, and possibly, xenoestrogens.
- If everything known about cancer prevention were practiced, up to two-thirds of cancers would not occur; thus cancer is largely a preventable disease.
- Only 5% to 10% of cancers are caused by genes that have been inherited. The genetic changes in body cells that result in cancer are not passed on to children, as these genetic changes have not occurred in sperm or egg.

- The treatments for cancer include: surgery; radiation; and chemotherapy. The goal of all three cancer treatments is the removal or destruction of as many cancer cells as possible.
- Recovery from cancer depends on good nutrition, positive attitudes, healing mental images, and medical treatment appropriate for the particular cancer. A healthy, active immune system also is an essential component in cancer prevention and recovery.
- Cigarette smoking is responsible for about one-third of all cancers, especially lung cancer.
- Dietary deficiencies or excesses are responsible for about one-half of all cancers.
- Overexposure to sunlight causes skin cancer, which is on the increase.
- Significantly reducing cancer requires major changes in people's lifestyles, including more attention to a healthy diet, elimination of tobacco use, limiting alcohol consumption, and reducing exposure to intense sunlight and chemical carcinogens.

Health and Wellness Online

The World Wide Web contains a wealth of information about health and wellness. By accessing the Internet using Web browser software, such as Netscape Navigator or Microsoft's Internet Explorer, you can gain a new perspective on many topics presented in *Health and Wellness, Seventh Edition*. Access the Jones and Bartlett Publishers Web site at http://www.jbpub.com/hwonline.

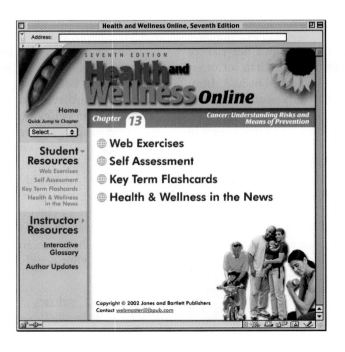

References

Albertsen, P. C. (1997, October 15). Prostate disease in older men:2. cancer. *Hospital Practice*, 159–181.

American Cancer Society (2000). *Cancer Facts and Figures, 2000.*

Bailar, J. C., and Gornik, H. L. (1997). Cancer undefeated. *New England Journal of Medicine, 336*, 1569–1574.

Byers, T. (2000). Diet, colorectal adenomas, and colorectal cancer. *New England Journal of Medicine, 342*, 1206–1207.

Chlebowski, R. T. (2000). Reducing the risk of breast cancer. *New England Journal of Medicine, 343*, 191–198.

Davis, D. L., and Bradlow, H. L. (1995, October). Can environmental estrogens cause breast cancer? *Scientific American*, 166–173.

Eckhardt, G. (1999, January 15). Angiogenesis inhibitors in cancer therapy. *Hospital Practice*, 63–84.

Eisen, A., and Weber, B. L. (1999). Prophylactic mastectomy—The price of fear. *New England Journal of Medicine, 340*, 137–144.

Eisenberg, L. (1995). Medicine—Molecular, monetary, or more than both? *Journal of the American Medical Association, 274*, 331–334.

Fackelmann, K. (1997). The birth of a breast cancer. *Science News, 151*, 108–109.

Fackelmann, K. (1998). Immune attack on cancer. *Science News, 153*, 380–381.

Foley, K. M. (2000, April 15). Controlling cancer pain. *Hospital Practice*, 101–112.

Holmes, M. D. et al. (1999). Association of dietary intake of fat and fatty acids with risk of breast cancer. *Journal of the American Medical Association, 281*, 914–919.

Hortobagyi, G. N. (1998). Treatment of breast cancer. *New England Journal of Medicine, 339*, 974–984.

Klopfer, B. (1957). Psychological variables in human cancer. *Journal of Prospective Techniques, 21*, 331–340.

Kramer, B. S., and Klausner, R. D. (1997). Grappling with cancer—Defeatism versus the reality of progress. *New England Journal of Medicine, 337*, 931–934.

Kuritzky, L. (1996, June 15). PSA: To screen or not to screen. *Hospital Practice*, 145–146.

Lichtenstein, P. et al. (2000). Environmental and heritable factors in the causation of cancer. *New England Journal of Medicine, 343*, 78–86.

Moon, M. A. (1997, May 1). Breast self-exams have yet to show benefit. *Internal Medicine News*, 38.

O'Leary, T. J. (2000). Molecular diagnosis of hereditary nonpolyposis colorectal cancer. *Journal of the American Medical Association, 282*, 281–282.

Safe, S. H. (1997). Xenoestrogens and breast cancer. *New England Journal of Medicine, 337*, 1303–1304.

Woolf, S. H. (2000). The best screening test for colorectal cancer—a personal choice. *New England Journal of Medicine, 343*, 1641–1643.

Suggested Readings

American Cancer Society. *Cancer Facts and Figures.* Published yearly by the American Cancer Society and available at any branch of the society. Contains the latest statistics on all forms of cancer.

Begley, S. (1997, February 24). Mammogram war. *Newsweek*, 55–58. Discusses the controversy over whether women in their 40s should get mammograms or not.

Frontiers in cancer research. (1997, November 7). *Science, 278.* A special issue devoted to the latest cancer research and prospects for prevention and more effective therapies.

Groopman, J. (2000, May 29). The prostate paradox. *The New Yorker*, 52–64. Discusses the new techniques for treating prostate cancer and the problems with choosing the right one for each patient.

Lerner, M. (1994). *Choices in Healing: Integrating the Best of Conventional and Complementary Approaches to Cancer.* Cambridge, Mass.: MIT Press. Discusses both conventional and alternative treatments for cancer.

Lewis, C. (2001, March–April). Online laetrile vendor ordered to shut down. *FDA Consumer*, 37–38, Laetrile was proven to be an ineffective cancer drug more than 20 years ago but is still marketed on the Internet. Buyer beware of unsubstantiated claims of cancer cures.

Specter, M. (2001, February 5). The outlaw doctor. *The New Yorker,* 48–61. Describes how a New York doctor successfully treats otherwise untreatable cancer patients with a severe regime of diet, pills, and enemas.

Weitzel, J. N. (1996, February 15). Genetic counseling for familial cancer risk. *Hospital Practice,* 57–67. Discusses the pros and cons of testing for inherited cancer genes for a number of different familial cancers.

Winawer, S. J., and Shike, M. (1996). *Cancer free: The comprehensive cancer prevention program.* New York: Touchstone. Describes a five-part program for healthy persons that will help them prevent cancer.

Study Guide and Self Assessment

Testing for Risk of Heart Disease

Health and Wellness Online

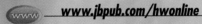 **www.jbpub.com/hwonline**

Chapter 14

Cardiovascular Diseases: Understanding Risks and Measures of Prevention

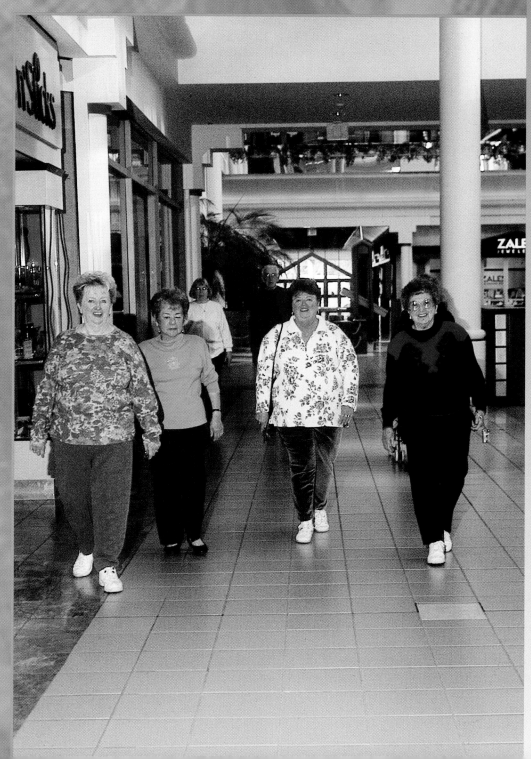

The human heart has long been a symbol of human love as it is expressed in poetry, stories, and everyday customs. Our language still reflects the idea that love and feelings reside in the heart. When love relationships collapse people refer to their "broken hearts" or the "heartlessness" of the former lover. People are described by the nature of their hearts—cruel, kind, warm, or cold; some are even referred to as having a heart of stone. When people refer to distressing experiences in life they talk of "heartache," and when they are happy, their heart may "leap with joy."

Today we know that emotions, thoughts, and feelings of every kind originate in the brain, not the heart. The heart's only function is to pump blood and circulate it throughout the body. The heart is an extraordinarily effective pump; it pumps slightly more than a gallon of blood per minute through approximately 60,000 miles of blood vessels in the body. In this gallon of blood are about 25 trillion red blood cells that carry oxygen from the lungs to all the body's cells and remove the carbon dioxide that is exhaled as waste. Each day about 200 billion new red blood cells are synthesized in bone marrow (the soft material at the center of large bones), and released into the circulation. Each day the heart expands and contracts (beats) 100,000 times and pumps about 2,000 gallons of blood. A healthy heart and blood vessels are essential for survival.

> Have a heart that never hardens
> A temper that never tires
> A touch that never hurts.
> CHARLES DICKENS

Understanding Cardiovascular Diseases

Cardiovascular disease refers to any of a number of conditions that damage the heart or the arteries that carry blood to and from the heart (Table 14.1). If the **coronary arteries** (the large blood vessels that carry blood to and from the heart) become diseased or blocked, a **heart attack** may result. If the cells of the heart do not receive a continual supply of blood and oxygen, the cells die, a condition known as an **infarction.** If the blood supply to the heart is only partially blocked, the process is known as **ischemia.**

According to current estimates, almost 60 million Americans have some form of cardiovascular disease (Heart and Stroke Statistical Update, 2000). More than 40% of all deaths each year in the United States result from cardiovascular diseases that lead to heart attacks and **strokes.** A stroke occurs when an insufficient supply of blood to brain cells causes them to die. While cardiovascular diseases tend to occur in the elderly, heart attacks can occur at any age, often without warning.

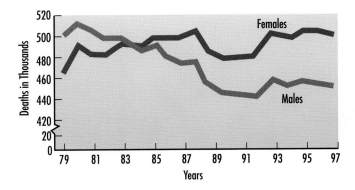

FIGURE 14.1 **Mortality from Cardiovascular Disease in the U.S. (1979–1997)** Death from heart disease has been declining for about 20 years but has increased again, especially among women.

Source: American Heart Association, Dallas, TX. Heart and Stroke Statistical Update, 2000.

The rate of death from cardiovascular diseases among men has been declining steadily in the United States for over 20 years but is increasing once again (Figure 14.1). Certainly public awareness of the risk factors in cardiovascular disease has been a major contributor to the overall decline. Less fat and cholesterol in the diet, less cigarette smoking, and more exercising have all contributed to reducing deaths from cardiovascular disease. Like cancer, most heart disease is preventable and is caused primarily by unhealthy lifestyles, poor diet, high blood pressure, and cigarette smoking.

The Heart and Blood Vessels

The human cardiovascular system consists of the heart (the pump) and the various blood vessels (Figure 14.2).

TABLE 14.1 **Categories of Cardiovascular Disease (CVD)**

Disease	Description
Atherosclerosis	Partial or complete blockage of one or more coronary arteries; the leading cause of heart attack and stroke
Arrhythmia	Heart rhythm disorders; includes atrial fibrillation and flutter
Cardiomyopathy	Inflammation and reduced function of the heart muscle
Endocarditis	Bacterial infection of the heart lining or valves
Congenital Heart Defects	Heart defects present at birth; about 30,000 babies are born each year with any one of three dozen different defects
Congestive Heart Failure	Occurs when the heart is unable to pump all the blood that is returned to it
Rheumatic Heart Disease	Damage to the heart caused by the immune system in response to certain bacterial infections occurring during childhood
Valvular Heart Disease	Results from defective heart valves, usually the aortic or mitral valves

Arteries carry oxygenated blood from the heart to all organs and tissues in the body. **Veins** return blood to the heart after oxygen and nutrients have been exchanged for carbon dioxide and waste products. **Capillaries** are tiny blood vessels that branch out from arteries and veins and circulate blood to all of the cells in the body. Blood vessels can be damaged by injury or by disease; this damage may obstruct the flow of blood carrying oxygen and nutrients.

The organ that keeps the blood circulating throughout the body is the heart, a highly specialized muscle about the size of an adult fist that pumps blood (Figure 14.3). The muscular wall of the heart is called the **myocardium.** If the blood supply to heart cells is blocked, cells begin to die and a heart attack results.

The heart consists of four separate chambers: the upper two chambers are called the left atrium and the right atrium; the lower two chambers are the right ventricle and the left ventricle. Blood that is depleted of oxygen returns to the heart via the right atrium and then flows to the right ventricle. From there blood is pumped to the lungs where it is reoxygenated and returned via the pulmonary veins to the left atrium. Finally, the fresh blood is pumped throughout the body's tissues from the left ventricle through the large artery called the **aorta.**

The heart contracts from 65 to 70 times a minute depending on the body's activity. The entire volume of blood in the body is recirculated almost once every minute. During an average lifetime of 70 years, the heart will pump between 30 to 40 million gallons of blood, and it will beat 2.5 billion times!

A healthy heart beats rhythmically at a pace initiated by the heart itself. In the right atrium a region called the **sinoatrial node** (pacemaker) generates an electric signal that causes the heart to contract and pump blood. The pace of the heartbeat, however, is also influenced by electrical signals from the brain, which explains how emotions, excitement, or stress can suddenly change the rhythm of the heartbeat.

The heartbeat also can be affected by nerve impulses that originate in areas of the heart other than the sinoatrial node. If these signals interfere with the normal heartbeat, causing different areas of the heart to beat independently of one another, the result is **fibrillation** (Figure 14.4). While fibrillation may precede a heart attack, many people have an irregular heartbeat without being at risk for a heart attack. Irregular heartbeat can be controlled by a **pacemaker,** a small electrical device that is implanted in a person's chest and provides a steadying electrical signal to the heart.

Regulating Blood Flow

To maintain uniform blood flow in the correct direction through arteries and veins, the cardiovascular system is equipped with one-way valves both in the chambers of the heart and in blood vessels (Figure 14.5). With every heartbeat, the valves in the heart open and close to allow blood to circulate in one direction. In rare cases, one or more of the heart valves may be defective at birth because of developmental abnormalities. With modern techniques of open-heart surgery, defective heart valves can be repaired or replaced with artificial valves that allow the heart to function normally.

Heart valves can also be damaged by childhood throat infections caused by *Streptococcus* bacteria. Repeated streptococcal infections can cause rheumatic heart disease (formerly called rheumatic fever), a serious inflammatory disease of the heart valves. In susceptible people, the immune system overreacts to the presence of the bacteria. Some proteins on the heart cells are similar in structure to proteins on the bacteria, so the immune system attacks heart valve cells as well as the infectious bacteria.

The mitral and aortic valves are particularly susceptible to damage by infections. Scar tissue forms and prevents the valves from opening and closing correctly. By listening to the heartbeat, a **cardiologist,** a physician who specializes in heart diseases, can detect abnormalities in the heart's valves. Because of potential heart problems, it is important that all "strep

Terms

cardiovascular disease: any disease that causes damage to the heart or to arteries that carry blood to and from the heart

coronary arteries: two arteries arising from the aorta that supply blood to the heart muscle

heart attack: death of, or damage to, part of the heart muscle caused by an insufficient blood supply

infarction: death of heart cells resulting from a blocked blood supply

ischemia: an insufficient supply of blood to the heart

stroke: an insufficient supply of blood to the brain, resulting in loss of muscle function, loss of speech, or other symptoms

arteries: any one of a series of blood vessels that carry blood from the heart to all parts of the body

veins: blood vessels that return blood from tissues to the heart

capillaries: extremely small blood vessels that carry oxygenated blood to tissues

myocardium: muscular wall of the heart that contracts and relaxes

aorta: the large artery that transports blood from the heart to the body

sinoatrial node: the region of the heart that produces an electrical signal that causes the heart to contract

fibrillation: rapid, erratic contraction of the heart

pacemaker: an electrical device implanted in the chest to control the heartbeat

cardiologist: a physician who specializes in diseases of the heart

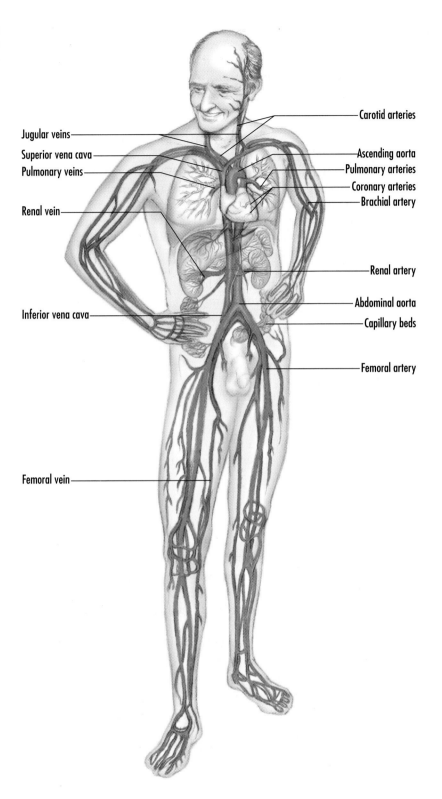

FIGURE 14.2 **Cardiocvascular System**
Includes the heart, arteries, and veins. The heart receives oxygenated blood from the lungs and pumps it to all tissues in the body.

Jugular veins

Superior vena cava

Pulmonary veins

Renal vein

Inferior vena cava

Femoral vein

Carotid arteries

Ascending aorta

Pulmonary arteries

Coronary arteries

Brachial artery

Renal artery

Abdominal aorta

Capillary beds

Femoral artery

throat" in children be treated with antibiotics to reduce the risk of developing rheumatic heart disease.

Another common, but less serious, defect of the circulation is in valves in the veins that cause **varicose veins.** These appear as unsightly, bluish bulges in veins, usually in the legs. Blood returning to the heart from the legs has to flow against the pull of gravity and one-way valves in the veins normally prevent the blood from draining downward. If the valves in the veins of the legs become weakened, blood tends to accumulate, distending the veins and producing visible varicose veins. The valve failures in the veins are not life-threatening and often can be corrected by surgical removal of the damaged areas.

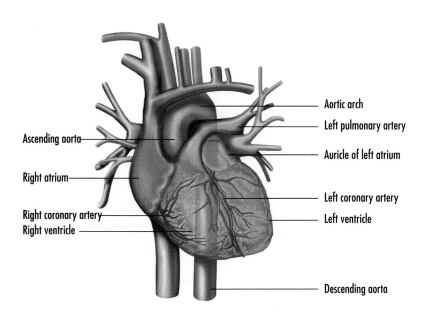

FIGURE 14.3   Heart and Major Arteries   Oxygenated blood is pumped through the arteries (red) and oxygen-depleted blood is returned to the heart via the veins (blue).

Aortic arch

Left pulmonary artery

Ascending aorta

Auricle of left atrium

Right atrium

Left coronary artery

Right coronary artery

Left ventricle

Right ventricle

Descending aorta

Effects of Atherosclerosis

Arteriosclerosis, which literally means hardening of the arteries, includes all kinds of diseases that damage the arteries. However, the one form of arteriosclerosis that is of primary concern is **atherosclerosis.** This arterial disease begins with damage to cells of the heart's arteries and leads to the formation of a fibrous, fatty deposit called **plaque.** The arterial plaque slowly increases in size until eventually the amount of blood flowing through the artery is greatly reduced or completely blocked (Figure 14.6). The current model of how atherosclerosis blocks arteries indicates that the plaque ruptures and flips up like a "trap door" to effectively block the flow of blood through the artery.

Obstruction of blood flow in an artery is very serious because heart cells are deprived of oxygenated blood and die. Oxygen is supplied to the heart by the coronary arteries, which are the first to branch from the aorta. Despite its relatively small size, the heart uses about 20% of the total oxygenated blood circulated through the body.

If the coronary arteries become partially blocked and the heart cells do not get enough oxygen, chest pain called **angina pectoris** results. The drug nitroglycerin dilates blood vessels and is used to relieve the pain

of angina. If a coronary artery becomes completely blocked, the person may have a fatal heart attack.

Diagnosis of a Heart Attack

Each year in the United States more than a million people are admitted to hospitals because of possible heart attacks. Tests eventually rule out a heart attack in about 50% of those admitted. Chest pains that mimic those of a heart attack can be brought on by severe indigestion (heartburn), panic, and stress.

Distinguishing between a heart attack and less serious causes of chest pain is crucial if appropriate treatment is to be started. At present, diagnosing a

Terms

varicose veins: swelling of veins (usually in the legs) resulting from defective valves

arteriosclerosis: hardening of the arteries

atherosclerosis: a disease process in which fatty deposits (plaques) build up in the arteries and block the flow of blood

plaque: deposit of fatty substances in the inner lining of arteries

angina pectoris: medical term for chest pain caused by coronary heart disease; a condition in which the heart muscle doesn't receive enough blood, resulting in chest pain

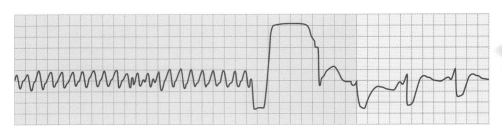

FIGURE 14.4   Recording of a Heart Beating   The first part shows the heart in fibrillation, with weak, irregular beats. The second part shows the heart returned to a normal heartbeat.

Source: Heart and Stroke Update, 2000. (Dallas, TX.: American Heart Association).

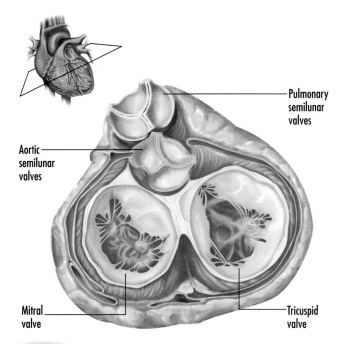

FIGURE 14.5 **Heart Valves** The heart's valves keep the blood flowing in one direction into and out of the chambers of the heart.

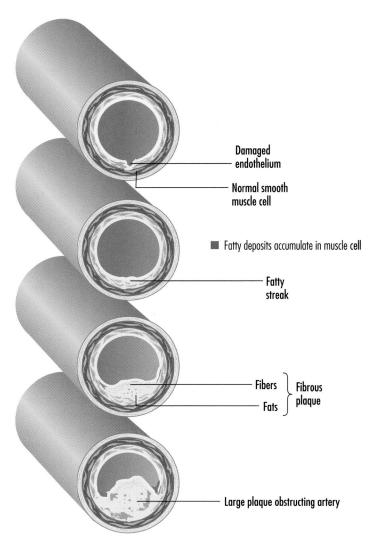

FIGURE 14.6 **Development of an Atherosclerotic Lesion (Plaque) inside an Artery** Plaque can eventually block blood flow, causing a heart attack or stroke. Many factors are suspected in the formation of a plaque, but none has been proven.

heart attack involves time-consuming and costly procedures. By the time a heart attack has been confirmed, it may be too late to save the patient. Tests that could quickly distinguish heart attack from other causes of chest pain would save many lives.

If a heart attack has occurred, the levels of certain proteins in the blood, such as creatine kinase, troponin, myoglobin, and myosin, begin to change. Tests are being developed that measure the levels of these proteins rapidly. This would allow physicians in emergency

Dollars and Health Sense

Defibrillators: Would Public Access Save Lives?

Each year about 250,000 Americans die from a sudden heart attack (cardiac arrest), usually within an hour of the onset of symptoms. Most cases of cardiac arrest are associated with ventricular fibrillation in which the heart suddenly begins to beat erratically. A defibrillator is an electrical device that can restore normal heart rhythm by delivering a series of electrical shocks to the heart; however, to improve chances of survival, defibrillation must be initiated within a few minutes of the heart attack. By the time a patient with fibrillation reaches the

emergency room, it is often too late for defibrillation. Thus, there is intense discussion among health policy organizations whether or not defibrillators should be made available to the general public and their use taught as part of a course in cardio-pulmonary resuscitation (CPR).

Strong arguments can be made on both sides. Arguments opposing deregulation of the sale and use of defibrillators include issues of safety, cost, and improper use, especially by untrained persons. On the other side of the argument is the fact that thousands

of lives could be saved by rapid implementation of defibrillation following cardiac arrest. However, this would only be effective if individuals were allowed to purchase defibrillators and to become proficient in their use. Still, experts wonder how the average person would know when someone truly was having a heart attack and when the use of defibrillation might save a life. Deregulation of defibrillators is a costly and controversial public health issue that is not easily resolved.

Managing Stress

Open Heart Meditation

Dr. Dean Ornish was able to show that the build-up of plaque along the inner linings of the coronary arteries can be reversed. Unlike others who created rehabilitation programs combining exercise and nutrition, Ornish added support group interaction and meditation to the exercise and nutrition formula with great success. Ornish believed that meditation was a crucial factor in reversing heart disease and was convinced there was a connection between the hardened arteries and one's level of anger or what he called a "hardened heart."

The following is a meditation exercise similar to that developed by Ornish. Its aim is to increase one's capacity for compassion and understanding and to forgive and let go of issues and feelings which contribute to anger and upset.

- Sit in a comfortable position, keeping your back straight.
- Begin to concentrate on your breathing by sensing the flow of air into your mouth or nose, down into your lungs, and begin to feel your stomach extend as you inhale and return as you exhale. Repeat this five times.
- Focus on your upper chest, specifically the middle of your upper chest.
- Now for each breath, feel as though you are taking air in through this area of your chest, breathing slowly and easily, comfortably slow and deep. Follow this with five more breaths and feel a sense of relaxation each time you exhale.
- Now imagine that just outside your chest bone (sternum) there is a bud of flower (you can use any image you wish, such as an elevator door, a book, a window, etc.). Visualize this flower bud and allow yourself to see the bud begin to open into a wonderfully beautiful flower. What color petals do you see? Imagine the petals grow and expand.
- Think of this flower (or your chosen symbol) as a symbol of compassion. Imagine what compassion feels like. If this feeling does not come easily, imagine holding a newborn puppy, or recreate the feeling of the happiest moment of your life. Think of the feeling in your mind, but feel it in your heart.
- As you breathe, continue to breathe through your chest and with each exhalation, feel the sensation of compassion.
- Once you have this feeling, think of someone you would like to share this feeling with (e.g., a friend, a parent, a child, a pet) and imagine a rainbow from your heart to theirs. Take five slow breaths, and with each breath think and feel this expression of compassion to that person as you exhale.
- Sharing love with someone you care for is wonderful, but it's also easy compared to sending compassion to someone whom you feel anger toward. Comb your mind for a moment and find someone with whom you are not at peace. Picture this person in front of you now. Realize that feelings of anger are toxic when left unresolved. Slowly take another deep breath through the heart area and as you exhale send a message of compassion to this person visualized in front of you. If it seems that a message of love is too difficult, you can begin with a message acknowledging his or her humanness.
- Remember to keep your symbolic image open as you send this thought and feeling to this person. And know that by opening up your heart you begin to release feelings associated with a hardened heart.

Try this meditation technique a couple of times per week. At first it may seem hard not to feel vulnerable, but with time you will find this exercise not only improves your emotional health, but your physical and spiritual health as well.

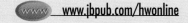 **www.jbpub.com/hwonline**

---

departments to quickly determine if a heart attack has occurred and to initiate appropriate treatment.

Even after extensive tests show that the heart and arteries are functioning normally, 15% to 30% of patients with severe chest pains continue to experience pain and symptoms of cardiovascular disease; these patients are defined as having Syndrome X (Kaski and Russo, 2000). In most of these patients, the angina pain can be controlled with medications, and they are not at any greater risk of a heart attack than persons without angina.

Repairing Blocked Arteries

When medical tests, such as an **angiocardiography,** a procedure for visualizing the flow of blood through the coronary arteries and chambers of the heart, confirm that one or several coronary arteries are blocked and that blood flow to the heart is restricted, additional tests or surgery are usually recommended.

A precise image of the flow of blood through the coronary arteries that supply blood to the heart is obtained by an invasive procedure called **arteriography** (also called cardiac catheterization). To visualize the blood flow, a thin tube is threaded from an artery in a leg or arm up into the coronary arteries. A dye is

Terms

angiocardiography: an x-ray examination of the coronary arteries and heart; produces a picture called an angiogram

arteriography (cardiac catheterization): visualization of blocked coronary arteries by injecting a dye and monitoring blood flow

Dollars and Health Sense

Think Twice before Undergoing Heart Surgery

High-tech surgical procedures, such as coronary bypass, angioplasty, and pacemaker implantation, have revolutionized the treatment of coronary heart disease (CHD). While these surgeries prevent some heart attacks and save lives, in many instances they are performed for heart conditions that do not warrant surgery. Many CHD problems such as angina (chest pain) can be controlled with medications.

In the 1950s, angina pain from partially blocked coronary arteries was relieved by an operation in which a chest artery was tied off in the hope that more blood would be supplied to the patient's heart. About 40% of the patients felt better following this operation. To determine whether the relief of angina pain was a placebo effect or actually resulted from the surgery, a number of mock operations were performed. (In the 1950s, informed consent was not mandatory in most hospitals.) Patients were given anesthesia, the chest was cut open, but nothing else was done to correct blood flow to the heart. Patients who underwent mock surgeries had just as much relief from angina as patients who had the chest artery tied off (Frank, 1975). As a result, this operation was abandoned.

In a similar fashion, coronary bypass operations may relieve angina as a result of the long period of rest and recuperation that patients undergo; lifestyle changes that people make also may contribute to their relief. A large part of the success of bypass surgery may be due to a placebo effect (see chapter 2).

The overuse of high-tech medical diagnostic and surgical procedures has greatly inflated the costs of American health care. Unnecessary medical procedures also cause risk to patients.

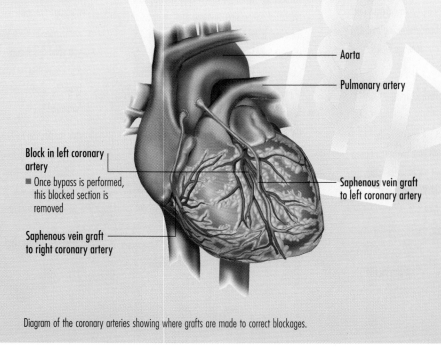

Block in left coronary artery
■ Once bypass is performed, this blocked section is removed

Saphenous vein graft to right coronary artery

Aorta

Pulmonary artery

Saphenous vein graft to left coronary artery

Diagram of the coronary arteries showing where grafts are made to correct blockages.

injected and high speed x-ray film records the flow of the dye in the arteries. Over a million cardiac catheterizations are performed each year in the U.S. on patients with suspected partial blockage of their coronary arteries.

In **coronary bypass surgery,** the diseased segment of an artery is cut out and a segment of a healthy vein or artery is grafted onto the damaged artery to restore normal flow of blood to the heart. If one graft is made into a blocked artery, the surgery is called a single coronary bypass; if four grafts are made it is called a quadruple bypass.

Coronary bypass surgery is a form of **open-heart surgery** and usually requires several months of recuperation. In open-heart surgery, while the heart is exposed and being repaired, the bloodstream is diverted through a heart-lung machine. More than half a million bypass surgeries are performed every year in the United States at an average cost of approximately $50,000. Although bypass surgeries are successful and save many lives, as many as half of bypass patients experience another arterial blockage within 5 years, especially if they do not modify their lifestyle to reduce the risk factors contributing to heart disease.

An alternative surgical approach to opening a blocked artery is **percutaneous transluminal coronary angioplasty** (PTCA), or simply, angioplasty. In this procedure, a thin wire is threaded from the femoral artery in the thigh up to the point of blockage in a coronary artery. Another thin tube containing a deflated balloon is then slipped over the wire and threaded up to the area of the arterial plaque. The balloon is inflated and pushes the plaque back into the wall of the artery, thereby opening it up. Angioplasty costs about half as much as a bypass operation, but the frequency with which the blockage recurs is quite high, making a repeat procedure necessary.

Overall, the number of cardiovascular operations and procedures has increased dramatically in recent years (see Figure 14.7). However, many physicians now question whether all the coronary bypass and PTCA surgeries really are necessary (Verghese, 2000). In Canada and Great Britain, where far fewer of these surgeries are performed, patients with cardiovascular disease live just as long. Like other aspects of American culture, coronary bypass surgery has become a "celebrity procedure." (David Letterman displayed his quadruple bypass on his TV show, direct from the hospital the day after surgery.) It also is a lucrative ($27 billion a year) industry that is extremely profitable for hospitals and surgeons. However, despite the glamour and profit, there is growing evidence that lifestyle changes and appropriate

medicines are more effective, safer, and less costly than surgery in treating cardiovascular disease.

Until recently, it was medical dogma that atherosclerosis was a progressive and irreversible disease. However, many clinical studies involving patients with partially blocked arteries have consistently shown that the blockages can be improved through lifestyle changes and that this entrenched medical view is incorrect (Ornish et al., 1998). Patients who are motivated and who change their lifestyle dramatically can improve the health of their arteries and avoid surgery. However, most patients with blocked arteries still opt for the quick fix of surgery, even though, for many, it is only a temporary solution to their cardiovascular problems. (Arteries often become blocked again within a few years after surgery.) Many physicians still feel obligated to recommend bypass surgery for fear of being sued for not recommending the standard and accepted medical treatment. Thus, heart and artery surgeries probably will continue to be performed excessively in our society until views change.

Stroke

Stroke is the third leading cause of death in the U.S., after coronary heart disease and cancer. As with the latter two diseases, stroke is, in most cases, a preventable disease. High blood pressure is the most important risk factor and plays a role in at least 70% of all strokes.

Stroke is a form of cardiovascular disease that affects arteries supplying blood to the brain. If a brain artery becomes blocked or ruptures, brain cells die within minutes from lack of oxygen. Parts of the body that depend on these damaged or dead cells in the brain for functioning also are affected. Thus, a person who has a stroke can lose the ability to speak, become

Terms

coronary bypass surgery: surgery to improve blood supply to the heart muscle; most often performed when narrowed coronary arteries reduce the flow of oxygenated blood to the heart

open-heart surgery: surgery performed on the opened heart while the blood supply is diverted through a heart-lung machine

percutaneous transluminal coronary angioplasty (PTCA): a procedure to open blocked arteries

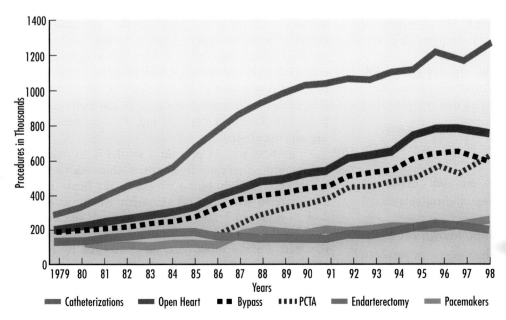

FIGURE 14.7   Increase in the Number of Cardiovascular Operations and Procedures in the United States in Recent Years

Source: American Heart Association, Dallas, TX. Heart and Stroke Statistical Update, 2000.

Catheterizations   Open Heart   Bypass   PCTA   Endarterectomy   Pacemakers

Risk factors for cardiovascular disease include being overweight, a sedentary lifestyle, smoking, and excessive alcohol consumption.

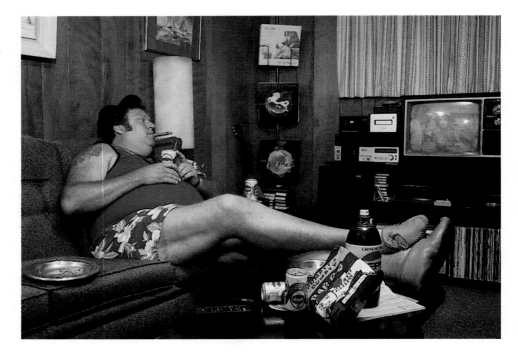

paralyzed in an arm or leg, or lose the use of one whole side of the body. Strokes can result from injuries to the head or from weak spots in the arteries called **aneurysms** that balloon out and rupture. Strokes also can result when the heart beat is weak and the heart does not pump enough blood through the arteries to the brain. The effects of strokes vary greatly, ranging from mild or unnoticed symptoms to sudden death.

Four kinds of strokes are defined medically; two are caused by the rupture and hemorrhage of an artery supplying blood to the brain, and two are caused by clots that block the flow of blood. Cerebral thrombosis and cerebral embolism are the most common types, accounting for about 70% to 80% of all strokes. These strokes are caused by clots that plug an artery. Cerebral and subarachnoid hemorrhages are caused by ruptured blood vessels. Although these types of strokes occur less frequently, they have a much higher fatality rate than strokes caused by clots.

The warning signs of a stroke are any of the following conditions that occur suddenly. Immediate medical attention is needed if any of the symptoms of stroke occur:

- Sudden weakness or numbness of the face, arm, or leg on one side of the body
- Sudden dimness or loss of vision, especially in one eye
- Loss of speech, difficulty understanding speech, or trouble talking
- Sudden, severe headaches with no known cause
- Unexplained unsteadiness, dizziness, or sudden falls, especially with one of the other symptoms

A small fraction of patients at risk for strokes may benefit from a surgical procedure called **carotid endarterectomy** that removes fatty deposits from the carotid arteries in the neck (see Figure 14.2). These arteries supply blood to the brain and, if they become blocked, may cause a stroke. Blocked neck arteries can be detected by listening to the blood flow with a stethoscope and confirmed by an ultrasound scan.

However, endarterectomies are still controversial and, although they have been increasing along with other cardiovascular surgeries in recent years, are not generally recommended except in special situations (Barnett and Meldrum, 2000). The principal danger of the surgery is that it will precipitate a stroke—the very thing that it is designed to prevent. Four large trials have been conducted to test the effectiveness of carotid endarterectomy in preventing strokes in both asymptomatic patients and in patients who have experienced a stroke. Only one of the four trials reported a statistically significant benefit. Unless other trials now in progress show a more positive result, use of this surgery to prevent strokes should be recommended only in carefully selected patients who meet certain high risk criteria following an initial stroke.

The best way to prevent a stroke is to reduce the risk factors. There are five controllable risk factors for a stroke: (1) high blood pressure; (2) heart disease; (3) cigarette smoking; (4) transient ischemic attacks; and (5) high red blood cell count, which thickens the blood and facilitates formation of a clot. These risk factors can, for the most part, be controlled by lifestyle changes and/or medications. Risk factors for a stroke that cannot be changed include: (1) increasing age; (2) being male; (3) race; (4) diabetes mellitus; (5) prior stroke; and (6) heredity.

Risk Factors for Cardiovascular Disease

What starts the development of plaque in arteries and leads to cardiovascular disease, heart attacks, and strokes? No one knows for certain. Arterial plaques are found in the hearts of healthy young people who die accidentally, suggesting that the disease process begins early in life in some individuals. Atherosclerosis is primarily a disease of modern, industrialized societies. Tribal people in New Guinea, Kung tribes in Africa, and Eskimos in Greenland have a low incidence of cardiovascular disease. Tarahumara Indians in Mexico have virtually no heart disease or high blood pressure as long as they consume their native diet. However, when researchers switched a group of Tarahumara Indian volunteers to a typical American diet, they gained weight and had dramatic increases in lipid and cholesterol levels in their blood (McMurry et al., 1991).

Although research has yet to uncover the specific factors that initiate formation of plaque in an artery, there is no shortage of candidates—environmental toxins, high blood pressure, dietary deficiencies and/or excesses, blood lipid levels, and infections by viruses and bacteria. Whether some or all of these factors are involved in plaque formation, there is general agreement that atherosclerosis is an inflammatory disease (Ross, 1999). And there is growing evidence that a particular bacterium, *Chlamydia pneumoniae*, may be responsible for the development of atherosclerosis in many patients (Benitez, 1999). These bacteria frequently infect the lungs and are a common cause of pneumonia, although in many people the symptoms may be too mild to be noticed. By age 30 about half of the population has been infected, and by age 70 more than 80% of people test positive for infection by *Chlamydia*. Clinical trials are in progress to determine if antibiotic treatment can reduce or eliminate *Chlamydia* infections and also reduce atherosclerosis and the risk of a heart attack.

The same factors that trigger changes in cells that lead to cancer may also be risk factors in cardiovascular disease. In particular, cigarette smoking, high

Terms

aneurysm: a ballooning out of a vein or artery

carotid endarterectomy: removal of fatty deposits in arteries in the neck to prevent a stroke

---

Wellness Guide

Risk Factors for Heart Disease

Major Risk Factors That Cannot Be Changed

- **Heredity:** Both heart disease and atherosclerosis appear to be linked to heredity. If your parents have had heart disease, or if you are an African-American, your risk of heart disease is greater than that of the population at large.

- **Sex:** Men have a greater risk of heart disease than women early in life. However, after women reach menopause, their death rate from heart disease increases. Research indicates the potential reason for this is the decrease in estrogen after menopause.

- **Age:** The majority of people who die from heart attacks are age 65 or older.

Major Risk Factors That Can Be Changed

- **Smoking:** People who smoke are twice as likely to have a heart attack as those who do not smoke. Cigarette smoking is the greatest risk factor for sudden cardiac death. Studies also indicate that chronic exposure to environmental tobacco smoke increases the risk of heart disease.

- **High blood cholesterol:** As your blood cholesterol level increases, so does your risk of coronary heart disease. A person's cholesterol level is affected by age, gender, heredity, and diet. With other risk factors such as high blood pressure and smoking, your risk of coronary heart disease increases even more.

- **High blood pressure (HBP):** High blood pressure is sometimes referred to as the "silent killer," because there are no specific symptoms or early warning signs. Eating properly, losing weight, exercising, and restricting sodium all will help reduce HBP. People with this factor should work with their doctor to control it.

- **Physical inactivity:** Physical inactivity is a risk factor for heart disease. Regular aerobic exercise plays a significant role in preventing heart disease; even modest levels of low intensity physical activity are beneficial if done regularly over the long term.

Other Contributing Factors

- **Diabetes:** More than 80% of people with diabetes die of some form of heart disease or blood vessel disease.

- **Obesity:** If you are overweight, overfat, or obese, you are more likely than a person of normal weight to have heart disease, despite the fact you may not have any other risk factors.

- **Individual response to stress:** There is some evidence of a relationship between coronary heart disease and stress, behavior, habits, and socioeconomic status.

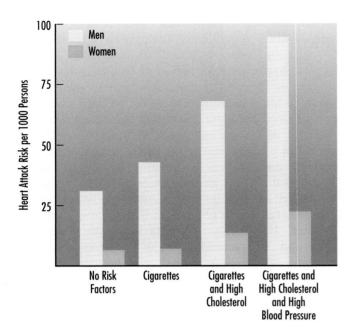

TABLE 14.2	Amount of Cholesterol in Various Foods
Food	*Cholesterol*
Lard, 1 tablespoon	12 mg
Cream, 1 oz.	20 mg
Cottage cheese, 1/2 cup	24 mg
Ice cream, 1/2 cup	27 mg
Cheddar cheese, 1 oz.	28 mg
Whole milk, 1 cup	34 mg
Butter, 1 tablespoon	35 mg
Oysters, salmon, 3 oz.	40 mg
Clams, tuna, 3 oz.	55 mg
Beef, pork, lobster, chicken, turkey, 3 oz.	75 mg
Lamb, veal, crab, 3 oz.	85 mg
Shrimp, 3 oz.	130 mg
Beef heart, 3 oz.	230 mg
Egg, one yolk	250 mg
Liver, 3 oz.	370 mg
Kidney, 3 oz.	680 mg
Brains, 3 oz.	1,700 mg

The most common source of cholesterol in the diet is egg yolk. Only about half of the consumed cholesterol is absorbed. Additionally, the human liver itself synthesizes 1,000 to 1,500 mg of cholesterol a day.

blood cholesterol levels, and high blood pressure are well documented risk factors that contribute to the development of both atherosclerosis and heart disease (Figure 14.8). Physical inactivity, stress, and high levels of glucose in the blood are additional factors that contribute to the risk of a heart attack once the blood supply to the heart has been restricted.

Cholesterol

Cholesterol is an essential component of body cells and is synthesized in the body as well as being obtained from food (Table 14.2). Cholesterol circulates in the blood mostly in the form of particles consisting of proteins, triglycerides (fats), and cholesterol. These particles are divided into two kinds. Called **high-density lipoproteins (HDL)** and **low-density lipoproteins (LDL)**, their functions are different and, in some sense, are opposite to one another. Other kinds of cholesterol-carrying particles also are found in the blood, but these are ultimately converted into LDL particles.

The cholesterol that gets deposited in plaques and blocks the arteries comes mainly from LDL particles. As LDL particles circulate in the blood, cholesterol is used by tissues to build new cells. Any excess cholesterol is processed in the liver and the cholesterol level in the blood is maintained by regulatory mechanisms in the liver. Receptor proteins on the surface of liver cells bind LDL particles and remove excess cholesterol. If the liver is overwhelmed with LDL particles, it may not be able to process all of them. When that occurs, too much cholesterol circulates in the blood

and may be deposited in the walls of the arteries. Because LDL particles carry the cholesterol that is deposited in plaques, they are often referred to as carrying "bad" cholesterol.

HDL particles are produced in the liver and intestines and are released into the bloodstream. As HDL particles circulate through the body, they pick up cholesterol and return it to the liver for removal. Thus, HDL particles scavenge excess cholesterol from the blood and arteries, thereby reducing the buildup of plaques. For these reasons, HDL particles are often referred to as carriers of "good" cholesterol.

People differ markedly in their ability to process excess cholesterol, just as they differ in other traits. The most dramatic example of cholesterol metabolism is that of an 88-year-old man who had eaten twenty-five eggs a day for over fifteen years and yet had completely normal blood cholesterol levels (Kern, 1991).

At the other extreme of the body's ability to process cholesterol are persons with a rare inherited disease called **familial hyperlipidemia (FH)**, which results in markedly elevated levels of cholesterol in the blood. People with this disease have two defective genes, one inherited from each unaffected parent. The normal forms of these genes are responsible for synthesizing LDL receptor proteins on liver cells that bind LDL particles and remove cholesterol from the blood. As a result of their defective genes, people with FH cannot synthesize these essential LDL receptor proteins. Cholesterol cannot be removed and processed in the liver, and it accumulates to exceptionally high levels in the blood. People with this disease usually have heart attacks at an early age. In a few cases, transplant of a normal liver has successfully reversed the effects of FH to a significant degree.

Measuring Cholesterol Levels Cholesterol and lipid levels in the blood are measured in various ways. Total cholesterol levels are measured in milligrams per deciliter (mg/dl) of blood. Generally, a cholesterol level below 200 mg/dl indicates relatively low risk of coronary heart disease (CHD); 240 mg/dl or higher doubles the risk of CHD. Blood cholesterol values between 200–239 mg/dl indicate moderate and increasing risk of CHD. However, the total cholesterol level may not be a reliable indicator of cardiovascular disease risk because the level of HDL in the blood is also important and can modify the risk inherent in high cholesterol levels.

For example, a cholesterol level of 240 might not be considered dangerous if your HDL level also was high. Generally, if the ratio of the total cholesterol divided by the HDL level is about 4.5, the risk is said to be average. A ratio above 4.5 increases the risk of heart disease; a ratio below 4.5 reduces it. The various numbers used to establish the risk of heart disease are quite confusing, but the general rules are explained in the wellness guide on interpreting blood cholesterol and lipid measurements.

Extensive research has shown a strong association between blood cholesterol levels and coronary heart disease; the higher the blood cholesterol level, the greater the risk of all forms of cardiovascular disease. However, many epidemiological studies show that diet is not always a good predictor of cholesterol levels.

For example, the French enjoy a diet laden with eggs, meats, and fats. They have cholesterol levels that, on average, are much higher than those of Americans. Yet the French die of heart disease at less than half the rate observed in the United States (sometimes called the "French paradox"). Nobody can give a satisfactory explanation for the discrepancy; some heart experts attribute it to drinking wine with meals (which may reduce stress) and eating more vegetables (which may be protective in some way).

Other epidemiological studies show that populations vary greatly in the level of cholesterol that constitutes a risk for CHD. People with a blood cholesterol level of 200 in the U.S. are five times as likely to die of CHD as people in Japan with the same cholesterol levels. People in southern Europe are also at a relatively low risk for a heart attack, even when their cholesterol level is above 250 mg/dl.

While there is no disagreement that high cholesterol levels are a major risk factor for cardiovascular disease, the level at which the risk begins to be significant is very controversial. In general, physicians in this country view cholesterol levels above 200 mg/dl as cause for intervention to lower them with dietary measures, drugs, or both. As with many aspects of health, individuals must decide whether their cholesterol levels constitute a risk of sufficient magnitude that taking cholesterol-lowering drugs is appropriate (Consumer Reports, 1998).

High Blood Pressure

Medical surveys indicate that one in every four Americans suffers from **hypertension,** blood pressure that is above the range that is considered normal. About one-third of these individuals is unaware of their hypertension, which contributes to stroke and heart and kidney disease. The cause of high blood pressure in 90% to 95% of cases is unknown; the medical term for this is **essential hypertension.**

The remaining cases of high blood pressure are symptoms of a recognizable problem, such as a kidney abnormality, congenital defect of the aorta, or adrenal gland tumor. This type of high blood pressure is called **secondary hypertension.** Generally, when the cause of secondary hypertension is determined and corrected, blood pressure returns to normal.

High blood pressure may be caused by psychosocial factors, although the mechanisms by which these factors could cause it are not understood. For example, people with low income and poor education are at higher risk for high blood pressure. Being poor or jobless may generate stress and raise blood pressure. Black and Hispanic Americans have a higher rate of high blood pressure than white Americans (Cooper, Rotimi, and Ward, 1999). The stress of being a member of a minority group may also increase the risk of high blood pressure and heart disease, although there is some evidence that being socially or economically disadvantaged contributes to hypertension. Hypertension is a disease of modern societies; even today tribes in New Guinea or the forests of Brazil do not develop hypertension when they grow old.

High blood pressure is a major risk factor for heart attacks and stroke because blood vessels in the heart

Terms

high-density lipoprotein (HDL): the carrier of cholesterol from tissues to the liver for removal from the circulation; carrier of "good" cholesterol

low-density lipoprotein (LDL): the carrier of "bad" cholesterol in blood

familial hyperlipidemia (FH): an inherited disease causing extremely high levels of cholesterol in the blood

hypertension: high blood pressure

essential hypertension: high blood pressure that is not caused by any observable disease

secondary hypertension: high blood pressure caused by a recognizable disease

Wellness Guide

How to Interpret Blood Cholesterol and Lipid Measurements

In evaluating your risk of heart and artery disease, the level of four different "fat" molecules are measured: cholesterol, high-density lipoprotein (HDL), triglycerides, and low-density lipoprotein (LDL). The range of values for each is indicated below.

Cholesterol
- Below 200 mg/dl: safe, unless the HDL level is below 35 mg/dl.
- 200 to 239 mg/dl: borderline high. If you have other risk factors for heart disease such as high blood pressure or an HDL level below 35 mg/dl, then you are at risk and some corrective action is needed.

- Above 240 mg/dl: high. Further tests are needed; dietary changes, as well as drugs to lower the level, may be recommended.

High-Density Lipoprotein
- 35 mg/dl: low. Exercise and other steps may be needed to raise the level. Women generally have higher levels of HDL than men.
- 35 to 60 mg/dl: considered protective, especially if cholesterol levels are below 240.

Triglycerides
- Below 200 mg/dl: considered normal range.
- 200 to 400 mg/dl: borderline high.

- Above 400 mg/dl: high. Dietary changes recommended.

Low-Density Lipoprotein
LDL is not measured directly, but levels are calculated according to the following formula:

$$LDL = Total\ cholesterol - HDL - (Triglycerides/5)$$

Using this formula, a LDL value below 130 is considered safe; a value above 160 is considered high, and lipid-lowering drugs may be prescribed. However, even this formula does not satisfy all the experts, some of whom believe that the ratio of LDL to HDL is the really significant measure of risk for heart disease.

---

or brain are more likely to rupture under increased pressure. Hypertension is often called the "silent killer" because it is a disease without symptoms until something serious occurs. As many as 50 million Americans have high blood pressure, which can occur even in young children.

Each time the heart contracts, blood is pumped through the arteries and exerts pressure on the arterial walls (Figure 14.9). In fact, there are two pressures that are measured. The maximum pressure in the arteries occurs when the heart contracts (**systole**), pumping blood from the heart to the lungs and body. Between contractions, the pressure falls (**diastole**) as blood flows from one chamber of the heart to another. Normal blood pressure is defined as a value less than 140/90 mm Hg (systole/diastole). Generally, the diastolic pressure is considered the more significant of the two with respect to health risk. A person with a diastolic pressure of 120 has double the risk of a heart attack or stroke compared to a person with a diastolic pressure of 90.

High blood pressure can be lowered by making certain changes in lifestyle. Obesity and excessive intake of calories are major risk factors that can be changed; increasing physical exercise also is required to reduce hypertension. Moderating salt and alcohol consumption also is beneficial. And ensuring that you

Prediction is very hard, especially when it's about the future.

YOGI BERRA

are obtaining an adequate amount of potassium (eat more bananas) will also reduce blood pressure.

Blood pressure is the result of two forces. The first is created by the heart as it pumps blood into the arteries, the second created by the arterial blood vessels as they resist blood flow from the heart. Tiny receptors in the walls of the arteries respond to changes in blood pressure. If blood pressure rises, these receptors send signals to the nerves to relax the arteries and to slow down

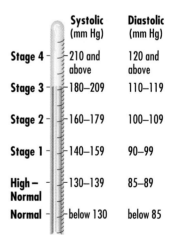

	Systolic (mm Hg)	Diastolic (mm Hg)
Stage 4	210 and above	120 and above
Stage 3	180–209	110–119
Stage 2	160–179	100–109
Stage 1	140–159	90–99
High – Normal	130–139	85–89
Normal	below 130	below 85

FIGURE 14.9   Stages of High Blood Pressure   According to current guidelines, normal blood pressure is 129/84 (systolic/diastolic) and high-normal is 139/89. High blood pressure (hypertension) is defined in four stages, the risk of heart disease being greater the higher the blood pressure. Weight loss, exercise, not smoking, and stress reduction are recommended ways to control hypertension at earlier stages; drugs may also be necessary at later stages.

the heartbeat, thus returning blood pressure to normal levels. However, these regulatory mechanisms can be overcome by signals from the brain. Arteries can be constricted and blood pressure raised by thoughts and emotions. Fear, tension, anger, and anxiety activate the sympathetic nervous system, which sends signals to the arteries causing them to constrict. If one's life is overly stressful or full of anger and frustration, arteries may stay constricted and blood pressure remain elevated.

While drugs are the most expedient (and profitable) means of controlling hypertension, mental relaxation techniques are also effective. By using biofeedback equipment that displayed blood pressure values, some people learned how to develop mental relaxation states that lowered their blood pressure. In fact, many studies demonstrate that a variety of relaxation techniques are effective in lowering blood pressure in hypertensive patients.

However, working with people to lower blood pressure through relaxation techniques is time-consuming and costly in a modern medical setting, so physicians prescribe antihypertensive drugs even though most of them have undesirable side effects (Consumer Reports, 1999). Everyone can start to control hypertension with diet, by exercising regularly, and by finding ways to reduce stress.

Cigarettes and Cardiovascular Disease

Smoking cigarettes is another major risk factor contributing to the development of cardiovascular disease, heart attacks, and strokes (Fichtenberg and Glantz, 2000). Smokers are at two to four times greater risk of dying from a heart attack than nonsmokers. The risk of heart disease from tobacco smoke extends to those who breathe second-hand smoke at work or at home (He et al., 1994). The more tobacco smoke a person is exposed to, the greater the risk of cardiovascular disease and a heart attack (Figure 14.10).

Cigarette smoke also damages the blood vessels that carry blood to the arms and legs, causing them to narrow and to lose elasticity. Heavy cigarette smokers are at risk for **gangrene,** the decay of tissue when the blood supply is obstructed. Gangrene is particularly common in smokers' legs and may lead to amputation. Cigarette smoke also decreases the level of HDL,

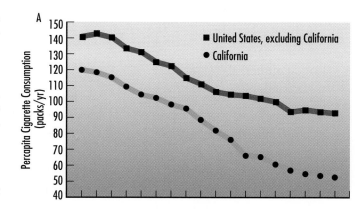

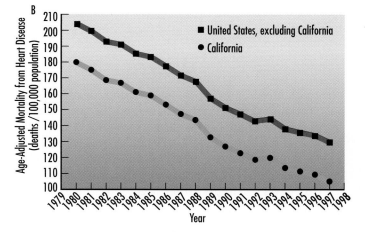

FIGURE 14.10 **Relation Between Cigarette Consumption and Death From Heart Disease** An aggressive anti-smoking campaign in California from 1989 to 1992 resulted in a significant decrease in cigarette consumption in the state as compared to the rest of the United States. Deaths from heart disease also were much lower in California than in the rest of the country in this period. These graphs show that the amount of cigarette smoking is directly related to deaths from heart disease.

which acts to protect blood vessels from damage, and reduces the survival and functioning of **platelets,** blood cells that are essential in the clotting process.

Stopping smoking at any time can reverse many of the harmful physiological effects of tobacco on the cardiovascular system. After several years of not smoking, ex-smokers have about the same risk of cardiovascular disease as nonsmokers. One key to protecting your heart is not smoking and not living or working in a smoke-filled environment.

Homocysteine Level

Just as a high blood cholesterol level serves as a predictor of increased risk of cardiovascular disease (CHD), an elevated level of homocysteine (an amino acid) in the blood also is a strong predictor of CHD risk (Hankey and Eikelboom, 1999). Levels of homocysteine in blood increase with age and are higher among men than in women. Other factors that increase homocysteine levels include: hereditary defects in certain

Terms

systole: the pressure in the arteries when the heart contracts (the higher number)

diastole: the pressure in the arteries when the heart relaxes (the lower number)

gangrene: decay of tissue when the blood supply is restricted

platelets: cells in the blood that are essential for clotting

---

Wellness Guide

Concussion to the Heart

Most everyone knows what a brain concussion is—a blow to the head that may cause unconsciousness, problems in mental functioning, and headaches for weeks or months after the concussion. Concussions are frequent in contact sports such as football, and NFL quarterbacks Troy Aikman and Steve Young were forced to retire after each suffered a series of concussions.

A blow to the left side of the chest caused by a punch, thrown baseball, hockey puck, or other object may cause a concussion to the heart that is medically known as *commotio cortis*. Such a blow, even a light blow, if delivered at a very precise moment during the rhythmic beating of the heart, can induce instant fibrillation (irregular heart beat) and sudden death. Cases of *commotio cortis* are rare, but at least 69 cases of sudden death in healthy young people due to being struck on the left side of the chest have been documented (Curfman,

1998). The sports carrying the highest risk of sudden death from *commotio cortis* are baseball, softball, and hockey.

Use of chest protectors and softer balls can reduce the risk of *commotio cortis* in some sports, especially among children and young athletes. Also, never punch or poke anyone in the chest.

---

enzymes, B vitamin deficiencies, kidney disease, and medications such as methotrexate and theophylline.

Since even high-normal levels of homocysteine are associated with increased CHD risk, it is advisable to reduce your homocysteine level if it is found to be high. Fortunately, most people can reduce their blood homocysteine level by simply taking B-vitamin supplements, especially folic acid. It also may help to supplement your diet with the antioxidant vitamins, vitamin C and vitamin E, especially if you are a fast-food junkie.

Stress

In the 1960s, two physicians, Meyer Friedman and Ray Rosenman, created a furor by suggesting that almost all heart disease is of behavioral origin. They claimed that in the absence of a pattern they called **type A behavior,** all the other risk factors would not cause cardiovascular disease. They argued that these other factors—smoking, lack of exercise, high cholesterol, hypertension—contribute to the development of heart disease, but that the main risk factor was stress caused by how people live and act.

Type A behavior is characterized by the following traits:

- Becoming irritated and impatient while waiting in lines
- Constantly feeling pressed for time
- Insisting that everything always be done on time
- Not letting other people finish what they are saying
- Always trying to show others how to do things correctly
- Playing games to win every time
- Not allowing time for relaxation

The association between type A behavior and heart attacks has been difficult to prove because of the difficulty in measuring the subjective behaviors associated with type A people. At least five large studies failed to find any connection between type A behavior and cardiovascular disease; however, other studies did find an association. Recent studies, using more sophisticated interviewing procedures, indicate that anger and hostility are key psychological factors associated with an increased risk of cardiovascular disease although these findings are still controversial (Iribarren, Sidney, Bild, et al, 2000). Whatever the scientific evidence for a connection between type A behavior and cardiovascular disease, all health research indicates that persistent stress is unhealthy. If the stress is accompanied by anger and hostility, high blood pressure and other unhealthy changes in the cardiovascular system may also occur.

Salt

One of the most controversial risk factors for cardiovascular disease and a stroke is dietary salt. As one reviewer of the salt controversy put it, "Indeed, the controversy over the benefits, if any, of salt reduction now constitutes one of the longest running, most vitriolic, and surreal disputes in all of medicine" (Taubes, 1998). For decades, Americans have been urged to reduce their consumption of salt—from an average of 10 grams per person per day to six grams or less. Many people find it difficult to reduce their salt intake because 80% of the salt consumed comes from processed foods. Because the taste of foods is determined by salt (and fat), food manufacturers are reluctant to reduce the amount of salt in their products.

Some of the problems in resolving the salt controversy include conflicting scientific studies, marginal effects one way or the other, and disagreement over the interpretation of the scientific results between health agencies and their critics. The primary reason

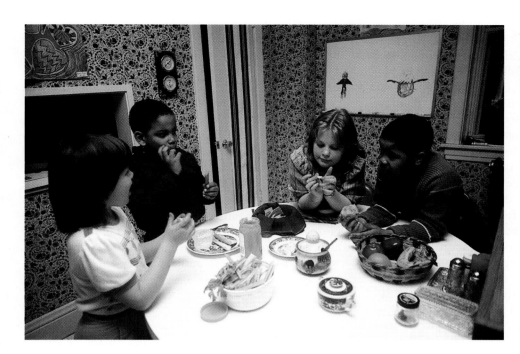

It's important to encourage children to eat heart-healthy snacks, so they won't have to break bad eating habits later in life.

for recommending reduced salt intake is its presumed effect in raising blood pressure. However, there is no compelling scientific evidence that reducing salt intake lowers blood pressure. One result of the salt controversy that everyone does agree with is that it has made the public much more skeptical of many nutritional recommendations. In our view, the best way to understand the salt controversy at present is to "take it with a grain of salt."

Diet and Cardiovascular Disease

As already mentioned, diet plays a major role in heart disease, especially as it contributes to being overweight and overfat and to elevated levels of cholesterol. However, certain foods and vitamins in the diet seem to provide some protection from cardiovascular disease.

Vitamin E

While the oxygen gas that we breathe is essential to life, uncombined oxygen atoms in cells can react with many substances and cause damage. For example, consider what happens to iron that is exposed to the oxygen in air under moist conditions; it quickly rusts and disintegrates. Body tissues also can be destroyed by oxygen atoms. The body has many mechanisms

for protecting cellular constituents from oxidation, among them the antioxidant action of vitamin C and vitamin E.

Vitamin E acts as an antioxidant in blood and reduces the amount of oxidized LDL that is formed. When volunteers took vitamin E supplements (800 IU), their LDL particles were more resistant to oxidation. Also, a study of 2000 patients with CHD found that those who took 400 to 800 IU of vitamin E every day for 2 years had a 37% lower risk of heart disease compared to a group of men who did not take the vitamin supplement (Rimm et al., 1993). A similar benefit from vitamin E was also reported for women.

B Vitamins

Other vitamins that protect against heart disease are three B vitamins, B_6, B_{12}, and folic acid (folate). As described above, high levels of the amino acid homocysteine are associated with atherosclerosis and heart disease. People with high levels of homocysteine in their blood also had low levels of the three B vitamins. On the other hand, people with low homocysteine levels had high levels of the B vitamins and were less likely to develop heart disease.

A man's worst enemies can't wish on him what he can think up himself
YIDDISH PROVERB

The key B vitamins can be obtained from food; however, many people do not obtain enough in their diets. The evidence that B vitamins do, in fact, protect against heart disease is now strong enough that some health authorities recommend taking them in a daily multivitamin supplement.

Terms

type A behavior: behaviors characterized by traits, such as anger or hostility, that contribute to the risk of heart disease

Vitamin C

For years, Nobel laureate Linus Pauling advocated using vitamin C (ascorbic acid) in megadoses to prevent or help minimize the effects of colds and cancer. Although the ability of vitamin C to ward off these illnesses has never been proven, vitamin C's value in protecting against cardiovascular disease is much greater. Like vitamin E, vitamin C is an antioxidant and can neutralize destructive oxygen atoms and other oxidizing substances called **free radicals.**

Free radical compounds in the blood may damage the elastic tissues in arteries that allow blood vessels to expand and contract. If a blood vessel is damaged and cannot relax, blood pressure rises. Vitamin C prevents such damage from occurring by eliminating the free radical compounds in blood. Taking up to a gram of vitamin C supplement a day is safe; any that is not used is excreted in urine. However, taking megadoses of vitamin C (10 grams a day) can cause serious side effects, such as stomach irritation and kidney stones.

Other studies that support the role of vitamin C in preventing heart disease were done with a group of hypertensive patients. These studies showed that people with the highest levels of vitamin C in their blood had the lowest blood pressure.

Calcium

Food profile studies indicate that half or more of all Americans of both sexes consume amounts of calcium that are less than the recommended amounts for bone development and health. Populations that are especially at risk are African Americans, pregnant women, obese persons, and elderly persons. Unless you consume foods that are high in calcium, such as milk and cheese, your daily calcium intake may be low.

Calcium deficiency is not only a risk factor for osteoporosis in women, it is also a significant risk factor for hypertension in persons of all ages. Calcium is readily obtained in the diet but levels can also be increased by taking calcium supplements, which cost much less and are much safer than antihypertensive medications.

Soy Products

Soybeans have been cultivated around the world for thousands of years; the Chinese name for soybean is *ta-tou*, which means "greater bean." Soy seems to boost the activity of LDL receptors in the liver, and thereby helps to remove cholesterol from the blood. Soy also seems to block oxidation of the LDL particles, which prevents them from sticking to the walls of arteries.

Wellness Guide

One Drink of Alcohol a Day Reduces the Risk of Heart Attacks

www.jbpub.com/hwonline

Alcohol is a drug to which more than 18 million Americans are addicted. Many alcoholics suffer from malnutrition, a diseased pancreas or liver, high blood pressure, and other problems (see chapter 18). Although the dangers of alcohol overuse are well documented, there may be benefits in limited amounts. A study of 44,000 male health professionals showed that those who reported having one-half to two drinks a day had a 26% *lower* risk of developing cardiovascular disease compared to people who rarely or never drank.

Moderate alcohol consumption seems to exert its beneficial effects by raising HDL levels in the blood. (High HDL levels counteract the effects of high cholesterol in the blood.) Although moderate drinking has some health benefits, the issue is very controversial, considering the many harmful effects of alcohol use.

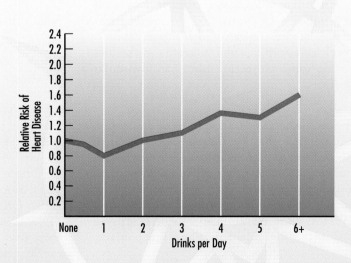

The relative risk of cardiovascular disease in white males aged 40–59 with varying amounts of alcohol consumption. Up to two drinks a day has a protective effect. More than two drinks a day, however, increases the risk, which rises appreciably with each added drink. (A drink is 1¼ oz. of 80 proof alcohol, a 12 oz. beer, or a 5 oz. glass of wine.)

Studies in which people ate 1 to 2 ounces of soy daily showed that both cholesterol and LDL levels dropped about 10%. Other studies indicate that soy is especially effective among people with cholesterol levels above 240 mg/dL. Soy products are available in a multitude of products, such as soy sauce, soy milk, soft and firm tofu, and tofu burgers.

Fish Oils

Populations that consume large amounts of fish in their diets—Greenland Eskimos and Japanese islanders—have lower rates of CHD than others. Americans who consume fish regularly in their diets also have healthier hearts (Daviglus et al., 1997). The protective effects of dietary fish have been ascribed to fish oils, in particular to n-3-polyunsaturated oils. In some studies, supplements of fish oil have reduced levels of cholesterol and blood pressure.

One of the best studies demonstrating the beneficial effect of fish was carried out in Tanzania among Bantu villagers. One group of Bantu lived on the shores of a lake, and people consumed about a pound of fish a day. The other Bantu population lived in nearby hills and had a diet that consisted primarily of vegetables. The Bantu people who ate fish had high levels of n-3-polyunsaturated oils in their blood. They also had lower levels of cholesterol and lipoproteins (Pauletto et al., 1996). Sardines, salmon, and mackerel have high levels of n-3-polyunsaturated oils, but all fish have some.

Tea

Both green and black tea contain antioxidant chemicals that help block oxidation of LDL particles in the blood; herb teas do not contain antioxidants. Consuming green or black tea helps protect the coronary arteries in a manner similar to that of the C and E antioxidant vitamins. Asian people drink green tea daily, which may contribute to their reduced risk of CHD.

Aspirin

A commonly used drug can significantly reduce the risk of CHD and heart attacks. Aspirin helps to "thin"

Terms

free radicals: oxidizing substances in the body that can damage blood vessels and tissues

blood and also acts to combat inflammation, which increases the risk of a heart attack. Hundreds of studies have been carried out in which aspirin was given to both healthy people and to people who had had a heart attack or stroke. In all studies, small amounts of aspirin (either a half tablet daily or a whole tablet taken every other day) reduced the risk of a heart attack.

It is now recommended that if you think you might be having a heart attack, first call 911 and then take a couple of aspirin, which will help prevent clotting. Whether healthy people who are at low risk of a heart attack should take aspirin on a regular basis is still an open question. As with vitamin supplements or drinking alcohol, each person must decide what is best for his or her health.

Alcohol

A large study of 275,000 middle-aged men showed that one or two drinks a day over 12 years reduced their risk of dying from a heart attack by about 20% in comparison to men who did not drink alcohol. Other studies show that moderate alcohol consumption also reduces the risks of stroke. However, more than two drinks a day *increases* the risk of both heart attack and stroke significantly. Women also experienced a benefit from a daily drink or two, but the small benefit to the heart is offset by a slight increased risk of cancer.

Although moderate alcohol drinking does have some health benefits, the issue of drinking is so controversial (and potentially harmful) that no recommendation can be made to drink because it may protect you from a heart attack. Many dietary and lifestyle changes are much more beneficial to your heart than drinking alcohol. On the other hand, persons who enjoy a drink occasionally need not feel guilty that they are damaging their health.

With the increased attention given to risk factors that cause cardiovascular disease, people are now armed with knowledge about reducing their chances of heart attacks and stroke. People should reduce consumption of foods containing large amounts of saturated fats and cholesterol. A diet rich in fresh fruits and vegetables helps protect your heart and arteries. Understanding the consequences of cigarette smoking should encourage smokers to quit. Also, taking supplements of vitamins C, E, B_6, B_{12}, and folic acid in the amounts present in a multivitamin tablet seems prudent. Cardiovascular disease can be prevented by adopting good health habits now!

Critical Thinking About Health

1. Black Americans as a group have higher blood pressure, on average, than white Americans. Various hypotheses have been advanced to explain the differences in blood pressure between the races, including genetic differences, social factors, economic factors, diet, and behavioral differences. Find out all that you can on racial differences in blood pressure (your local branch of the American Heart Association is a good place to start for information). Then write a report giving your views as to why the blood pressure discrepancy exists among races and ethnic groups in our society.

2. Using Table 14.1 (on page 302) as a guide, try to determine approximately how much cholesterol you consume in an average week. Then try to construct a diet for yourself, either by reducing amounts of certain foods or by eliminating them altogether, that will reduce your average weekly cholesterol intake by at least 20%. Can you construct a diet that satisfies you and that contains 50% less cholesterol? Write up your findings in a report. If you need more accurate information on the cholesterol content of foods, consult any nu-

trition textbook or handbook that lists the components of foods. Also most canned and packaged foods list the cholesterol content on the nutrition label.

3. Make a list of all the factors discussed in this chapter that increase the risk of cardiovascular disease, heart attacks, and stroke. How many of the risk factors do you have? Among the risk factors that can be changed, discuss how you would go about reducing them in your life to improve your cardiovascular health now and for the future.

4. People in Japan or Southern European countries have one half to one third the risk of dying from heart disease in comparison to people from the U.S. or Northern Europe, even when their cholesterol levels, on average, are the same. A person with a cholesterol level of 250 mg/dl in Denmark has a two to three times greater risk of a fatal heart attack compared with an Italian with the same cholesterol level. Develop arguments to explain this difference that seem reasonable to you and organize your facts and ideas in the form of a hypothesis.

Health in Review

- The heart is a pump that maintains blood circulation in the arteries and veins. The arteries carry oxygen and nutrients to cells, and the veins carry carbon dioxide back to the lungs.
- Damage to the heart or arteries is called cardiovascular disease, which is the leading cause of death in the United States.
- Major risk factors of heart disease that cannot be changed are: heredity, gender, and age.
- Major risk factors of heart disease that can be changed are: cigarette or tobacco use, high blood cholesterol, high blood pressure, physical inactivity, and poor diet.
- Other factors that contribute to heart disease are: diabetes, obesity, and stress.

- Various surgeries are performed to repair clogged arteries. These include coronary bypass surgery and angioplasty.
- Vitamins E, C, B_6, and B_{12}, and folic acid all help protect against heart disease.
- One aspirin tablet every other day may reduce the risk of cardiovascular disease.
- Calcium, soy products, fish oils, and green tea all help keep the heart healthy.
- Heart disease is caused by modern lifestyles and can be prevented. Making changes in your diet, smoking, and exercise behaviors while you are young can help keep the heart and arteries healthy throughout life.

Health and Wellness Online

The World Wide Web contains a wealth of information about health and wellness. By accessing the Internet using Web browser software, such as Netscape Navigator or Microsoft's Internet Explorer, you can gain a new perspective on many topics presented in *Health and Wellness, Seventh Edition*. Access the Jones and Bartlett Publishers Web site at http://www.jbpub.com/hwonline.

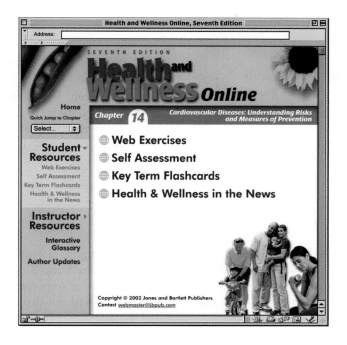

References

Barnett, H. J. M., Meldrum, H. E. (2000). Appropriate use of carotid endarterectomy. *Hospital Practice*, November 15, 53–62.

Benitez, M. (1999). Atherosclerosis: An infectious disease? *Hospital Practice*, September 1, 79–90.

Cholesterol drugs. (1998). *Consumer Reports*, October, 54–56.

Cooper R. S., Rotimi, C. N., Ward, R. (1999). The puzzle of hypertension in African-Americans. *Scientific American*, February, 56–63.

Curfman, G. D. (1998). Fatal impact—concussion of the heart. *New England Journal of Medicine, 338,* 1841–1843.

Daviglus, M. L. et al. (1997). Fish consumption and the 30-year risk of fatal myocardial infarction. *New England Journal of Medicine, 336,* 1946–1052.

Fichtenberg, C. M., Glantz, S. A. (2000). Association of the California tobacco control program with declines in cigarette consumption and mortality from heart disease. *New England Journal of Medicine, 343,* 1772–1777.

Frank, J. D. (1973). *Persuasion and healing.* Baltimore: Johns Hopkins University Press.

Hankey, G. J., Eikelboom, J. W. (1999). Homocysteine and vascular disease. *The Lancet, 354,* 407–412.

He, Y., Lam, T. H., Li, L. S. (1994). Passive smoking at work a risk factor for coronary heart disease in Chinese women who never have smoked. *British Medical Journal, 308,* 6925.

Heart and stroke statistical update (2000). Dallas, Tex.: The American Heart Association Publications.

Hypertension: What works? (1999). *Consumer Reports*, May, 60–62.

Iribarren, C., et al. (2000). Association of hostility with coronary artery calcification in young adults. *Journal of the American Medical Association, 283,* 2546–2551.

Kaski, J. C., Russo, G, (2000). Cardiac syndrome X: An overview. *Hospital Practice*, February, 75–94.

Kern, F. (1991). Normal plasma cholesterol in an 88–year-old man who eats 25 eggs per day. *New England Journal of Medicine, 324,* 13.

Marmot, M. (1994). The cholesterol papers. *British Medical Journal, 308,* 6925.

McMurry, M. P., Cerqueira, M. T., Connor, S. L., and Connor, W. E. (1991). Changes in lipid and lipoprotein levels and body weight in Tarahumara Indians after consumption of an affluent diet. *New England Journal of Medicine, 325.*

O'Malley, P. G. et al. (2000). Lack of correlation between psychological factors and subclinical coronary artery disease. *New England Journal of Medicine, 343,* 1298–1304.

Ornish, D. et al. (1998). Intensive lifestyle changes for reversal of coronary heart disease. *Journal of the American Medical Association, 280,* 2001–2007.

Pauletto, P. et al. (1996). Blood pressure and atherogenic lipoprotein profiles of fish-diet and vegetarian villagers in Tanzania: The Lugalawa study. *Lancet, 348,* 784–788.

Ross, R. (1999). Atherosclerosis—an inflammatory disease. *New England Journal of Medicine, 340,* 115–126.

Stephens, N. G. et al. (1996). Randomized controlled trial of vitamin E in patients with coronary disease. *Lancet, 347,* 781–790.

Taubes G. (1998). The (political) science of salt. *Science, 281,* 898–907.

Verghese, A. (2000). Bypass nation. *Talk,* March, 105–154.

Verschuren, W. M. et al. (1996). Serum total cholesterol and long-term coronary heart disease mortality in different cultures. *Journal of the American Medical Association, 274,* 131–136.

Suggested Readings

American Heart Association (AHA). *Heart and stroke facts, 2000.* Published yearly and obtainable from any AHA office. Contains the latest information on cardiovascular diseases, treatments, and statistical data.

Cooper, R. S., Rotimi, C. N. and Ward, R. (1999, February). The puzzle of hypertension in African-Americans. *Scientific American,* 56–63. Discusses both the genetic and environmental factors that have been investigated in order to explain why black Americans have a much higher prevalence of hypertension as compared to white Americans.

Ornish, D., et al. (1998). Intensive lifestyle changes for reversal of coronary heart disease. *Journal of the American Medical Association, 280,* 2001–2007. A report documenting that the blockages in arteries can be reversed by changes in lifestyle and that the beneficial changes persist for years.

Pickering, T. (1996). *Good news about high blood pressure.* New York: Simon and Schuster. Explains the risk factors for hypertension and how to control hypertension without drugs, if possible.

Taubes, G. (1998). The (political) science of salt. *Science, 281,* 898–907. Overconsumption of salt has been blamed as one of the risk factors for hypertension, stroke, and death from cardiovascular disease. However, despite hundreds of studies, claims and counter claims, this conclusion is still highly controversial. Read all about it!

Verghese, A. (1999, March). Bypass nation. *Talk,* 105–107. Discusses why coronary bypass surgeries are so common and the financial and social pressures that favor surgery over equally effective, safer, and cheaper procedures.

Learning Objectives

1. Identify and describe several congenital birth defects.
2. Identify and describe several chemical substances that cause birth defects.
3. Explain what a hereditary disease is.
4. Discuss the importance of genes in health and disease.
5. Explain prenatal testing for genetic diseases and discuss the importance of genetic counseling.
6. Describe how some hereditary diseases can be treated.
7. Describe several kinds of genetic discrimination.
8. Explain genetic testing and gene therapy.

Study Guide and Self Assessment

Health and Wellness Online

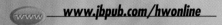 **www.jbpub.com/hwonline**

Chapter 15

How Genes Affect Health

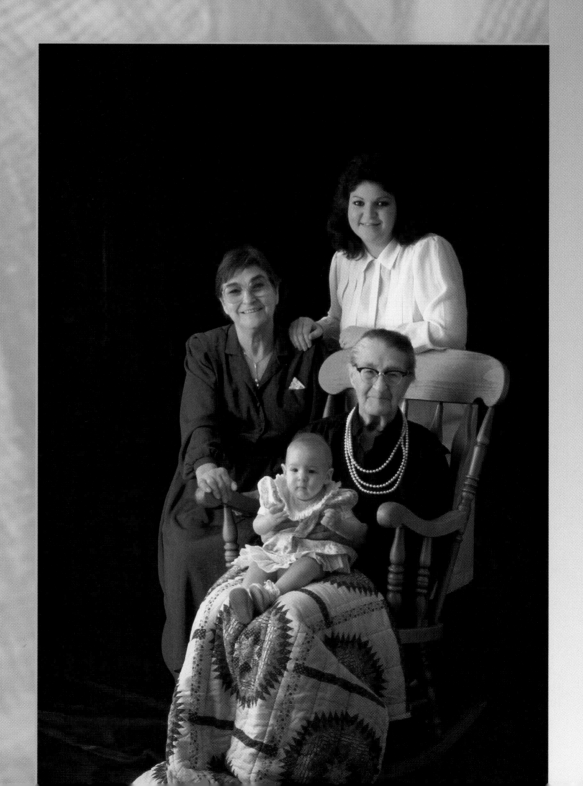

When the sperm from your father joined with the egg from your mother when you were conceived, the genes in both cells began to direct the development of a new individual—you. You inherited about 40,000 different genes from each of your parents that directed the formation of all of your tissues and organs, including your brain and its wiring to all parts of your body. The instructions for all of the chemical reactions in all of the cells in your body are determined by your genes. Occasionally, a chemical error in a gene can alter the body's biochemistry and cause a person to be born with an inherited disease, a physical or mental abnormality, or with a susceptibility to heart disease or cancer later in life. The genes we inherit play a crucial role in determining our health and even how long we will live.

Most babies are born healthy; however, in about 1 in every 50 births in the U.S., a physical abnormality is observable when the baby is examined at birth. In addition to observable physical abnormalities, approximately 3% of all newborns have mental defects that will not become noticeable until later in life. It has been determined that defects in more than 300 different human genes can cause some degree of mental retardation.

Birth defects can also be caused by environmental factors, such as toxins or drugs that affect the normal development of the fetus. In many cases of birth defects, it is difficult to sort out the relative contributions of the genetic and the environmental factors. However, using a variety of medical tests, about half of all birth defects are found to be caused by defective genes that were passed to children from one or both parents.

An explosion of new information pertaining to human hereditary disorders is beginning to reveal how certain defective genes cause particular inherited disorders and disease susceptibilities. But the extraordinary advances in diagnosis of inherited disorders in both adults and developing fetuses have also generated complex personal, social, and ethical problems for individuals and society (Holtzman, 1998).

Ethical and personal problems always arise when genetic analyses indicate that the fetus has a serious inherited disease. Prospective parents must decide whether to abort the pregnancy or to continue it, knowing the child will be born with a handicap, or to take some other medical step. As more and more defective genes can be detected in the fetus, the decisions become more and more difficult. For example, in the near future, a pregnant woman may be able to find out if the fetus she is carrying is at risk for alco-

> *In nature there's no blemish but the mind, None can be called deformed but the unkind.*
> SHAKESPEARE
> *TWELFTH NIGHT*

holism, obesity, or violent behavior. Such knowledge is bound to affect parents' decisions both to have that child and also how the child is raised after birth.

Testing both adults and fetuses for defective genes is highly controversial, but it emphasizes why people need to understand what genes are and how they function in determining health and susceptibility to disease. Only with some understanding of genes and how hereditary diseases are passed on can you become a knowledgeable consumer of the new genetic tests and gene therapies that are being developed.

Congenital Defects

Each newborn is examined immediately after birth for any observable physical abnormalities, which are called **congenital defects.** Such defects are not necessarily inherited, although defective genes passed on from parents may play some role. Most congenital defects are caused by a complex interaction of genes and environmental factors. Examples of congenital defects are cleft lip, cleft palate, and spina bifida (cleft spine), which result from developmental abnormalities in the formation of the oral cavity and the spine, respectively (Figure 15.1).

Cleft lip has been known to occur in only one of a pair of identical twins, so environmental factors other than genes must contribute to this abnormality. The importance of environmental factors during fetal development also is borne out by the observation that even though identical twins share identical genes, they usually are born with different birth weights. This shows that identical twins are affected differently by environmental factors even during development in the same uterus.

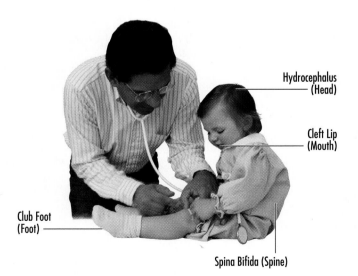

Hydrocephalus (Head)

Cleft Lip (Mouth)

Club Foot (Foot)

Spina Bifida (Spine)

FIGURE 15.1   Congenital defects arise during fetal development and are detected at birth.

Managing Stress

The Art of Acceptance

Sometimes we encounter major stressors in our lives. One such case is having a hereditary disease. How do we learn to cope with such a situation? Those who consider themselves most successful in coping are those who have learned how to accept their situation and get on with their lives. Perhaps it was said best by Reinhold Niebuhr in the now famous Serenity Prayer: *"Lord, grant me the serenity to change the things I can, accept the things I cannot change, and the wisdom to know the difference."*

When people hear the word "acceptance," there is often a sense of resignation. There is also a sense of anger and victimization. "Why me? Why did this have to happen to me? What did I do to deserve this?" Unconditional acceptance is an understanding of the existing conditions, a receptivity to the things that cannot be changed, and a discarding of the feelings of pity. True acceptance is not giving up; rather it is a recognition of the particular situation. In the stage of acceptance, there is no trace of anger or pity, no feelings of victimization. Unconditional acceptance allows you to move on with your life. With acceptance may come hope and the conviction that it will all work out.

As we are now learning, not all symptoms of hereditary diseases are evident at birth. Many surface in the second, third, or fourth decades of life. In terms of spiritual wellness, roadblocks on life's path may actually be the path itself. Stressors, like hereditary diseases or a significant injury of some kind, are not a punishment. Rather, they may be an opportunity to learn about life from a different perspective. Unfortunately, many people facing major health problems in their lives feel anger and frustration. Rather than trying to overcome the obstacle, they may become immobilized by it.

Some of our greatest role models are people born with great odds against them. They not only overcome adversity, but do it with great distinction. Consider the physicist Stephen Hawking, author of *A Brief History of Time*. Recognized as a genius at an early age, he was struck with a crippling disease in his twenties. Although he was unable to use his body, he never stopped exercising his mind. Now recognized as one of the world's leaders in cosmology and physics, Hawking shows that roadblocks in life can be overcome.

The art of acceptance is not a skill acquired overnight. It takes practice over a lifetime. Nor do all problems go away once we accept them. But when we learn the skill of unconditional acceptance, we learn to direct energy where it will serve the highest good. In the words of Richard Bach, author of *Illusions*, "There is no such thing as a problem without a gift for you in its hands. You seek problems, because you need their gifts."

Spina bifida is a congenital defect that affects 1 of every 1,000 newborns. It occurs when one or more spinal vertebrae fail to close and the spinal cord and nerves bulge through the cleft, forming an easily damaged, fluid-filled sac. The protruding spinal nerves are vulnerable to paralysis-causing damage and also to life-threatening infections. The most serious congenital defect of the nervous system is *anencephaly*, which refers to very abnormal brain development; affected babies are either stillborn or die soon after birth. Surgery can repair some of the damage resulting from spina bifida; however, nothing can be done for anencephaly.

Supplementing the diet of pregnant women with the vitamins folic acid (folate) and B_{12} has been shown to dramatically reduce the risk of spina bifida and other birth defects. Folic acid is the most effective of the B vitamins in preventing birth defects and should be taken during the first few weeks of pregnancy.

Women who plan on becoming pregnant should take folic acid (400 micrograms per day) before and after becoming pregnant. Flour and cereals have been supplemented with folic acid for the past several years. As a result, the incidence of spina bifida birth defects has decreased significantly in the United States.

Any environmental agent that causes a defect in a developing fetus is called a **teratogen** (Table 15.1). Many environmental agents, such as prescription and illegal drugs, viral and bacterial infections, alcohol consumption, and smoking cigarettes, act as teratogens (from the Greek; to produce a monster) during pregnancy and may cause abnormal development in a fetus. With a little care, many teratogens can be avoided, thereby increasing the likelihood of a healthy baby. In particular, smoking cigarettes and drinking alcohol should be avoided by any woman who is pregnant or attempting to become pregnant. Alcohol is concentrated in crossing the placenta so that even one or two drinks can lead to high alcohol levels in the fetus and affect its development.

Thalidomide

Thalidomide is a sleeping pill that also was once used to quell morning sickness early in pregnancy. It was

Terms

congenital defect: any physical or biological abnormality observed in a newborn

teratogen: any environmental agent that causes abnormal development of a fetus

considered safe and was widely prescribed in Europe in the early 1960s. It had been tested in animals and no teratogenic effects were discovered; however, the drug was not approved for distribution in the United States. By 1961, it was clear that thalidomide was causing serious birth defects. Thalidomide interferes with the normal development of the bones of the arms and legs of the fetus and causes other developmental abnormalities. Between 1960 and 1962, in many countries, several thousand babies were born with deformed arms and legs before the teratogenic effects of the drug were established. Aside from its teratogenic effects in pregnant women, thalidomide is a very safe drug and is still being used to treat certain diseases today.

DES

In the 1950s and 1960s, the synthetic hormone DES (diethylstilbestrol) was prescribed to help prevent

TABLE 15.1   **Teratogens**
Environmental agents (e.g., infectious viruses and other microorganisms, chemicals, medicines) can act as teratogens and cause birth defects. Many agents in addition to those listed below are suspected of causing abnormal development of the fetus.

Environmental agent	Effects
Accutane (acne drug)	Spontaneous abortion, stillbirth, malformation of the brain and heart
Alcohol	Growth deficiencies, mental retardation
Antithyroid drugs	Thyroid defects
Carbamazepine	Neural tube defects
Cocaine	Fetal death, nervous system and genital abnormalities
Cytomegalovirus, herpes simplex virus, varicella zoster virus	Growth deficiencies, mental retardation
Diethylstilbestrol (DES)	Masculination of female, abnormalities of vagina and cervix, risk of vaginal cancer
Ionizing radiation	Growth deficiencies, mental retardation, organ malformation (depending on dose)
Lithium carbonate	Heart and blood vessel defects
Methotrexate and etretinate	Prescription drugs that cause severe birth defects
Nonsteroidal anti-inflammatory drugs	Circulation defects
Phenytoin	Central nervous system defects
Polychlorinated biphenyls	Growth deficiencies, pigment abnormalities
Poor nutrition during fetal development	Growth deficiency, mental retardation
Rubella virus (German measles)	Heart and eye abnormalities, mental retardation
Tetracycline (antibiotic)	Teeth and bone abnormalities
Thalidomide	Limb malformation
Tobacco smoke	Growth deficiencies, increased risk of sickness and death soon after birth
Warfarin	Central nervous system defects

miscarriage. DES was not identified as a teratogen until the 1970s. Many daughters of women who took DES before or during pregnancy discovered that they had abnormalities in their reproductive organs when they tried to become pregnant. These daughters also have a higher risk of developing vaginal cancer. Although the drug did not cause abnormalities in all children of DES mothers, the risk is sufficiently great that most DES women carry the psychological burden of their potential for reproductive problems and cancer.

Accutane

Isotretinoin is an analog of vitamin A and is sold as a drug called Accutane that is used to treat severe acne and other skin disorders. Accutane was tested in laboratory animals and labeled a teratogen because it caused birth defects when administered to pregnant mice and rats. The drug was finally released with the warning that it should not be used during pregnancy. However, during the 1980s, hundreds of babies with congenital defects were born to women who became pregnant while taking Accutane for skin problems. In some cases, the women may have become pregnant by accident while taking the drug; in others, the desire to improve their skin condition may have caused them to disregard the warning. This points out a dilemma that is faced by the Food and Drug Administration (FDA), the government agency that regulates drugs. Should an effective drug that is known to be a teratogen be released with a warning or should it be banned entirely?

Alcohol, Drugs, and Pregnancy

Chronic use of alcohol during pregnancy may cause the newborn to be affected with fetal alcohol syndrome (FAS), which is characterized by abnormal facial features and mental retardation. Although most babies with FAS are born to women who consume large amounts of alcohol during pregnancy, studies show that even moderate drinking during pregnancy may increase risk.

The drinking of alcohol by pregnant women who give birth to a handicapped child raises questions about individual rights. Does a mother have a right to do with her body as she sees fit even if it means harming the baby? Does society have the right to regulate the consumption of alcohol and other harmful substances by a pregnant woman? Some people argue that a pregnant woman who irresponsibly takes drugs during pregnancy should be imprisoned while pregnant so that her use of dangerous substances can be controlled. The ethical and legal questions surrounding pregnancy and drugs, including alcohol, are very complex.

Many congenital defects could be prevented if women took more care with their diet and drug use during pregnancy. Smoking cigarettes and drinking alcohol should be eliminated, because they greatly increase the risks of spontaneous abortion, low birth weight, and congenital defects. The most critical period of development for the fetus is the first months of pregnancy, so if a pregnancy is anticipated, the consumption of alcohol and cigarettes should be discontinued. Use of over-the-counter and prescription drugs also should stop if possible.

Human Heredity

Hereditary Diseases

A **hereditary (genetic) disease** results from the following sequence of events. A defective gene (one whose chemistry has been altered in chromosomes of sperm or eggs) is passed on to a child from one or both parents. As a result of inheriting the defective gene or genes, a protein is produced that is abnormal or a protein may be missing completely. For example, if an essential muscle protein is defective or missing in a fetus, muscle tissues develop abnormally. Several forms of *muscular dystrophy* are inherited in this way. If a protein necessary for bone formation is defective, short stature, or *dwarfism*, results.

If the defective protein is an enzyme, an essential chemical reaction in the body will be affected and some aspect of metabolism will be abnormal. For example, in *hemophilia*, an enzyme called Factor VIII, required for normal blood clotting, is defective as a result of an altered gene on an X chromosome. *Phenylketonuria* (PKU) is an inherited disease caused by a defect in an enzyme that is needed to digest the amino acid phenylalanine, which is present in food. If excess phenylalanine in the blood is not broken down, it accumulates in tissues and causes abnormal brain development and mental retardation.

Sickle cell disease is caused by a defect in hemoglobin proteins present in all red blood cells. Hemoglobin molecules pick up oxygen as blood circulates through the lungs. In sickle cell disease, the defective hemoglobin proteins change the shape of red blood cells so that they tend to clog small blood vessels. As a result, essential oxygen cannot reach tissues and organs.

Hereditary diseases are *always* caused by defective chromosomes or genes that change body structure or chemistry in some way. However, determining if a disease or physical abnormality is inherited is not a simple matter. As indicated, many birth defects are caused by infections, teratogens, or other environmental factors, as well as by defective genes.

Sometimes a disease is said to "run in the family," which means that several members of a family have the same disease. Children of parents who suffer from certain diseases are at higher risk of developing these diseases as compared to the average risk in the general population (see Table 15.2). Allergies, obesity, or alcoholism may run in the family, but this does not mean that these diseases are inherited or are caused by defective genes. Families share many environmental factors as well as genes. For example, families share the same water, food, and air, any one of which may contain harmful or toxic substances. When parents have a poor diet, children usually do also. To appreciate the difference between an inherited disease and one that "runs in the family" consider these examples. Being a Protestant or a Catholic runs in families as does being a Republican or a Democrat, but these traits clearly are not determined by any genes that have been inherited. Only a physician trained in medical genetics can determine if a disease or defect is a result of inherited genes, environmental factors, or a combination of both.

> *Love is a great exaggeration of the worth of one individual over the worth of everybody else.*
> GEORGE BERNARD SHAW

TABLE 15.2   **Increased Risk of Certain Diseases and Disorders Among Children in Whom One Parent is Affected**
Although genes probably are involved to some degree, the number of genes conferring risk, or extent of the genetic contribution, is basically unknown. In all cases, environmental factors also are involved.

	Lifetime risk	
	General population	One parent affected
Alcoholism (men)	10%	40%
Alcoholism (women)	3% to 5%	12% to 20%
Alzheimer's	5% to 10%	10% to 20%
Colon cancer	6%	12% to 18%
Diabetes, type 2	3% to 7%	10% to 15%
Depression, bipolar	1% to 3%	9% to 27%
Dyslexia	5% to 10%	30% to 60%
Psoriasis	1% to 2%	25%
Rheumatoid arthritis	1%	5%
Schizophrenia	1%	10%

Terms

hereditary (genetic) disease: any disease resulting from the inheritance of defective genes or chromosomes from one or both parents

TABLE 15.3   Chromosomal Abnormalities

Some genetic diseases are associated with an extra or missing chromosome. Most abnormalities in chromosome number (more or less than the normal 46) are incompatible with long-term survival; in most cases, affected babies die before birth. However, abnormalities in chromosome 21, X, or Y are compatible with survival but usually produce physical and mental abnormalities.

Genetic disease/disorder	Chromosomal defect	Incidence per live births	Symptoms
Turner's syndrome (female)	Missing X	1/1000	Absence of ovaries, short stature, underdeveloped breasts
Klinefelter's syndrome (male)	Extra X	1/1000	Small, undeveloped testes, sterility, mental retardation
Down syndrome (male or female)	Extra chromosome 21	1/700	Physical abnormalities, mental retardation, heart defects
XXX syndrome (female)	Extra X	Uncertain (1/1000)	No clinical abnormalities, height above average, possible mental retardation
XYY (male)	Extra Y	Uncertain (1/1000)	No clinical abnormalities, height above average, controversy over "criminal" tendency

Chromosomes

Each person carries 23 pairs of chromosomes (46 total) in every cell of his or her body. Men and women differ only in a pair of chromosomes called the sex chromosomes; men have an XY pair and women have an XX pair. In both men and women, the chromosomes that were present in the fertilized egg are also present in skin, brain, heart, lung, or liver cells. Half of each parent's chromosomes is passed on to progeny in the sperm and egg that join during fertilization. Occasionally, errors are made when the chromosomes are distributed to sperm or egg, resulting in too few or too many chromosomes; these cause hereditary diseases (Table 15.3). About 20% of all human conceptions have a chromosomal abnormality of some kind. The majority of fetuses with chromosomal abnormalities are aborted spontaneously (Sluder and McCollum, 2000).

Human chromosomes have a characteristic size, shape, and banding pattern that shows up when they are stained with dyes. In this way, each of the 23 different chromosomes can be distinguished and identified. Human chromosomes are visualized under the microscope and then are photographed and arranged in pairs in a standardized display called a **karyotype.** Visualization of chromosomes in cells removed from a fetus, child, or adult can identify chromosomal abnormalities, such as the extra chromosome 21 that causes *Down syndrome* (Figure 15.2).

This serious inherited birth defect occurs in about one in every 700 babies born in the United States. However, the rate increases dramatically in women over age 35 who bear a child. Because of the increase in Down syndrome with increased maternal age, all pregnant women over age 35 are advised to undergo genetic tests of fetal cells (see section on prenatal testing) to determine if they are carrying a fetus with Down syndrome. If the tests are positive, women can elect to have an abortion or continue the pregnancy, knowing that they will deliver a child with Down syndrome.

The extra chromosome 21 carried in all cells of individuals with Down syndrome causes heart defects, altered facial features, and mental retardation. With modern medical care, the life expectancy of a person with Down syndrome is 40 to 50 years. However, caring for a Down syndrome person beyond childhood is taxing on families both emotionally and financially. Eventually, most individuals with Down syndrome are placed in special living situations with trained caregivers.

Genes

Genes are present in chromosomes in a chemical substance called **DNA (deoxyribonucleic acid).** Each chromosome, depending on its size, contains hundreds or thousands of different genes. Together the 46 human chromosomes contain about 200,000 genes, the combination of which determines a unique human being. Since chromosomes occur in pairs, each person carries two copies of each gene; these may be identical or slightly different from one another. When the chemistry of a gene is significantly different from that found in healthy people, the defective gene usually alters a chemical reaction in the body and causes an inherited disease.

Almost all of the different human genes direct the synthesis of uniquely different proteins. Some of these proteins are used to construct the bones and muscles of

---

Terms

karyotype: visual display of all of a person's chromosomes that can detect chromosomal abnormalities characteristic of inherited diseases

DNA (deoxyribonucleic acid): the chemical substance in chromosomes that carries genetic information

enzymes: proteins in cells that carry out and speed up chemical reactions

genetic counseling: information to help prospective parents evaluate the risks of having or delivering a genetically handicapped child

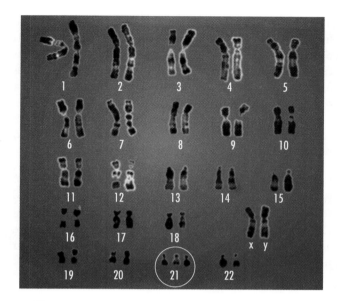

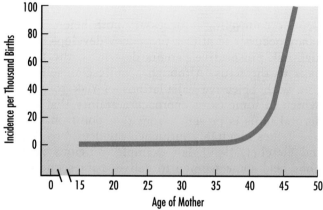

FIGURE 15.2   Karyotype of Individual with Down Syndrome   Note three copies of chromosome 21. Frequencies of children born with Down syndrome are shown in relation to the age of the mother. At age 35 the risk of this particular chromosomal defect begins to rise sharply.

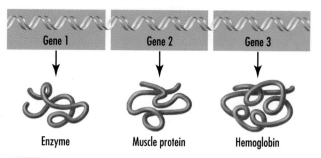

FIGURE 15.3   DNA in Chromosomes   Genes direct the synthesis of proteins in cells. Each gene in a chromosome codes for a different protein. Most proteins are enzymes that speed up chemical reactions in cells. Other proteins are used to construct bone, muscle, hair, and nails. Genes consist of sequences of chemical substances called bases in DNA. Proteins consist of sequences of amino acids that fold and twist to form specific shapes that determine the protein's function.

the body. However, most genes direct the synthesis of special proteins called **enzymes** (Figure 15.3). Enzymes catalyze (speed up) the thousands of different chemical reactions in cells that keep them (and us) alive.

Preventing Hereditary Diseases

Prenatal Testing

An important goal of modern medicine is preventing inherited diseases caused by defective genes or chromosomes. Genetic counseling of couples who are at risk for having a child with a hereditary disorder can help prevent them from having a handicapped child by counseling them before and during pregnancy. Genetic counseling can provide useful information for parents, but in the end the parents make the decisions. Prenatal

Wellness Guide

Determining If You Are at Risk for Bearing a Genetically Handicapped Child

Prenatal testing and **genetic counseling** are advised if a person falls into any one of the risk categories listed below:

- Maternal age over 35 years (risk of Down syndrome)
- High or low levels of alphafetoprotein during pregnancy (risk of neural tube defect).
- Woman had a previous child with a chromosomal abnormality or neural tube defect.

- Woman had a previous stillbirth or neonatal death.
- Woman or mate carries a previously diagnosed chromosomal or genetic abnormality.
- Woman carries a previously diagnosed defective gene.
- Woman and mate carry the same previously diagnosed defective gene.

- Close relatives have a child with an inherited disorder.
- Woman has been exposed to a teratogenic agent during pregnancy.
- Woman has recently been infected by rubella (measles) virus or cytomegalovirus.

testing is not advised or necessary for all pregnant women or couples planning to have a child. Only those who are at higher-than-average risk for bearing a child with a hereditary defect are advised to undergo prenatal testing and genetic counseling.

Hundreds of single gene defects that cause hereditary diseases now can be detected *in utero* with a prenatal surgical procedure called **amniocentesis** (Figure 15.4). In this procedure, fetal cells are obtained by removing a sample of amniotic fluid from the womb around the fifteenth week of pregnancy. Although amniocentesis is very safe, there is still a small risk of harming the fetus or inducing a miscarriage. The physician should discuss the risks and benefits of the procedure as part of the genetic counseling. Amniocentesis is performed so that prospective parents can decide whether to continue the pregnancy or abort the fetus. The decision is generally made after discussion with their physician and a counselor.

The fetal cells obtained by amniocentesis are grown in the laboratory and tested for biochemical and genetic abnormalities. Examination of the chromosomes in the karyotype analysis also identifies the sex of the fetus, but this information is only provided if the pregnant woman specifically requests it. (While most people in American society are joyful at the birth of either a boy or a girl, in many other countries, male children are still considered more desirable. In fact, determination of a female fetus by amniocentesis and karyotype analysis is the most common cause of elective abortion in many countries of the world, particularly in India.)

Another prenatal procedure called **chorionic villus analysis** can be performed as early as 8 weeks after conception. This earlier test provides information regarding the health of the fetus, allowing the parent(s) to make an earlier decision with respect to terminating the pregnancy.

A noninvasive form of prenatal testing is **ultrasound scanning** which is used to visualize the developing fetus (Figure 15.5). Ultrasound scans use high frequency sound waves that bounce back from the various tissues in the fetus with different intensities. The sound waves reflected from the fetus are displayed on a screen, and the image is interpreted by a physician trained in the use of this technique.

Ultrasound scans are used to detect multiple fetuses and to determine the location of the placenta, which is important if amniocentesis is to be performed. The scans can gauge the fetus' head size, thereby providing determination of the age of the fetus. Abnormal brain development and neural tube defects also can be diagnosed with an ultrasound scan. Despite the safety of these tests, pregnant women are advised not to have an ultrasound scan unless their health or that of the fetus requires one.

Genetic Counseling

Genetic counseling is necessary both before a pregnancy occurs and after a pregnancy develops to help high-risk prospective parents determine the genetic risks to the fetus. Although genetic counseling begins with objective calculations of risk to a fetus (which in some cases approach certainty that an abnormal fetus is present), from that point on subjective values inevitably influence the decisions (Wertz and Fletcher, 1989). For example, religious convictions lead some women to deliver babies known to have Down syndrome.

Although genetic counselors strive to be objective, the counseling process is subtle and counselors may inadvertently convey personal opinions. For example, prospective parents who carry certain genes can be told that any child that they bear will have one chance in four of being abnormal, or they can be told that the odds are three to one that the child will be normal. Both statements express the same truth about the probabilities, but the prospective parents may well interpret the two statements differently.

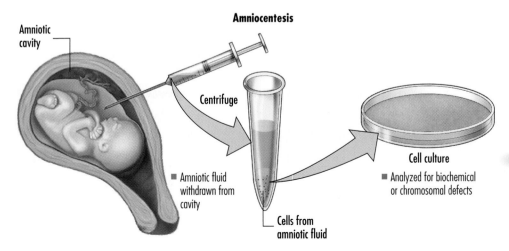

Amniocentesis

Amniotic cavity

Centrifuge

■ Amniotic fluid withdrawn from cavity

Cells from amniotic fluid

Cell culture
■ Analyzed for biochemical or chromosomal defects

FIGURE 15.4   Amniocentesis In the diagnostic procedure called amniocentesis, a sample of the fluid that surrounds the developing fetus is collected. Both the fluid and the fetal cells it contains are then analyzed for biochemical or chromosomal defects.

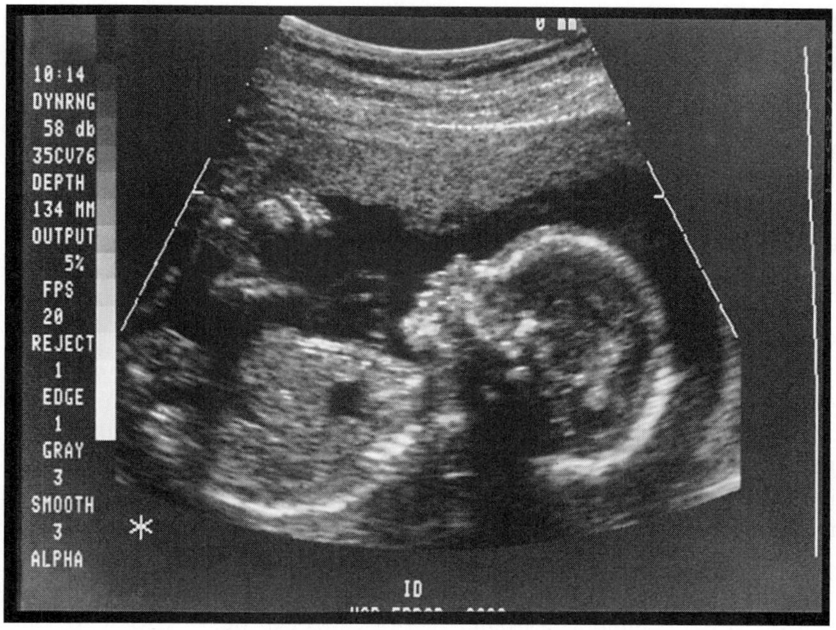

FIGURE 15.5   Ultrasound Scanning
Image of a fetus obtained by ultrasound scanning. Such ultrasound scans reveal the position of the fetus and may also indicate certain physical abnormalities.

Giving advice or making recommendations that affect the life of another person inevitably necessitates moral decisions—decisions that are influenced by many factors. Ideally, the personal views of the genetic counselor should not influence the families' decisions. Clients should arrive at their own decision after careful consideration of all medical options that have been explained to them.

Treating Hereditary Diseases

Very few of the thousands of known hereditary diseases can be treated effectively. Phenylketonuria (PKU) is an exception; it can be managed if the affected newborn is diagnosed at birth. Because PKU is treatable and because the test is accurate and inexpensive, all newborns in the United States are tested for PKU. The amino acid phenylalanine is present in any normal diet and, if it is eaten by a child with PKU, it accumulates in the blood, brain development is affected, and mental retardation follows. A person with PKU lacks an enzyme that is essential for the chemical breakdown of phenylalanine present in most proteins, including proteins in milk. Thus, any baby with PKU is immediately put on a phenylalanine-free diet, which must be maintained at least until and often beyond puberty.

Another genetic disease that can be treated successfully is hemophilia, which is caused by a defect in the blood-clotting protein called Factor VIII. The normal factor VIII protein is now manufactured by biotechnology companies, and hemophiliacs take the drug to prevent bleeding. Another important drug produced by biotechnology is human growth hormone (HGH). Individuals who inherit a defective gene that causes dwarfism can now be treated with HGH during childhood and will grow to near normal height.

Gene Therapy

Thousands of human disorders are caused by the inheritance of a gene that is defective in some way. Because genes contain the information for making proteins, inheriting a defective gene means that a defective protein is synthesized; the result is some abnormality in body chemistry that is manifested as a disease. For example, the gene that makes an essential clotting protein called Factor VIII is defective in people with *hemophilia*. People with *sickle cell anemia* inherit a defective gene for hemoglobin synthesis. In *cystic fibrosis*, the defective protein is in cell membranes that determine how chemicals enter and exit cells. And in *muscular dystrophy*, proteins that are used to build muscle are defective. The problem for medical science is how to treat or cure these inherited diseases.

Occasionally the defective protein can be manufactured and injected into patients in order to replace the missing one, as in the treatment for hemophilia. In other cases, drugs are used to lessen the severity of symptoms, as in cystic fibrosis and sickle cell anemia.

Terms

amniocentesis: a procedure in which amniotic fluid is removed from the uterus and tested to determine if genetic or anatomical defects exist in the fetus

chorionic villus analysis: a prenatal procedure used to determine if genetic or anatomical defects exist in a fetus; an alternative to amniocentesis

ultrasound scanning: use of sound waves to visualize the fetus in the womb

However, because a fundamental gene is defective in all of the cells in a person's body, these kinds of treatments do not permanently cure the patient. That is the goal of **gene therapy.**

As more and more human genes are isolated and cataloged by laboratories around the world, the normal genes corresponding to the defective ones become available for gene therapy. Once a normal human gene has been purified, it can be inserted into affected patients by a variety of medical techniques. The hope is that the normal gene will function once it is in the cells, and that the protein will be produced in sufficient quantity to permanently cure the inherited disease.

> *People through finding something beautiful think something else unbeautiful.*
> *Through finding one man fit judge another unfit.*
> LAO-TZU

The logic of gene therapy is sound; however, in practice it has proved exceptionally difficult to overcome the technical and biological obstacles, and to actually cure inherited or any other kind of disease. Despite thousands of clinical trials of gene therapy since 1990 in people with inherited diseases or with cancer, significant success so far has been reported in just two patients (Anderson, 2000).

Gene therapy is the only hope for treating incurable hereditary diseases and incurable cancers, but experiments are proceeding slowly and cautiously because some gene therapy trials resulted in the premature death of patients. It is expected that with more time, experience, and experiments, gene therapy eventually will become a safe and accepted medical treatment (Eck, 1999).

Genetic Testing

Now that the Human Genome Project is essentially complete, hundreds of genes that underlie human health problems, behavioral disorders, and inherited diseases are being discovered. Once a gene is discovered and its DNA sequence is deciphered, it becomes possible to construct a genetic test that can determine if a person carries a "normal" copy of the gene or one that predisposes the individual to a health problem, such as a higher risk of cancer or heart disease, or one that may cause an inherited disease if passed on to children. Genetic testing to determine whether individuals carry "healthy" or "unhealthy" genes offers both potential benefits and potential harm.

One of the major goals of genetic testing is to alert parents to their degree of risk for passing on an inherited disease. Sometimes a single altered gene is

Wellness Guide

Is There a Gay Gene?

In modern American society the word *gay* has come to be equated with a homosexual male. Historically, the word *gay* meant "mirthful, high-spirited"; later, it began to be associated with sexual conduct as in the term "gay blade." But how the word *gay* came to be associated with male homosexuals is still not clear (Dynes, 1990).

In recent years, two scientific researchers claimed to have uncovered evidence pointing to a biological explanation of male homosexuality, and more specifically the presence of a "gay gene" on the X chromosome. However, other studies have failed to confirm the existence of a gay gene (Wickelgren, 1999). Looking at all the evidence gathered over the years, it seems unlikely that a single gene is responsible for homosexuality. Sexual

orientation is most likely determined by hundreds (thousands) of genes and environmental factors that we are exposed to during development both as a fetus and after being born.

Research on the genetic basis of homosexuality is exceptionally controversial both within the scientific community and among the general public. In the past, homosexual individuals have been forced to undergo sometimes brutal treatments to change their sexual orientation; homosexuality was regarded medically as a pathological condition such as cancer or heart disease. That extreme view has changed in America and other societies, but *homophobia* (an irrational fear or hatred of homosexuality and homosexual individuals) still exists in this country and elsewhere around the world.

Anthropological evidence indicates that homosexuality has existed in all human cultures past and present and that homosexual individuals constitute between 2% and 4% of any human population. Ethicists argue that any research aimed at establishing a genetic basis for homosexuality can only reinforce homophobia and may lead to yet another form of genetic discrimination (Schüklenk et al., 1997). If a genetic influence on the development of homosexuality were found and a genetic test became available, it is not hard to imagine people using such a test to determine the suitability of a marriage partner or to justify the abortion of a fetus carrying such a gene.

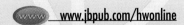 **www.jbpub.com/hwonline**

Dollars and Health Sense

Genetic Tests May Lead to Genetic Discrimination

One of the undesirable consequences of genetic testing is the possibility of discrimination against a person because he or she carries a particular defective gene. We all understand what discrimination based on sex or race means, and laws have been passed to prevent such discrimination in housing, employment, restaurants, and the armed forces. Although rarely described in genetic terms, racial and sexual discrimination is actually genetic discrimination because these traits are determined solely by the genes that one happens to inherit from parents. To hate someone because of his or her skin color is to hate the genes that determine skin color. Expressed in this way, racial discrimination sounds pretty stupid—and is.

Employers and insurance companies are the organizations most interested in knowing what genes a person carries. Companies would prefer not to hire someone who is likely to acquire a serious disease after working for several years; this would prove costly to the company in terms of both lost work and higher costs for health benefits. A company's health insurance might even be canceled if the payments for seriously ill individuals were considered to be too costly.

Health and life insurance companies also would like to have information about a person's genetic profile, so that they could select members who are the best risk from an insurance standpoint and reject those who are at high risk of a medical condition that will cost them money. Insurance companies can make these profit-driven decisions only if they are allowed access to a person's medical records and genetic testing information.

Because of the potential for such genetic discrimination, approximately 15 states have passed laws prohibiting genetic discrimination in employment. However, despite these laws, many people have lost their jobs when their employers found out they had a serious genetic disease or carried a gene that would cause disease later in life (Bingham, 1998). Currently, there is no federal legislation to protect people from genetic discrimination in employment or in obtaining health and life insurance. Until this vital social and health problem is solved, individuals who are unfortunate enough to have inherited a "bad" gene may become victims of genetic discrimination.

---

sufficient to cause an inherited disorder; sometimes it requires two altered genes, one from each parent. If parents are concerned that they may be carrying a defective gene because of their family history, they can be tested to ascertain their risks. (Not all couples are at risk but may benefit from genetic tests.) This can bring relief in knowing that there is no risk. This may also alert them to the risk, so that they can take precautions if they do not wish to have a child with a serious inherited disease.

Genetic tests are most useful when they can be used to prevent the passing on of an inherited disease. Some common inherited diseases for which genetic tests already exist include: cystic fibrosis, Duchenne muscular dystrophy, hemophilia A, sickle cell anemia, Fragile X syndrome, Huntington's disease, and many more. People who are concerned about inherited diseases in their family should consult their physicians about what tests are available and how to obtain genetic counseling (Motulsky, 1999).

Despite the expected boom in genetic tests in the near future, not all medical experts agree as to the wisdom or usefulness of widespread genetic testing as expressed in the following statement.

It would be revolutionary if we could determine the genotypes of the majority of people who will get common diseases. The complexity of the genetics of common diseases casts doubt on whether accurate prediction will ever be possible. Differences in so-cial structure, lifestyle, and environment account for much larger proportions of disease than genetic differences. Those who make medical and science policies in the next decade would do well to see beyond the hype.

—*Holtzman and Marteau, 2000*

Any person who is contemplating being tested for defective genes that may affect that individual's health or the health of offspring should talk to a genetic counselor before deciding to be tested. Knowing what your disease risks are can change the course of your life forever. Many people decide that, in some cases, "not knowing" is the healthiest way to live.

Genetically Modified Foods

Another widespread use of genetic engineering that may have profound effects on human health is in the manufacture of **genetically modified foods (GMFs).** Genetically modified foods refer to plants or animals into which genes from other organisms ("foreign

Terms

gene therapy: a technique for replacing defective genes with normal ones in certain tissues of a person affected with a hereditary disease

genetically modified food (GMF): any edible plant or animal that carries one or more genes derived from a different organism (foreign genes)

Dollars and Health Sense

How GMF Companies Twist the Truth

When "golden rice," a genetically modified (GM) rice, was announced, it was hailed as the solution to solving a major health problem among impoverished children around the world. The leading cause of blindness in underdeveloped countries is a lack of vitamin A in the diet. Throughout Asia and other impoverished areas of the world, people subsist on rice when other foods are not available or affordable; this leads to malnourishment and vitamin deficiencies.

Golden rice was genetically engineered to contain a gene (transferred from daffodils) that produces beta-carotene, a substance that is converted to vitamin A in the body. The company that developed the rice, Zeneca Corporation, announced that it was going to donate the rice seeds to poor countries to "help prevent blindness and infection in millions of children" with vitamin A deficiency. Who could argue with that? It appeared

that GM foods finally had achieved a moral victory by showing both the value of the technology for improving health and the altruism of companies who manufacture GM foods. *Time* magazine celebrated the announcement with a front page story. But is there more than meets the eye in this GM food?

An investigative reporter uncovered the following facts, which did not appear in nationwide stories or in company propaganda (Pollan, 2001).

- The beta-carotene level in the current strain of golden rice means that a typical child would have to eat 11 pounds of golden rice a day to get enough vitamin A to prevent blindness.
- Beta-carotene is only effectively converted to vitamin A if sufficient fat and protein also are present in the diet—an unlikely situation for people who are starving or severely undernourished.
- Convincing Asian people to eat anything but

white rice may be an insurmountable problem. Brown rice, which is nutrient-rich, is shunned by Asians who prefer heavily processed white rice for religious and cultural reasons.

Low-tech solutions already exist for eradicating the vitamin A deficiency in malnourished children. The most effective solution is to provide children with vitamin A supplements that cost only pennies. Aid groups that work in underdeveloped countries advocate this solution; they claim that solving the vitamin A blindness problem simply requires political will and money.

The company that plans to donate the golden rice seeds to impoverished countries has budgeted $50 million to advertise its good deeds. This amount of money in itself could probably buy enough vitamin A supplements to prevent blindness in most of the world's children.

genes") have been introduced by genetic engineering to improve the plant or animal in a desired way. For example, a gene has been introduced into corn, soy, and other plants in order to make them resistant to a commonly used herbicide called Roundup. Fields of such genetically engineered crops can be sprayed with Roundup to control weeds, but the crop will not be harmed. The problem is that people who eat the corn or soy or other such plant also are eating the protein that makes the plant resistant to herbicides.

Although the U.S. government considers GMFs to be as safe and as healthy as their unmodified counterparts, many other countries—in Europe especially—have banned GMFs because of environmental and health concerns (Wolfenberger and Phifer, 2000). Large food companies such as Gerber, H.J. Heinz, and Iams (manufacturer of pet foods) have pledged not to use any GMFs in their products. Archer Daniels Midland, a giant food processing company, has asked its suppliers to separate GM grains from unmodified ones, but this may prove to be impossible.

Planting of GM crops is already so widespread in the United States and other countries in Latin America

and Asia that it soon may be impossible to find an unadulterated supply of corn and soy (Barboza, 2001). Corn products have already been recalled because the manufactured products were found to contain small amounts of the "herbicide resistant" protein.

Genetic engineering can modify virtually any trait in a plant or animal by removing or introducing genes and creating novel organisms never produced by nature. Because of this, opponents of GMFs have labeled them "Frankenfoods." There is no doubt that many useful (and profitable) changes can be made in the foods that people eat. In fact, this is the argument that the industry advances; malnourishment can be abolished and health improved by the widespread use of GMFs. Foods can be produced more cheaply and with less pesticide spraying. However, the GMF industry has, so far, failed to convince consumers of the value of its products. Even in cases where the GMF in question seems to offer prospects for improved nourishment and health, as in the case of "golden rice," GM companies still are being deceptive (see "Dollars and Health Sense").

Critical Thinking About Health

1. A woman friend who is about 25 years old has just learned that she is pregnant. The woman smokes cigarettes and likes to party on weekends. Based on what you have learned about the causes of congenital defects in this chapter, make a list of all the behavioral, dietary, and lifestyle changes you would recommend to your friend to help ensure that she gives birth to a healthy child. Discuss the rationale for each of your recommendations.

2. Abortion is one of the most controversial issues in American society. At one end of the spectrum of views are people who think that all abortions should be prohibited for any reason whatsoever, even if the life of the pregnant woman is in jeopardy. At the other extreme are people who believe that each pregnant woman should have complete freedom to do whatsoever she chooses with respect to her pregnancy, since it is her body. Evaluate these two views of abortion and present your own views in as much detail as possible. Substantiate each of your views with scientific facts, religious statements, or other information that has led you to your present views.

3. You and your spouse decide now is the time to begin a family. Your spouse has a younger brother who is mentally handicapped and you have an older sister who was born with a cleft palate that was corrected by surgery. Do you believe that your risks of having a child with a congenital defect or inherited disorder is higher than average? Based on what you have learned in this chapter, are there any precautions that you should take or any genetic tests that you think

would be appropriate to reduce any anxiety about becoming pregnant? Make a list of questions that you both would like to discuss with your physician regarding things that you should know or tests that you should take to help ensure giving birth to a healthy child.

4. A few years ago, the U.S. military ordered all service personnel to have a blood sample taken so that the DNA of each individual's cells could be analyzed and the pattern placed on file, much as the FBI keeps files of fingerprints of criminals and others. The reason the military wants each person's DNA analyzed is so that remains can be positively identified in case that person dies in a future conflict. One soldier refused to give a blood sample in violation of a direct order and was ordered to stand before a court martial. The soldier argued that he had no assurance that his DNA information would be kept private and could be used for purposes of discrimination or to his detriment in other ways.

   a. Do you think the military is justified in wanting each person's DNA on file?
   b. In what ways might the DNA information be used to the detriment of the soldier either in the military or after his release from military service?
   c. Discuss the pros and cons of having the DNA profile of every person in the U.S. on file in a federal agency so that any person could be positively identified by law enforcement authorities, government agencies, or other organizations, should the need arise.

Health in Review

- Congenital defects are observed at birth in about 1 out of 50 newborn babies in the United States. Abnormal development of the fetus during pregnancy can be caused by environmental factors, chemically defective genes that were passed on from one or both parents, or a combination of both.

- Ultrasound, amniocentesis, and chorionic villus analysis are prenatal diagnostic procedures that can determine if fetal development is normal or if there is a physical or biological defect.

- Taking prescription or illegal drugs, drinking alcohol, or becoming infected by viruses during

pregnancy also can harm the fetus. If drugs or alcohol are used by a pregnant woman, especially in early pregnancy, the fetus may abort spontaneously or the newborn may suffer growth deficiencies, mental retardation, or other problems.

- Couples who are at higher-than-average risk for having a genetically handicapped child should undergo genetic counseling before and after pregnancy is established.

- Modern genetic diagnostic tests can detect hundreds of different hereditary diseases; however, only a few can be treated successfully.

- Genetic discrimination may occur when people find out that they or others carry genes that predispose them to diseases and disorders.
- Gene therapy is a promising new method of treating genetic diseases.

- Genetically modified foods are already in the food supply but may not be better or healthier than genetically unmodified foods.

Health and Wellness Online

The World Wide Web contains a wealth of information about health and wellness. By accessing the Internet using Web browser software, such as Netscape Navigator or Microsoft's Internet Explorer, you can gain a new perspective on many topics presented in *Health and Wellness, Seventh Edition*. Access the Jones and Bartlett Publishers Web site at http://www.jbpub.com/hwonline.

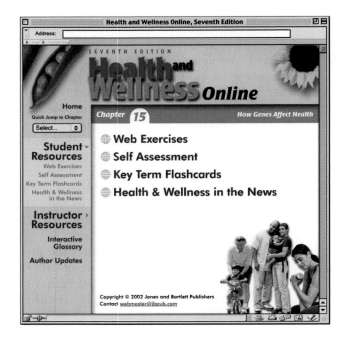

References

Anderson, W. F. (2000). The best of times, the worst of times. *Science, 288,* 627–629.

Barboza, D. (2001, June 10). As biotech crops multiply, consumers get little choice. *New York Times,* 1–6.

Bingham, E. (1998). Ethical issues of genetic testing for workers. In *Biomarkers: Medical and workplace applications,* eds. M. L. Mendelsohn, L. C. Mohr, and J. P. Peters. Washington, D.C.: Joseph Henry Press. 415–422.

Dynes, W. R. (Ed.). (1990). *Encyclopedia of homosexuality,* New York: Garland Publishers.

Eck, S. L. (1999, October 15). The prospects for gene therapy. *Hospital Practice,* 67–75.

Holtzman, N. A. (1998, January 15). Bringing genetic tests into the clinic. *Hospital Practice,* 107–128.

Holtzman, N. A., and Marteau, T. M. (2000). Will genetics revolutionize medicine? *New England Journal of Medicine, 343,* 141–144.

Motulsky, A. G. (1999). If I had a gene test, what would I have and who would I tell? *Molecular Medicine, 354,* 35–37.

Pollan, M. (2001, March 4). The great yellow hype. *New York Times Magazine,* 15–16.

Schüklenk, U., Stein, E., Kerin, J., and Byne, W. (1997, July-August). The ethics of genetic research on sexual orientation. *Hastings Center Report.*

Sluder, G., and McCollum, D. (2000). The mad way of meiosis. *Science, 289,* 254–255.

Wickelgren, I. (1999). Discovery of "gay gene" questioned. *Science, 284,* 571.

Suggested Readings

Collins, F. S., and McKusick, V. A. (2001). Implications of the Human Genome Project for medical science. *Journal of the American Medical Association,* 540–545. Discusses what the human genome project means for medicine and treatments in the 21st century.

Council for Responsible Genetics (www.genewatch.org). A watchdog organization that evaluates ethical and health concerns of genetically engineered drugs and foods. Also publishes a monthly magazine, *GeneWatch.*

Genetically modified foods: Are they safe? (2001, April). *Scientific American,* 51–65. A series of articles exploring how genetically modified foods are made and whether they are safe to eat.

Motulsky, A. G. (1999). If I had a gene test, what would I have and who would I tell? *Molecular Medi-cine, 354,* 35–37. A famous geneticist discusses a few examples of the implications and problems with genetic testing.

Spector, M. (1999, January 18). Decoding Iceland. *The New Yorker,* 40–51. The Icelandic government gives a company permission to put all of its citizens' genetic information into a database in the hopes of identifying disease-causing genes. Is this a good idea? The author explores both sides of the question.

Zallen, D. T. (1997). *Does it run in the family? A consumer's guide to DNA testing for genetic disorders.* New Jersey: Rutgers University Press. Explains the genetic tests that are available and presents case studies of families trying to decide what to do.

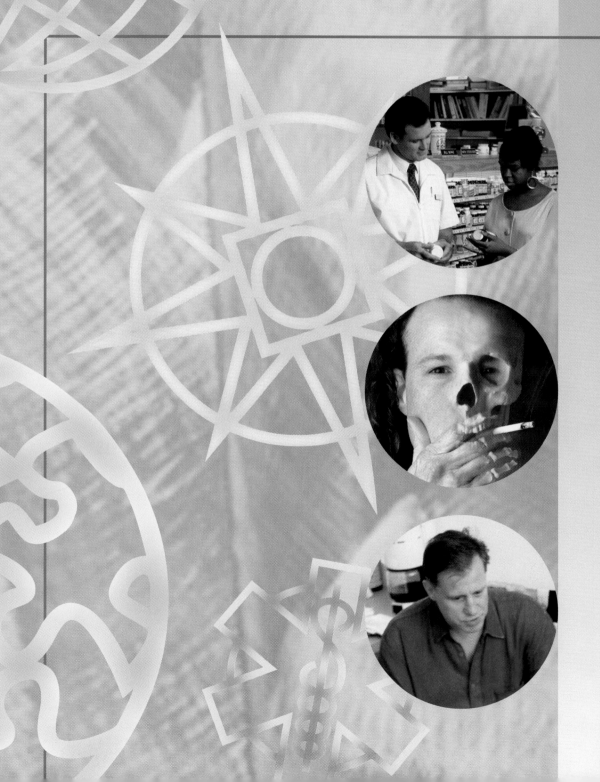

Part 5

Explaining Drug Use and Abuse

1. Explain the difference between a drug and a medicine.
2. Explain the concept of a drug receptor and its relation to drug side effects.
3. Describe the logic of a double-blind drug effectiveness study.
4. Give examples of the overuse of legal drugs in American society and the influences of drug advertising on drug use.
5. Define the terms addiction, physical dependence, habituation, tolerance, and withdrawal.
6. Describe the different effects of the major classes of psychoactive drugs: stimulants, depressants, marijuana, hallucinogens, PCP, and inhalants.
7. Describe the health hazards of using anabolic steroids.

Study Guide and Self Assessment

The Drugs You Take
Be a Knowledgeable Consumer

Health and Wellness Online

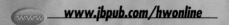 **www.jbpub.com/hwonline**

Chapter 16

Using Drugs Responsibly

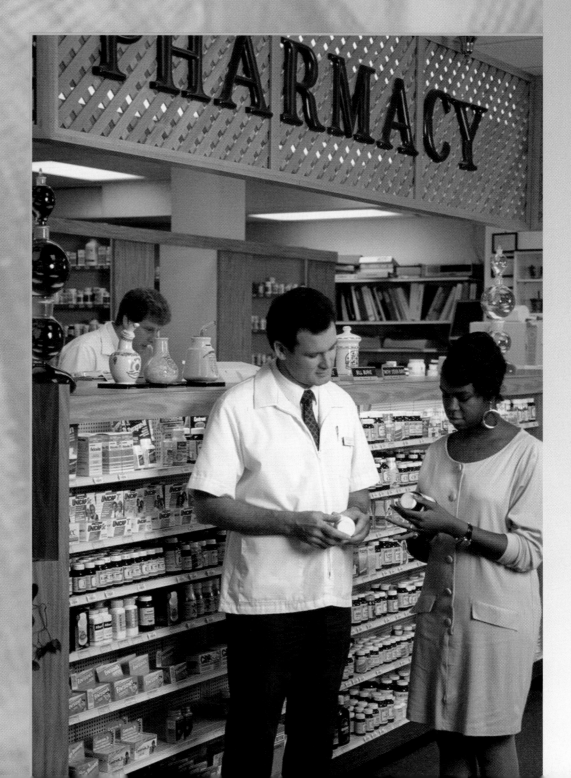

For thousands of years, people have been ingesting substances to heal themselves, change consciousness, produce sleep, drive out evil spirits, and promote tribal and family harmony. For most of that time, such substances were obtained by chewing the leaves of a particular plant, brewing a tea from a plant's bark or roots, or mixing a potion made up of plant and animal materials, as the three witches in Shakespeare's *Macbeth* did when they concocted "eye of newt and toe of frog, wool of bat and tongue of dog." Today, some healing substances are still obtained by ingesting plant and animal tissues or their extracts directly, whereas others are single, chemically pure substances that are manufactured by modern chemical and biological technologies.

> Drugs become useful or dangerous depending on how we view them and how we use them.
> ANDREW WEIL, M.D.

No matter how they are obtained, many substances are of enormous value in relieving pain, preventing disease, and facilitating healing. However, indiscriminate or inappropriate use and overuse of drugs also are major problems in our society. For example, in 1997, the combination of phentermine and fenfluramine ("phen/fen"), taken by millions of people to control body weight, was found to cause heart valve damage, and the drugs were banned. Overuse of antibiotics has led to the creation of antibiotic-resistant organisms, against which no antibiotic drugs are effective (see chapter 12). Alcohol and the use of other drugs are associated with a greater risk of homicide and suicide (Rivara et al., 1997). And everyone has heard of the "war on drugs," which is concerned with the social and legal problems associated with the use of cocaine, heroin, and other illegal substances.

The use of drugs in our society has become so commonplace and accepted that many people automatically turn to drugs to solve their physical, mental, and emotional problems, failing to understand the dangers and health hazards. When people have symptoms of headache, backache, fatigue, stomach upset, colds, or allergies, many believe that taking drugs is the *only* source of relief. Although many medicines are extremely valuable, reliance on drugs to solve life's problems opens the way for chemical dependency. Many people do not consider the possible consequences of drug use, which often have a negative impact on well-being.

What Is a Drug?

A **drug** is a single chemical substance in a medicine that alters the structure or function of some of the body's biological processes. The alteration can start,

---

Dollars and Health Sense

Fast Track Drug Approvals May Be Dangerous

A major responsibility of the Food and Drug Administration (FDA) is to protect consumers from unsafe and useless drugs. Because the testing of new drugs is both expensive and time consuming, new drugs can get "fast track" approval if they meet certain criteria. However, fast track approval is not without consequences. Between 1997 and 2000, ten different drugs given fast track approval by the FDA were later withdrawn from the market because they were found to be harmful and, in some cases, lethal. One of these drugs was troglitazone, an anti-diabetes drug that the FDA banned in early 2000. There had been 88 cases of liver failure and 61 deaths linked to troglitazone use.

Controversy has swirled around troglitazone since it was approved for use in the United States in 1997. The drug potentially could cause liver damage, and it already had been banned in the United Kingdom and Japan for this reason. To counteract the concern that people taking the drug risked fatal liver damage, proponents of troglitazone said the risk could be managed if doctors who prescribed the drug tested patients periodically for liver damage; if any damage appeared, the patients could be taken off the drug. This strategy failed, however, because less than 30% of doctors even knew to do the tests and fewer still ordered them.

At the FDA approval hearings for troglitazone, the committee was split. Five members voted for approval, and five voted against approval. The committee chairperson voted against approval, but troglitazone was approved anyway. An FDA medical officer subsequently was fired because of his opposition to approval of the drug. In 1994, a research scientist said that she was "coerced" to downplay liver problems in two patients on whom she tested troglitazone prior to FDA approval. In 1999, an FDA medical officer had to ask the U.S. Congress to pressure administrators at the FDA to remove troglitazone from the market.

In 2001, the *Los Angeles Times* newspaper reported that highly placed officials at the FDA had leaked information to executives at the drug company that developed and sold troglitazone. At the behest of the drug company, FDA officials fired the staff person who opposed troglitazone's approval and also pressured other staff members not to speak publicly about troglitazone's effects on the liver.

The troglitazone situation has raised serious questions about the influence of the pharmaceutical industry on the FDA's drug approval process—something all consumers should be concerned about.

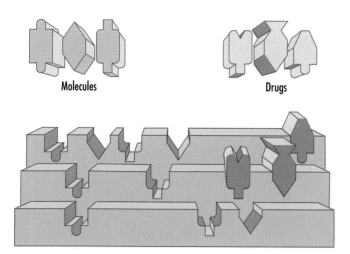

FIGURE 16.1   Bindings of Drugs to Cellular Receptor Sites The molecular structures of many drugs are similar to molecules normally produced in the body. The drugs compete for receptor sites on cells and alter the physiological functioning of organs and tissues.

stop, speed up, or slow down a process, depending on the specific drug and its effect. A **medicine** is a drug (or combination of drugs) that is intended to: (a) prevent illness, as vaccines do; (b) cure disease, as antibiotics do; (c) aid healing, as ulcer medications do; or (d) suppress symptoms, as pain relievers do. Not all drugs —for example, alcohol and nicotine—are medicines.

Drugs are usually classified according to the particular biological process they affect rather than by their chemical properties. For example, all substances that increase urine production, regardless of their chemical structure, are called **diuretics;** those that reduce pain are **analgesics;** and those that produce nervous system excitation are stimulants.

How Drugs Work

Many drugs act by binding to **receptors** on the surface of, or within specific cells in the body. A drug-receptor interaction is akin to a key (the drug) fitting into a lock (the receptor) (see Figure 16.1). When a drug binds to a cell's receptor, it alters one or more biological processes of the cell. Frequently, a drug may chemically resemble a natural body component, such as a hormone or a neurotransmitter, which interacts with the receptor as part of normal functioning. The drug binds to the receptor in place of the natural substance and thereby alters physiology.

For example, the receptors for many antibiotics are on structures within bacteria that are responsible for manufacturing vital bacterial proteins. When an antibiotic binds to its receptor in a bacterium, it blocks the manufacture of bacterial proteins, the bacteria do not reproduce, and the infection stops. The receptors for many antidepressant drugs are located in the brain on cells that utilize the neurotransmitter serotonin. When an antidepressant binds

to its receptor, serotonin transport into those cells is blocked, and depression is relieved.

Unintended Harmful Effects of Drugs

Even though a drug may be intended to have a single effect, it often has more than one, because it binds to a variety of receptors in or on different cells. Unintended drug actions are called **side effects** (Figure 16.2), which may be minor or severe. Some side effects include allergic reactions (**drug hypersensitivity**); harm to developing embryos and fetuses (**teratogen**); or physical dependence.

Drug side effects can be quite dangerous. One study estimated that, each year in the U.S., drug side effects are responsible for injury and illness in over 2 million hospitalized patients (Lazarou et al., 1998). Furthermore, drug side effects are responsible for the deaths of 100,000 hospitalized patients per year, making them the sixth leading cause of death in the U.S. These adverse drug reactions are caused by the unintended effects of the drugs and not to errors in prescribing or dosing, drug abuse, or accidental poisoning. This means that in the present climate of heavy drug advertising, it is necessary for good health to remember and respect that drugs are potent biological agents with both benefits and potentially fatal drawbacks.

In addition to side effects, a drug also may be harmful if the drug-taker has a condition that is aggravated by that drug. A medical reason for not taking a drug is called a **contraindication.** For example, a history of blood vessel disease is a contraindication for taking birth control pills. The need to screen for contraindications is one reason why many medicines are available only by prescription.

Medical practitioners should be knowledgeable about the side effects and contraindications of drugs,

Terms

drug: a single chemical substance in a medicine that alters one or more of the body's biological functions

medicine: drugs used to prevent, treat, or cure illness; aid healing; or suppress symptoms

diuretics: drugs that increase urine production

analgesics: drugs that relieve pain

receptor: protein on the surface or inside a cell to which a drug or natural substance can bind and thereby affect cell function

side effects: unintended and often harmful actions of a drug

drug hypersensitivity: an allergic reaction to a drug

teratogen: a drug that affects the development of a fetus, causing birth defects

contraindication: any medical reason for not taking a particular drug

Common side effects of drugs of abuse

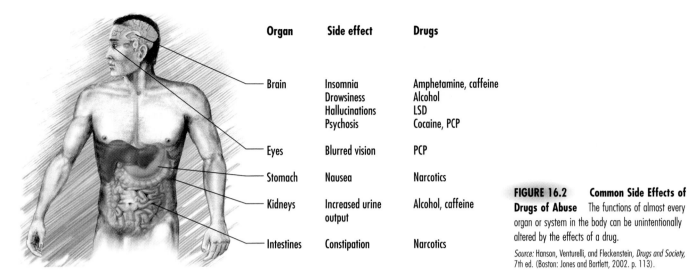

Organ	Side effect	Drugs
Brain	Insomnia	Amphetamine, caffeine
	Drowsiness	Alcohol
	Hallucinations	LSD
	Psychosis	Cocaine, PCP
Eyes	Blurred vision	PCP
Stomach	Nausea	Narcotics
Kidneys	Increased urine output	Alcohol, caffeine
Intestines	Constipation	Narcotics

FIGURE 16.2 **Common Side Effects of Drugs of Abuse** The functions of almost every organ or system in the body can be unintentionally altered by the effects of a drug.

Source: Hanson, Venturelli, and Fleckenstein, *Drugs and Society,* 7th ed. (Boston: Jones and Bartlett, 2002. p. 113).

but sometimes these are overlooked. About one-third of hospital stays are needlessly extended because inappropriate medications are administered or managed improperly by medical staff. The United States Institute of Medicine estimates that 7,000 Americans die each year from medication errors. Consumers of medications should learn as much as they can about the intended use and side effects of their drugs, and they should ask their medical providers to explain the rationale for the medications prescribed (Table 16.1).

Routes of Administration

Drugs can be taken by mouth, inhalation, or injection into the muscles, under the skin (from which they diffuse into surrounding tissues and blood) or directly into the bloodstream. Drugs also can be absorbed through the skin and the mucous membranes of the nose, eyes, vagina, and anus. Regardless of the route of entry, most drugs remain active in the body for several hours.

Once in the body, drugs are degraded or destroyed by the liver and the lungs. Drugs are also filtered by the kidneys and eliminated from the body in urine. Drugs such as inhalatory anesthetics or nitrous oxide are eliminated in expired air.

Terms

dose: amount of drug that is administered

double-blind: when neither the person receiving the drug nor the person administering the drug know whether it is a placebo or the real drug

Effectiveness of Drugs

The **dose** of a drug is the amount that is administered or taken. The effectiveness of a particular dose of a drug is influenced by a person's body size, how rapidly the drug breaks down and is eliminated, and sometimes, by the presence of other drugs and foods recently consumed (Table 16.2). A drug's effectiveness also depends on the person's expectations of the drug's efficacy (placebo effect) (see chapter 3) and the

TABLE 16.1 **Latin Terms Commonly Used in Prescriptions**

Latin	Abbreviation	Meaning
ante cibum	ac	before meals
bis in die	bid	twice a day
gutta	gt	drop
hora somni	hs	at bedtime
oculus dexter	od	right eye
oculus sinister	os	left eye
per os	po	by mouth
post cibum	pc	after meals
pro re nata	prn	as needed
quaque 3 hora	q 3 h	every 3 hours
quaque die	qd	every day
quater in die	qid	four times a day
ter in die	tid	three times a day
†, ††, or †††		1, 2, or 3 (of the dosage form, such as tablets)

TABLE 16.2   Drug and Food Interactions That Should Be Avoided

If you take	Avoid	Because
Erythromycin or penicillin-type antibiotics	Acidic foods; pickles, tomatoes, vinegar, colas	These antibiotics are destroyed by stomach acids
Tetracycline-type antibiotics	Calcium-rich foods: milk, cheese, yogurt, pizza, almonds	Calcium blocks the action of tetracycline
Antihypertensives (to lower blood pressure)	Natural licorice (artificial is OK)	A chemical in natural licorice causes salt and water retention
Anticoagulants (to thin blood)	Vitamin K: green leafy vegetables, beef liver, vegetable oils	Vitamin K promotes blood clotting
Antidepressants (monoamine oxidase inhibitors)	Tyramine-rich foods: colas, chocolate, cheese, coffee, wine, avocados	Tyramine elevates blood pressure
Diuretics	Monosodium glutamate (MSG)	MSG and diuretics both increase water elimination
Thyroid drugs	Cabbage, brussels sprouts, soybeans, cauliflower	Chemicals in these vegetables depress thyroid hormone production

person's mental state. For example, when stressed or anxious, many people require higher doses of analgesics to relieve pain than when they are relaxed. Most drugs have a narrow range of effectiveness, i.e., doses that produce intended results. In excess, many drugs are toxic and some are lethal. If the dose is too low, insufficient therapeutic effect may result.

The effects of a drug or medicine are often determined scientifically by performing double-blind clinical trials, which involve administering the drug and a look-and-taste-alike placebo to matched groups of patients. Neither the people administering the drug nor the patients know who is receiving the drug and who is receiving the placebo (thus the expression **double-blind**). Only after the trial is the code revealed that tells which patients received the drug. What is most remarkable about many of these drug trials is not that drugs show a therapeutic effect, but that placebos often come very close to giving the same relief or results as do the drugs (see chapter 2).

In 1984, ibuprofen was introduced into the over-the-counter (OTC) market. Because aspirin and acetaminophen compounds commanded over 90% of the pain-reliever market, manufacturers of ibuprofen advertised heavily in medical journals to get physicians to recommend or prescribe the new drug. One advertisement showed that, after 4 hours, Nuprin, the trade name for an ibuprofen drug, relieved headaches about 8% more effectively than acetaminophen (Figure 16.3). From a holistic health perspective, however, the more significant result is that 40% of headache sufferers got the same relief with a placebo. Thus, 4 out of 10 headache sufferers found relief simply by believing that they had taken a pain-relief medicine.

An even more remarkable placebo effect is shown by the ability of balding men to stimulate hair growth simply by believing that they are using a hair-stimulating drug called Rogaine. The Upjohn Company, manufacturer of Rogaine, advertises extensively in the most prestigious medical journals and on TV. In

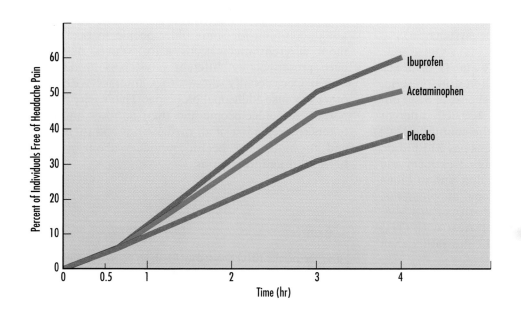

FIGURE 16.3   A Study of the Effectiveness of Ibuprofen versus Acetaminophen in Relieving Headaches   Note that 40% of headache sufferers get relief with no drug at all.

More over-the-counter drugs are available in the United States than anywhere else in the world.

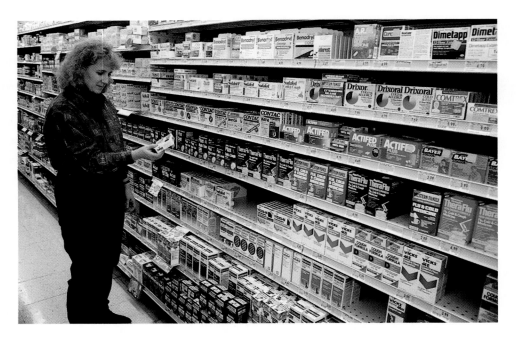

these ads, the company emphasizes the effectiveness of Rogaine compared to a placebo solution applied to the scalp. Rogaine produces minimal to moderate growth of new hair in 33% of patients receiving the drug. However, a placebo containing no active ingredient produces minimal to moderate hair growth in 20% of patients. While this fact is ignored by the advertising, it means that one out of five men who have pattern baldness (an inherited trait) can stimulate new hair growth simply because they believe they are using a drug. How the mind changes physiology to accomplish this is unknown. The point, however, is never to underestimate the power of your mind to act like a drug and help you to heal an injury or illness.

The Overmedicating of Americans

Americans consume an enormous quantity of drugs. In the United States, about two billion drug prescriptions are filled each year at an annual cost of $120 billion. In addition, there are about 100,000 different kinds of nonprescription, or **over-the-counter (OTC) drugs,** purchased, for which Americans pay $15 billion a year. Millions of people ingest herbal extracts and teas for their purported medicinal value, and millions more take vitamins, not as nutritional supplements, but as medicine. Indeed, when Americans are sick, four times out of five times they self-treat with OTC drugs and so-called alternative medicines rather than visit a medical doctor.

More than one-fourth of the legal drugs sold in the U.S. are **psychoactive,** i.e., they alter thoughts, feelings, and sensations. Psychoactive drugs include tranquilizers, sleeping pills, and mood modifiers. About 100 million Americans use alcohol regularly, another 53 million smoke cigarettes or chew tobacco for the stimulant effects of nicotine, and more than one-third of adult Americans ingest caffeine daily for its stimulatory effects. In addition, about 12 million Americans regularly use illegal drugs (e.g., marijuana, cocaine, LSD, heroin) for the drug experience, to fit in socially, to self-medicate, or to ward off the misery of not taking a drug to which one is addicted.

As a group, older persons tend to take the most drugs, usually because they have a variety of chronic medical complaints. Two-thirds of those over age 65 take one drug per day; one-fourth of people over age 65 take three or more drugs per day (Williams, 1997). It is not uncommon for some older people to take 10 or more different medications daily, which may have been prescribed by different physicians at different times. Occasionally these drugs interact with each other to cause additional problems. That's why it's important for older people and their families and caretakers to keep a list of all medications and their doses and to inquire of health providers about possible harmful drug interactions.

Terms

over-the-counter (OTC) drugs: drugs that do not require a prescription

psychoactive: any substance that primarily alters mood, perception, and other brain functions

In American society, the belief that drugs are legitimate and desirable solutions to life problems is pervasive. Consider this ad that appeared in a medical journal in 1997: A middle-aged man sits at a table in a restaurant on which there's a bowl of chili, a plate of fried food, and a bottle of hot sauce. The man's face signals discomfort and his right hand is placed on his obviously upset stomach. The headline in the ad says "OH, MY GERD," referring to the man's recurring problem with heartburn (called "gastroesophageal reflux disease" in medical language). The ad, of course, is for a drug that relieves the symptoms of heartburn. No mention is made of the possibility that avoiding foods that cause this man to be so miserable (the ones on the table before him) is another way for him to feel better.

About half of all doctor visits are for nonmedical or mental health problems that manifest as fatigue, lethargy, gastrointestinal upset, aches and pains, and sleeplessness. Often patients expect health care providers to prescribe a medicine, and just as often, health care providers feel obligated to offer some remedy, even if a medically legitimate one does not exist. The answer to this dilemma is provided by pharmaceutical companies that manufacture and advertise mood-altering drugs. If a person is anxious, drug ads suggest offering a tranquilizer; for depression, an antidepressant; for sleep problems, a sedative or hypnotic.

In some cases, the tranquilizer or sleeping pill may help temporarily. Sometimes people become so depressed or upset over a life situation that they cannot muster the clear thinking and action necessary to deal with the problem. In such instances, a sleeping medication, tranquilizer, or antidepressant may help achieve a calmer psychological state in which appropriate action can be taken. Unfortunately, too many people and their doctors mistakenly assume that the drug itself will solve the problem; whereas, it may, instead, substitute for proper help and treatment.

Many physicians recognize this problem. They would prefer to deal only with physically ill people—the patients whose problems they were educated to treat. But many patients resist the suggestion that they do not have a disease for which there is a diagnosis and insist that they receive a drug; this is a serious form of drug abuse. As people become more informed and aware of the undesirable consequences of taking drugs and how infrequently drugs are really necessary, they will elect to cope with stress and anxiety in ways that do not involve drugs.

Being healthy means, among other things, being responsible for the drugs you use. You do not have to resort to "chemical coping" for emotional problems. You can resist being pushed into "pill popping" by drug company advertising. Seeking alternatives to prescription or over-the-counter drug use may be the most healthful action you can take (see chapter 20).

Drug Company Advertising

Through advertising to both consumers and health care providers, drug companies encourage drug-taking. Because most drug sales come from prescription medications, the heaviest drug company advertising is directed toward physicians. Drug companies spend more than $10,000 per year per physician trying to persuade them to prescribe the drugs that they manufacture (Wazana, 2000). Drug companies send sales representatives to doctors' offices, hospitals, and health maintenance organizations (HMOs) to inform them of the company's products and to leave free samples. Drug companies sponsor seminars and courses often accompanied by free lunches or vacations to update health care providers on the diagnosis and treatment of particular diseases (for which the company manufactures a drug). And drug companies deluge physicians with pharmaceutical "junk" mail; one doctor received more than 500 pounds of drug company junk mail in one year.

Pharmaceutical companies spend more than $11 billion each year promoting their products in a variety of ways. Consider the antibiotic Zithromax, which was marketed to doctors and parents using a doll-mascot, Max the Zebra (remember that the name of the product is ZithroMAX). Pediatricians were given stuffed zebras to give to their patients; the drug's manufacturer donated a zebra to the San Francisco Zoo (guess the animal's name); a season of "Sesame Street" was sponsored by the drug's manufacturer, and the "Sesame Street" character Elmo helped to promote the drug. This marketing scheme is intended to influence doctors to prescribe and parents to demand Zithromax for the treatment of otitis media, an inner ear infection that is common among children. However, a study commissioned by the Centers for Disease Control and Prevention reported that Zithromax is not a particularly effective treatment for ear infections and that a different antibiotic (amoxicillin), which has been used for years, is still the best treatment. A standard course of treatment with amoxicillin costs less than $10. The same treatment with Zithromax is about $30. Because the FDA approved Zithromax for ear infections, the manufacturer is doing nothing illegal by promoting the drug to doctors and parents.

In addition to physicians and other health care professionals, consumers also are targets of prescription drug advertising. In 1996, the FDA relaxed its regulations regarding the advertising of prescription medications directly to consumers, and pharmaceutical

Dollars and Health Sense

Profits and Medicines Sometimes Don't Mix

Americans were fortunate that the 2000–2001 flu season was mild, because there was a shortage of the flu vaccine. The companies that make the flu vaccine had to curtail vaccine production in some of their manufacturing plants because the FDA found those facilities to be out of compliance with FDA manufacturing standards. With the plants closed down, there was less vaccine for distribution.

Health officials knew of the shortage months before flu season arrived, and they tried to get what supplies were available to people most at risk (e.g., the elderly and children) and health care workers. The healthy adult population was supposed to wait until sufficient supplies of the vaccine became available. However, on hearing that the vaccine was being rationed, businesses, colleges, and other organizations purchased large quantities of the vaccine for their members, and many individuals offered to pay high prices to be vaccinated by their doctors. Distributors of the flu vaccine were happy to comply with the intense demand by raising the price of the vaccine by as much as 1000%.

Many doctors and health officials accused the pharmaceutical distributors of price gouging. They also were critical of the vaccine manufacturers who were out of compliance with FDA regulations for failing in their social obligation to be sure that the production facilities in which the vaccine was made conformed to FDA standards of safety.

Besides the flu vaccine, several other drugs that doctors depend on have been rationed because of production shortages. For example, in 2001, one of the two manufacturers of the tetanus vaccine stopped production because it considered that vaccine unprofitable. The same manufacturer discontinued a drug used in eye surgery for the same reason. Because the FDA has no authority to force a company to manufacture a particular vaccine or drug, the country's drug supply is theoretically at risk. The fear is that companies will develop and market only drugs with high profit potential and limit or stop altogether production of drugs that no longer contribute sufficiently to profits.

---

companies quickly found that **direct-to-consumer (DTC) advertising** is very profitable. One example is the allergy medication Claritin, which was not a big seller until TV personalities and athletes were featured in TV commercials for the drug. Within a short period of time, sales of Claritin skyrocketed. Another example is the cholesterol-lowering drug Lipitor, sales of which rose 56% in 1999 after its manufacturer increased DTC advertising for the drug from $7.8 million to $55.4 million. The success of DTC advertising is confirmed by the fact that in the year 2000, the pharmaceutical industry spent nearly $2 billion on it, and 25 of the most frequently advertised drugs accounted for more than 40% of drug sales.

Direct-to-consumer advertising is designed to encourage consumers to demand advertised drugs from their health care providers in the belief that the drugs they see in advertisements are superior, while unadvertised, lesser-known generic drugs are inferior. This creates pressure on health care providers to prescribe advertised drugs, even if another (or generic) medication is available and less expensive. Many doctors are "rated" for customer service by the HMOs that pay them, so they do not want to make patients angry. If no harm is done medically, sometimes it is easier for a physician to say "yes" rather than argue with a patient who is determined to obtain a specific drug. To make it easier to say "yes," pharmaceutical companies provide large cost reductions for their advertised drugs to pharmacies run by HMOs in exchange for the HMO allowing doctors to exclusively prescribe the advertised drugs.

A subtle form of DTC drug advertising involves famous retired athletes revealing in interviews on TV news and talk shows that they have or are currently battling a serious illness. What is usually not disclosed in these interviews is that the retired celebrity is being paid by a pharmaceutical company to participate in the interview to help sell a drug. For example, Bart Conner, a retired gymnast, was paid to talk about the drug Celebrex as a treatment for his osteoarthritis. Athletes Dorothy Hamill and Bruce Jenner did the same thing to help sell the arthritis drug Vioxx. Unlike other commercial endorsements by well-known athletes and coaches, these interviews are presented both to journalists and the public as news stories and not commercials; the financial arrangement between the ex-athlete and the pharmaceutical company is generally kept secret.

The Internet plays into DTC advertising, too. If consumers go to a Web site that supposedly offers information about a health issue (say, sleep problems),

Terms

direct-to-consumer advertising: the marketing of prescription drugs to consumers in order to stimulate demand for a drug

drug abuse: persistent or excessive use of a drug without medical or health reasons

addiction: physical and psychological dependence on a drug, substance, or behavior

and they fill out a form to get more information, they may soon find in their mailbox a $5 coupon for a prescription sleep medication—a product of the pharmaceutical company that sponsored the sleep-problem Web site.

Proponents of DTC marketing (besides drug companies and their stockholders) say it benefits consumers by making them more aware of both illness and medications. Opponents of DTC advertising argue that it can make it difficult for doctors to prescribe appropriate medications and that it creates a demand for drugs in lieu of non-drug treatments and prevention. One problem with this barrage of advertising is that it reinforces the general message that a drug is the first-line answer to a medical condition. The United States is the only industrialized country in the world that permits DTC advertising of prescription medications.

Consequences of Drug Use

The human body is capable of tolerating and eliminating small quantities of virtually any substance or drug with no permanent harmful effects. However, it may be harmful to ingest large doses or to use a drug often even in small quantities. Generally, using any drug to the point where health is adversely affected or the ability to function in society is impaired can be defined as **drug abuse.**

Drug abuse refers not to the type or amount of a drug taken but to whether or not the person taking the drug is personally or socially impaired. If a drug is used to mask anxiety or facilitate undesirable behaviors, it is being abused. If a drug is used continually to combat the effects of stress, it is being abused. If pleasure is experienced only when a drug is taken, the drug is being abused. If a person cannot control the use of a drug, it is being abused.

Most of the commonly abused drugs are psychoactive substances that affect thoughts, perceptions, feelings, and moods; in other words, they change consciousness (Table 16.3). Consciousness is the state of being aware of one's mental processes. Each of us has a "normal" state of consciousness, although many people would have difficulty describing what they mean by "normal." However, everyone knows when his or her state of consciousness deviates from normal—for example, when drunk, extremely angry, sad, or depressed. A high fever can alter consciousness even to the point of hallucinations.

There are numerous activities not generally regarded as consciousness-altering that produce changes in consciousness comparable in many respects to those produced by psychoactive drugs. Long-distance runners may experience a change of consciousness that is described as a "runners' high"; dancing can produce psychic "highs" and even ecstatic states of consciousness, which is the goal of the whirling dervishes who practice particular forms of Sufi dancing. Fasting can produce profound changes in consciousness, which is why prolonged fasts are often part of religious training. Many "thrill" activities, such as riding on roller coasters, shooting the rapids on river rafts, or bungee-jumping, change consciousness and presumably are enjoyed for that reason. Put into this perspective, ingesting psychoactive drugs is only one of many ways people use to change consciousness.

Taking psychoactive drugs to alter consciousness is particularly dangerous because the cognitive, emotional, and behavioral processes that the drugs alter are required for harmonious adaptation to one's environment. Drugs that induce pleasant emotions can give a false sense of benefit. Drugs that block uncomfortable emotions (e.g., sadness, fear, pain) can impair useful defenses. Furthermore, regular use of psychoactive drugs can alter the biology of the brain to the point that drug-using becomes a goal in itself, irrespective of any desire to alter thoughts and emotions.

> *Freedom's just another word for nothing left to lose.*
> JANIS JOPLIN

Addiction

One of the many dangers of drug abuse is **addiction,** which is a progressive, chronic, primary disease that is characterized by:

- Compulsion: An overwhelming preoccupation, desire, or drive to use a psychoactive drug, which can include obsessive thinking about a drug and drug-seeking and drug-hoarding behavior
- Loss of control: The inability to control use of a drug or loss of control over one's behavior because of taking a drug (e.g., impulsive actions, verbal or physical violence, impulsive sexual behavior)
- Continued drug use despite adverse consequences: The tendency not to stop drug use in the face of arrest, job loss, family breakdown, and health problems
- Distortions in normal thinking: Not admitting that problems are the result of drug-taking (denial)

Addiction is chronic and progressive: It tends to get worse over time, not better. Family members who wait for an addicted family member to "get better" generally are severely disappointed. Addiction is classified as a primary disease because, from a medical point of view, addiction has certain characteristics and treatments regardless of the substance to which a person is addicted.

Physical Dependence

Addiction is often associated with **physical dependence** (also called tissue dependence), which is biological adaptation to long-term exposure to a drug. First-time or infrequent use of a psychoactive drug causes intoxication because the drug upsets the biological balance in the brain. With continued use of a psychoactive drug, actual physical changes take place in brain tissues to adapt to the continual presence of the drug (Figure 16.4).

TABLE 16.3   Classifications of Drugs That Affect the Central Nervous System

Drug classification	Common or trade name	Medical uses	Effects of average dose	Physical dependence	Tolerance develops
Narcotics	Codeine Demerol Heroin Methadone Morphine Opium Percodan	Analgesic (pain relief)	Blocks or eases pain; may cause drowsiness and euphoria; some users experience nausea or itching sensations	Marked	Yes
Analgesics	Darvon Talwin	Pain relief	May produce anxiety and hallucinations	Marked	Yes
Sedatives	Amytal Nembutal Phenobarbital Seconal Doriden Quaalude Halcion	Sedation, tension relief	Relaxation, sleep; decreases alertness and muscle coordination	Marked	Yes
Minor tranquilizers	Dalmane Equanil/Miltown Librium Valium Xanax	Anxiety relief, muscle tension	Mild sedation; increased sense of well-being; may cause drowsiness and dizziness	Marked	No
Major tranquilizers (phenothiazines)	Mellaril Thorazine Prolixin	Control psychosis	Heavy sedation, anxiety relief; may cause confusion, muscle rigidity, convulsions	None	No
Alcohol	Beer Wine Liquor	None	Relaxation; loss of inhibition; mood swings; decreased alertness and coordination	Marked	Yes
Inhalants	Amyl nitrite Butyl nitrite Nitrous oxide	Muscle relaxant, anesthetic	Relaxation, euphoria; causes dizziness, headache, drowsiness	None	?
Stimulants	Benzedrine Biphetamine Desoxyn Dexedrine Methedrine Preludin Ritalin	Weight control, narcolepsy; fatigue and hyperactivity in children	Increased alertness and mood elevation; less fatigue and increased concentration; may cause insomnia, anxiety, headache, chills, and rise in blood pressure; organic brain damage after prolonged use	Mild to none	Yes
Cocaine	Cocaine hydrochloride	Local anesthetic, pain relief	Effects similar to stimulants	Marked	No
Cannabis	Marijuana Hashish	Relief of glaucoma, asthma, nausea accompanying chemotherapy	Relaxation, euphoria, altered perception; may cause confusion, panic, hallucinations	None	No
Hallucinogens	LSD PCP Mescaline Peyote Psilocybin	None	Altered perceptions, visual and sensory distortion; mood swings	None	Yes
Nicotine	(In tobacco)	None	Altered heart rate; tremors; excitation	Yes	Yes

Both legal and illegal drugs can cause physical dependence. The legality of a drug is more a function of social, political, and economic considerations than the drug's toxicity or pharmacology. From a personal and community health standpoint, alcohol causes far more harm than all other drugs combined, yet it is legal.

The legal status of drugs changes with social customs and people's beliefs. In the 1920s and 1930s, alcohol was illegal in the United States but marijuana was legal. During the early twentieth century, opium, morphine, and cocaine were openly advertised and sold in the form of tonics and cough syrups. Coca-Cola, concocted by a Georgia pharmacist in 1886, was sold as both a remedy and an enjoyable drink. "Coke" contained cocaine until 1906, when the cocaine was replaced by caffeine.

Tolerance

Tolerance is an adaptation of the body to a drug so that larger doses are needed to produce the same effect. Thus, the longer one uses a drug, the more of that drug must be consumed to produce the desired effect. Because not all parts of the body become tolerant to a drug to the same degree, these higher doses may be dangerous. For example, a heroin or barbiturate user can become tolerant to the psychological effects of the drug, but the user's respiratory center in the brain, which controls breathing, does not. If the person takes a high dose of heroin or barbiturate to overcome the tolerance to the drug's psychological effects, the brain's respiratory center may cease to function as a result of the overdose, and the person may stop breathing.

Withdrawal

A consequence of physical dependence is the experience of withdrawal (or abstinence syndrome), which occurs when the body adapts to the absence of a drug on which it has become physically dependent. Withdrawal is often uncomfortable, and it may be fatal. For example, someone physically dependent on heroin may experience anxiety, pain, sweating, muscle cramps, frightening hallucinations, and fatal seizures when deprived of the drug. Indeed, for those who have experienced withdrawal, the fear of experiencing it again may become a greater motivator to continue drug use than the effects of the drug itself.

With many drugs, **withdrawal symptoms** are the opposite of the drug's primary effects. In general, withdrawal from central nervous system depressants, such as alcohol, opiates, tranquilizers, and sedatives, leads to symptoms such as hyperexcitedness, anxiousness, irritability, and susceptibility to seizures. Withdrawal from stimulants, such as cocaine, amphetamines, and caffeine, on the other hand, can produce sleepiness, depression, and loss of consciousness.

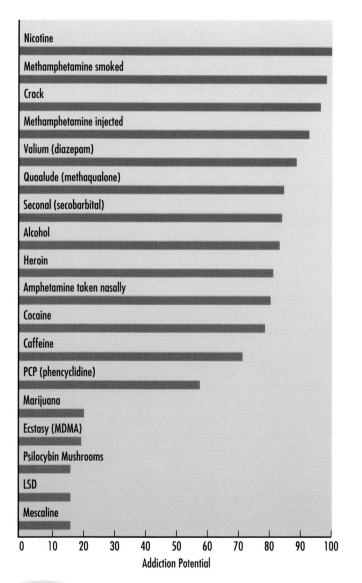

FIGURE 16.4   Health experts' ratings of how easy it is to become addicted and how difficult it is to stop using the following drugs, with 100 being the highest addiction potential. Note that both legal and illegal drugs can be highly addictive.

Source: Hanson and Venturelli, Drugs and Society, *6th ed. (Boston: Jones and Bartlett, 2001), p 95.*

Terms

physical dependence: a physiological state that depends on the continuous presence of a drug; absence of the drug may cause discomfort, nervousness, headaches, and sweating (withdrawal symptoms) and sometimes death

tolerance: a condition in which increased amounts of a drug or increased exposure to an addictive behavior are required to produce desired effects

withdrawal symptoms: uncomfortable and sometimes dangerous reactions that occur after a person stops taking a physically addicting drug

Managing Stress

Meditation

It's fair to say that most people experiment with drugs as a result of curiosity, peer pressure, or a combination of the two. What may begin as an innocent experiment, however, can become a struggle for self-sovereignty.

People who have given up drugs give a number of reasons, the most common being that although the trips may have been exciting, the side effects were horrendous, if not tragic. This was the case with the Beatles, who found that drug use stifled rather than promoted their creative efforts. Seeking a way to gain passage through the door to objective reality, they met Maharishi Mahesh Yogi, the founder of transcendental meditation (TM). And so began a journey of exploration of human consciousness, natural highs, and profound revelations without the unwanted baggage of side effects and addiction.

Today we know that there are many ways to meditate. What is important is to find a style that's right for you. The standard definition of meditation is increased concentration leading to increased awareness, and indeed, with repeated practice, some experiences may occur that surpass any drug-induced high.

Meditation isn't so much thinking about something as it is *not* thinking about anything. Meditation is a way to clear the thoughts from your mind and deactivate the censoring process of the ego to open the way for new insights, wisdom, intuition, or enlightenment that otherwise go unnoticed in the course of a hectic day.

The steps to meditation are easy. They require nothing more than (a) a quiet environment, (b) a comfortable body position, (c) a passive attitude, and (d) a meditative object (such as your breathing or the sound of ocean waves.)

After accomplishing the first three steps, try this exercise:

Imagine yourself standing in a cylinder, about four feet in diameter, made of concrete blocks. As you look up, you see the walls are high, too high to climb. The walls represent the walls of your ego. Each block has etched in it a description of an issue you are dealing with or an unresolved conflict with another person. The way out is not through physical means, but rather through your mental, emotional, and spiritual energies. First, you take a few slow deep breaths to relax your mind and body. By trying to address each issue in your mind (e.g., patience, detachment, forgiveness, acceptance), you slowly see the walls begin to descend, eventually to a point where you are no longer held captive by your thoughts and feelings of anger and anxiety. You are free of the limitations of your own mind. As these walls disappear, what do you see in front of you, and all around you? What do you experience? Take a moment to sense all that you can.

This is just one of many types of meditation exercises to help you shift your way of thinking and explore the realms of consciousness without the aid or complications of drugs.

Psychological Dependence

Besides physical dependence, drugs can create **habituation** or **psychological dependence**, which are manifested as an intense craving for the drug. Habituation becomes injurious when a person becomes so consumed by the need for the desired drugged state that all of that person's energy is siphoned into compulsive drug-seeking behavior. Physically addicting drugs like heroin, alcohol, and nicotine often produce habituation. As a consequence of compulsive drug-seeking behavior, relationships, jobs, and families may be destroyed.

Stimulants

Stimulants are substances that increase the activity of the central nervous system. These drugs include cocaine, amphetamine, amphetamine-like drugs, and caffeine. Their main effects are an increase in mental arousal and physical energy and production of a state of euphoria, which is why they are referred to as "uppers." Stimulants also can cause restlessness, talkativeness, and difficulty sleeping. Long-term use of stimulants tends to produce physical and psychological dependence.

Cocaine

Cocaine is obtained from the leaves of the coca shrub, *Erythroxylum coca*, a plant indigenous to the Andes. For thousands of years, inhabitants of Peru, Bolivia, and Colombia have chewed coca leaves to obtain a

Terms

habituation: psychological dependence arising from repeated use of a drug

psychological dependence: dependence that results because a drug produces pleasant mental effects

stimulants: substances that increase the activity of the central nervous system

cocaine: a stimulant drug, obtained from the leaves of the coca shrub, that causes feelings of exhilaration, euphoria, and physical vigor

amphetamines: synthetic drugs that stimulate the central nervous system and sometimes produce hallucinogenic states

moderate stimulant effect intended to overcome fatigue. After the Spanish conquest of the Inca empire in the sixteenth century, coca leaves were introduced to Europe and later to North America. In the late nineteenth century, Angelo Mariani, a Corsican, received a medal from the pope for manufacturing an extract of coca leaves that "freed the body of fatigue, lifted the spirits, and induced a sense of well-being." In the United States in the 1880s, Atlanta pharmacist J. C. Pemberton mixed extracts of coca leaves and kola nuts to produce Coca-Cola, claimed at the time to be not only refreshing but also "exhilarating, invigorating, and a cure for all nervous afflictions." Today, of course, Coke no longer contains cocaine, although cocaine-free extracts of coca leaves are still used for flavoring. Sigmund Freud extolled the use of cocaine as a mood elevator, a possible antidote to depression, and a treatment for morphine addiction. However, witnessing a friend's severe and terrifying psychotic reaction to cocaine tempered Freud's enthusiasm for the drug.

As an illegal recreational drug, cocaine is most commonly taken into the body by sniffing ("snorting") it as a white powder, injecting it directly into the bloodstream (an obvious risk factor for AIDS), or smoking "free base" or "crack" cocaine. Each of these methods rapidly produces euphoria, a sense of power and clarity of thought, and increased physical vigor. The drug's effects last from minutes to an hour, depending on dose and the route of administration into the body. After the initial "high," users tend to experience a letdown ("crash") and an intense craving for more of the drug.

Cocaine increases heart rate and blood pressure. Continued use of the drug can result in appetite and weight loss, malnutrition, sleep disturbance, and altered thought and mood patterns. Frequent cocaine sniffing can inflame the nasal passages and cause permanent damage to the nasal septum. An overdose can cause seizures or death. Pregnant women who ingest cocaine risk giving birth to cocaine-addicted babies, who may be permanently handicapped or even die in infancy.

Cocaine does produce tolerance, physical dependence, and withdrawal. The potential for psychological dependence is great, probably the greatest among all psychoactive drugs. Some people develop such a strong craving for the drug that their lives are consumed by their cocaine habit.

Amphetamines

Amphetamines are manufactured chemicals that stimulate the central nervous system. The most common amphetamine substances are dextroamphetamine, methamphetamine, dextromethamphetamine, and amphetamine itself. Amphetamines are usually taken orally but they can also be injected ("mainlined") and smoked. The effects of an oral dose usually last several hours. Slang terms for amphetamines include dexies, footballs, orange, bennies, peaches, meth, speed, and ice.

Although amphetamines may be used medically to treat narcolepsy and attention-deficit hyperactivity disorder, they are principally used (illegally) to produce feelings of euphoria, increased energy, and greater self-confidence; an increased ability to concentrate; increased motor and speech activity; a perception of improved physical performance; and weight loss. Besides being used by those wishing to experience an amphetamine high, these drugs are frequently abused by people who fight sleep, such as students cramming for exams, entertainers, and truck drivers.

Excessive amphetamine use can cause headaches, irritability, dizziness, insomnia, panic, confusion, and delirium. The user often experiences a "crash," which occurs when the stimulants wear off, during which he or she usually is very depressed and tired and sleeps for long periods.

Prolonged use of amphetamines can lead to tolerance, especially for the euphoric effects and for appetite suppression. Amphetamines can cause mild physical dependence, and create a psychological dependence and a particular pattern of use called the "yo-yo," which is a cycle of amphetamine use for the stimulatory effect followed by use of a depressant in order to sleep, followed by more amphetamines the next day to get going. Chronic use can cause an amphetamine psychosis, consisting of auditory and visual hallucinations, delusions, and mood swings.

A particularly dangerous form of amphetamine is "ice"—a smoked form of pure methamphetamine hydrochloride. The inhaled drug reaches the brain almost immediately, producing a high that can last for several hours. Because the drug can be so easily inhaled, the potential for compulsive use, tolerance, and abuse is also very great. This amphetamine is manufactured at clandestine laboratories; the purity of the drug varies considerably from one laboratory to another, which adds to the risks of abusing it.

Ecstasy

Ecstasy is *3-4 methylenedioxymethamphetamine*, or MDMA. Some of its common nicknames are "Adam," "XTC," "Clarity," and "Essence." Ecstasy is a man-made chemical; that is, it does not occur naturally in plants. The substance has a chemical structure similar to the stimulant methamphetamine and the hallucinogen mescaline, and it can produce both stimulant and psychedelic effects. Ecstasy is most often available in tablet form and is taken orally. It also is available as a powder; it is

Wellness Guide

Risk Factors for Addiction

Risk factor	Leading to this effect
Biologically Based Factors (e.g., genetic, neurological, biochemical)	
• A less subjective feeling of intoxication	• More use to achieve intoxication (warning signs of abuse absent)
• Easier development of tolerance; liver enzymes adapt to increased use	• Easier to reach the addictive level
• Lack of resilience or fragility of higher (cerebral) brain functions	• Easy deterioration of cerebral functioning, impaired judgment, and social deterioration
• Difficulty in screening out unwanted or bothersome outside stimuli (low stimulus barrier)	• Feeling overwhelmed or stressed
• Tendency to amplify outside or internal stimuli (stimulus augmentation)	• Feeling attacked or panicked; need to avoid emotion
• Attention deficit hyperactivity disorder and other learning disabilities	• Failure, low self-esteem, or isolation
• Biologically based mood disorders (depression and bipolar disorders)	• Need to self-medicate against loss of control or the pain of depression; inability to calm down when manic or to sleep when agitated
Psychosocial and Developmental "Personality" Factors	
• Low self-esteem	• Need to blot out pain, gravitate to outsider groups
• Depression rooted in learned helplessness and passivity	• Need to blot out pain; use of a stimulant as an anti-depressant
• Conflicts	• Anxiety and guilt
• Repressed and unresolved grief and rage	• Chronic depression, anxiety, or pain
• Post-traumatic stress syndrome (as in veterans and abuse victims)	• Nightmares or panic attacks
Social and Cultural Environment	
• Availability of drugs	• Easy, frequent use
• Chemical-abusing parental model	• Sanction; no conflict over use
• Abusive, neglectful parents; other dysfunctional family patterns	• Pervasive sense of abandonment, distrust, and pain; difficulty in maintaining attachments
• Group norms favoring heavy use and abuse	• Reinforced, hidden abusive behavior that can progress without interference
• Misperception of peer norms	• Belief that most people use or favor use or think it's "cool" to use
• Severe or chronic stressors, as from noise, poverty, racism, or occupational stress	• Need to alleviate or escape from stress via chemical means
• "Alienation" factors: isolation, emptiness	• Painful sense of aloneness, normlessness, rootlessness, boredom, monotony, or hopelessness
• Difficult migration or acculturation with social disorganization, gender or generation gaps, or loss of role	• Stress without buffering support system

Source: Hanson, Venturelli, and Fleckenstein, *Drugs and Society,* 7th ed. (Boston: Jones and Bartlett, 2002. p. 95).

sometimes snorted and occasionally smoked, but rarely injected.

Ecstasy stimulates the release of the neurotransmitter serotonin from brain neurons, producing a high that lasts from several minutes to an hour. The drug's rewarding effects vary with the individual taking it, the dose, purity, and the environment in which it is taken. Ecstasy can produce stimulant effects, such as an enhanced sense of pleasure and self-confidence and increased energy. Its psychedelic effects include feelings of peacefulness, acceptance, and empathy. Users claim they experience feelings of closeness with others and a desire to touch them. Because Ecstasy engenders feelings of closeness and trust and has a short duration of action, some clinicians claim that the drug is potentially valuable as a psychotherapeutic agent. However, Ecstasy is classified by federal regulators as a drug with no accepted medical use.

The risks associated with using Ecstasy are similar to those found with the use of amphetamines and cocaine:

- confusion, depression, sleep problems, drug craving, severe anxiety, and paranoia during and sometimes weeks after taking the drug
- muscle tension, involuntary teeth clenching, nausea, blurred vision, rapid eye movement, faintness, and chills or sweating
- increases in heart rate and blood pressure
- long-term damage to serotonin-producing nerve cells in the brain
- liver damage with long-term use

Ecstasy-related fatalities have been reported; still, ecstasy is the fastest-growing illegal drug in America (Klam, 2001). The stimulant effects of the drug, which enable the user to dance for extended periods, combined

TABLE 16.4   Caffeine Content of Beverages and Chocolate

Beverage	Caffeine content (mg)	Amount
Brewed coffee	90–125	5 oz.
Instant coffee	14–93	5 oz.
Decaffeinated coffee	1–6	5 oz.
Tea	30–70	5 oz.
Cocoa	5	5 oz.
Coca-Cola	45	12 oz.
Pepsi-Cola	30	12 oz.
Chocolate bar	22	1 oz.

Source: Hanson, Venturelli, and Fleckenstein, *Drugs and Society,* 7th ed. (Boston: Jones and Bartlett, 2002, p. 287).

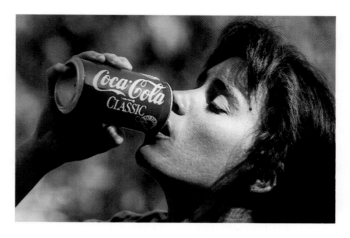

Most Americans consume more soft drinks than glasses of water. This can mean a significant daily intake of caffeine.

with the hot, crowded conditions usually found at raves, or parties, can lead to dehydration, hyperthermia, and heart or kidney failure.

A content analysis of Ecstasy pills collected anonymously from people attending raves and other events in several American cities showed that 63% contained some "Ecstasy" or a close chemical relative, 21% contained the cough suppressant chemical dextromethorphan, 8% contained either caffeine, pseudoephedrine, ephedrine, or aspirin, and 9% contained no identifiable drug (Baggott, 2000). The amount of dextromethorphan in fake "Ecstasy" pills was 2–4 times the amount recommended for cough suppression, which could produce toxic symptoms including lethargy, hyperexcitability, racing heart rate, dizziness and loss of balance, and PCP-like psychosis. MDMA and dextromethorphan block the drug-degrading system in the liver, which increases the risk of toxicity.

Caffeine

Caffeine is a natural stimulant found in a variety of plants used in coffee, tea, chocolate, and soft drinks (Table 16.4). These beverages and foods are an integral part of American eating habits and may be enjoyed partly for their psychoactive properties.

The effects of caffeine are familiar to most people. They include decreased drowsiness and fatigue (especially when performing tedious or boring tasks), faster and clearer flow of thought, and increased capacity for sustained performance (for example, typists work faster with fewer errors). In higher doses, caffeine produces nervousness, restlessness, tremors, and insomnia and it may have a negative effect on performance of complex tasks. In very high doses (10 grams, or 60 cups of coffee), it can produce convulsions, which can be fatal.

In the past, caffeine was prescribed for a variety of complaints, but it is rarely used medically any more.

However, it is still a key ingredient in over a thousand over-the-counter drugs. For example, many "energizers" and "stay-awake" products are pure caffeine. Pain relievers, cough medicines, and cold remedies contain caffeine to counteract the drowsiness produced by other ingredients in these medications. Caffeine is also put into weight control and menstrual pain products because it increases urine output and water loss.

Psychological dependence may result from chronic use of caffeine, and tolerance to the stimulant effect may gradually develop. Mild withdrawal symptoms, such as headache, irritability, restlessness, and lethargy, may occur when caffeine use is stopped.

Ephedrine (Ephedra)

Ephedrine is an amphetamine-like substance that acts as a central nervous system and cardiovascular stimulant. Ephedra, also known by the Chinese name *ma huang,* is the herbal form of ephedrine, derived from the plant *Ephedra sinica. Ma huang* has been used in China for thousands of years to treat nasal congestion and the common cold.

Pharmaceutical-grade ephedrine is available over the counter to treat nasal congestion and asthma. Herbal ephedra is sold in dietary supplements for weight loss ("herbal fen-phen"), building muscle, and boosting energy. There is no scientific evidence to substantiate claims for its ability to foster weight loss or increase muscle strength.

Ephedra also is sold as "herbal ecstasy" to alter consciousness. Users describe feeling relaxed, tingly,

Term

caffeine: a natural stimulant found in a variety of plants; commonly found in tea, coffee, chocolate, and soft drinks

ephedrine: an amphetamine-like stimulant

and energetic. Calling the product "herbal" to make it seem natural and therefore "healthful" should not mask the fact that the product contains a drug.

Because the FDA does not routinely test and regulate herbals, ephedra-containing supplements may contain very different amounts of ephedrine than are listed on the product label. Many ephedra-containing supplements also contain caffeine, which increases their excitatory properties. A jury in Alaska awarded a woman $13.3 million because she suffered a stroke after taking an ephedrine-containing weight loss product.

Millions of people use ephedrine-containing products safely. However, since 1994 the FDA has received and investigated more than 800 reports of adverse reactions associated with the use of ephedrine-containing products. These range from episodes of high blood pressure, heart rate irregularities, insomnia, nervousness, tremors, and headaches to seizures, heart attacks, and strokes. Deaths from cardiac arrest have been reported for people taking herbal ephedrine and coffee.

Ephedrine should not be used by pregnant women, people with elevated blood pressure or heart disease, prostate enlargement, glaucoma, pheochromocytoma, diabetes, Graves' disease or other hyperthyroid conditions, insomnia, anxiety, or suicidal tendencies. Ephedrine should not be combined with caffeine, monamine oxidase inhibitors, cardiac glycosides, or ergot or its derivative ergotamine.

Depressants

Depressants comprise a vast number of drugs whose common effects include a reduced level of arousal, motor activity, and awareness of the environment and increased drowsiness and sedation. The depressants include alcohol (see chapter 18), and drugs that affect sleep, sedatives, hypnotics, and opiates. A number of other drugs, such as antihistamines and some medications used in the treatment of high blood pressure or heart disease may also act as depressants. In low doses, depressants produce a mild state of euphoria, reduce inhibitions, or induce a feeling of relaxation. In high doses, they may impair mood, speech, and motor coordination.

Depressants are dangerous. All carry the potential for physical and psychological dependency, tolerance, unpleasant withdrawal symptoms, and toxicity from continual use or overuse. Acute overdoses may produce coma, respiratory or cardiovascular collapse, and even death. Aggravating the potential for lethal overdose are the synergistic actions of depressants. That is, when taken together, two or more different depressants can produce a much stronger effect than the sum of both drugs. The most common synergistic effect occurs when people drink alcohol while taking depressant medications, such as barbiturates or tranquilizers.

Sedative and Hypnotic Drugs

A **sedative** is a drug that promotes mental calmness and reduces anxiety. A **hypnotic** is a drug that promotes sleep or drowsiness. Because of their potential for inducing dependence, almost all sedatives and hypnotics are highly regulated and are available only by prescription. Nevertheless, sedative-hypnotics are among the most widely used drugs in the U.S.

The most common sedative-hypnotics are drugs called benzodiazepines, more popularly known as **tranquilizers.** Medically, these drugs are used to relieve anxiety, promote relaxation, induce sleep, alleviate muscle spasm and lower back pain, treat convulsive disorders, and lessen the discomfort of alcohol and opiate withdrawal. Benzodiazepines are most helpful when used on a short-term basis (a few weeks) as an adjunct to psychotherapy or medical therapy. Long-term use (more than 4 months) increases the risk of both dependence and of not confronting and overcoming issues and symptoms for which the benzodiazepines were originally prescribed.

Rohypnol (flunitrazepam) is a benzodiazepine with the nicknames "Ropies," "Roofies," and "Rope." The drug is illegal in the United States, but it is legal in some other countries, from which it is smuggled into the U.S. Rohypnol has been dubbed "the date-rape drug" for its purported effect of reducing a woman's level of consciousness and, therefore, her resistance to sexual assault. Several victims of sexual assault have apparently been intoxicated with the drug—in some instances because it was given to

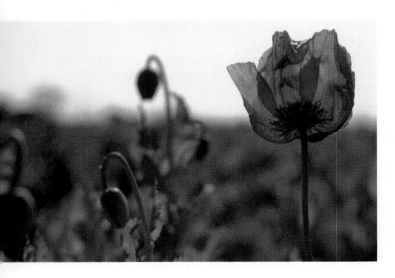

Opium poppies (Papaver somniferum) *from which morphine is obtained.*

them without their knowledge or consent—before the attack.

Another extremely dangerous "date-rape drug" is gamma hydroxybutrate (GHB) and its chemical derivatives. This drug is colorless and can be mixed in water bottles; an unsuspecting person may drink from the water bottle and die from a drug overdose, which has happened to several young persons (Nordenberg, 2001). GHB was sold in health food stores in the 1960s as a dietary supplement and was used by bodybuilders to stimulate muscle growth. However, by the 1990s, its use had become more widespread and dangerous. Hundreds of emergency room visits due to GHB poisoning have been reported to the FDA by hospitals. In 1999, four young men in Michigan were charged with the poisoning death of a ninth-grade student. They had slipped some GHB into her Mountain Dew at a party. Young people should be cautioned against sharing water bottles and drinks at parties, especially if drugs are being used by others.

Barbiturates are sedative-hypnotic drugs that include barbituric acid and its derivatives: amobarbital (Amytal), pentobarbital (Nembutal), phenobarbital (Luminal), secobarbital (Seconal), and Tuinal (50% amobarbital plus 50% secobarbital). Because they are less safe than benzodiazepines, barbiturates tend not to be prescribed for medical conditions that call for sedative-hypnotic drug therapy.

Opiates

The **opiates** are a group of chemically related drugs that depress the central nervous system. These substances cause physical dependence, habituation, and tolerance and produce serious withdrawal symptoms. Opiates are derived from the opium poppy, *Papaver somniferum*, extracts of which have been used for thousands of years in a variety of cultures to produce euphoria, to relieve pain, and to treat various diseases.

Medically, opiates are used for pain relief, cough suppression, and treatment of diarrhea. They can be taken by mouth, injection, snorting, and smoking. Heroin is converted to morphine in the body, and the

morphine is eventually excreted in urine, saliva, sweat, and the breast milk of lactating women (which means that nursing infants can become addicted). Because morphine crosses the placenta, a developing fetus may become addicted even before birth and may experience withdrawal symptoms after it is born.

Opiates are commonly abused substances, taken for their pain-relieving and psychoactive effects. The psychological sensations produced by opiates include feelings of warmth and belonging, relaxation, and mellowness. Regular use of opiates can produce tolerance to the psychological effects, constipation, loss of appetite, depression, loss of interest in sex, constriction of the pupil of the eye, disruption of the menstrual cycle, and drowsiness. Very large doses or prolonged use can be fatal because of respiratory failure.

Marijuana

Marijuana is another name for the plant *Cannabis sativa*, which grows in temperate climates all over the world. Species of this plant have been cultivated for thousands of years as a source of hemp fiber used to make clothing and rope or for a substance that, when ingested, produces euphoria, a sense of relaxation, mood elevation, and altered perceptions of space and time.

The principal psychoactive ingredient in marijuana is a chemical called *delta-9-tetrahydrocannabinol* (THC). This substance is found in the plant's leaves, buds, seeds, and resins. THC can be ingested by smoking the dried and crushed flowers and leaves or by eating food that has been prepared with marijuana as a minor ingredient.

Hashish (a resin generally smoked in a special pipe) is a highly potent derivative of marijuana obtained from the sticky resin found on the flowers and leaves of marijuana plants. *Ganja*, another derivative of marijuana, consists of the dried tops of female plants. *Bhang* (called "ditch weed") is made from parts of the plant that contain lesser amounts of THC. *Sinsemilla* (from the Spanish word "without seeds") is a potent form of marijuana derived exclusively from female plants. All male plants are removed from the plot to prevent seed formation and to allow more of the female plant's energy to be directed into the growth and formation of psychoactive compounds.

Besides its intended psychoactive effects, marijuana ingestion may evoke confusion, anxiety, panic, hallucinations, and paranoia. Speech and short-term memory may be impaired, which may be interpreted as humorous changes in one's normal mental state. However, because perception, motor coordination, and reaction time are also impaired, driving a car or

Terms

sedatives: CNS depressants used to relieve anxiety, fear, and apprehension

hypnotics: CNS depressants used to induce drowsiness and encourage sleep

tranquilizers: central nervous system depressants that relax the body and calm anxiety

opiates: CNS depressants derived from the opium poppy

marijuana: a psychoactive substance present in the dried leaves, stems, flowers, and seeds of plants of the genus *Cannabis*

hashish: the sticky resin of the *Cannabis* plant

operating other machines while intoxicated with THC is unsafe. Marijuana use may also aggravate an existing mental health problem or negative mood.

Some of the possible health dangers of long-term marijuana use include the risk of bronchitis caused by marijuana smoke, increased heart rate and blood pressure, and possibly a slight depression of immune system functions. Long-term use of highly potent marijuana may produce tolerance and a mild physical dependence. Marijuana smoke, like tobacco smoke, contains carcinogens (see chapter 13). Research has not yet ascertained whether long-term use contributes to a syndrome of lack of motivation and reduced productivity (*amotivational syndrome*). Contrary to what was once popular belief, marijuana does not turn users into crazed murderers and rapists nor does it cause genetic damage.

Since 1996, voters in several states have approved the use of marijuana for medical purposes. In 1999, the U.S. National Academy of Sciences' Institute of Medicine (IOM) reported that "there are some limited circumstances in which we recommend smoking marijuana for medical uses." The IOM report concluded that marijuana's active chemical components are potentially effective in treating pain, nausea, the anorexia of AIDS, and other symptoms, and should be tested rigorously in clinical trials. Such trials should be carried out in tandem with the development of new delivery mechanisms for the drug that are safe, fast-acting, and reliable but do not involve inhaling smoke.

Too much of a good thing is wonderful.
                              MAE WEST

The IOM report found little support for the contention that marijuana is an effective treatment for glaucoma. Smoked marijuana can reduce some of the eye pressure associated with glaucoma, but only for a short period of time. Also, with the exception of muscle spasms in multiple sclerosis, there is little evidence of its potential for treating movement disorders like Parkinson's disease or Huntington's disease.

Terms

hallucinogens: psychoactive substances that alter sensory processing in the brain; produce visual or auditory sensations that are not real (i.e., that are hallucinatory)

LSD: a powerful hallucinogenic chemical; ingestion alters brain chemistry and produces a variety of hallucinogenic and behavioral effects

phencyclidine (PCP): drug that, depending on the route of administration and dose, can be a stimulant, depressant, or hallucinogen; originally developed as an animal anesthetic

inhalants: vaporous substances that, when inhaled, produce alcohol-like intoxication

TABLE 16.5   Substances Considered to Be Hallucinogenic or Psychedelic

Substance or active ingredient	Common name
D-lysergic acid diethylamide	LSD
Trimethoxyphenylethylamine	Mescaline (peyote)
2,5-Dimethoxy-4-methyl-amphetamine	STP
Dimethyltryptamine	DMT
Diethyltryptamine	DET
Tetrahydrocannabinol	Marijuana (cannabis)
Phencyclidine	PCP
Psilocybin	Mushrooms

This federally funded IOM report urged the government to give patients and physicians access to medical marijuana. Prior to 1992, the U.S. government allowed certain patients access to medical marijuana under a "compassionate use" program. However, in 1999 the federal government rejected the IOM report and declared it would prosecute any patient using marijuana for any reason. The U.S. government grows marijuana in a closely guarded plot and processes the plants' THC into a drug called Marinol. Marinol can be prescribed for nausea and vomiting associated with cancer chemotherapy, as well as for anorexia and weight loss associated with AIDS. However, most patients report little relief of symptoms from using Marinol, as compared to smoking marijuana. Most physicians are reluctant to prescribe marijuana for a medical condition because they fear federal prosecution and possible loss of their medical licenses.

Hallucinogens

The **hallucinogens** comprise a variety of chemical substances derived from as many as 100 kinds of plants as well as by chemical synthesis in the laboratory (Table 16.5). Despite their chemical differences, hallucinogens share the ability to alter perception, thought, mood, sensation, and experience. The similarity of their effects to psychotic hallucinatory experience is one reason they are called hallucinogens, but in many respects the psychedelic drug experience is not the same as a psychotic hallucination. Psychotic hallucinations are generally auditory and frightening, and the hallucinator believes them to be real. Drug-induced hallucinations tend to be visual, usually are enjoyable, and the individual is aware that the experience is unusual and is not part of his or her normal state of consciousness.

Hallucinogens are most often ingested orally, either by eating the plant itself or by ingesting powder containing the active chemical. Normally, a hallucinogenic drug begins to take effect in 45 to 60 minutes. The first effects are physical: sweating, nausea, increased body temperature, and pupil dilation. These symptoms eventually subside, and the psychological effects become manifest within an hour or two of ingestion. Depending on the particular substance and the amount ingested, the "trip" lasts anywhere from 1 to 24 hours. Perhaps the most commonly used hallucinogen is **LSD** (D-lysergic acid diethylamide), commonly called "acid."

A common feature of the hallucinogenic experience is the suspension of the normal psychic mechanisms that integrate the self with the environment. The distortion of self-environment interactions makes the user extremely open to conditions in the surroundings. For this reason, experience in any particular drug episode is highly influenced, for better or worse, by the environmental setting in which the trip takes place and by the "psychic set"—the expectations and attitudes—of the user.

Phencyclidine (PCP)

Phencyclidine, also known as **PCP,** angel dust, hog, crystal, and killer weed, was developed originally for medical use as an animal anesthetic. But because of the drug's many adverse effects, it was removed from legal sale and became an illegal recreational drug. In the 1960s, phencyclidine was called the PeaCePill—a serious misnomer in view of the drug's effects.

The effects of PCP are variable: depending on the dose and the route of administration, it can be a stimulant, a depressant, or a hallucinogen. Some of the intended effects are heightened sensitivity to external stimuli, mood elevation, relaxation, and a sense of omnipotence. Some of the common unintended effects are paranoia, confusion, restlessness, disorientation, feelings of depersonalization, and violent or bizarre behavior. In high doses, the drug can cause coma, interruption of breathing, and psychosis.

Many admissions to psychiatric emergency rooms are for PCP intoxication. The drug impairs perception and muscular control, and users are prone to accidents such as falling from heights, drowning, walking in front of moving vehicles, and collisions while driving under the influence of the drug. PCP does not induce tolerance or physical dependence, but because it is eliminated slowly from the body, chronic users may experience the drug's effects for an extended period.

The effects of PCP are unpredictable and frequently unpleasant, if not terrifying and life-threaten-ing. PCP produces more unwanted and dangerous symptoms of drug intoxication than any other psychoactive substance. Drug dealers often surreptitiously mix PCP with marijuana or cocaine or sell PCP while claiming it to be LSD, DMT, or some other drug. Because PCP is relatively easy to manufacture, it is one of the more readily available and dangerous of the illegal recreational drugs.

Inhalants

Inhalants are a wide variety of chemical substances that vaporize readily and when inhaled produce various kinds of depressant effects similar to those of alcohol. Like alcohol, inhalants are depressants of the central nervous system. Generally, their intended effect is loss of inhibition and a sense of euphoria and excitement. Unintended effects include dizziness, amnesia, inability to concentrate, confusion, impaired judgment, hallucinations, and acute psychosis.

Inhalants commonly used for recreational purposes include:

1. Commercial chemicals, such as model airplane glue, nail polish remover, paint thinner, and gasoline, and substances such as acetone, toluene, naphtha, hexane, and cyclohexane.
2. Aerosols—found in aerosol spray products.
3. Anesthetics, such as amyl nitrite, nitrous oxide ("laughing gas"), diethyl ether, and chloroform.

Because they are vaporous, these substances enter the body rapidly. The fumes are usually inhaled from plastic bags. The intoxicant effects are often felt

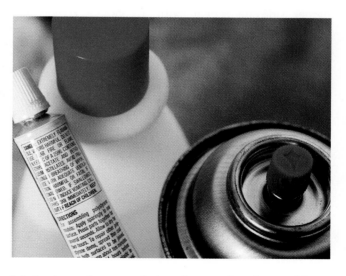

Inhalants are dangerous but, unfortunately, often readily available to kids looking for a "rush."

within minutes, and the high lasts less than an hour. Regular users tend to be preteens and others without the money to buy other drugs. Some adults use amyl nitrite ("poppers") during sexual relations, believing that the drug enhances the sexual experience. Some medical personnel are frequent users of nitrous oxide or "laughing gas" because it is easily available.

The inhalant chemicals do not produce tolerance or withdrawal, nor do they induce physical dependence. However, they are dangerous. In addition to any harm resulting from uncontrolled behavior (such as driving while intoxicated), these chemicals damage the kidneys, liver, and lungs and can upset normal rhythmic heartbeat. Some users have suffocated while inhaling the fumes from plastic bags, and the potential for explosion is always present.

Anabolic Steroids

Characteristics and Use

Anabolic steroids are synthetic derivatives of the male hormone testosterone. These derivatives of testosterone promote the growth of skeletal muscle and increase lean body muscle. Anabolic steroids were first abused by elite athletes seeking to improve performance. Today, athletes and nonathletes use steroids to enhance performance and also to change physical appearance.

Anabolic steroids are taken orally or injected, typically in cycles of weeks or months rather than continuously. Users frequently combine several different types of steroids to maximize their effectiveness while minimizing negative side effects, a process known as stacking. Anabolic steroids produce increased lean muscle mass, strength, and ability to train longer and harder. Side effects of anabolic steroid use include liver tumors, jaundice, fluid retention, high blood pressure,

severe acne, and trembling. Shrinking of the testicles, reduced sperm count, infertility, baldness, and development of breasts have been observed in males. In females, growth of facial hair, changes or cessation of menstrual cycle, enlargement of the clitoris, and deepened voice are among the side effects.

Reducing Drug Use

Almost everyone takes drugs of one kind or another at one time or another. People take drugs to relieve headaches, heartburn, tension, cramps, fatigue, and anxiety. Drugs are used to get to sleep and to stay awake. They are used for body problems and emotional problems. When used appropriately, drugs can play a vital role in the treatment and prevention of disease.

However, as a society we are overmedicated and overly dependent on drugs. The healthiest approach is to be as free of drugs as possible. Wellness is not achieved by taking drugs. No drug should ever be taken casually, whether prescribed, over-the-counter, or offered in a social setting. Each person should learn when drugs are necessary to maintain or restore health and when the benefits of the drug outweigh the risks.

All drugs are dangerous, and illegal recreational drugs are especially so, since you cannot be sure of either the quality or the strength. The use of most recreational drugs is illegal, and if caught, users and sellers are prosecuted as criminals. Still, many people in American society, especially young people, experiment with one or more illegal drugs. Experimenting with drugs is just that: you are taking a chance of getting caught, or getting high and causing an accident, or getting the wrong dose and dying.

Critical Thinking About Health

1. The graph below shows the results of a test of a new drug. Four groups of patients were involved. Group 1 received placebo; Group 2, 20 mg of the drug; Group 3, 40 mg; and Group 4, 80 mg.
   a. Do the data support the hypothesis that the drug is effective? Why or why not?
   b. What percentage of people get well without the drug? What's a likely explanation?
   c. What's the maximum percentage of people that can be expected to get well from taking the drug?
   d. If 80 mg produces the desired effect in the largest number of people, why didn't the experimenters report the effects of 100 mg?

2. Bob Kozlo came home from work early one day. Upon hearing his dad's car pull up in the driveway, Jamie, Bob's 16-year-old son, quickly disposed of the joint he and his friend Max were sharing. Mr. Kozlo, who as a teenager also had experimented with marijuana, smelled the telltale odor and knew immediately what Jamie and Max had been up to.
   a. Should Mr. Kozlo ignore this situation or take some kind of action, and if so, what should he do?
   b. Should he tell Max's parents?
   c. What is your opinion of teenagers experimenting with marijuana or any other drugs, including alcohol and tobacco?

3. Why are some drugs illegal? What characteristics distinguish a legal drug from an illegal one? If you had unlimited power and resources, what would you do to solve the illegal drug problem in the U.S.?

4. In what ways has substance use and abuse touched your life?

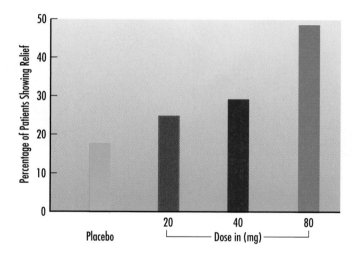

Health in Review

- People have been ingesting drugs throughout recorded history for a variety of reasons, including curing illness and facilitating social interaction.
- A drug is a chemical substance capable of producing a change in physiology. Most drugs react by binding to receptor sites in or on cells, which alters biological activity.
- Legal or illegal, medical or nonmedical, drug use in the United States is widespread. Drug use is encouraged by extensive advertising by the pharmaceutical industry.
- Drug abuse is the overuse of a drug, often to the point of loss of control. Many drugs of abuse are psychoactive, meaning that they alter thoughts,

feelings, and perceptions. Many psychoactive drugs cause physical dependence; some cause psychological dependence.

- Tolerance is the adaptation of the body to repeated drug use so that ever increasing doses of the drug are required to produce an effect.
- The most commonly used psychoactive drugs in the United States include stimulants (cocaine, amphetamine, caffeine); depressants (sedatives, tranquilizers, hypnotics); opiates; marijuana; hallucinogens; cocaine and ecstasy.
- The medical use of marijuana has been legalized in several states.

Health and Wellness Online

The World Wide Web contains a wealth of information about health and wellness. By accessing the Internet using Web browser software, such as Netscape Navigator or Microsoft's Internet Explorer, you can gain a new perspective on many topics presented in *Health and Wellness, Seventh Edition.* Access the Jones and Bartlett Publishers Web site at http://www.jbpub.com/hwonline.

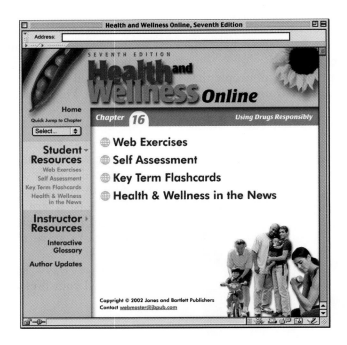

References

Baggott, M. et al. (2000). Chemical analysis of ecstasy pills. *Journal of the American Medical Association, 284,* 2190.

Hanson, G., Venturelli, P. J., and Fleckenstein, A. (2002). *Drugs and Society.* (7th ed.). Boston: Jones and Bartlett Publishers.

Klam, M. (2001, January 21). Experiencing ecstasy. *New York Times Magazine,* 38–79.

Lazarou, J., Pomeranz, B. H., and Corey, P. N. (1998). Incidence of adverse drug reactions in hospitalized patients. *Journal of the American Medical Association, 279,* 1200–1205.

Nordenberg, T. (2000). The death of the party. *Consumer Reports, 34,* 14–17.

Rivara, F. P. et al. (1997). Alcohol and illicit drug abuse and the risk of violent death in the home. *Journal of the American Medical Association, 278,* 569–575

Wazana, A. (2000). Physicians and the pharmaceutical industry. *Journal of the American Medical Association, 283,* 373–380.

Williams, R. D. (1997, April). Medication and older adults. *FDA Consumer,* 17–21.

Suggested Readings

Angell, M. (2000). The pharmaceutical industry—to whom it is accountable? *New England Journal of Medicine, 342,* 1902–1904. The distinguished former editor of the *New England Journal of Medicine* analyzes the threat to health care represented by the economic power of the pharmaceutical industry.

Graedon, J., and Graedon, T. (1997). *Deadly drug interactions.* New York: St. Martin's Griffin. Explains how most commonly used drugs interact with foods, other drugs, vitamin and mineral supplements, herbs, and alcohol.

Graedon, J. and Graedon, T. (2001). *The People's Pharmacy: Guide to Home and Herbal Remedies.* New York: St. Martin's. A compendium of the pros and cons of common drugs and herbals.

Gray, M. (2000). *Drug Crazy: How We Got Into This Mess and How We Can Get Out.* Routeledge. A scathing account of America's decades-long war on drugs, which has benefited only two groups of people: professional anti-drug advocates and drug lords.

Griffith, H.W. (2001). *The complete guide to prescription and non-prescription drugs* (15th ed.). NY: Perigee. A complete encyclopedia for the average person.

Iversen, L. L. (2000). *The Science of Marijuana.* Oxford University Press. A well-known neuropharmacologist summarizes the historical and recent research on marijuana.

Prevention Online (Prevline). The Substance Abuse and Mental Health Service Administration's National Clearinghouse for Alcohol and Drug Information on preventing alcohol and drug abuse in families, schools, and the workplace. (http://www.health.org)

Public Citizen Health Research Group. A nonprofit organization that publishes a monthly magazine, *Worst Pills—Best Pills,* that warns of dangerous prescription drugs. The organization also reports on FDA actions and the drug industry. (www.citizen.org/hrg)

U.S. National Institute of Drug Abuse. A division of the National Institutes of Health dedicated to improving drug abuse and addiction prevention, treatment, and policy. (http://www.nida.nih.gov)

Learning Objectives

1. Describe the hazards of cigarette smoking.
2. Identify and explain the physiological effects of tobacco.
3. Describe the hazards of smokeless tobacco use.
4. Discuss the short-term and long-term health-related and social consequences of tobacco use.
5. Discuss the effects of smoke on nonsmokers, including children.
6. Explain why some people smoke.
7. Identify ways to quit smoking.
8. Describe the various ways tobacco companies promote their products to young people.

Study Guide and Self Assessment

Commit to Quit

Health and Wellness Online

 www.jbpub.com/hwonline

Chapter 17

Eliminating Tobacco Use

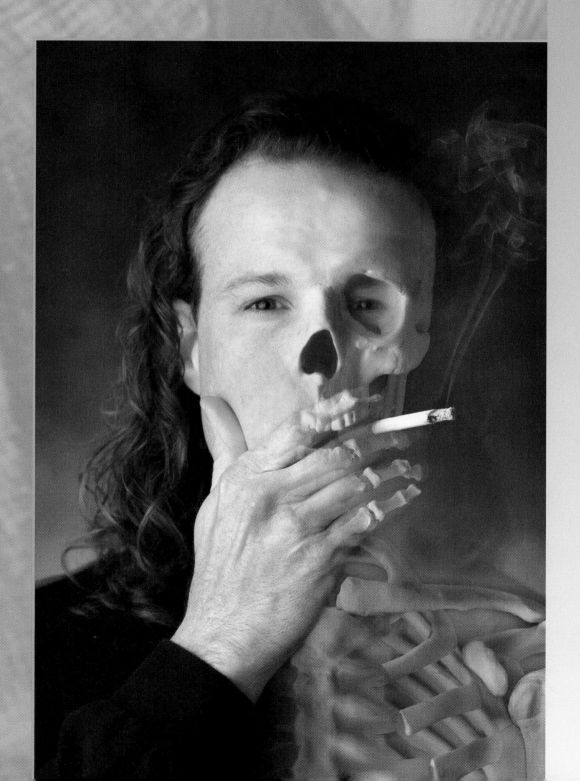

"Warning: The Surgeon General Has Determined That Cigarette Smoking is Dangerous to Your Health." By now, this message and other warnings about the dangers of smoking have reached just about everyone. Despite the warnings, however, about 62 million Americans aged 12 and older are cigarette smokers, making nicotine the most used addictive drug in the United States.

The health costs of smoking are staggering. Ten million people have diseases caused or made worse by smoking, including chronic obstructive lung disease, heart disease, stroke, erection problems, high blood pressure, and cancer of the lung, breast, esophagus, larynx, mouth, bladder, cervix, pancreas, and kidney. Each year about 430,000 Americans die as a result of smoking (see Figure 17.1); this accounts for one in five deaths in the United States annually. Included in this total are approximately 1,300 children who die from in-home fires caused by cigarettes. Worldwide, about 4 million people die from smoking each year. On average, smokers die about seven years earlier than nonsmokers. Tobacco use is the single most preventable cause of death in the United States (see Figure 17.2).

> *Cigarettes are the only legal product that, when used as intended, cause death.*
>
> LOUIS W. SULLIVAN
> former secretary of Health and Human Services

The economic costs of smoking are staggering as well. Cigarette smoking costs the United States more than $100 billion in health care costs and lost productivity annually. About $30 billion of those costs are covered by smokers themselves in the form of cigarette taxes, direct costs, and health insurance. The remaining $70 billion in smoking-related costs is borne by nonsmokers. On average, each pack of cigarettes sold costs American society about four dollars in smoking-related health expenses.

Tobacco Use in the United States

About 24 million American men and 22 million American women smoke cigarettes. The prevalence of smoking among adult Americans has declined in the past 35 years as the social views of cigarette smoking have become more and more negative (see Figure 17.3).

About one-third of American college students use tobacco at least occasionally (Rigotti, Lee and Wechsler, 2000); about half of student smokers smoke one to ten cigarettes per day while 12% smoke one or more packs of cigarettes a day. Cigar smoking accounts for about 8% of tobacco use among college students, mostly among men, and smokeless tobacco accounts for about 4%, also mostly among men.

Smoking among young people (under age 18) increased by nearly 50% during the 1990s (see Figure 17.4). Each day, 3,000 young Americans begin to smoke cigarettes. Smoking among youth is particularly troublesome, because adolescence is when regular use and dependence on tobacco begin. Among people who smoke daily, 71% had done so by age 18.

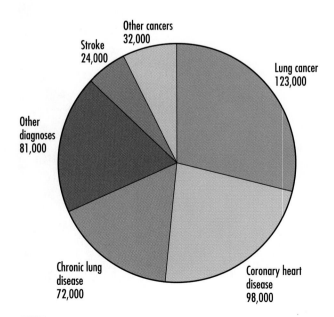

FIGURE 17.1   **430,000 Annual Deaths Attributable to Cigarette Smoking in the United States**
Source: Centers for Disease Control and Prevention.

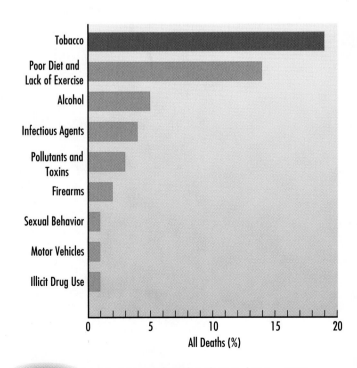

FIGURE 17.2   **Actual Causes of Death in the United States, 1990**
Source: McGinnis, J.M., & Foege, W.H. (1993). Actual causes of death in the United States. *Journal of the American Medical Association, 270,* 2207–2212.

Wellness Guide

Stop Your Financial Future From Going up in Smoke!

The smoking habit costs smokers a lot of money. A pack-a-day smoker spends about $1,275 a year just for cigarettes (estimated per pack cost plus taxes = $3.50). If that money were invested at an 8% annual return, before taxes it would total:

- After 1 year. . .$1,377
- After 5 years. . .$7,494
- After 10 years. . .$18,506

- After 20 years. . .$58, 506
- After 30 years. . .$144,416

Source: Hugh's Calculators
(http://www.interest.com/hugh/calc/smoking.cgi)

What is Tobacco?

Tobacco used for smoking, chewing, or snuff is the processed product of the leaves of the plant *Nicotinia tabacum*. This plant is indigenous to the Western Hemisphere, where it grows best in semitropical climates.

Tobacco was introduced to European societies in the sixteenth century by the Spanish returning from voyages to the Americas. The Spanish had learned about smoking from Native Americans, who used tobacco much as it is used today. In fact, the word "tobacco" is an Indian word referring to the pipe used to smoke the minced or rolled leaf of the tobacco plant.

The smoking habit spread quickly in Europe, fueled by tobacco imports from Spain's colonies. By the nineteenth century, changing social customs had caused tobacco smoking to be replaced largely by tobacco chewing; even more popular was the habit of sniffing tobacco in the form of snuff. Not until the 1880s, when the cigarette-making machine was invented in the United States, did cigarette smoking become the predominant form of tobacco use worldwide. Camel cigarettes, introduced in 1913, ushered in the modern era of smoking in the United States. By

coincidence, the American Cancer Society was established in the same year.

Processing tobacco for consumption involves harvesting the tobacco leaves and curing them by any one of several drying methods. The cured tobacco leaves are shredded, and various types of leaves are blended into commercially desirable mixtures. Often flavorings and colorings are added, as well as chemicals that facilitate even burning. Finally, the mixture is used to manufacture cigarettes, pipe tobacco, and chewing tobacco, or is wrapped in specially cured tobacco leaves to make cigars.

The most familiar chemical constituent of tobacco is **nicotine,** but when tobacco is burned, approximately 4,000 other chemical substances are released and carried in the smoke. These chemicals include acetone, acrolein, carbon monoxide, methanol, ammonia,

Terms

nicotine: an addicting chemical in tobacco that produces rapid pulse, increased alertness, and a variety of other physiological effects

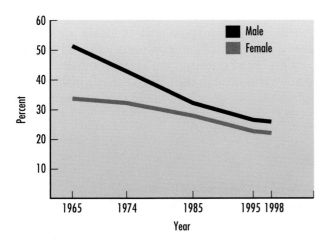

FIGURE 17.3   **Percentage of the U.S. population that smokes cigarettes.**
Source: National Center for Health Statistics.

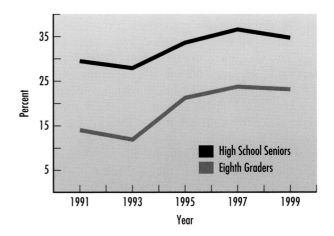

FIGURE 17.4   **Percentage of high school seniors and eighth graders who smoke cigarettes.**
Source: National Institute on Drug Abuse.

Global Wellness

Beyond the Clouds—Tobacco Smoking in China

Whereas the prevalence of smoking among adults in the United States has remained unchanged since the early 1990s, on a global scale the picture is very different. In developing countries, cigarette smoking is rising by 3% per year, and the number of deaths attributable to smoking is expected to be 10 million by the year 2020 (Brundtland, 2000).

China is the world's largest tobacco-producing country and has the most smokers—more than 400 million. Each year, 1.8 trillion cigarettes are smoked in China. Smoking in China has increased rapidly since the 1980s. If current smoking patterns continue, about 100 million Chinese eventually will die of tobacco use.

China has been proactive with regard to tobacco use prevention by establishing the Chinese Association on Smoking and Health in 1990, and in 1995, banning all cigarette advertising in print and electronic media. In some major cities, smoking has been banned in public places. China was also the first country to ban smoking on all domestic air flights.

Tobacco use prevention and control efforts have been intensified in China, as they take on the challenge of an ever-increasing population (predicted to rise from 1.25 billion to 1.513 billion by 2025), and an estimated two million deaths annually from smoking.

nitrous dioxide, hydrogen sulfide, traces of various mineral elements, traces of radioactive elements, acids, insecticides, and other substances. Besides these chemical compounds, tobacco smoke also contains countless microscopic particles that contribute to the yellowish brown residue of tobacco smoke known as **tar,** a documented cause of lung cancer. Forty-three of the chemicals in tobacco are known to cause cancer.

Bidis—hand-rolled cigarettes from India—are falsely believed to be less harmful than commercial American cigarettes. Whereas *bidis* contain about half the tobacco content of a standard cigarette, they contain 25% more nicotine per gram of tobacco. One *bidi* does deliver less tobacco smoke and nicotine than a standard American cigarette, but as with smokers of "light" cigarettes, *bidi* smokers are likely to make up the difference by smoking more cigarettes.

Physiological Effects of Tobacco

Most of the physiological effects of tobacco smoking are attributable to the pharmacological effects of nicotine. The most prominent effects include increased heart rate, increased release of adrenaline, and a direct stimulatory effect on the brain, which combine to produce the mild "rush" cigarette smokers may experience when they light up. It also lowers skin temperature and reduces blood flow in the legs and feet. Nicotine is also responsible for the nausea and vomiting experienced by most beginning smokers. Addiction to nicotine is largely responsible for perpetuating a smoker's habit.

Some harmful cardiovascular effects of cigarette smoking probably result from nicotine and carbon monoxide, which are believed to contribute to the development of heart and blood vessel disease. A host of other harmful chemicals contribute to the development

of cancer and diseases of the respiratory tract. Among these chemicals are benzoapyrene, aza-arenes, N-nitrosamines, and radioactive polonium. Polonium is a product of the breakdown of radioactive lead, a natural constituent of soil. Radioactive particles in the soil become deposited on sticky tobacco leaf hairs and eventually become part of tobacco smoke. Radon, a radioactive gas, is also present in tobacco smoke inhaled both by the smoker and nonsmoker via second-hand smoke. These radioactive substances can become trapped in tiny air sacs in the lungs, where they induce cancerous changes in lung tissue.

Smokeless Tobacco

Smokeless tobacco is available in two main forms: **chewing tobacco** and **snuff.** Chewing tobacco is processed into three different forms: loose leaf, firm/moist plug, and twist/rope chewing tobacco. A portion of chewing tobacco is either chewed or placed in the mouth and held in place between the lower lip and gum. Snuff is made from powdered or finely cut tobacco leaves and is available in two forms, dry and moist. In many European countries dry snuff is inhaled through the nose. However, in the United States a pinch of snuff is placed in the mouth and held in place between the

Terms

tar: the yellowish brown residue of tobacco smoke

chewing tobacco: a form of shredded smokeless tobacco; chewed or placed in mouth between lower lip and gum

snuff: a form of smokeless tobacco; made from powdered or finely cut leaves

moist snuff: a form of snuff made from air- and fire-cured tobacco leaves; most hazardous form of smokeless tobacco

cheek and gum, referred to as "snuff dipping." Dipping snuff is highly addictive and exposes the body to levels of nicotine equal to those of cigarettes. **Moist snuff** is made from air- and fire-cured tobacco leaves that are processed into fine particles, flavored, and packaged in moist form in round, flat containers. Moist snuff is considered the most hazardous form of smokeless tobacco because of the methods used in processing it.

History of Smokeless Tobacco

Tobacco for chewing and sniffing has been used for many centuries. Smokeless tobacco use by both men and women flourished until the end of the nineteenth century. At this time, scientists discovered that tuberculosis bacillus and other harmful organisms could survive in saliva and be spread by air. Spitting into spittoons and onto barroom floors became unacceptable and even unlawful in many public places. Cigarettes replaced chew and snuff. Chewing became a habit retained mainly by older men.

Chewing tobacco became fashionable again in the 1970s when the dangers of cigarette smoking became clear. Cigarettes were publicized as carcinogenic, and advertisers promoted smokeless tobacco as being a healthy alternative to cigarette smoking. Currently, about 9% of Americans use smokeless tobacco.

Smokeless tobacco is not a safe alternative to smoking. Smokeless tobacco mixes with saliva, and the nicotine and other chemicals are absorbed into the bloodstream. Tobacco in this form leads to nicotine addiction just as cigarette smoking does. Smokeless tobacco causes various kinds of oral cancer. It also causes other diseases of the mouth, such as hard white patches on the gums (leukoplakia) and inflammatory lesions of the gum (gingivitis). The majority of these lesions are benign, but about 2% to 6% of cases develop into cancer. Some users show a marked increase in blood pressure, which is a major factor in heart disease.

Smokeless tobacco has also been linked to other health problems. Taste-enhancing sugars and sweeteners found in loose chewing tobacco may lead to tooth decay. Abrasive ingredients found in tobacco cause receding gums in areas where the tobacco is held for long periods between the teeth and lower lip or the teeth and the cheek. Tobacco users often experience halitosis or a loss of taste and smell.

Social consequences for using smokeless tobacco include yellow and brown stains on the teeth, clothing, and automobile; the tobacco may cling to teeth, lips, tongue, and clothing. Spitting tobacco juice disgusts others.

Reducing Smokeless Tobacco Use

The health risks of smokeless tobacco have become increasingly apparent, and various steps have been taken to alert the public to this problem. Federal legislation has been enacted to help combat smokeless tobacco use.

In 1986, the Comprehensive Smokeless Tobacco Health Education Act was passed. This bill banned all smokeless tobacco ads on television and radio, and mandated that health hazard warnings be placed on all tobacco packages. However, advertisements in print media and at car races and rodeos have increased the use of smokeless tobacco among young people.

Cigars

Americans consume far fewer cigars annually as compared with 470 billion cigarettes. Cigar packages are not required to say anything about health hazards, and cigar smokers generally don't inhale, making the health dangers appear negligible. Despite the fact that we really don't know how many deaths are attributable to cigars, we do know that tobacco smoke is a carcinogen, whether it comes in the form of a cigarette or a cigar, and that there is no safe level of exposure.

Smoking and Disease

Almost from the beginning of tobacco use in Europe and America, people have been concerned about the possible harmful effects of smoking (Figure 17.5). Several articles in the medical literature of the eighteenth and nineteenth centuries claimed tobacco smoking as a cause of cancer of the lip, tongue, and lung. Modern research on the health consequences of cigarette smoking has provided overwhelming evidence that, among smokers as a group, the incidence of certain diseases is greater, sometimes much greater, than among nonsmokers. Smoking has been established as a factor in the development of coronary artery disease; lung cancer; bronchitis; emphysema; cancer of the larynx, lip, and oral cavity; cancer of the bladder and stomach; duodenal ulcer; and allergies.

Overwhelming data demonstrate that the death rate from cancer, heart disease, and respiratory diseases is higher among cigarette smokers than among nonsmokers. In fact, smoking decreases a person's life expectancy by an average of 7 years. Smokers between the ages of 35 and 70 have death rates three times higher than those who have never smoked.

Effects of Parental Smoking on Children

Parental smoking harms children beginning in pregnancy and continuing throughout a child's life. Smoking is a risk factor for spontaneous abortion, death among newborns, and sudden infant death syndrome

FIGURE 17.5   "A custom loathsome to the eye, hateful to the nose, harmful to the braine, dangerous to the lungs, and in the blacke, stinking fume thereof, nearest resembling the horrible Stigian smoke of the pit that is bottomlesse." So concluded James I of England in his *Counterblaste to Tobacco*, published in 1604. Sir Walter Raleigh had promoted and popularized the habit of smoking in the court of Queen Elizabeth of England in the late sixteenth century. But James I, who became king when Elizabeth died in 1603, was strongly opposed to the habit. He eventually had Raleigh beheaded for political reasons, but perhaps Raleigh also had smoked too much in the king's presence.

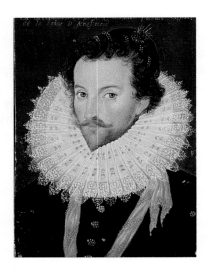

(SIDS). A pregnant woman exposed to environmental tobacco smoke (ETS) risks giving birth to a low-birth-weight infant. Compared to children raised in a non-smoking environment, children exposed to environmental tobacco smoke have a higher risk of bronchitis, pneumonia, and other respiratory tract infections. They also are at higher risk for asthma and ear infections.

Long-Term Health Effects of Tobacco Use

Smoking kills more people than AIDS, poor diet and sedentary lifestyles, car accidents, alcohol, homicides, illegal drugs, suicides, and fires combined (McGinnis & Foege, 1993). It contributes substantially to deaths from cancer (especially cancers of the lung, esophagus, oral cavity, pancreas, kidney, and bladder), cardiovascular disease (i.e., coronary disease, stroke, and high blood pressure), lung disease (i.e., chronic obstructive pulmonary disease and pneumonia), burns, and problems in infancy caused by low birth weight.

> *There are two ways of being disappointed in life; one is not to get what you want and the other is to get it.*
> GEORGE BERNARD SHAW

Lung Cancer

Lung cancer is responsible for more deaths among men and women than any other type of cancer. Each year approximately 171,000 persons receive a diagnosis of lung cancer and about 160,000 people die of this disease. Smoking is responsible for almost 90% of lung cancers among men and more than 70% among women (1998). The number of men dying of lung cancer has increased steadily since 1940. While the rate of increase among men is beginning to decline because fewer men are smoking cigarettes, the rate of increase among women is rising because more women have been smoking during the last three decades. In 1987,

for the first time in U.S. history, lung cancer passed breast cancer as the leading cancer-related cause of death in women.

The increase in lung cancer deaths is the principal reason that the overall cancer death rate continues to rise. If lung cancer death rates are excluded from the statistics, the death rate from cancer has been falling steadily for many years, principally because of preventive efforts and improved diagnosis and treatment of cancers. This situation is ironic as well as tragic, for lung cancer is one of the most preventable of all diseases. People simply need to stop (or never start) smoking cigarettes.

A full biological explanation of how smoking causes lung cancer (and contributes to cancer at other sites) is not yet available. There are 43 known **carcinogens** found in tobacco smoke that are thought to cause the cellular changes leading to cancer.

Heart Disease

Smoking cigarettes increases the risk of heart disease. Smoking can increase tension in the heart muscle walls, speed up the rate of muscular contraction, and increase the heart rate. As the heart's workload increases, so does the need for oxygen and other nutrients. Smoking also reduces the amount of high-density lipoprotein (HDL) cholesterol (i.e., the "good" cholesterol), facilitating plaque formation and blood clotting.

Bronchitis and Emphysema

Bronchitis and **emphysema** are respiratory diseases sometimes classified with asthma as **chronic obstructive pulmonary diseases (COPD).** Each of these diseases is associated with breathing difficulty caused by obstruction or destruction of some part of the respiratory system. Often persons suffer from more than one of these conditions at the same time. Cigarette smoking is responsible for more than 65,000 deaths due to COPD.

The Respiratory system

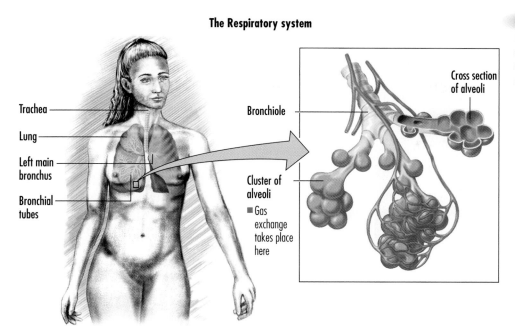

Trachea

Lung

Left main
bronchus

Bronchial
tubes

Bronchiole

Cluster of
alveoli

▪ Gas
exchange
takes place
here

Cross section
of alveoli

FIGURE 17.6   Respiratory System
Provides oxygen and removes carbon dioxide. Oxygen enters and carbon dioxide leaves via tiny air sacs in the lungs called alveoli. The rest of the respiratory system facilitates gas exchange in the alveoli.

Bronchitis is an inflammatory condition of the upper part of the respiratory tract, principally the **trachea,** the main airway. Bronchitis is characterized by excessive production of mucus by cells that line the airways, which causes the major symptoms of bronchitis—such as a continual cough (smoker's cough) and the production of large amounts of sputum. Some affected people also experience shortness of breath, particularly during exertion.

Apparently, excessive production of mucus by the glands of the bronchi is a reaction to irritation caused by cigarette smoke.

Fortunately, the pathology that produces the symptoms of bronchitis can be almost completely reversed by quitting smoking, reducing exposure to polluted air, or both. However, many people "live with" their persistent cough for many years and are not concerned with the message their body is giving them. If the disease is left to run its course, sufferers increase their vulnerability to other respiratory illnesses, and the airways may become irreversibly damaged.

Smoking is the primary cause of emphysema, which results from the destruction of the tiny air sacs deep in the lungs called **alveoli** (Figure 17.6). Each lung contains millions of alveoli; across their thin membranes the function of breathing is accomplished—the exchange of the respiratory gases, oxygen and carbon dioxide.

Emphysema is a disabling condition in which the walls of the air sacs in the lungs lose their elasticity and are gradually destroyed. The lungs' ability to obtain oxygen and remove carbon dioxide is impaired, requiring the heart to work harder, which results in the heart becoming enlarged. Emphysema involves a slow, irreversible process of alveolar destruction; as the disease progresses, affected people have greater and greater trouble breathing.

As with lung cancer, the exact mechanism by which tobacco smoking or air pollution contribute to emphysema is unknown. One hypothesis suggests that cells in the lung (macrophages and leukocytes produced by the immune system) (see chapter 12) normally engaged in the destruction of material foreign to the body release enzymes that inadvertently destroy lung tissue, thereby causing emphysema. Normally, a protein called **alpha-1-antitrypsin (AAT)** inhibits the activities of destructive enzymes in the lungs. The inhibitory protein blocks the action of the enzyme elastase, which, if not properly regulated, destroys alveoli and results in emphysema. Some people have low levels of the inhibitor due to a defective gene, and they

T e r m s

carcinogens: substances that can cause cancer in people and other animals

bronchitis: inflammation of the bronchi of the lungs as a result of irritation; often accompanied by a chronic cough

emphysema: a progressive degeneration of the lung alveoli, causing breathing and oxygen assimilation to become more and more difficult

chronic obstructive pulmonary diseases (COPD): diseases that restrict the ability of the body to obtain oxygen through the respiratory structures (bronchi and lungs); including asthma, bronchitis, and emphysema

trachea: upper part of respiratory tract

alveoli: tiny air sacs in the lungs that exchange oxygen and carbon dioxide

alpha-1-antitrypsin (AAT): a protein that inhibits destructive enzymes implicated in causing emphysema

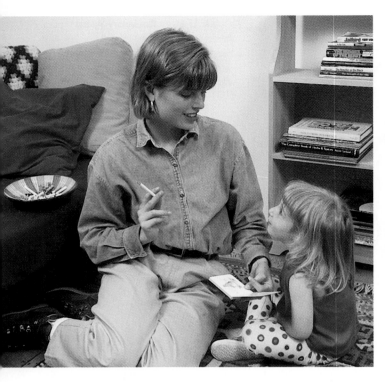

Children who live in homes where adults smoke have more respiratory problems than children who are raised in smoke-free environments.

are particularly at risk for emphysema. Rarely, an inherited AAT deficiency may cause cases of emphysema before age 50.

Tobacco Smoke's Effects on Nonsmokers

Nonsmokers who are exposed to tobacco smoke run a significant health risk. People who work or live in environments heavily laden with tobacco smoke inhale the same smoke-borne substances as do smokers. In fact, about two-thirds of the smoke from a burning cigarette enters the environment.

Environmental tobacco smoke (ETS) contains the same 4,000 chemicals that inhaled tobacco smoke does, but the concentration is greater because ETS is unfiltered. Annually, about 3,000 nonsmoking American adults die of lung cancer and about 50,000 die from heart disease as a result of exposure to ETS. Also, breathing ETS increases the severity of asthma in nearly 1 million American children and is responsible for several hundred thousand cases of bronchitis and pneumonia in children less than 18 months old.

A nonsmoker in a smoke-filled room can inhale in one hour the equivalent of a cigarette's worth of nicotine, carbon monoxide, and carcinogenic substances. Also, many people are allergic to tobacco smoke, which can produce eye irritation, headache, cough, nasal congestion, and asthma. Nonsmokers forced to inhale tobacco smoke for long periods, such as workers in enclosed smoke-filled workplaces, can suffer

impaired lung function equivalent to that of smokers who inhale while smoking 10 cigarettes a day. A study of the risks of passive smoking found that spouses of smokers had a 30% higher cancer mortality rate compared with spouses of nonsmokers.

Why People Smoke

Most people begin to smoke in their teen years, emulating parents, others who smoke, or cigarette ad models. Teenagers also smoke to attain acceptance in their peer group. About half of those who experiment with smoking continue the habit into adulthood. There must be some very compelling reasons that people continue to smoke despite the unpleasant taste, the initial adverse physiological reactions to smoke and nicotine, and the knowledge—now widespread—that tobacco smoke causes cancer and other life-threatening diseases.

According to the American Cancer Society, the motivations of smokers fall into six general categories:

- **Stimulation.** Some people experience a psychological lift from smoking. They say that smoking helps them to wake up in the morning and organize their energies. They often report that smoking increases their intellectual capacities.
- **Handling.** Some people enjoy the mere handling of cigarettes and smoking paraphernalia, such as lighters.
- **Pleasurable relaxation.** Some smokers say they smoke simply because they like it. Smoking brings them true pleasure and relaxation and is often practiced to enhance other pleasurable sensations, such as the taste of food and alcoholic beverages. However, smoking actually dulls the tastebuds.
- **Reducing negative feelings (crutch).** Approximately one-third of smokers say they smoke because it temporarily helps them deal with stress, anger, fear, anxiety, or pressure.
- **Craving.** Some people crave cigarettes and have no other explanation for their habit except that they have a frequent need to smoke, regardless of the tension-relieving effects that smoking might bring.
- **Habit.** Some smokers light up only because of habit. They no longer receive much physical or psychological gratification from smoking; often they smoke without being aware of whether or not they really want the cigarette.

The question that still eludes a definitive answer is: What distinguishes people who smoke from those who do not? The list of suggested answers includes a biological susceptibility to dependence on nicotine; a variety of personal, sociological, and environmental traits; and a need to deal with stress. In the final analysis, however, smoking, like any other habitual, health-threatening behavior, is a matter of choice. In the case of smoking, the choice can ultimately be—and often is—fatal.

Quitting Smoking

There's an old joke among smokers: "It's easy to quit. I've done it fifty times!"

Whereas the little joke is intended to show how difficult stopping smoking can be, it also confirms research that shows stopping smoking is a process, not an event. Often, people think about stopping for a period of time before they even consider trying, and sometimes people go through one or more cycles of stopping for a while before they quit permanently. These tries and re-tries are part of the stopping process (see "Wellness Guide" on page 376).

The smoking habit is part biological (dependence on nicotine), part mental (smoking alters mood and provides pleasure), and part social (smokers smoke with other smokers). Because smoking involves several parts of a smoker's life, quitting successfully generally requires examining how smoking is integrated into one's life, then planning and adopting alternative experiences that meet the biological, mental, and social needs that smoking satisfies.

Most smoking cessation plans center on a **quit date**—the day that the smoker stops smoking completely. Prior to the quit date, the smoker prepares for stopping by:

- cutting back on the number of cigarettes smoked each day
- identifying which cigarettes will be the hardest to give up (e.g., first of the day; after a meal) and planning alternative activities for after the quit date
- identifying and preparing to do without the benefits of smoking and finding alternative activities to meet the needs that smoking provides (e.g., stress management)
- asking friends and family to offer support while quitting
- planning to stay away from smoking stimuli (e.g., not going to bars, not hanging out with friends who smoke, not smoking at breaks with co-workers, not smoking in the car)
- investigating the possibility of using **nicotine replacement therapy** (nicotine patch, gum, or nasal spray) to lessen the effects of nicotine withdrawal and *buproprion*, a prescription drug that lessens the urge to smoke

People stop smoking for a variety of reasons: to reduce the risk of early death from heart or lung disease; to enjoy, once again, the unpolluted taste of food; to please nonsmoking loved ones; to eliminate the ever-present ashes and smell of cigarette smoke from their homes and cars; and to fulfill a simple, yet important, commitment to be healthy. Frequently, a positive change in other aspects of life leads to cessation of smoking. For example, many people who take up meditation, t'ai chi ch'uan, jogging, or other physical activity lose the desire to smoke and stop smoking.

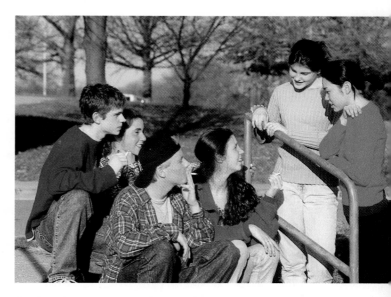

Smoking begins at an early age when peer acceptance is highly sought after.

It is never too late to quit. The sooner smokers quit, the more they can reduce their chances of getting cancer and other diseases. Within 20 minutes of smoking the last cigarette, the body begins a series of regenerating changes. After 20 minutes, blood pressure drops to normal. After 48 hours, nerve endings start regrowing, and the ability to smell and taste is enhanced. In one to nine months, coughing, sinus congestion, fatigue, and shortness of breath decrease and cilia regrow in the lungs. After five years, the lung cancer death risk decreases by almost half. After 15 years, the risk of coronary heart disease is that of a nonsmoker's, and the risk of dying from lung cancer is only slightly higher than that of a nonsmoker's. The

> *A good plan executed right now is better than a perfect plan executed next week.*
> GEORGE S. PATTON

Terms

quit date: the day a smoker designates as the one on which she or he will stop smoking completely

nicotine replacement therapy: using nicotine-containing gum, skin patch, nasal spray, or inhaler to temper the symptoms of nicotine withdrawal when quitting smoking

Wellness Guide

Stages of the Quitting Process

Quitting smoking is a process involving five stages. The more one knows about the quitting process the more likely one is to stop smoking and to have the confidence to remain tobacco-free. The five stages of the quitting process are:

Precontemplation Stage

Smokers in the precontemplation stage spend little time thinking about their smoking and may not see it as a problem. They see more negatives about quitting than positives, resulting in low motivation for stopping, even though they know that smoking carries serious health risks.

Contemplation Stage

Smokers in the contemplation stage are aware of the benefits of stopping and think about their smoking—and even about quitting—but they feel ambivalent about actually stopping. They may think about the negative aspects of smoking and the positive aspects associated with quitting, yet doubt that the long-term benefits associated with quitting will outweigh the short-term costs. Such ambivalence is a normal part of the quitting process and may last several months or even years.

Preparation

Smokers in the preparation stage have made the decision to quit and are taking steps to get ready to stop smoking. They see the cons of smoking as outweighing the pros and say things like "I've got to do something about this—this is serious," or "Something has to change. What can I do?"

Action Stage

Smokers in the action stage are actively trying to stop smoking. They may try several different techniques, believe they have inner strength to quit, and tend to seek help and support. They develop plans to deal with both personal and external pressures that may lead to slips, and they use short-term rewards to sustain their motivation.

Maintenance Stage

Smokers in the maintenance stage have learned to anticipate and handle temptations to smoke. They remain aware that what they are striving for is personally worthwhile and meaningful and are patient with themselves, recognizing that it often takes a while to let go of old behavior patterns and adopt new ones. They see "slipping" not as failure but as a learning experience and remind themselves of how much progress they have made.

---

extent to which these risks are reduced depends on the total amount the person has smoked, the age that the person started smoking, and the amount of inhalation.

The War of Words

A longstanding war of words exists between public health professionals and the tobacco industry (tobacco growers and other businesses involved in the production and sale of smoking products). At stake is influencing the behavior of millions of smokers and prospective smokers, especially teens. The health groups try to persuade people not to smoke; the tobacco industry encourages them to smoke more and more.

The health war of words takes place in relative obscurity compared with tobacco advertising. Each year in the United States the tobacco industry spends billions of dollars to promote its products and to recruit new smokers. Perusal of many major magazines and newspapers reveals that cigarette advertising relies heavily on imagery portraying smoking as enjoyable and smokers as attractive, sexy, slim, and of high social status. Many magazines depend heavily on the income from cigarette advertising. When cigarette advertising was banned from radio and television in 1971, tobacco companies shifted their advertising to newspaper and magazine ads. They also developed costly promotional campaigns (such as the Virginia Slims Tennis Tournament) in an attempt to associate smoking cigarettes with health, fun, and fitness. Tobacco companies began to support health research, exotic travel excursions, rock concerts, and major athletic events to promote smoking.

Smoking in Films and on TV

Films and TV promote cigarette smoking. When actors smoke cigarettes on screen, they give viewers the message that smoking and smokers are cool (see Table 17.1). More than 85% of films contain tobacco use (Sargent et al., 2001). Tobacco use is present in one third of films rated for adolescent audiences and 20% of films rated for children. In 1998, the film industry imposed a ban on itself on accepting money from tobacco companies to have their products appear in films. This was after the disclosure that Sylvester Stallone had accepted $500,000 to smoke a particular brand of cigarettes in three of his movies. Tobacco companies even paid to have their brands of cigarettes placed in *Who Framed Roger Rabbit* and *The Muppet Movie*.

To determine the extent and type of tobacco use in movies, the American Lung Association asked more than 200 teenagers to review the top 50 box office movies annually between 1991 and 1998 (American Lung Association, 1998). Teen reviewers found

Dollars and Health Sense

Making Money by Making Others Sick

In 1996, the American Medical Association resolved that "all physicians, health professionals, medical schools, hospitals, public health advocates and citizens . . . divest of any tobacco holdings (stocks) including mutual funds that include tobacco holdings; and that all life and health insurance companies and HMOs divest of any tobacco holdings."

An analysis of 1999 stock holdings of some insurance companies showed that Prudential had invested $892 million in tobacco companies, MetLife, $62.1 million, and Cigna, $42.7 million (Himmelstein, 1999). Showing that investors who would not wish to invest actively in tobacco stocks nevertheless may do so passively through mutual funds, the same analysis revealed that several

popular mutual funds invest in tobacco stocks: Vanguard, about $1.2 billion; Fidelity, about $6.6 billion; Sanford Bernstein, about $1 billion, and TIAA/CREF, about $800 million. The researchers comment: "A life insurer or health insurer that buys tobacco company stock positions itself to profit from both life and death. The insurers who increasingly govern health care seem driven only by money."

---

that more than half of the 350 movies reviewed included pro-tobacco messages. One fourth of the movies showed scenes in which tobacco use could be interpreted as sexy, exciting, powerful, sports-related, sophisticated, celebratory; one-third of the movies included scenes in which tobacco use could be considered relaxing. Fourteen percent of the movies showed scenes in which tobacco use demonstrated independence or rebellion. Men lit up nearly twice as often as women. Exposure of the Marlboro brand was ten times as high as any other brand of tobacco. One fourth of the movies included anti-tobacco messages, including no-smoking signs (4%), comments by actors (16%), and visual clues such as coughing or waving smoke away (8%).

The U.S. government plays a paradoxical role in the smoking war. It supports both sides. Through the Department of Agriculture, the government provides price supports and other financial aids to tobacco growers and the tobacco industry. Through the Department of Health and Human Services, the govern-

ment supports antismoking educational programs and finances research into the health effects of smoking. The pluralistic nature of our governmental system allows this dichotomy, which illustrates why it would be foolish to depend entirely on the federal government—or on any other organization—to be the guardian of your personal health.

Stopping Tobacco's Damage to Society

In 1998, 46 states and seven large tobacco companies (Philip Morris Inc., R.J. Reynolds Tobacco Company, Brown and Williamson Tobacco Corporation, British American Tobacco Company, Lorillard Tobacco Company Inc., American Tobacco Company Inc., and the United States Tobacco Company) settled the states' lawsuits to recover their tobacco-related health care costs. The settlement, called The Master Settlement Agreement (MSA), totaled $206 billion, to be paid to the states over 25 years.

In addition to the MSA payments, the cigarette companies will pay $5.15 billion over 12 years into a trust fund to compensate tobacco farmers and others for anticipated financial losses resulting from the implementation of the MSA. The states also signed a separate agreement with the leading smokeless tobacco company, United States Tobacco, that contains many of same public health provisions as the MSA.

The MSA provides numerous restrictions and prohibitions on the tobacco industry including bans on:

- the use of cartoons in tobacco advertisements
- the targeting of youth in advertising, promotions, or marketing including free sampling
- the use of most outdoor advertisements including billboards and signs and placards in arenas, stadiums, shopping malls, and video game arcades
- the distribution of apparel and merchandise with brand-name logos

TABLE 17.1 Cigarette Smoking in Films, 1991–1998

Year	Percentage of tobacco use in all films	Average number of incidents of smoking per PG-rated Film	Percentage of main actors smoking
1997/98	88	18	74
1996/97	76	17	62
1995/96	68	16	48
1994/95	74	6	54
1993/94	94	11	74
1992/93	76	14	48
1991/92	86	6	74

Source: American Lung Association

Wellness Guide

Women and Cigarette Advertising

For more than 50 years tobacco company ads have tried to entice women to smoke cigarettes by emphasizing sexiness, slimness, elegance, and fun. The success of such ads over the years in getting women to smoke is borne out by the current number of lung cancer deaths among women smokers. Currently, about 22 million American women smoke cigarettes. Between 1935 and 1999 the percentage of women who smoked increased from 18% of all women to 22%. (During the same interval the percentage of men who smoked decreased from 52% to 28%.)

About 140,000 women die from cigarette-caused diseases each year. Lung cancer has surpassed breast cancer as the leading cause of cancer deaths among women. Smoking also increases women's chances of heart disease and cervical cancer. And if that's not enough, the beauty editor of *Harper's* magazine points out that "smokers' skin wrinkles up to 10 years sooner than that of nonsmokers." As long as tobacco is legal,

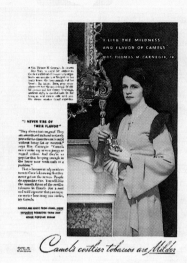

companies have a right to advertise. You also have the right to not smoke, which is one of the single most important health decisions you can make.

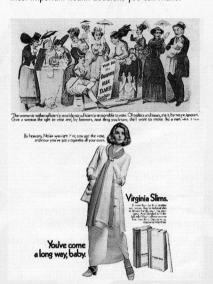

- payments to promote tobacco products in films, TV, and theater productions
- distributing free samples of cigarettes any place where underage persons may be present
- tobacco company lobbying against any proposed laws that limit youth access to tobacco
- tobacco industry attempts to limit or suppress research on the health effects of smoking

Tobacco industry secret documents have revealed that for more than 40 years, tobacco companies misled and lied to the public about the harmful, addictive effects of tobacco. It is clear that they targeted and manipulated young people into starting smoking. And, despite the MSA, they continue to do so. In 2001, R. J. Reynolds was sued by the states of Arizona and California for mailing free cigarettes. The MSA prohibits tobacco companies from giving away free samples where children might gain access. In 1999, the United States Tobacco Company, the largest distributor of smokeless tobacco, was sued by the state of California for advertising with a discount coupon for one of its

products in the San Diego State University student newspaper. Moreover, after the MSA, cigarette advertising increased in 19 magazines for which youth readers (between 12 and 17 years old) make up at least 15% of the readership (Massachusetts Department of Public Health, 2000). These magazines included *Sports Illustrated*, *TV Guide*, *Rolling Stone*, *Glamour*, and *Vogue*. Advertising for Marlboro, by far the most popular brand of cigarette among youth, increased by 25% in such magazines. In 1999, the advertising of tobacco products on billboards was banned, but tobacco companies simply moved their ads inside retail stores and increased giveaways of branded objects like clocks and other items.

Because 90% of new smokers begin the habit before reaching age 18, the tobacco industry targets youth with its advertising and promotional messages. The tobacco industry knows that "today's teenager is tomorrow's potential regular customer." As the Campaign for Tobacco-Free Kids points out, the tobacco industry is addicted to advertising to children.

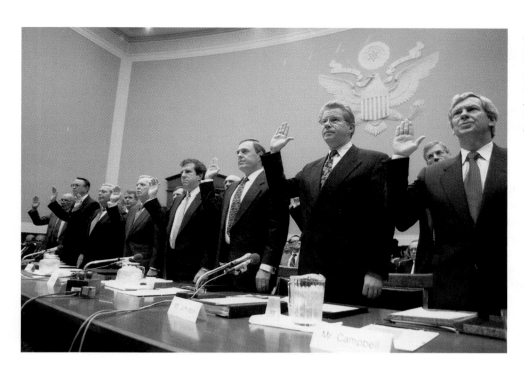

In the mid-1990s, the chief executives of the seven major U.S. tobacco companies were called before Congress to explain their business practices. Each of the executives testified under oath, "I do not believe smoking is addicting."

Critical Thinking About Health

1. Smoking takes a toll on everyone—those who smoke and those who do not. Government officials estimate that cigarette smoking costs the nation about $100 billion a year in health care costs and lost productivity. These costs are borne equally by nonsmokers and smokers.
   a. Should nonsmokers pay for the health care expenses of people who smoke? Why or why not?
   b. Should cigarettes be taxed by the government to cover their full cost to society, which could lessen tobacco consumption, put tobacco growers out of business, and drastically reduce tobacco companies' profits?
2. Purchase a popular magazine and count the number of cigarette ads in that issue. Review each ad and respond to the following questions:
   a. Who is the ad targeting? (e.g., women, men, young, old)
   b. How is the ad appealing to its target audience? (e.g., sex, friends)
   c. Besides the warning label (which is required by law) does the ad mention any negative side effects of smoking?
   d. What does the ad imply will happen if you smoke their brand of cigarette?

3. Over the last three decades cigarettes have been shown to be hazardous to one's health. Smokeless tobacco was once thought to be a substitute for cigarette smoking, and its popularity increased during the 1970s and 1980s. Cigars are now very popular with cigar parlors being established in cities across the United States. You have been asked to return to your high school to discuss the negative consequences of tobacco.
   a. Identify two primary reasons for a young person not to begin using tobacco products.
   b. Respond to the following young athlete's question: "I don't smoke cigarettes because they are nasty. I use chew instead—my grandpa told me it wasn't bad. What can happen to me? I'm not inhaling tobacco."
4. Visit or call your local health department and ask them for a list of restaurants in your community that are smoke-free.
   a. What percentage of your community's eating establishments are smoke-free?
   b. What can you do to promote smoke-free eating establishments within your community?
   c. Should all public places—indoor and outdoor—be smoke-free?

Health in Review

- No public health message is disseminated as widely as that on every package of cigarettes and in every cigarette advertisement: "Warning: The Surgeon General Has Determined That Cigarette Smoking Is Dangerous to Your Health."
- Despite the overwhelming evidence that cigarette smoking is associated with higher death rates from cancer, heart disease, and respiratory diseases, approximately 46 million American adults smoke. Smoking also is associated with a higher risk of emphysema and bronchitis.
- Cigarette smoking is responsible for 430,00 American deaths per year, far more than AIDS, auto accidents, and drug use combined. Smoking increases the risk for heart disease, lung cancer, respiratory diseases, and cancers of all kinds.
- Smoking tobacco comes from the processed leaves of *Nicotinia tabacum*. Tobacco smoke contains more than 4,000 chemicals, including nicotine—which is responsible for many of tobacco's drug effects including physical dependence—and 43 others that are known to cause cancer.
- Smokeless tobacco is not a healthy alternative to smoking tobacco; it causes cancers of the lip and mouth. Cigar smoking also is harmful.
- Children are harmed by breathing parents' tobacco smoke. Pregnant women who smoke risk the health of their babies.
- Environmental tobacco smoke contains the same 4,000 chemicals and 43 carcinogens that inhaled tobacco smoke does, thus affecting the health of nonsmokers.
- People smoke cigarettes because of physical dependence on nicotine and a variety of psychological and social rewards that come from smoking.
- Smokers can stop smoking either on their own or with the help of a stop-smoking program.
- The advertising of cigarettes largely is aimed at young people and contributes to recruiting them to the smoking habit. In 1998, 46 states won a $206 billion settlement (Master Settlement Agreement) with the tobacco industry. This settlement is intended to help pay for smoking-related health costs and forbids tobacco companies from promoting tobacco products to youths under age 18.

Health and Wellness Online

The World Wide Web contains a wealth of information about health and wellness. By accessing the Internet using Web browser software, such as Netscape Navigator or Microsoft's Internet Explorer, you can gain a new perspective on many topics presented in *Health and Wellness, Seventh Edition*. Access the Jones and Bartlett Publishers Web site at http://www.jbpub.com/hwonline.

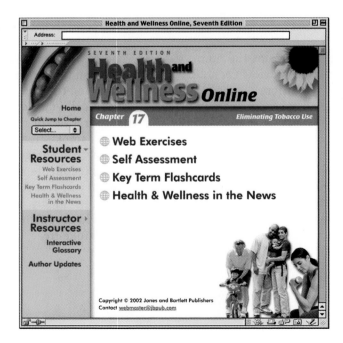

References

American Lung Association (1998). Thumbs up! Thumbs down! (http://www.lungusa.org/events/tutd/results_redux.htm)

Brundtland, G. H. (2000). Achieving worldwide tobacco control. *Journal of the American Medical Association, 284,* 750–751.

Himmelstein, D.U. et al. (2000). Investment of health insurers and mutual funds in tobacco stocks. *Journal of the American Medical Association, 284,* 697.

Massachusetts Department of Public Health (2000). Cigarette advertising expenditures before and after the Master Settlement Agreement.

McGinnis, M., and Foege, W. (1993). Actual causes of death in the United States. *Journal of American Medical Association, 270*(18), 2207–2212.

Rigotti, N. A., Lee, J. E., and Wechsler, H. (2000). U.S. college students' use of tobacco products. *Journal of the American Medical Association, 284,* 699–705.

Sargent, J. D. et al. (2001). Brand appearances in contemporary cinema films and contribution to global marketing of cigarettes. *Lancet, 357,* 29–32

Suggested Readings

Davis, R. M. (1998). Exposure to environmental tobacco smoke: Identifying and protecting those at risk. *Journal of the American Medical Association, 280,* 1947–1949. An overview of the health effects of environmental tobacco smoke.

National Cancer Institute. Smoking facts and tips for quitting. http://rex.nci.nih.gov/NCI_Pub_Interface/Smoking_Facts/facts.html

U.S. Centers for Disease Control Tobacco Information and Prevention Source (TIPS). Everything you ever wanted to know about smoking and tobacco use. http://www.cdc.gov/tobacco/

U.S. Department of Health and Human Services (2000). Reducing tobacco use: a report of the Surgeon General. Discusses all aspects of the tobacco issue.

Yang, G. et al. (1999). Smoking in China. *Journal of the American Medical Association, 282,* 1247–1253. An analysis of the effects of the coming health catastrophe on citizens of the world's largest producer and consumer of cigarettes.

1. Discuss the prevalence of drinking, types of drinking, reasons for drinking, and attitudes toward drinking among college students.
2. Explain the effects of alcohol on the body.
3. Describe how alcohol is absorbed into the body and how this absorption relates to blood alcohol concentration.
4. Discuss the effects of alcohol on behavior, including sexual behavior.
5. Describe the long-term effects of alcohol overconsumption.
6. Define alcohol abuse, alcohol addiction, and alcoholism.
7. Explain the phases of alcoholism.
8. Describe how alcohol affects one's significant others and the help that is available for both the family and the alcoholic.

Study Guide and Self Assessment

How to Cut Down on Your Drinking

Health and Wellness Online

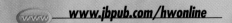 www.jbpub.com/hwonline

Chapter 18

Using Alcohol Responsibly

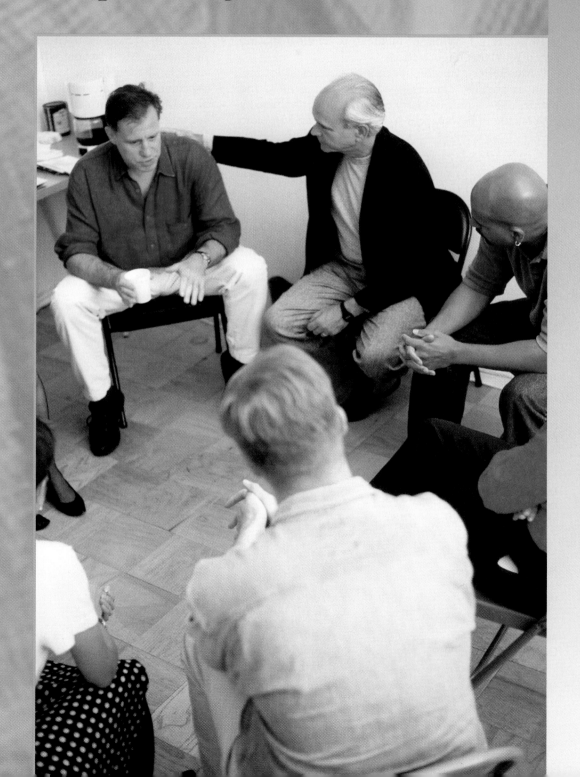

Alcohol abuse is one of the most significant health-related drug problems in the United States and in many other countries. Although cocaine and other illegal drugs receive much more attention from governments and the news media, these drugs affect far fewer people and cause far fewer health problems than alcohol. Each year, over 100,000 deaths are alcohol-related, many resulting from automobile fatalities, and alcohol abuse in the United States is responsible for approximately $150 billion in health and social costs. Excessive alcohol use is also associated with thousands of divorces, perhaps as many as 80% of the incidents of family violence, and millions of hours of school and job absenteeism. In addition, alcohol abuse is linked to a long list of medical, psychological, and social problems (Figure 18.1).

Alcohol use has long been a part of social events, such as parties, dinners, weddings, ball games, and picnics. The liquor industry encourages alcohol use by advertising in newspapers and magazines, and on radio and television. No direct link between advertising alcoholic products and alcohol abuse has been established. However, public health authorities and organizations such as the American Medical Association are concerned that advertising that associates drinking with athletic prowess, material wealth, social prestige, and sex encourages irresponsible drinking behavior. Breweries and liquor distributors are especially active on college campuses, spending millions of dollars each year on advertising in campus newspapers and promoting their products by sponsoring "pub nights," giving away items with product logos, and underwriting some of the costs of college athletic events.

Alcohol's positive public image makes many people doubt that they need to learn about alcohol use and abuse. Most people who drink believe that they can "hold their liquor" and that alcoholic beverages, especially beer, are no more harmful to health than soft drinks. As with so many other aspects of health, for most people responsible and moderate alcohol con-

Diseases and disorders associated with alcohol abuse

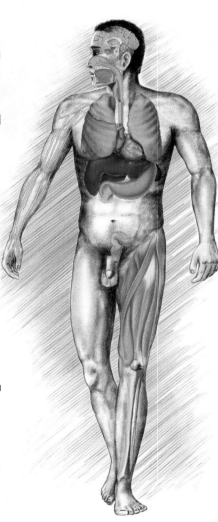

Brain Wernicke's syndrome, an acute condition characterized by ataxia, mental confusion, and ocular abnormalities; Korsakoff's syndrome, a psychotic condition characterized by impairment of memory and learning ability, apathy, and degeneration of the white brain matter

Esophagus Esophageal varices, an irreversible condition in which the person can die by drowning in his own blood when the varices open

Liver An acute enlargement of the liver, which is reversible, as well as irreversible alcoholic's cirrhosis of the liver

Muscles Alcoholic myopathy, a condition resulting in painful muscle contractions

Blood and bone marrow Coagulation defects and anemia

Eyes Tobacco-alcohol blindness; Wernicke's ophthalmoplegia, a reversible paralysis of the muscles of the eye

Pharynx Cancer of the pharynx is increased tenfold for drinkers who smoke

Heart Alcoholic cardiomyopathy, a heart condition

Lungs Lowered resistance is thought to lead to greater incidences of tuberculosis, pneumonia, and emphysema

Spleen Hypersplenism

Stomach Gastritis and ulcers

Pancreas Acute and chronic pancreatitis

Rectum Hemorrhoids

Testes Atrophy of the testes

Nerves Polyneuritis, a condition characterized by loss of sensation

FIGURE 18.1 Medical, Psychological, and Social Problems Associated with Alcohol Abuse

TABLE 18.1   Criteria for Moderate and At-Risk Alcohol Use*

Moderate drinking

Men: ≤ 2 drinks/day

Women: ≤ 1 drink/day

Over 65 (men and women): ≤ 1 drink/day

At risk drinking

Men: > 14 drinks/week, or > 4 drinks/occasion

Women: > 7 drinks/week, or > 3 drinks/occasion

Alcohol abuse

Significant impairment or distress in a 12-month period including

- failure to meet obligations at work, school, or home
- recurrent use of alcohol in hazardous situations
- legal problems related to alcohol
- continued use despite alcohol-related social or interpersonal problems

Alcohol dependence

Significant impairment or distress in a 12-month period including

- tolerance to alcohol
- withdrawal symptoms with abstinence from alcohol
- use of larger amounts over a longer period than intended
- persistent desire for alcohol (craving)
- unsuccessful attempts to cut down or control use
- important social, occupational, or recreational activities given up because of drinking
- use despite knowledge of alcohol-related problems (denial)

*One drink = 12 g of alcohol, which is the equivalent of 180 ml (6 oz) of wine, 360 ml (12 oz) of beer, or 45 ml (1.5 oz) of 90-proof distilled spirits.

Source: U.S. National Institute on Alcohol Abuse and the American Psychiatric Association.

sumption is more desirable than overzealous adherence to a single course of action. Everyone can benefit from knowing more about the effects of alcohol.

History of Alcohol Use

It is likely that humans have been drinking alcohol since someone accidentally noticed the psychological effects of drinking fermented liquids. Archaeological evidence indicates that Stone Age people drank the fermented juice of berries. Perhaps this first fruit wine was produced when some berry juice was left too long in a covered earthen jar and yeasts began fermentation, converting the sugar in the juice to alcohol. The first recorded use of alcohol dates from the Mesopotamian agrarian cultures of around 2000 B.C.

Through the ages, drinking fermented grains (beer); fermented berries, grapes, and fruits (wine); and the distilled products of natural fermentation ("hard" liquors) has become commonplace in many human societies. Alcohol is used in some religious ceremonies,

is taken as medicine, is used to seal contracts, agreements, and treaties, and is offered to display hospitality. Alcohol consumption has been an integral part of American life since the landing of the *Mayflower* at Plymouth Rock. Yet over the years, many people have come to regard drinking as a social evil and drunkenness as a sin. The United States government tried to legislate alcohol use out of American lives in 1919 by the Volstead Act, a constitutional amendment that prohibited

> *O God, that men should put an enemy into their mouths to steal away their brains!*
> *That we should with joy, pleasure, revel, and applause, transform ourselves into beasts.*
> SHAKESPEARE
> TWELFTH NIGHT

the sale and consumption of alcoholic beverages. This attempt to control alcohol consumption failed, however, and in 1933, Prohibition was repealed by another amendment to the Constitution.

Today, alcoholic beverages are available in many varieties. Not only are there the old standbys of beer, wine, and traditional hard liquors, but beverage manufacturers also market a variety of premixed cocktails, often sweetened with sugar and containing various flavors; wine coolers; and malt liquors.

Approximately 63% of U.S. adults are currently drinkers, 16% are former drinkers, and 22% are lifetime abstainers. Most of those who consume alcohol engage in moderate drinking. Approximately 9% of the U.S. population's drinking behavior puts them at risk for alcohol-related health and social problems (Table 18.1).

Drinking on Campus

Each year several college students die from ingesting massive quantities of alcohol. In its coverage of these tragic occurrences, the national media reminds Americans that drinking is as much a part of going to college as is going to class. Indeed, American college students spend more money on alcoholic beverages each year than they do on textbooks and soft drinks combined (Cohen, 1997).

Whereas it is true that many students drink to excess and that, by virtue of being underage, they drink illegally, it is wrong to assume that college campuses are taverns in disguise. On the contrary, college students are only a bit more likely to drink alcohol than their age peers who are not attending college (Gfroerer et al., 1997).

Given the extraordinary efforts of manufacturers of beer and other alcoholic beverages to market their products to college students, it's a wonder that so

Dollars and Health Sense

Alcohol and Lemonade—A Cool Way to Make Money

Everyone loves lemonade. Selling lemonade at a homemade wooden stand used to be the way a child made his first nickel. Mike's Lemonade Co. of San Francisco has found a way to make really big money from lemonade—add alcohol to it. Mike put together a drink containing lemon juice, sugar, malt liquor and carbonation. It was so popular that Mike sold 7 million cases in 2000. Mike's Lemonade is now marketed nationally. And while no one will admit it, the drink clearly is aimed at teenage drinkers, many of whom do not like the taste of beer or wine.

Hard sodas actually were introduced in England years ago by Bass, a large beer brewer. Their malt lemonade was called Hooper's Hooch and was such a hit that other British brewers soon introduced their own hard lemonades with catchy labels. United States brewers followed suit but stoutly deny that their hard lemonades are for underage drinkers; Anheuser-Busch claims that its "Doc" Otis drink is intended only for adults that want an alternative drink.

Critics argue that all this denial is just big business subterfuge. Teenagers who love sodas will quickly find out which ones pack a kick. Just as teens have no trouble obtaining cigarettes, they have no trouble getting hard sodas. Masking the taste of alcohol with sugar and lemon makes it easy for teenagers who hate the taste of beer and liquor to drink alcohol and "enjoy" its effects.

Beverage companies that claim they are not contributing to the underage drinking problem and helping to develop a new generation of alcoholics are doing just what the cigarette companies did for decades—deny everything as long as the product is legal and profitable.

---

many college students drink responsibly. A typical campus newspaper usually contains advertisements for alcoholic beverages and bar events. Slogans such as "Think when you drink," "Know when to say when," and "Friends don't let friends drive drunk" only masquerade as responsible drinking messages. Their real message is to drink as much as you can and institute back-up precautions for when you are drunk.

Although the majority of college students drink responsibly (or not at all), some engage in drinking behaviors that are dangerous. About 40% of students engage in **binge drinking,** which is defined as consuming five drinks in a row for men or four drinks in a row for women (Wechsler et al., 1999). A drink is defined as a 12-ounce serving of beer, a 4-ounce glass of wine, or a 1.5-ounce "shot" of distilled liquor in a mixed drink. Frequent binge drinking is associated with a number of alcohol-related problems. For example, compared with non–binge drinkers, binge drinkers are much more likely:

If you drink, don't park; Accidents cause people.
ANONYMOUS

- To miss class
- To get behind in schoolwork
- To do something they regret
- Not to use protection when engaging in sex
- To engage in unplanned sexual activity
- To get into trouble with campus police
- To damage property
- To get injured
- To engage in dangerous driving behaviors

- To disturb, insult, quarrel with, or assault others
- To require care from others while being sick from drunkenness

Compared to non-athletes, college athletes are much more likely to engage in both heavy and binge drinking (Nelson and Wechsler et al, 2001). Because athletes are so visible on campus, their drinking behaviors contribute to the overall campus atmosphere regarding drinking and students' perceptions and expectations of campus norms regarding alcohol use.

The behaviors of binge drinkers can affect non-binge drinkers and alcohol-abstainers. So-called **secondhand binge effects** include:

- Being interrupted while studying
- Being awakened at night
- Having to take care of a drunken fellow student
- Being insulted or humiliated by a drunken student
- Being pushed, hit, or assaulted by a drunken student
- Being the victim of sexual assault or date rape

In general, the cultural attitude of the campus regarding alcohol use has a tremendous influence on student drinking behavior. A campus culture that encourages legal and responsible alcohol use and discourages underage drinking, binge drinking, and alcohol-induced anti-social behavior promotes responsible behavior among the students (Haines & Spear, 1996). The opposite is true for a campus that has few or no student alcohol-use policies and at which students perceive that just about anything goes with regard to alcohol use. College students who drink heavily tend to view campus attitudes toward drinking as liberal

(Baer, Stacy, & Larimer, 1991). Students with the most enthusiastic attitudes toward drinking are typically the heaviest drinkers.

To reduce the degree of heavy and binge drinking, college campuses are changing the campus climate around alcohol use. Irresponsible drinking is not viewed as a rite of membership in campus organizations (e.g., clubs, athletic teams, fraternities, sororities), as an acceptable way to lessen social anxiety in party or other social situations, as the definition of partying, as an acceptable means to deal with academic stress, or as a rite of passage to adulthood and independence from parental control.

How Alcohol Affects the Body

Composition of Alcoholic Beverages

The alcohol in beverages is a chemical called **ethyl alcohol (ethanol).** There are many other kinds of alcohol, such as **methyl alcohol** and **isopropyl alcohol.** Most alcohols are poisonous if ingested in small amounts. In large amounts, even ethanol is toxic, but the body has ways to detoxify and eliminate it, given enough time.

The amount of ethanol in a commercial alcoholic product usually is listed on the product label (beer is the exception). The amount of alcohol in beer and wine is usually given as the percentage of the total volume. Beer, for example, is generally about 4% alcohol, although some beers contain more or less (socalled light beers have nearly the same alcohol content as regular beers). Wine is about 12% alcohol. The amount of alcohol in distilled liquors (e.g., scotch, vodka, bourbon, tequila, rum) is given in terms of **proof,** a number that represents twice the percentage of alcohol in the product. Thus, an 80-proof whiskey is 40% alcohol; 100-proof vodka is 50% alcohol.

Most standard portions of alcoholic drinks contain about one-half ounce of ethanol. For example, a

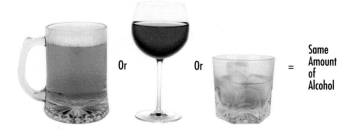

FIGURE 18.2   A mug of beer, glass of wine, and a mixed drink have about the same amount of alcohol. So don't be fooled by the type of drink.

12-ounce can of beer that is 4% alcohol contains 0.48 ounce of alcohol. The same amount of alcohol is contained in a 4-ounce glass of wine. The alcohol content of a cocktail mixed with one shot (1 ounce) of a 100-proof bourbon is 0.5 ounce. So, a can of beer, a glass of wine, and a highball contain approximately the same amount of alcohol (Figure 18.2).

How Alcohol Is Absorbed, Excreted, and Metabolized

After alcohol is ingested, it is readily absorbed into the body through the gastrointestinal tract. About 20% of ingested alcohol is absorbed by the stomach and the rest by the small intestine. The alcohol is then carried through the bloodstream to all the body's tissues and organs. Although not strictly a food (it contains no protein, vitamins, or minerals), alcohol does contain calories—in fact, 7 calories per gram (almost twice as many calories per gram as sugar).

Several factors affect the rate at which alcohol is absorbed into the body tissues. For example, food in the stomach—especially fatty foods or proteins—slows the absorption of alcohol. Nonalcoholic substances in beer, wine, and cocktails can also slow absorption of alcohol. The presence of carbon dioxide in beverages, such as champagne, sparkling wines, beer, and carbonated mixed drinks, increases the rate of alcohol absorption. That is why people feel intoxicated more quickly when drinking champagne or beer, especially on an empty stomach. The higher the alcohol content in a drink, the faster it is absorbed.

The concentration of alcohol in the blood is called the **blood alcohol content (BAC),** which is measured in grams of alcohol per deciliter of blood. A simple way to estimate BAC is to assume that ingesting one standard drink per hour (one beer, one glass of wine, one mixed drink), which contains approximately one-half ounce of ethyl alcohol, produces a BAC of 0.02 in a 150-pound male. Thus, the BAC of an average-sized man who drinks five beers during the first hour at a party will be 0.10; this level of alcohol in the blood violates the drinking-and-driving laws of most

Terms

binge drinking: ingesting five (men) or four (women) or more drinks on one occasion

secondhand binge effects: negative experiences caused by another's binge drinking

ethyl alcohol (ethanol): the consumable type of alcohol that is the psychoactive ingredient in alcoholic beverages; often called grain alcohol

methyl alcohol: wood alcohol or methanol

isopropyl alcohol: rubbing alcohol, sometimes used as an anesthetic

proof: a number assigned to an alcoholic product that is twice the percentage of alcohol in that product

blood alcohol content (BAC): the amount of alcohol in the blood

states. This shorthand method of approximating BAC changes depending on a person's body size, body composition (e.g., muscle, fat), and sex. All other things being equal, the BAC of a large person is less than that of a smaller person because the alcohol is diluted more in the large person's tissues. Women tend to have a higher BAC from the same number of drinks as men because they generally weigh less than men, have proportionately more body fat (which does not absorb alcohol as readily as muscle and other tissues), have sex hormones that tend to increase alcohol absorption and decrease its elimination, and tend to absorb more alcohol from the stomach.

Alcohol is eliminated from the body in two ways. About 10% is excreted unchanged through sweat, urine, or breath (hence the use of breath analyzers to test for drinking). The portion of alcohol that is not excreted (about 90%) is broken down primarily by the liver (metabolized), ultimately winding up as carbon dioxide and water. The liver detoxifies alcohol at a rate of about one-half ounce per hour; there is no way to speed up the process. Sobering-up remedies, such as drinking a lot of coffee, taking a cold shower, or engaging in vigorous exercise, do not accelerate the rate at which the liver removes alcohol from the body.

> You never know what is enough unless you know what is more than enough.
> WILLIAM BLAKE
> THE MARRIAGE OF HEAVEN AND HELL

The Hangover

An occasional consequence of drinking alcohol is a **hangover,** which may involve stomach upset, headache, fatigue, weakness, shakiness, irritability, and sometimes vomiting after drinking too much. The frequency and severity of hangovers vary. The particular factors in alcohol that cause a hangover are unknown, but several causes have been suggested:

- When alcohol is present in the body, normal liver functions may slow in order to break down the alcohol. This slowdown may reduce the amount of sugar the liver releases into the blood, resulting in temporary hypoglycemia and its resultant fatigue, irritability, and headache.
- Alcohol may inhibit REM sleep, resulting in fatigue, irritability, and trouble concentrating.
- **Congeners,** which are chemical substances in an alcoholic beverage or the breakdown products produced in the liver may cause a hangover.
- **Acetaldehyde,** a toxic substance produced when the liver breaks down alcohol, may be responsible for hangover symptoms.

The best way to deal with a hangover is to sleep, to drink juice to replace lost body fluid and blood sugar (alcohol increases urine output), and perhaps to take an analgesic for a headache. Ingesting more alcohol will only prolong the hangover symptoms.

The Effects of Alcohol on Behavior

Pharmacologically, alcohol acts as a central nervous system depressant, which means that it slows certain functions in some parts of the brain. In moderate amounts, alcohol may affect the parts of the brain that control judgment and inhibitions, which is why many people have a drink or two at a party to help "loosen up" or to become less shy and more able to interact freely with others. While some people may talk or laugh more than usual, others may become boisterous, argumentative, irritable, or depressed.

TABLE 18.2   Behavioral Effects of Alcohol in a 150-Pound Male

Number of drinks	Ounces of alcohol	BAC* (g/dl)	Approximate time for removal	Effects
1 beer, glass of wine, or mixed drink	½	0.02	1 hour	Feeling relaxed or "loosened up"
2½ beers, glasses of wine, or mixed drinks	1¼	0.05	2½ hours	Feeling "high"; decrease in inhibitions; increase in confidence; judgment impaired
5 beers, glasses of wine, or mixed drinks	2½	0.10	5 hours	Memory impaired; muscular coordination reduced; slurred speech; euphoric or sad feelings
10 beers, glasses of wine, or mixed drinks	5	0.20	10 hours	Slowed reflexes; erratic changes in feelings
15 beers, glasses of wine, or mixed drinks	7½	0.30	15–16 hours	Stuporous, complete loss of coordination; little sensation
20 beers, glasses of wine, or mixed drinks	10	0.40	20 hours	May become comatose; breathing may cease
25–30 beers, glasses of wine, or mixed drinks	15–20	0.50	26 hours	Fatal amount for most people

*BAC, blood alcohol content.

Wellness Guide

One Student's DUI Experience

Early in the morning last summer, I was arrested for driving under the influence of alcohol.

It's not easy to recall what actually happened—I see it through a fog, as if I was watching someone else.

The actual arrest is the blurriest. I was running for those few moments on pure adrenalin and fear. For awhile, I don't even think I was breathing.

It's hard to explain the exact emotions.

It's hard to explain what it feels like to want more than anything to be sober.

It's hard to explain losing complete control of your life for even a short time.

It is hard to explain the feeling of handcuffs.

It's hard to explain what it feels like to sit in a holding cell and bite your lip in the hope of not going to sleep.

One thing for sure is that when those flashing lights appeared in my rearview mirror, all the rationalizations that got me into that car vanished. "It's just around the corner," "I need to get a friend home," or "No one is on the road at this hour"— none of them mean a thing—zero.

At the jail, it took what seemed like days to be fingerprinted and photographed and to fill out the required forms. Each step was just a little more humiliating than the last.

I am still overwhelmed at how a single, incredibly poor judgment could affect so many parts of my life.

The ramifications will be with me in various ways for the next 3 years—which is as far ahead as I have ever cared to plan.

These shock waves include probation for 3 years, an exorbitant increase in the cost of my car insurance, a restricted driver's license for 90 days (which was agreed upon in lieu of 2 days in jail), and a $600 fine, to name a few.

Many of the ramifications cannot be quantified. There was the call home, a couple of days of generally feeling lousy, and the unshakable sense that I had proven myself a fool.

Through all of it, however, I have some things to be thankful for.

On the top of that very short list is the fact that I didn't kill anyone.

Having struggled to come to terms with the arrest, it is impossible to imagine . . . for that there is no atonement.

Also on that list is the discovery of some very supportive people in my life, all of whom said not that what happened was okay, but that I was going to be okay. I turned to my parents and friends for help, and no one turned away—I am thankful.

Whether this column will keep anyone from driving drunk is doubtful. If I had read this column before my arrest, I would have thought of a hundred reasons why it would never have applied to me— but I would have been wrong.

Source: The Aggie (April 10, 1990). University of California, Davis.

Drinks (2-hour period)

Weight	$1\frac{1}{2}$ oz. liquor or 12 oz. beer											
100	1	2	3	4	5	6	7	8	9	10	11	12
120	1	2	3	4	5	6	7	8	9	10	11	12
140	1	2	3	4	5	6	7	8	9	10	11	12
160	1	2	3	4	5	6	7	8	9	10	11	12
180	1	2	3	4	5	6	7	8	9	10	11	12
200	1	2	3	4	5	6	7	8	9	10	11	12
220	1	2	3	4	5	6	7	8	9	10	11	12
240	1	2	3	4	5	6	7	8	9	10	11	12

☐ **Be careful driving**
BAC = up to 0.05%

☐ **Driving will be impaired**
BAC = 0.05% – 0.08%

☐ **Do not drive**
BAC = 0.08 – 0.10%

Effects of Drinking on Driving

The behavioral effects of alcohol depend on the BAC (Table 18.2). At a BAC of 0.02, the "loosening-up" effects of alcohol become manifest. At a BAC of 0.10, the depressant effects of the drug become pronounced, the person may become sleepy, and motor coordination is affected. Speech may become slurred and postural instability may become noticeable.

Alcohol's effects on motor skills, judgment, and reaction times make driving after drinking extremely dangerous. Even after just one or two drinks, although an individual may not be legally drunk, reaction time, perception, and judgment are impaired. Approximately 40% of the nearly 40,000 highway fatalities each year involve people who are intoxicated. Highway accidents are among the 10 leading causes of

Terms

hangover: unpleasant physical sensations resulting from excessive alcohol consumption

congeners: flavorings, colorings, and other chemicals present in alcoholic beverages

acetaldehyde: a toxic substance produced when the liver breaks alcohol down

death in the United States. One-third of male college students and nearly one-fourth of female college students report driving after having consumed alcohol (Douglas et al., 1997).

Each year there are over 120 million episodes of alcohol-impaired driving in the United States (Liu et al., 1997). Men in the 21 to 34 age group have the highest frequency of alcohol-impaired driving; men in the 18 to 20 age group have the second-highest frequency, despite the fact that all states prohibit drinking for persons under age 21. By contrast, the rate of alcohol-impaired driving among women in the same age groups is one-fourth that of their male peers. The frequency of alcohol-impaired driving declines as people become middle-aged.

Besides impaired driving, alcohol consumption contributes to arguments, fights, jeopardized relationships, employee absenteeism, school failure, and lost jobs. According to the National Institute on Drug Abuse, 30% of all drinkers aged 18 to 25 reported that they had become "aggressive" while drinking; 19% had been in "heated arguments"; and 11% had been absent from school or work as a result of drinking. More than three-fourths of incidents of domestic violence are alcohol-related (Brookoff et al., 1997).

Sexual Behavior

The effects of alcohol on sexual desire and performance vary from person to person, and depend on the BAC. In some individuals, small amounts of alcohol may dispel uncomfortable feelings about sex and may facilitate sexual arousal. Higher amounts of alcohol (a BAC of 0.10 or more) may cause problems for males, such as getting and maintaining an erection or ejaculating, and for females, such as inadequate vaginal lubrication and difficulty reaching orgasm. Even at moderate BACs, some individuals are too intoxicated to effectively give and receive sexual pleasure.

Alcohol consumption may contribute to a variety of undesired consequences of sexual behavior. While intoxicated, people can forget to use a birth control method or simply ignore the practice altogether and thus become unintentionally pregnant. Not using condoms or having sex with a stranger increases the risk of transmission of STDs and AIDS. Alcohol can blur one's judgment and can lead to unintended sexual experiences.

Acquaintance rape has been linked to alcohol consumption on college campuses (see chapter 23). A sexual assault study revealed that 26% of men who acknowledged committing sexual assault on a date reported being intoxicated; 29% reported being slightly intoxicated. In this same study, 21% of the women who were victims of sexual aggression on a date reported being intoxicated; 32% were slightly intoxicated. A woman's alcohol consumption may prevent her from realizing that her friendly behavior is being perceived as seductive; men may be inclined to perceive friendly cues from a woman as a sign of sexual interest.

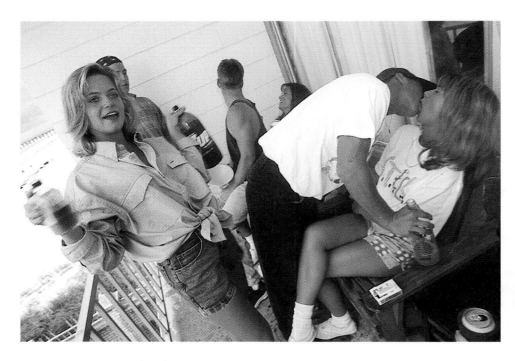

Drunkenness at parties can lead to actions and feelings that one regrets the next day—and sometimes for much longer.

Other Effects of Alcohol

Alcohol can impair the functioning of body organs other than the brain. Alcohol can irritate the organs of the gastrointestinal (GI) tract—the esophagus, stomach, intestine, pancreas, and liver—causing upset or irritability, nausea, vomiting, or diarrhea. Alcohol can also dilate arteries and cause bloodshot eyes. Dilation of arteries in the arms, legs, and skin can cause a drop in blood pressure and decrease body heat, explaining why people occasionally feel flushed when they drink. Giving people alcohol to "warm them up" actually produces the opposite physiological effect.

Alcohol should not be ingested simultaneously with other central nervous system depressants such as tranquilizers, sedatives, and antihistamines, which are found in cold medicines. In many instances, the depressant effects of alcohol and the other drug interact so that the combined effects of the two drugs is greater than the simple additive effects of either drug taken separately. Seemingly reasonable amounts of alcohol taken with another depressant drug can dangerously suppress brain function and respiration (Table 18.3).

Long-Term Effects

Long-term heavy drinking can affect the immune, endocrine, and reproductive functions and can cause neurological problems, including dementia, blackouts, seizures, hallucinations, and peripheral neuropathy. Various cancers associated with heavy drinking include cancers of the lip, oral cavity, pharynx, larynx, esophagus, stomach, colon, rectum, tongue, lung, pancreas, and liver. Long-term heavy drinking can also increase the risk of chronic gastritis, hepatitis, hypertension, cirrhosis of the liver, and coronary heart disease.

Chronic alcoholic men may become "feminized," with breast enlargement and female body hair patterns. Chronic alcoholic women may experience menstrual disturbances, loss of secondary sex characteristics, and infertility. Women who drink heavily experience more gynecological problems and have surgery more often than women who do not.

Fetal Alcohol Syndrome

Alcohol can harm the health of anyone, man or woman, young or old. Even a fetus can be damaged by alcohol. Over the last 10 years, evidence has accumulated showing that numerous kinds of birth defects

TABLE 18.3 Alcohol and Drugs That Don't Mix
Alcohol should NOT be consumed when taking drugs such as these.

Drug	Dangerous interaction
Acetaminophen (Tylenol, Anacin-3)	Moderate use plus alcohol can cause liver damage.
Aspirin (Anacin, Excedrin)	Heavy use plus alcohol can cause bleeding of stomach wall and GI tract.
Antihistamines (Chlor-Trimeton, Benadryl)	Drowsiness and loss of coordination increased by alcohol.
Tranquilizers, sedatives (Valium, Dalmane, Miltown)	Alcohol increases their effects.
Painkillers (codeine, Percodan, morphine)	Alcohol increases sedation and reduces ability to concentrate.
Barbiturates (Amytal, Seconal, phenobarbital)	Potentially FATAL. NEVER use with alcohol.

and mental retardation may result from ingestion of alcohol by pregnant women—a condition known as **fetal alcohol syndrome** (see chapter 15). Fetal alcohol syndrome is estimated to be the third leading cause of birth defects and mental retardation among newborns. Since the harmful effects on the fetus are believed to occur during the first few weeks or months of prenatal development, a time during which much of the nervous system is being formed, women should refrain from drinking if they are trying to become pregnant or if they suspect they are pregnant. Studies have also shown that the level of alcohol in the fetus' blood may be ten times greater than the BAC of the mother. This explains why even a couple of drinks early in pregnancy can endanger normal fetal development.

Health Benefits of Alcohol

A variety of studies have shown an association between consuming a small amount of alcohol (about a drink per day) and a lower risk of heart disease and stroke (LeBuono, 2000). The benefits of alcohol consumption were first reported among people in France, where it was noted that despite a diet high in fat, the rate of heart disease is low. This anomaly became known as the "French Paradox." At first the French Paradox was explained by the fact that red wine is widely consumed in France, and that substances in red wine, called flavonoids, were antioxidants that produced the heart-healthy effects. However, several studies have shown that the healthful effects of drinking are not specific to the type of drink, and hence it is concluded that such effects are due to ethanol.

The enzyme responsible for detoxifying alcohol in the body is called *alcohol dehydrogenase*. It comes in three different forms, depending on a person's genetic

Terms

fetal alcohol syndrome: birth defects and mental retardation caused by ingestion of alcohol during pregnancy

makeup. The people who have the slow oxidizing form of the enzyme experience the benefits of moderate alcohol consumption in preventing heart attacks (Hines et al., 2001), so moderate drinking is not necessarily beneficial for everyone.

Alcohol Abuse and Alcoholism

Alcohol abuse is the principal drug problem in the United States. Approximately 14 million Americans of different ages, religions, races, educational backgrounds, and socioeconomic status have problems with alcohol. Over 3 million American teenagers between ages 14 and 17 have a drinking problem. More than a third of all suicides involve alcohol. Approximately 6 million adults have personal and health problems associated with alcohol that are severe enough to warrant the label **alcoholic** and be said to have **alcoholism.** These people exhibit an intense craving for alcohol, are unable to control their drinking, are physically dependent on alcohol, and may experience withdrawal symptoms, including **delirium tremens (DTs),** characterized by hallucinations and uncontrollable shaking, when deprived of alcohol.

> *I don't even know what street Canada is on.*
> AL CAPONE

Problem drinking can cause numerous negative consequences. Job and school performance can be impaired, family relationships and friendships can be destroyed, and drunk driving may cause financial problems, injuries, legal problems and fatalities. Because alcohol supplies calories, alcoholics are rarely hungry. They may have vitamin deficiency syndromes, which result in mental confusion and loss of muscular coordination.

The cause or causes of problem drinking and alcoholism are unknown, although hypotheses abound.

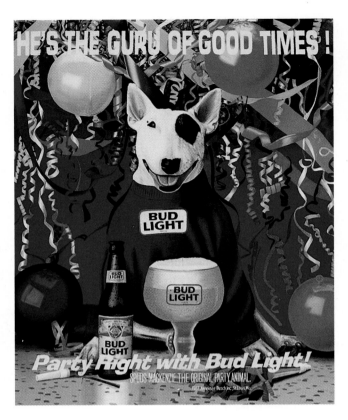

Alcohol advertisements, like cigarette ads, emphasize the connections among drinking, sex, and fun.

Before the advent of modern psychology and medicine, alcohol abuse was thought to be a manifestation of immorality and irreligiousness. Some people still hold that view, but many professionals (and problem drinkers) interpret alcohol abuse as a behavioral disorder or a medical disease. For example, some people may drink in order to feel better about themselves or to try to cope with life's adversities. Instead, they may add a drinking problem to their other problems.

Managing Stress

Breaking Addictive Behaviors

It's a little known fact, but it was psychologist Carl Jung who inspired the Alcoholics Anonymous program. Frustrated with a client unable to change his alcoholism, Jung suggested that his only hope for recovery was to purposefully have a spiritual experience to rid himself of this addictive habit. So, Roland H. did just that. After conquering his addiction, he went on to share this experience with Edwin T., then Bill W., who then went on to co-found Alcoholics Anonymous.

In response to a letter from Bill W., Jung wrote, "His craving for alcohol was the equivalent, on a low level, of the spiritual thirst of our being for wholeness, expressed in medieval language: the union with God. You see alcohol in Latin is *spiritus*, and we use the same words for the highest religious experience as well as for the most depraving poison. The helpful formula therefore is: *Spiritus contra spiritum.*" (Spiritual crises require spiritual cures).

Wellness Guide

Are You a Problem Drinker?

The CAGE Questionaire is a diagnostic tool for alcohol problems.

C = Concern by the person that there is a problem
A = Apparent to others that there is a problem
G = Grave consequences
E = Evidence of dependence or tolerance

Answer these questions:

1. Have you ever felt that you should Cut down on your drinking?
2. Have you ever become Annoyed by criticism of your drinking?
3. Have you ever felt Guilty about your drinking?
4. Have you ever had a morning Eye opener to get rid of a hangover?

One "yes" response indicates possible alcohol abuse.

Some evidence indicates that, at least for some people, alcoholism may have a biological basis, either because people metabolize alcohol differently or because their brains respond differently to alcohol. Some experts resist considering alcohol abuse a disease because doing so may remove the sense of personal and social responsibility for problem drinking. Others argue that calling alcohol abuse a "disease" fosters successful treatment because it removes the stigma, lessens guilt, and offers a supervised and presumably scientifically based plan for treatment.

The Phases of Alcoholism

Alcoholism usually develops from a prealcoholic stage of needing to drink to relieve tensions and anxieties. The prealcoholic phase may last for years, during which tolerance to alcohol gradually develops. Progression to a state of alcoholism is characterized by three phases:

- **The warning phase.** In this first stage of alcoholism, problem drinkers increase tolerance for alcohol and become more preoccupied with drinking. For example, when invited to a party they may ask what alcoholic beverages will be served rather than who is going to be there. In this stage problem drinkers may sneak drinks often and may deny that they are drinking too much. **Blackouts** may also occur. Blackouts are periods in which others observe the drinker as behaving normally or abnormally, but the drinker has no recall of events that happened while drinking.

- **The crucial phase.** This phase of alcoholism is characterized by loss of control over how much alcohol is consumed. The person may not drink every day, but cannot control the amount of alcohol consumed once drinking has begun. In this stage, the problem drinker may rationalize drinking behavior and actually believe that there are good reasons for heavy drinking. Alcoholics may still carry out responsibilities (e.g., housework, job, schoolwork) for some time, and they may employ a series of strategies to keep the family from rejecting them, including promises to stop drinking. Often alcoholics' extravagant measures to prove they do not have a drinking problem appear successful, but eventually they begin drinking heavily again. At this point the problem with alcohol is sometimes blamed on the kind of drinks preferred or on the usual place of drinking; as a result, problem drinkers may change to a different form of alcoholic beverage or to a different place in which to drink.

- **The chronic phase.** In this phase, the alcoholic is dependent on the drug, and drinking behavior consumes all aspects of life. Friends and family have resigned themselves to the problem and may be angry or ignore the alcoholic. At this stage of alcoholism the person may miss work or school occasionally. The health consequences of alcohol abuse may intensify and the person may need medical attention and even hospitalization. When physical addiction to alcohol occurs, continual drinking is needed to prevent withdrawal symptoms. Drinking for days at a time (a **bender**) may take place. The great majority of alcoholics do not wind up on "skid row," but instead struggle with their problem within their families and communities.

Terms

alcohol abuse: frequent, continued use of alcohol; binge drinking

alcoholic: a person dependent on alcohol

alcoholism: loss of control over drinking alcohol

delirium tremens (DTs): hallucinations and uncontrollable shaking sometimes caused by withdrawal of alcohol in alcohol-dependent individuals

blackout: failure to recall normal or abnormal behavior or events that occurred while drinking

bender: several days of binge drinking

The Effects of Alcoholism on the Family

Alcoholism can severely disrupt marital and family relationships. One family member's drinking problem can put stress on all the other members, causing them mental and emotional suffering and sometimes financial hardship. Alcoholism is costly to many people, not just the alcoholic. Seventy-six million Americans, about 43% of the population, have been exposed to alcoholism in the family.

Close relatives of a problem drinker can experience a variety of emotions, ranging from joy and relief when the problem drinker stops drinking for a time to feelings of failure and depression when the problem drinker begins drinking again. In between the highs and lows, family members can feel anger, shame, guilt, pity, and constant anxiety. They may try to cope with the situation in different ways. Some may try to assume responsibility for the problem; others may be designated as scapegoats and blamed for it, while some family members blame others (i.e., other family members, other people) for the drinker's problem. Some may withdraw in silence while others try to maintain their sense of humor. These behaviors are all defense mechanisms against the family's psychological pain.

Like the problem drinker, family members may deny the problem, try to rationalize it, isolate themselves from friends and relatives, and, in some cases, actually feel responsible for the other's drinking problem. This **enabling,** or protection process, keeps the alcoholic from feeling responsible for his or her drinking—which is part of the paradox experienced by families of alcoholics. In their attempts to protect the alcoholic, family members may unwittingly contribute to the drinking problem; they may try to protect the alcoholic from serious social consequences of excessive drinking, for instance, making excuses for absenteeism from work or school.

Family members of alcoholics may attend Alanon, an organization that helps spouses, families, and friends of alcoholics. Alateen is a similar organization that helps children of alcoholics. Alanon and Alateen help family members understand how alcoholism has affected their lives and help them to explore the family relationships that contribute to the alcohol problem. Family therapy (with or without the problem drinker's participation) may help a family find ways to cope with the problem and regain harmony in their family life.

Children of Alcoholics

The National Clearinghouse for Drug and Alcohol Information estimates that there are 28 million children of alcoholics (COAs) in the United States, 11 million of whom are under the age of 18. Adult children of alcoholics (ACOAs) and COAs grew up in families in which one or both parents had a drinking problem. As children, many of these individuals experienced neglect, emotional deprivation, an unstable family environment, and sometimes violence and abuse. As a result, they may have developed ways of thinking and behaving that impair personal and relationship harmony in adulthood. Children of alcoholics are at a high risk of becoming alcoholics themselves.

To numb the emotional pain stemming from parental alcoholism, many ACOAs learn as children to block from their awareness the truth of their situation—both the fact of a parent's alcoholism and also the emotional pain resulting from it. This tendency is referred to as **denial.** The consequences of denial by the ACOA go beyond issues of parental alcoholism to become a generalized way of approaching life. As adults, many ACOAs are constricted in their capacities to see the world as it really is and also to experience emotional fulfillment.

Denial gives many ACOAs a negative self-image and a tendency to be hypercritical of themselves. Rather than face the painful truth, many ACOAs, when children, believed themselves to be the cause of their parent's erratic, violent behavior. Indeed, sometimes the troubled parents reinforced this assumption by blaming their children for their problems. The children not only come to believe themselves to be "bad," but they also tend to believe they are responsible for everyone else's emotions. Thus, they become very other-focused, a behavior called **codependency.**

Another consequence of growing up in an alcoholic family is the tendency to try to control situations and other people. Because family life was unstable and painful, many ACOAs come to believe that their interpersonal environment is likely at any moment to become emotionally painful, violent, or disruptive. Thus, ACOAs tend to be constantly anxious and hypervigilant for signs of danger. To minimize the threat (experienced as criticism, abandonment, or abuse), ACOAs tend to be compliant and agreeable and actively try to please. Believing that others cannot be trusted and that the world must be made safe, ACOAs also try to be totally self-reliant and in control of their lives.

Denial, a negative self-image, the tendency to take responsibility for others, the need to control oneself

---

T e r m s

enabling: denial of, or excuses for, the excessive drinking by an alcoholic to whom one is close

denial: refusal to admit you (or someone else) have a drinking problem

codependency: a relationship pattern in which the nonaddicted family members identify with the alcoholic

and the environment, and other characteristics help an ACOA survive childhood in an alcoholic family. Unfortunately, in adulthood these same "survival" mechanisms limit the opportunity to grow and develop unique individual qualities and to experience healthy interpersonal relationships. Fortunately, these self-limiting beliefs and behaviors can be changed through counseling, 12-step programs, such as Codependents Anonymous, and various spiritual practices.

Seeking Help: Treatment Options

The situation of problem drinkers and alcoholics is serious but not hopeless. Recovery is possible if the person is strongly motivated to stop drinking. Moreover, as in other aspects of health, "an ounce of prevention is worth a pound of cure."

Sometimes the motivation to stop drinking comes in the form of a threat—a drinking-related legal problem or illness, severe disruption of family life, the loss of a job. The motivation to stop drinking can also come from the person's own resolve to stop his or her self-destructive behavior and to stop feeling helpless, hopeless, and confused.

Alcoholics Anonymous (AA), the worldwide nonprofit self-help organization, has assisted many people to get on the road back to wellness and enjoyment of life. AA bases its program on total sobriety, anonymity, and a step-by-step program of recovery. The environment at AA meetings is relaxing, caring, and open. Members share their experiences, strengths, and hopes with each other, with the goal of helping new and old members identify and learn more about their own problems with alcohol. Practical tips on how to remain sober are shared, and telephone numbers are exchanged so that a member can contact another member if stressful situations arise that previously led to drinking.

Alcoholics Anonymous emphasizes that sobriety is a state of mind, which means that recovering from a drinking problem involves changing values, attitudes, and lifestyles. The AA program helps problem drinkers honestly examine their feelings, recognize their limitations, and accept responsibility for past wrongs. For problem drinkers, remaining sober is an ongoing process, which involves finding new ways to satisfy emotional, spiritual, and social needs.

Besides AA, problem drinkers can receive help from individual and group psychotherapy. Many therapists are trained specifically to help problem drinkers and their families recover. Also, certain medicines may help. Disulfuram ("Antabuse") causes uncomfortable physical and mental feelings when alcohol is ingested. Naltrexone ("ReVia") can help reduce the craving for alcohol.

Responsible Drinking

Each person has the option of drinking or abstaining from alcohol. Each of you has the responsibility for determining the occasions for drinking and the amounts of alcohol that you consume. If you are one of the millions of people who already enjoy drinking, here are some guidelines to remember:

- Make sure that alcohol use improves your social interactions and does not harm or destroy them.
- Drink slowly and avoid mixing alcohol with other drugs.
- Be sure that using alcohol enhances your general sense of well-being and does not make either you or other persons feel disgusted with your actions.
- If you plan to drink, decide beforehand that you will not drive and designate someone who will not drink to be the driver.

In addition to being responsible for your own drinking habits, you can also help others to drink responsibly. Respect the wishes of the person who chooses to abstain from drinking and don't push drinks on people at parties. If you are giving a party, be sure to provide alternatives to alcohol. You may also offer places to sleep for those who have been drinking and should not drive home. Remember to eat when you drink and to provide food at your parties.

There is no evidence to indicate that total abstinence from alcohol is necessary for health and wellness. On the other hand, there is a great deal of evidence showing that excessive alcohol use can destroy personal health and family relationships, can cause traffic deaths and suicides, and can produce birth defects in newborns. We believe that you can significantly improve your health and happiness by developing responsible drinking habits while you are young and maintaining moderate drinking habits throughout life.

Critical Thinking About Health

1. After about a month it was clear that inviting Chris to be their roommate had been a brilliant move. With a 3.9-plus GPA, Chris was a fountain of help with every subject from history to chemistry. Getting into law school was a forgone conclusion. The real question was how to get Chris on "Jeopardy!"

   When mid-term exams rolled around, the roommates noticed that Chris was coming home every day with a 12-pack of beer—six cans would disappear before dinner and the rest disappeared as the night's studying progressed. Although Chris showed no signs of impairment from ingesting this quantity of alcohol, the roommates were concerned.

   a. What concerns might the roommates have? If you were Chris' roommate, would you be concerned?

   b. Given Chris' obvious success in school and the fact that Chris shows no outward sign of impairment, would you agree or disagree that Chris has a problem with alcohol?

   c. Do you think Chris' roommates should try to change Chris' drinking behavior, or is it none of their business?

2. "I don't like alcohol all that much. And it's never fun to wake up and find that you vomited all over yourself and don't remember doing it. There have been times I don't know how I got home, and I only hope that whoever drove the car wasn't as wasted as I was. Still, you need it. There's no better way to de-stress after a hard week of school. And you need to drink so you can be loose at a party. No one wants to dance with a dweeb, much less have sex with them."

   What's your opinion on this person's attitude? If you disagree with this student's philosophy, explain your reasons.

3. Every summer, State U. invites the parents of incoming students to "Parents' Day," a chance to visit the campus and talk to faculty, students, and administrators. Last summer, Dr. Meredith, one of the university's newest faculty members, gladly volunteered to give a "sample lecture" on paleontology to the parents and to chat with them at the luncheon in the Faculty Dining Room.

   A father of an incoming female student engaged Dr. Meredith in conversation about his daughter's likely experiences living in the college dormitory and swimming on the swim team.

   "My daughter's never been away from home before," said the father. "I want to be sure she'll be OK."

   Dr. Meredith silently gulped hard, for he knew that the dormitories had the reputation for massive illegal drinking during the first month or two of the school year, and that the swim coach would drink beer with the team members after swim meets.

   a. Does the father have anything to be concerned about?

   b. Should Dr. Meredith tell the father about alcohol use at the college?

   c. To avoid having to encounter another parent with similar concerns, Dr. Meredith vowed never again to help out at Parents' Day. What else could Dr. Meredith do to avoid such unpleasant experiences? Remember that Dr. Meredith is new at the university and without tenure.

   d. What is the campus climate toward tolerating alcohol use among students on your campus?

4. A college needs an electronic scoreboard for its football stadium, and a beer company is willing to buy it in exchange for exclusive advertising rights on the scoreboard and in the football game programs. The college president is against this deal, arguing that it promotes drinking on campus. However, the athletic director and the president of the alumni association favor it, arguing that it's vital to have the new scoreboard and besides, "beer and college always have gone together and always will, and there's nothing wrong with it."

   a. Do you favor or object to the scoreboard deal?

   b. Do you agree or disagree with the college president about the fact that advertising promotes drinking?

   c. Do you agree or disagree with the athletic director and alumni president that beer and college always have and always will go together?

Health in Review

- Alcohol abuse is the major drug problem in the United States. Consumption of alcohol is responsible for almost half of all highway fatalities and for numerous social, family, and health problems.
- Alcoholic beverages contain ethyl alcohol, which is produced by the action of yeast on sugar (fermentation) in grains and the juices of berries and fruits. Beer and wine are direct products of fermentation; "hard" liquor, such as whiskey, vodka, rum, and brandy, is made from distilled fermented liquids. Most standard portions of alcoholic beverages contain one-half ounce of ethyl alcohol.
- Social and normative influences on drinking behavior are evident in specific drinking patterns among college students. Drinking on campus increases the risk of violence, including sexual assault.
- Alcohol enters the bloodstream within minutes after ingestion. The physical and behavioral effects of alcohol depend on the blood alcohol content (BAC). A BAC of 0.02 produces a "loosening up" effect. A BAC of 0.10 seriously impairs motor coordination and judgment; in most states it is illegal to drive with a BAC of 0.10.
- Frequent and constant use of alcohol can lead to physical dependence and tolerance for the drug (alcoholism). Alcoholism develops in stages, starting with the inability to control drinking and advancing to complete physical dependence.
- Alcoholics may encounter severe health problems and their personal lives, family relationships, and friendships may be disrupted. Millions of children who grew up in families where one or both parents were alcoholics experience, as adults, personal problems, which stem from their childhoods.
- Organizations, such as Alcoholics Anonymous, and individual or group psychotherapy can help people recover from problem drinking and alcoholism. Alcohol abuse can be prevented by taking responsibility for one's drinking behavior.

Health and Wellness Online

The World Wide Web contains a wealth of information about health and wellness. By accessing the Internet using Web browser software, such as Netscape Navigator or Microsoft's Internet Explorer, you can gain a new perspective on many topics presented in *Health and Wellness, Seventh Edition.* Access the Jones and Bartlett Publishers Web site at http://www.jbpub.com/hwonline.

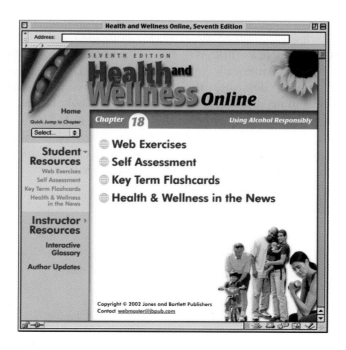

References

Baer, J. S., Stacy, A., and Larimer, M. (1991). Biases in the perception of drinking norms among college students. *Journal of Studies of Alcohol, 52* (6), 580–586.

Brookoff, D. et al. (1997). Characteristics of participants in domestic violence. *Journal of the American Medical Association, 277,* 1369–1373.

Cohen, A. (1997, September 8). The endless binge. *Time Magazine,* 54–56.

Douglas, K. A. et al. (1997). Results from the 1995 national college health risk behavior survey. *Journal of American College Health, 46,* 55–64.

Gfroerer, J. C., Greenblatt, M. S., and Wright, D. A. (1997). Substance use in the US college-age population. *American Journal of Public Health, 87,* 62–65).

Haines, S., and Spear, S. F. (1996). Changing the perception of the norm: A strategy to decrease binge drinking among college students. *Journal of American College Health, 45,* 134–140.

Hines, L. M. et al. (2001). Genetic variation in alcohol dehydrogenase and the beneficial effect of moderate alcohol consumption on myocardial infarction. *New England Journal of Medicine, 344,* 549–555.

Liu, S. et al. (1997). Prevalence of alcohol-impaired driving. *Journal of the American Medical Association, 277,* 122–125.

LeBuono, C. (2000, March 15). Dealing with the alcohol controversy. *Patient Care,* 211–225.

Nelson, T. E. and Wechsler. H. (2001). Alcohol and college athletes. *Medicine and Science of Sport and Exercise, 33,* 43–47.

Thun, M. J. et al. (1997). Alcohol consumption and mortality among middle-aged and elderly U.S. adults. *New England Journal of Medicine, 337,* 1705–1714.

Wechsler, H. et al. (1999). College binge drinking in the 1990s: A continuing problem. Harvard School of Public Health College Alcohol Study (http://www.hsph.harvard.edu/cas/rpt2000/CAS2000rpt2.htm).

Suggested Readings

Ashworth, M., and Gerada, C. (1997). ABC of mental health. Addiction and dependence II: alcohol. *British Medical Journal, 315,* 358–360. This article explains alcohol addiction.

Brown, S. (1996). *Treating adult children of alcoholics: A developmental perspective.* New York: Wiley. This book, written by one of America's best known alcohol-treatment therapists, describes the psychological problems that occur in people who grew up in alcoholic families and effective ways to recover.

O'Brien, C. P. (1997). A range of research-based pharmacotherapies for addiction. *Science, 278,* 66–70. This article reviews modern pharmacological approaches to the treatment of addiction, including alcoholism.

O'Connor, P. G., and Schottenfeld, R. S. (1998). Patients with alcohol problems. *New England Journal of Medicine, 338,* 592–602. This article reviews patterns of alcohol use in the United States, and the health consequences and medical treatment of alcohol abuse.

Schuckit, M. A. (2000). Alcohol and Alcoholism. *Medscape.* The author, a world-renowned researcher in alcohol issues, presents a concise overview of the effects of alcohol abuse.

Vallee, B. L. (1998, June). Alcohol in the Western world. *Scientific American,* 80–85. A distinguished scientist examines the history of the role of alcohol in Western civilization.

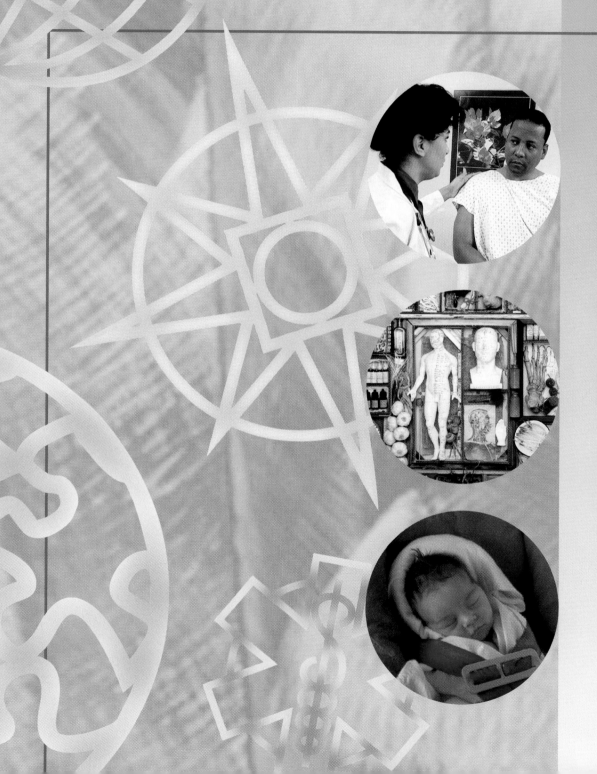

Part 6

Making Healthy Choices

Study Guide and Self Assessment

Intelligent Health Consumer Profile

Health and Wellness Online

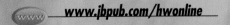 **www.jbpub.com/hwonline**

Chapter 19

Making Decisions about Health Care

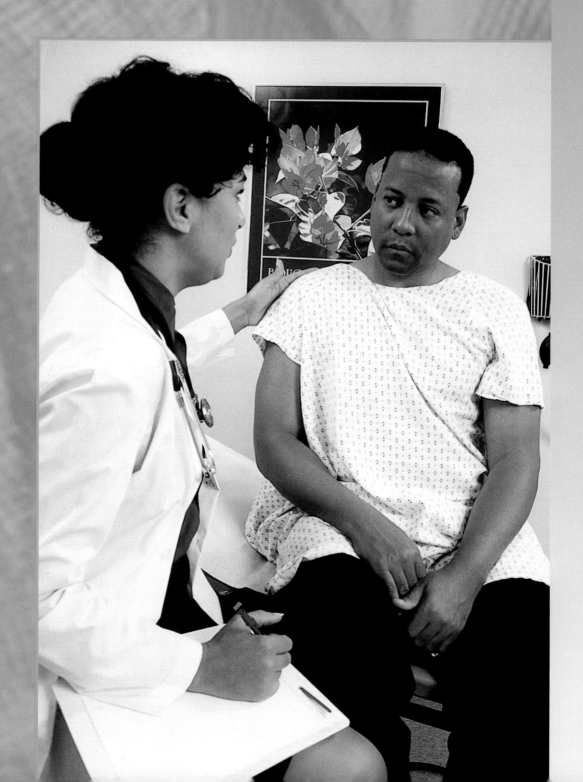

Everyone will need health care at some time. People need to go to health care professionals for vaccinations, physical exams, and diagnostic tests and for assistance when they are not feeling well. Occasionally people need to be hospitalized for serious illness, injury, or surgery. Health care and the cost of medical services are among people's most important concerns. Both state and federal governments have been trying to ensure that all citizens have some form of health insurance and can receive health care when needed, but millions of people in this country still do not have access to health care services or cannot afford health insurance.

Brief History of Medicine.
2000 BC: Here, eat this root.
1000 AD: That root is heathen. Here, say this prayer.
1850 AD: That prayer is superstition. Here, drink this potion.
1940 AD: That potion is snake oil. Here, swallow this pill.
1985 AD: That pill is ineffective. Here, take this antibiotic.
2001 AD: That antibiotic doesn't work anymore. Here, eat this root.

Modern medicine has become highly technical and expensive. The consumer of health care services must be able to evaluate the risks and benefits of diagnostic tests, treatments, recommended drugs, or surgery if he or she is to maintain control of decisions that affect health. Understanding your rights as a patient and knowing how to communicate your concerns and needs to health professionals will help you stay healthy and help in the healing process when you become sick.

Being a Wise Health Care Consumer

Making wise decisions about your health is part of self-care and self-responsibility. As health care consumers, we make important decisions about the health products we purchase, the health services we select, and the information we receive.

Behaviors that can help protect you from health fraud and unnecessary medical procedures include:

- Being well informed and knowing how to make healthy decisions
- Seeking reliable sources of information
- Being skeptical about health information appearing in news media or advertising
- Being wary of unlicensed practitioners and undocumented claims by health practitioners
- Selecting practitioners with great care and asking questions about fees, diagnoses, treatments, and alternative treatments
- Reporting health care fraud and wrongdoing to government regulating agencies

Good health care should be a partnership between you and the health care provider. The quality and cost of health care depend both on you and your doctor. Being a wise health care consumer starts with three basic principles: (1) working in partnership with your health care provider; (2) sharing in health care decision making; and (3) becoming skilled at obtaining health care.

Communication is extremely important in a physician-patient relationship. As a partner in your own health care, you are responsible for managing minor health problems at home. At the first sign of a health problem, you should observe and record symptoms to share with your health care provider, so that you and your health care provider can better manage problems. When visiting your health care provider, be prepared; you only have a limited time with them. Prepare a checklist of questions you want to ask, as well as a list of your symptoms. During your visit state your concerns, describe the symptoms, and ask questions regarding prescribed drugs, the diagnosis, and treatment recommendations.

The second principle in being a wise health care consumer is shared decision making. In partnership with your health care provider you should actively participate in every medical decision. You have this right except in the emergency room, where informed consent is not necessary. There are numerous ways to share in health care decisions: (1) let your doctor know what you want; (2) do your own research; (3) ask why a test or treatment is recommended; (4) ask about alternatives; (5) consider watchful waiting; (6) state your health care preferences; and (7) accept responsibility.

Being skilled at obtaining health care is the third principle. By communicating and partnering with your health care provider, you can become skilled in purchasing health care services. There are many ways to cut the cost of health care without affecting the quality: (1) exercise self-care and self-responsibility; (2) seek health care from a primary health care provider; (3) reduce unnecessary medical tests; (4) reduce drug use; (5) use specialists only when necessary; (6) use emergency services only for real emergencies; and (7) use hospitals only when required.

Selecting a Health Care Practitioner

The self-care movement became strong in the United States in the 1970s when health care costs began increasing and Americans became more interested in wellness and healthier lifestyles. However, self-care is not always appropriate and can be dangerous in some situations. Today's health care system is extremely

TABLE 19.1   Selected Medical Specialties

Specialty	Specific focus
Anesthesiology	Administration of drugs to prevent pain or to induce unconsciousness during surgical operations or diagnostic procedures
Cardiology	Diagnosis and treatment of diseases of the heart and blood vessels, including such problems as heart attacks, hypertension, and stroke
Dermatology	Diagnosis and treatment of skin diseases
Endocrinology	Deals with medical problems that result from abnormalities in the endocrine (hormone) system in the body
Family practice	General medical services for patients and their families
Geriatrics/gerontology	Concerned with problems of the elderly
Internal medicine	Diagnosis and nonsurgical treatment of internal organs of the body
Neurology	Diagnosis and nonsurgical treatment of diseases of the brain, spinal cord, and nerves
Obstetrics and gynecology	Care of pregnant women and treatment of disorders of the female reproductive system
Oncology	Diagnosis and treatment of all forms of cancer
Ophthalmology	Medical and surgical care of the eye, including prescription eyeglasses
Orthopedics	Diagnosis and treatment of abnormalities in bone and muscle, especially injuries resulting from sport activities
Pathology	Examination and diagnosis of organs, tissues, body fluids, and excrement
Pediatrics	Medical care of children, usually up to teenage years
Preventive medicine	Prevention of disease through immunization, good health care, and concern with environmental factors
Psychiatry	Treatment of mental and emotional problems
Public health	Subspecialty of preventive medicine that deals with promoting the general health of the community
Radiology	Use of radiation for the diagnosis and treatment of disease
Urology	Treatment of male reproductive system and urinary tract and treatment of female urinary tract

icine, one must pass a national or state examination. Because the range of medical knowledge is so broad, many medical school graduates choose to become specialists, which requires 3 or more years of specialty training (Table 19.1). Medical specialty boards have high standards of performance and training. Successful specialty training applicants are board certified. Many states and specialty boards require physicians to participate in continuing education programs to maintain their license and specialty license, respectively.

The doctor of medicine (M.D.) and the doctor of osteopathy (D.O.) provide both primary and specialty care. Many states have a single licensing board for doctors of medicine and doctors of osteopathy; others have separate boards for each profession. The training of these two physician groups is similar, except that doctors of osteopathy place greater emphasis on musculoskeletal diagnosis and treatment.

Dentists

Dentists are licensed in every state and hold either a doctor of dental surgery (D.D.S.) or a doctor of medical dentistry (D.M.D.) degree. Dental schools require at least 2 years of college; however, most entering dental students have a baccalaureate degree. Dental school takes 4 years with at least 2 or more years of training for a dental specialty (Table 19.2).

Podiatrists

Doctors of podiatric medicine (D.P.M.) are engaged in the diagnosis, prevention, and treatment of foot problems. Education includes at least 3 years of undergraduate work and 4 years of study at one of seven accredited colleges of podiatric medicine in the United States. The American Podiatric Medical Association

complex, with numerous medical, dental, and allied health professionals addressing consumers' health care needs. Deciding which health care professional to choose can be confusing. All physicians practice conventional, Western, or modern medicine. This type of medicine is based on principles of modern science and clinical experience and trials. Practitioners of alternative medicine include chiropractors, homeopaths, and naturopaths, who rely on alternative methods of healing, which may, or may not, be based on scientific research. People often use alternative medicines to complement the treatments they receive from their physicians.

Medical Doctors

Physicians must have at least 3 years of undergraduate work and 4 years of training at an accredited medical or osteopathic school. To be licensed to practice med-

TABLE 19.2   Dental Specialties

Specialty	Specific focus
Endodontics	Prevention and treatment of diseases of the root pulp and related structures
Oral and maxillofacial surgery	Tooth extraction; surgical treatment of diseases, injuries, and defects of the mouth, jaw, and face
Oral pathology	Diagnosis of tumors, other diseases, and injuries of the head and neck
Orthodontics	Diagnosis and correction of tooth irregularities and facial deformities
Pediatric dentistry	Dental care of infants and children
Periodontics	Treatment of diseases of the gums and related structures
Prosthodontics	Treatment of oral dysfunction through the use of prosthetic devices, such as crowns, bridges, and dentures
Public health dentistry	Prevention and control of dental disease and promotion of community dental health

(APMA) estimates that there are approximately 13,800 practicing podiatrists in the United States, treating corns, bunions, calluses, and malformations of the foot.

Seeing the Doctor

The majority of people who go to a doctor have minor complaints, have come for a routine follow-up of some chronic problem, or may simply need some kind of reassurance. In general, patients fall into three categories: (1) those who think they are sick and are; (2) those who think they are well but are actually sick; and (3) the "worried well" who come for reassurance that they are not sick. This last group may account for as many as half of all patients who are seen by family practice physicians.

Although some physicians encourage annual checkups, most studies show that frequent medical exams for people who are basically healthy are unnecessary. How often you see a physician depends on your personal needs, but many people go to a physician for minor complaints and illnesses that usually do not require medical attention (Table 19.3). Often people are asking more from their doctors than just medicine.

Patient satisfaction with health care usually depends on what occurs in the physician's office. The quality of health care depends to a great degree on the interaction between the physician and the patient. Often, anxiety about what may be wrong, long waits to see the physician, and a seemingly endless number of tests can contribute to patients' stress. You can increase the chance of a successful encounter with your health care provider or hospital if you have a clear understanding of what you want to accomplish during your office visit or hospital stay.

The medical profession recognizes that medical education needs to be about more than providing medical facts. Learning to listen, asking questions, and expressing empathy with patients also need to be part of medical education. A few medical schools have tried to help medical students understand how to relate better with patients. Communication skills can be learned. As wise health care consumers you need to select physicians who meet not only your health care needs but your communication needs as well.

Diagnosis is separate and distinct from any agreement you make about treatment. In any illness, there are two important choices: first, admitting that you are sick and finding out what is wrong, which is the process of the **diagnosis;** and second, deciding what is the best course of treatment, based on the diagnosis.

For example, suppose you have had a slight pain in your chest and the diagnostic tests indicate that you have partial blockage of a coronary artery. One physician might recommend dietary changes, exercises, and a drug to control the pain. Another physi-

Wellness Guide

How to Have a Successful Interaction with Your Physician

- You should choose a physician you trust and in whose medical skills you have complete confidence. Take the time to find a primary care physician who can satisfy your medical needs. He or she should be someone to whom you can openly express your health concerns.

- Clear and open communication between you and your physician is essential. You should understand the nature of your medical problems and the reasons for any tests that are ordered. You should feel free to ask about different treatment options. You are entitled to all the information pertaining to your condition in language you can understand.

- You should feel confident enough to share with

your physician any emotional problems you may have or any stress in your life. This information may be important in arriving at an accurate diagnosis and treatment recommendation. If you are upset in your interaction with a physician, the art of healing is not being practiced.

- Before going to a physician's office, try to relax your mind and body by practicing a meditation or image visualization exercise. This will help calm you when you are discussing your problems with the physician.

- Always remember how suggestible your mind is during a medical consultation. What the physician says about your condition can be as important in the healing process as the treatment. If the

physician is positive and encouraging, the likelihood of a cure is increased.

- While negative statements made by the physician cannot be ignored, try not to let your mind be unduly influenced by them. For example, statements regarding complications, adverse effects, chance of permanent disability, and probable duration of the sickness are general comments derived from statistical data collected from thousands of patients. You are not a statistic but an individual and averages need not apply to you. Negative statements that are believed tend to produce negative effects on the body.

TABLE 19.3   The 20 Most Common Complaints, Problems, or Symptoms for Doctor Visits
One in eight persons go to the doctor without any complaint or symptom.

Rank	Complaint	Rank	Complaint
1	Progress visits	11	Gynecological exam
2	Physical exam	12	Visit for medication
3	Pain, etc.—lower extremity	13	None
4	Pregnancy exam	14	Headache
5	Throat soreness	15	Fatigue
6	Pain, etc.—upper extremity	16	Pain in chest
7	Pain, etc.—back region	17	Well-baby exam
8	Cough	18	Fever
9	Abdominal pain	19	Allergic skin reaction
10	Cold	20	All other symptoms

cian might insist on immediate surgery to correct the condition. Only by obtaining as much information as possible can you make a decision that feels right to you.

Hospitals

At some time in your life you will need to use a health care facility, whether a hospital for planned surgery, an emergency room, or as you, your parents, or friends become older, nursing home facilities. To make wise decisions concerning health care facilities, it is important to understand the types of facilities available and whether they meet your needs.

Most Americans will be admitted to a hospital at some time during their lives. For many people the hospital experience is confusing and frightening. To cope with this unpleasant reality, one should understand a hospital patient's rights.

On admission to a hospital, a patient is required to sign a consent form delegating all decisions regarding his or her care to the hospital and physicians. In most instances, physicians obtain informed consent for any invasive procedure, either diagnostic or therapeutic, before proceeding. But the amount of information that is given to the patient and how well a patient understands the proposed treatment usually depend on many factors that affect communication between the patient and the physician. The American

Hospital Association publishes a Patient's Bill of Rights covering the situations and questions most often encountered by hospital patients. You are entitled to ask for a list of patients' rights in that hospital.

The most frustrating and anxiety-producing situations for a patient are not understanding what is going to happen and, even worse, not knowing what is happening while being subjected to unfamiliar and uncomfortable procedures. Except in the case of a life-threatening emergency that demands immediate action, you have the right to be fully informed of all

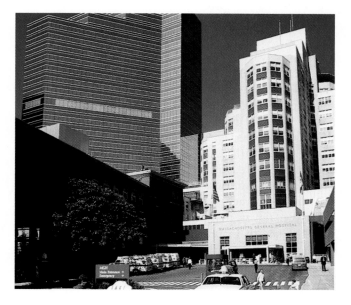

For many people, the hospital is an impersonal and confusing place. Developing good communication with health care providers and knowing your rights as a consumer can help combat those feelings.

Terms

diagnosis: the cause of a disease or illness as determined by a physician

Wellness Guide

Caring for and Preventing Back Pain

Back pain, especially acute pain in the lower back, is one of the most common complaints for which people seek help from physicians, chiropractors, massage therapists, or other healers. Diagnosing the cause of back pain is crucial for proper treatment. If no injury or disease of the spine is detected by X rays or other medical tests, muscle strain and/or tension is the probable cause of the pain.

For back pain caused by strain, poor posture, or muscle tension, the accepted medical treatments are bed rest or back extension exercises. In general, studies comparing bed rest, exercises, and continuing with one's daily activities as much as

possible show that continuing with normal activities is the best choice, as long as one is careful not to worsen the condition. Most back pain caused by strain or tension clears up without treatment, although many sufferers get relief from chiropractic manipulation or massage. However, lifting heavy objects, including children, is not advised while recovering from back pain. Sleeping on a firm, flat surface can help.

Simple back care exercises can help prevent tension, strain, and pain in the back. One helpful exercise involves standing flat against a wall. Try to press your head, heels, shoulders, and butt flat

against the wall. If there is a space between the small of your back and the wall big enough to insert your hand, your back is overarched. To correct this, slide your feet forward, bend your knees slightly, and try to press the small of your back against the wall. Try to hold this posture as you slide your back up the wall. Make sure the small of your back is as close to the wall as possible. Slowly walk away from the wall holding your back in this new position. Repeat the exercise several times each day until your posture improves and your back feels stronger.

God heals and the doctor takes the fee.
BEN FRANKLIN

medical procedures and the reasons for them. As a patient, you have the responsibility for deciding what you want done. Once you have made that decision, you should understand how to cooperate fully to gain the most benefit.

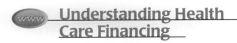

Understanding Health Care Financing

In various ways, the United States has attempted to make health care available to Americans. Some employers have provided health care for their employees and dependents; the federal government has provided health care for members of the armed services and their dependents, war veterans, and government employees; and with assistance from local and state governments, the federal government has provided health care for poor families. Nevertheless, a program to ensure universal access and equity in health care services has never materialized. There are three basic types of health insurance plans available: private insurance, health maintenance organizations (HMOs), and preferred provider organizations (PPOs).

Private Insurance

Fee-for-service or private health insurance is the traditional type of health care plan in the United States. Fee-for-service plans generally have a deductible the insured person pays before receiving benefits. Most

plans pay some physician and hospital expenses; most do not cover preventive health care, such as annual physicals or immunizations.

Health Maintenance Organizations

Health maintenance organizations (HMOs) are prepaid health insurance plans that are an alternative to private insurance. The growth of HMOs has surged during the last two decades. In 1998, more than 42 million Americans were enrolled in HMOs. HMOs are characterized by four principles defined by Congress in the Health Maintenance Organization Assistance Act of 1973: (1) an organized system of health care that accepts the responsibility to provide health care; (2) an agreed-upon set of comprehensive health maintenance and treatment services; (3) a voluntarily enrolled group of people in a specific geographic region; and (4) reimbursement through a prenegotiated and fixed payment schedule on behalf of the enrollee. An example of a large, successful HMO is the Kaiser-Permanente Medical Care Program, in which physicians emphasize early detection and disease prevention.

HMOs and other organizations that deliver medical services of various kinds provide what is known as **managed care.** In 1999, more than 90 percent of Americans with health insurance were enrolled in a managed care health organization. The simplest definition of managed care is a system that attempts to reduce the cost of health care. The escalating cost of health care in the U.S. results from many factors: excessive use of expensive diagnostic tests, treatments on demand, unnecessary visits to specialists, high-tech procedures and long stays in hospitals.

Despite certain benefits, HMOs have also experienced severe criticism. In contracts between physicians and HMOs, physicians often are prohibited from recommending certain expensive procedures that are not covered by the HMO; they also may receive bonuses for not recommending referrals or for other services. Physicians also are prohibited from disclosing the conditions of their contracts; this so-called "gag rule" has been severely criticized and has generated a backlash against some HMOs. Although managed health care is well established in the U.S., some health care analysts believe that eventually health care will have to evolve into some form of more equitable, universal coverage for all Americans (Ginzberg, 1997).

Choosing the best HMO for your needs is difficult, especially if choices are limited by your place of employment or financial resources. However, some guidelines may help. Some independent organizations attempt to rate the quality of HMOs. Check carefully what each HMO offers, especially for emergency care or for chronic conditions. If you are enrolled in an HMO, find a physician that you trust and with whom you can communicate freely. If you are not satisfied with a diagnosis or treatment, consult another doctor or ask for a second opinion.

Preferred Provider Organizations

Preferred provider organizations (PPOs) are a combination of the traditional fee-for-service health care plan and an HMO. Employers or insurance companies negotiate low fee-for-service rates with selected hospitals and health care providers in a specific geographic region. Participants in PPOs must use one of the "preferred" providers if they want their medical bills paid. If a participant opts for care from a nonprovider, he or she will be charged a substantial fee. Group health

Terms

health maintenance organization (HMO): an organization (either nonprofit or for-profit) of physicians, hospitals, and support staff that provides medical services to members

managed care: systems of health care in which the primary goal is to reduce costs

preferred provider organization (PPO): physicians who belong to the organization provide medical care at reduced costs that are negotiated by the organization

Wellness Guide

Health Care Insurance Terminology

Terminology to be familiar with when purchasing health insurance

Coinsurance	Arrangements by which the insurer and the insured share, in a specific ratio, payment for losses covered by the policy after the deductible is met
Comprehensive medical expense insurance	Form of health insurance that in one policy provides protection for both basic hospital expenses and major medical expense coverage
Coordination of benefits (COB)	Method of integrating benefits payable under more than one health insurance plan so that the insured's benefits from all sources do not exceed 100% of allowable medical expenses or eliminate appropriate patient incentives to contain costs
Deductible	Amount of covered expenses that must be incurred by the insured before benefits become payable by the insurer
Health insurance	Coverage providing for payment of benefits as a result of sickness or injury; includes insurance for losses from accident, disability, medical expense, or accidental death and dismemberment
Managed care	Those systems that integrate the financing and delivery of appropriate health care services to covered individuals by means of • Arrangements with selected providers to furnish a comprehensive set of health care services to members • Explicit criteria for the selection of health care providers • Formal programs for ongoing quality assurance and utilization review • Significant financial incentives for members to use providers and procedures associated with the plan
Maximum benefit	Highest amount an individual may receive under an insurance contract
Reasonable and customary charges (R&C)	Amounts charged by health care providers that are consistent with charges from similar providers for identical or similar services in a given locale
Utilization	Patterns of usage for a single medical service or type of service (hospital care, prescription drugs, physician visits). Measurement of utilization of all medical services in combination usually is done in terms of dollar expenditures. Use is expressed in rates per unit of population at risk for a given period, such as the number of annual admissions to a hospital per 1000 persons over age 65.
Utilization review	Program designed to reduce unnecessary hospital admissions and to control the length of stay for inpatients through the use of preliminary evaluations, concurrent inpatient evaluations, or discharge planning.

Dollars and Health Sense

Marketing Managed Care in Latin America

As managed care came under attack in the United States in the 1990s for excluding certain expensive procedures from coverage and for rewarding physicians who referred fewer patients to specialists, managed care organizations and insurance companies began to market managed care to countries in Latin America.

Managed care organizations can operate in Latin America with far fewer restrictions than in the United States. For example, use of financial incentives to physicians who limit care and referrals usually are not questioned as much in Latin American countries. And the managed care organizations often receive support from government officials who may be rewarded with stock or other benefits. Also, physicians' salaries and other costs are significantly lower.

In 1996, Aetna Insurance Company made a profit of $1.2 billion in Brazil from their managed care operation (Stocker, Waitzkin, & Iriart, 1999). Other multinational corporations also have reported making hundred of millions of dollars from for-profit health care plans introduced in Latin America.

Exporting health care plans is part of the new global economy. It offers the opportunity for companies to make considerable profits. It also has the potential to improve the health of people in Latin America. However, in the view of one health expert who has followed the export of managed care to Latin America:

These developments could represent a major advance for the health of the people of Latin America—if they lead to the establishment of health systems that emphasize the coordination of care and are committed to promoting medical education and research. Unfortunately, that is not the current situation, which resembles more closely a new corporate imperialism in health care (Perez-Stable, 1999).

---

insurance costs are reduced for both an HMO and PPO in exchange for a guaranteed pool of patients.

Federal Government Support: Medicare and Medicaid

Only in the last 50 years has the federal government become involved in providing health care coverage. Resulting from a concern for the social conditions of the economically disadvantaged and the elderly, Congress passed legislation in 1965 establishing Medicare and Medicaid.

Medicare is a federal health insurance program for Americans over age 65, for certain disabled Americans under age 65, and for people of any age with permanent kidney failure. The basic purpose of Medicare is to provide health care for all eligible older persons. All eligible beneficiaries, on reaching age 65, automatically are enrolled in Medicare, Part A, which covers hospital costs, rehabilitation in a skilled nursing facility, and hospice care for the terminally ill. Enrollment in Medicare, Part B, is voluntary, but most beneficiaries choose to enroll. Part B pays for 80 percent (after a $100 deductible) of physicians' services, emergency room visits, laboratory fees, diagnostic tests, and other medical expenses.

Medicare is an extremely popular government program, but it is expected to run out of money in the

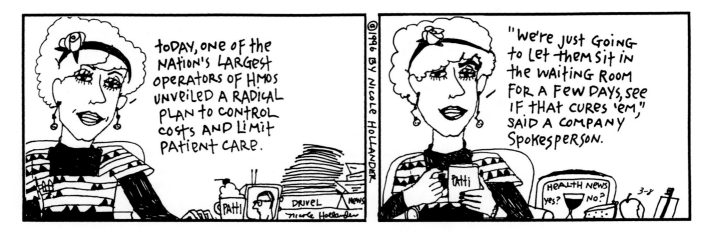

Source: SYLVIA © 1996 by Nicole Hollander.

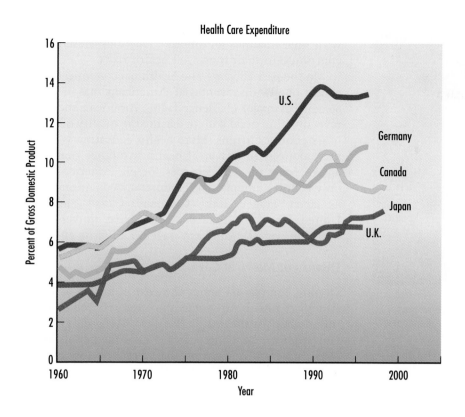

Health Care Expenditure

FIGURE 19.1 Health care expenditures in the major industrialized nations expressed as a percent of their gross domestic product (GDP). Although all countries spent approximately the same percent of their GDP on health care in 1960, by 2000, the United States was spending far more than any of the other major industrialized nations.

near future due to escalating costs and as the number of older people in the population increases. In its first year of operation in the 1960s, Medicare spent $21.5 billion; in 1997, the amount had increased to $214.6 billion, and it is still rising rapidly (Iglehart, 1999).

Medicaid provides health insurance for certain poor people in the United States. To be eligible for Medicaid benefits, an individual must be on welfare, have dependent children, or receive supplementary security income for the aged, blind, or disabled. In addition, Medicaid covers nursing home care for many elderly Americans.

 ## Health Care Issues Today

Rising Health Care Costs

Anyone who has been to a physician, filled a prescription, paid a health insurance premium, or been admitted to a hospital realizes how expensive medical care in the United States has become. In 1994, the cost of medical care exceeded $1 trillion; that was the year former President Clinton tried and failed to pass comprehensive health care legislation that would have reformed the health care system, expanded Medicare and Medicaid coverage, and restrained cost increases. However, agreement could not be reached, and the legislation failed to pass in Congress. Since then, the

problems and costs of health care in the United States have continued to escalate.

Many factors contribute to the dramatic increases in the costs of health care in the United States: physician fees, cost of prescription drugs and malpractice insurance, cost of hospital rooms and emergency services, and cost of health insurance. Another significant factor is the aggressive marketing of medical technologies, drugs, and tests to physicians and also directly to patients. The overzealous use of diagnostic and therapeutic technologies is largely what distinguishes U.S. medical care from that in other major industrialized countries; it also continues to drive up the costs of health care (see Figure 19.1). The United States leads the world in organ and bone marrow transplants, coronary bypass surgeries, and **magnetic resonance imaging (MRI)** use. While MRI is an important diagnostic tool for many medical problems, ownership of an expensive MRI machine by a hospital demands frequent use to pay for it. Also, to stay competitive, almost every

Terms

magnetic resonance imaging: use of a strong magnetic field to produce images of internal parts of the body; especially useful for soft tissues

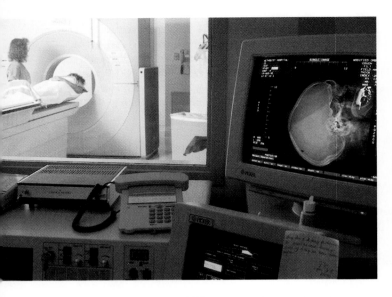

Computed tomographic (CT) scans and magnetic resonance imaging (MRI) help physicians make the correct diagnosis of an injury or disease.

hospital must have one. For example, Orange County, California has more MRI machines than are in all of Canada (Doyle, 1999).

Americans are paying more out-of-pocket for their health care than citizens of other countries. Americans pay over 20% of their health care costs, not including health insurance premiums. Another factor affecting health care costs is that more Americans are living longer. As the population ages, so does its risk for chronic and acute illnesses.

> At one time I had ambitions, but I had them removed by a doctor in Buffalo.
>
> TOM WAITS

Other factors contributing to high health care costs are lifestyle behaviors. Many health conditions that strain our health care system are preventable. Cancer due to smoking, heart disease due to obesity, automobile accidents due to drinking and driving—all are caused by behaviors that we choose. They cost us billions of dollars each year.

Inequities in Health Care

Socioeconomic status and race play crucial roles in health and health care (Freeman and Payne, 2000). Level of education, amount of income, and type of job all contribute to a person's health. A 1993 study showed that people earning less than $9,000 a year died at a rate three to seven times greater than those earning more than $25,000 a year. Black and Hispanic Americans generally have lower incomes than white Americans, experience more health problems, and are less likely to receive medical care. Poor people smoke more cigarettes, drink more alcohol, use more illegal drugs, and are exposed to violence more than people with high incomes and more education; these factors contribute to their increased health risks.

In the past 20 years, the health of economically and educationally disadvantaged Americans has declined steadily. A major challenge facing American society is reversing this trend and increasing the quality of health of its poorest citizens. More health education is necessary, along with universal health insurance that guarantees basic medical services for all. America is the only country among major industrialized nations, such as Japan, France, Italy, Germany, Canada, and the United Kingdom, that does not have universal (or nearly universal) health coverage for all of its citizens.

Quality of Medical Care

Despite complaints about the cost of health care, the American health care system is often referred to as being the best in the world. But is it? According to several studies, the United States falls far behind most other industrialized nations based on a variety of measures (Starfield, 2000). Based on child survival to 5 years of age, disparities across social groups in access to health care, expenditures for health care, and life expectancy, the World Health Organization ranked the United States 15th among 25 industrialized nations. The United States ranks near the bottom for low birth-weight babies and neonatal deaths and for years of potential life lost (excluding accidents and other external causes). While the United States excels at high-technology medicine, such as organ transplants, coronary bypass and angioplasty procedures, eye surgeries (LASIK), and cosmetic surgeries (liposuction, breast implants, face lifts, etc.), it does not meet many basic health needs as well as other countries that spend far less on health care.

Even more serious shortcomings of American medicine were documented in a report from the Institute of Medicine (IOM) entitled "To Err Is Human." This detailed study, which received wide coverage in various media, came to the following conclusions (Brennan, 2000):

- 12,000 deaths a year result from unnecessary surgery
- 7,000 deaths a year result from errors in medications in hospitals
- 20,000 deaths a year result from other hospital errors
- 80,000 deaths a year result from nosocomial (hospital acquired) infections (see chapter 12)
- 106,000 deaths a year result from adverse effects on patients of medications that were not given in error

Thus, the study found that more than 200,000 deaths occur each year in the United States from drug, hospital, or medical errors. Bear in mind that these numbers do not include adverse effects of errors that result in disability or suffering but not in death. To put these number of deaths in perspective, medical and hospital errors and adverse drug effects actually are the third leading cause of death after cardiovascular disease and cancer. The message from this study by the IOM is that the health care system in the United States is in need of a thorough overhaul. Another message is that paying more than twice as much as other countries does not guarantee the overall quality of health care.

The term "quality of life" refers to the physical, mental, and social aspects of health that are interrelated with the quality of medical care. Measuring the quality of life of a person can be done with a variety of questionnaires, and the results can be quantified (Testa and Simonson, 1996). Many health professionals believe quality of life should be measured both before and after treatment.

For example, testing for and treating prostate cancer is extremely controversial. Most prostate cancers are very slow-growing and do not cause death. However, a diagnosis of prostate cancer can lead to surgery that severely erodes the patient's quality of life. Prostate surgery often causes loss of sexual function, incontinence, depression, and other symptoms. For many people confronting serious disease, quality of life is more important that quantity of life, especially among the elderly.

While quality medical care can prevent and cure many forms of illness and prevent suffering, even the best and most costly medical care cannot protect us from health-destroying behaviors. The Centers for Disease Control and Prevention estimate that at least 50% of premature sickness could not be prevented by improved access to medical care (Foster, 1997). Half of the American population becomes sick because of behavioral factors: tobacco use, unsafe sex, poor nutrition, sedentary lifestyle, alcohol and drug abuse, and violent and risk-taking behaviors. We need to accept more responsibility for our behaviors and not expect health to be delivered to us by health care professionals.

Critical Thinking About Health

1. If you are old enough to have had a family physician who ran his or her own office and was not a member of any HMO or PPO, evaluate the health care that you had from them compared with the type of health care that you receive now. Describe what form of health insurance you have now and what form of insurance (if any) you had before.

2. Have you ever been hospitalized for an illness or injury? Describe the condition that caused you to be hospitalized, and discuss the care and tests that you experienced in the hospital. What things were the most positive and healing in the hospital? What things were the most distressing and unhealthy about your hospital experience? Suggest ways (based on your experience) that hospitals might improve the care they provide to patients.

3. The Medicare program, like the Social Security program, will face a fiscal crisis in the near future. The money that is collected by these two federal programs will not cover their costs unless they are restructured. Congress has proposed a new Medicare system for retired persons in which each worker would be required to put away a percentage of earnings during working years to pay for medical needs after retirement. This means that workers would now have to contribute a portion of wages to both Social Security and Medicare. Discuss whether you think this is the proper solution to solve Medicare's financial problems. Can you propose any other alternatives to provide the Medicare program with the money that is needed and that you think would be fair? Or do you think the federal government should not be involved in providing health care for retired persons at all?

4. Joe Windam is in the hospital with liver failure. Joe is only 32 years old but has been a heavy drinker most of his life, just like his father. He also contracted a hepatitis C infection several years ago that has contributed to his liver disease. Joe has been out of work for over a year and does not have any health insurance. The only hope that Joe has is a liver transplant; without a new liver, Joe will probably die in a few months. Do you think Joe should be given a high priority for a liver transplant because of his young age? Who should pay the several hundred thousand dollars in hospital and doctor bills? How should the priority for liver transplants be assigned, since there are not enough livers available for all the patients who need them?

Health in Review

- Everyone needs medical care at some time in his or her life. Knowing what to ask and what to expect from your physician is essential.
- The physician's responsibility is to find the cause of illness. The patient's responsibility is working in partnership with the health care provider, sharing in health care decision making, and becoming skilled at obtaining health care.
- Admission to a hospital is often an unsettling experience. Patients should be aware of their rights and ask questions that will ease their concerns.

- Health care is increasingly provided by large organizations of physicians and hospitals, called preferred provider organizations or health maintenance organizations.
- The costs of medical care in the United States have grown so rapidly that some form of health care reform is needed. Millions of citizens lack health insurance and access to health care.
- "Quality of life" refers to physical, mental, and social aspects of health that may be affected by medical care.

Health and Wellness Online

The World Wide Web contains a wealth of information about health and wellness. By accessing the Internet using Web browser software, such as Netscape Navigator or Microsoft's Internet Explorer, you can gain a new

perspective on many topics presented in *Health and Wellness, Seventh Edition*. Access the Jones and Bartlett Publishers Web site at http://www.jbpub.com/hwonline.

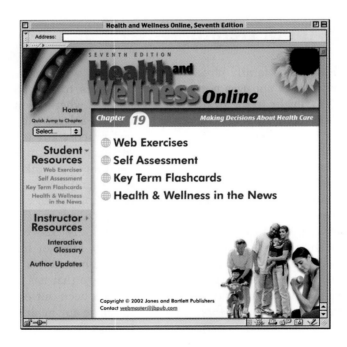

References

Brennan, T. A. (2000). The Institute of Medicine Report on medical errors—Could it do harm? *New England Journal of Medicine, 342*, 1123–1125.

Doyle, R. (1999, April). Health care costs. *Scientific American, 36.*

Dudley, R. A., and Luft, H. S. (2001). Managed care in transition. *New England Journal of Medicine, 344*, 1087–1092.

Fein, R. (1992, November). Health care reform. *Scientific American.*

Foster, H. W. (1997). The enigma of low birth weight and race. *New England Journal of Medicine, 337*, 1232–1233.

Freeman, H. P., and Payne, R. (2000). Racial injustice in health care. *New England Journal of Medicine, 342*, 1045–1047.

Ginzberg, E., and Ostow, M. (1997). Managed care—A look back and a look ahead. *New England Journal of Medicine, 336*, 1018–1020.

Holden, C. (1996). New populations of old add to poor nations' burdens. *Science, 273*, 46–48.

How good is your health plan? (1996). *Consumer Reports, 61*, 28–42.

Iglehart, J. K. (1999). The American health care system. *New England Journal of Medicine, 340*, 327–332.

Perez-Stable, E. J. (1999). Managed care arrives in Latin America. *New England Journal of Medicine, 340*, 1110–1112.

Starfield, B. (2000). Is the U.S. health really the best in the world? *Journal of the American Medical Association, 284*, 483–485.

Stocker, K., Waitzkin, H., and Iriart, C. (1999). The exportation of managed care to Latin America. *New England Journal of Medicine, 340*, 1131–1136.

Testa, M. A., and Simonson, D. C. (1996). Assessment of quality of life outcomes. *New England Journal of Medicine, 334*, 835–840.

Suggested Readings

Gawande, A. (1999, February 1). When doctors make mistakes. *The New Yorker*, 40–53. A doctor's firsthand account of how even good doctors make mistakes or are not prepared to deal with unforeseen medical emergencies.

How good is your health plan? (1996, August). *Consumer Reports*, 18–42. Explains and evaluates the country's biggest managed care plans.

Iglehart, J. K. (1999). The American health care system. *New England Journal of Medicine, 340*, 327–332. A discussion of the problems with Medicare, Medicaid, and the American health care system and what might be done to fix them.

Merck manual of medical information—Home edition. (1997). New York: Merck Publishing Group. A very helpful guide to understanding diseases and drugs. This book is based on the book doctors use when they leave the examining room to figure out what is going on.

Miller, M. S. (Ed.). (1997). *Health care choices for today's consumer.* New York: Wiley. A proactive guide to all the the various healthcare options available to consumers.

Study Guide and Self Assessment

Alternative Therapies Checklist

Health and Wellness Online

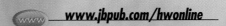 **www.jbpub.com/hwonline**

Chapter 20

Exploring Alternative Medicines

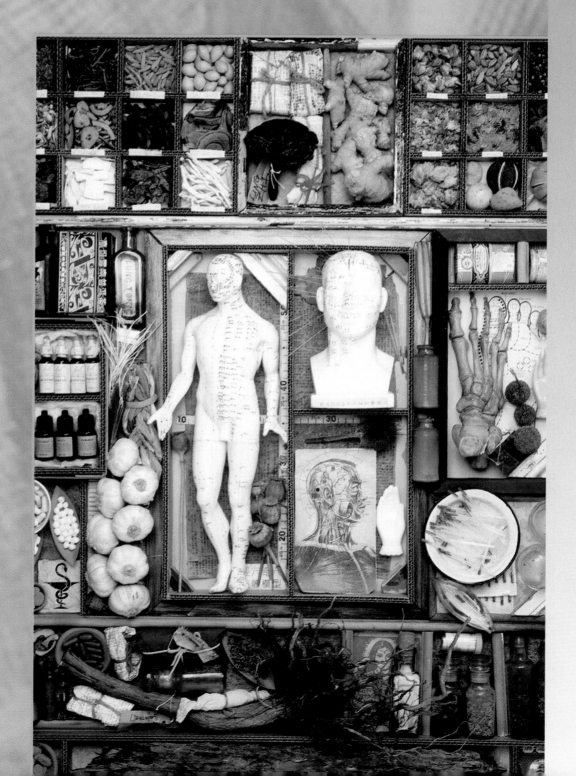

Although most people in the U.S. elect to visit a physician when they are sick, many seek alternatives to modern medicine for a variety of reasons. One reason may be cultural: persons raised in cultures that rely on herbal remedies and tribal healers to treat sickness often continue to use their own remedies even if they live in a foreign country.

Another large group that seeks healing alternatives are those persons for whom modern medicine has little to offer to relieve their suffering or to cure their disease. People who have terminal cancer for which no further treatments are available will often seek any help that offers hope. People with chronic diseases, such as arthritis or allergies, that do not respond satisfactorily to medical care or drugs often find relief in alternative therapies.

The medical profession is just beginning to acknowledge the importance of alternative therapies, often referred to as **alternative medicine,** in the lives of many of their patients. Some people prefer the term *complementary medicine* to emphasize that both approaches facilitate healing. A 1990 survey found that at least one third of patients with serious medical problems were using some form of alternative medicine. A follow-up study found that the use of alternative medicine had increased substantially seven years later (Eisenberg et al., 1998). The alternative medicines that increased the most were herbal remedies, folk remedies, massage, megavitamins, self-help groups, energy healing, and homeopathy. Partly in response to patients' preferences, some physicians are beginning to practice **integrative medicine,** the goal of which is to combine the best practices of both conventional and alternative medicine and to emphasize self-healing.

> *A desire to take medicine is perhaps the great feature which distinguishes man from other animals.*
>
> SIR WILLIAN OSLER, M.D.

In 1997 patients sought alternative medicine practitioners almost twice as often as they went to physicians; 629 million visits versus 386 million visits, respectively. The most common problems for which people turned to alternative medicine for relief were back problems, allergies, fatigue, arthritis, headaches, and cancer.

Despite the dramatic increase in the use and acceptance of alternative medicine, it still has many critics, especially among influential physicians. For example, some herbs are dangerous and have caused serious illness, most alternative therapies have not been scientifically tested and proven to be safe and effective, and some practitioners of alternative medicine are untrained and unlicensed. In the view of two physicians:

> It is time for the scientific community to stop giving alternative medicine a free ride. There cannot be two kinds of medicine—conventional and alternative. There is only medicine that that has been adequately tested and medicine that has not, medicine that works and medicine that may or may not work . . . assertions, speculation, and testimonials do not substitute for evidence. Alternative treatments should be subjected to scientific testing no less rigorous than that required for conventional medicine (Angell & Kassirer, 1998).

In recognition of the growing use of alternative medicine, Congress established the Office of Alternative Medicine (OAM) in 1992. The task of OAM was to fund experiments that would test the validity and effectiveness of many alternative medicine treatments such as acupuncture, massage, hypnosis, biofeedback, yoga, macrobiotic diets, and others. Most scientists condemned the OAM for being biased toward alternative medicine and for funding poorly designed studies. In 1999, a new director was named, and the OAM was changed to the National Center for Complementary and Alternative Medicine (NCCAM). The new director, Stephen Straus, is a highly regarded scientist whose goal is to "bring scientific rigor to a field many of his peers would just as soon see disappear" (Stokstadt, 2000).

Even if scientific studies "prove" certain alternative therapies to be of no value, it is not certain that the public will heed the results. For example, the very principles of homeopathy (discussed later) preclude its being tested scientifically, and most of its medicines contain no active ingredients. Yet homeopathy is being used more and more around the world, and millions of people attest to its therapeutic value in treating many diseases.

TABLE 20.1   Partial List of Alternative Medicines and Healing Methods

Physical and nutritional	Mental and spiritual
Acupuncture	Ayurveda
Alexander technique	Biofeedback
Ayurveda	Christian Science
Feldenkrais technique	Co-counseling
Herbal medicine	Guided imagery
Kinesiology (touch for health)	Hypnosis
Macrobiotics	Meditation
Massage	Past lives therapy
No nightshade diet	Primal scream therapy
Qigong	Progressive relaxation
Reflexology	Psychic healing
Shiatsu	Magnetic therapy
T'ai chi ch'uan	Psychodrama
Yoga	Rebirthing

Defining Alternative Medicine

Alternative medicine can be divided into four broad categories based on the method of healing or intervention: (1) spiritual, psychic, or mental approaches, including prayer, meditation, hypnotherapy, and faith healing; (2) nutritional therapies, including change in diet, fasting, and the use of supplements; (3) therapies using herbs or other substances derived from natural sources, such as homeopathy, herbal medicine, or immune system boosters; and (4) physical therapies, such as chiropractic, acupuncture, massage, and yoga. Table 20.1 presents a partial list of the hundreds of different kinds of alternative medicine.

Some alternative medicines, such as acupuncture and herbal remedies, have been used for thousands of years and would not have survived if people had not benefited. Other alternative medicines, such as homeopathy and chiropractic, are of recent origin and emerged partly as a response to the extraordinarily harsh practices of conventional medicine in the eighteenth and nineteenth centuries. (Some would argue that certain modern medical practices, such as bone marrow transplants, spinal surgeries, and chemotherapy, are still extremely harsh and only marginally successful.)

Before this century, irritants of all kinds were used to purge the body of unknown causes of illness. Bleedings, cuppings, leechings, enemas, and emetics (vomiting inducers) were all commonly used by doctors to treat diseases of which they had no real understanding. These treatments generally weakened the patient and usually interfered with the processes of healing.

Today, patients with chronic diseases and pain still seek treatments that offer the promise of relief and which do little harm. The problem for the health consumer is knowing what alternative medicines might be of help and which ones are safe. To help you understand how to choose an alternative medicine, some of the more widely used alternative medicines are described below.

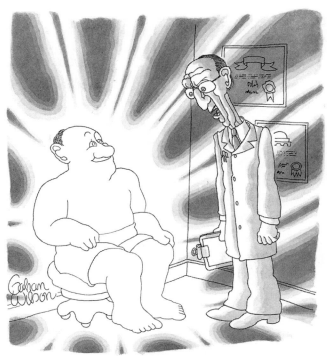

"You've been fooling around with alternative medicines, haven't you?"

Drawing by Gahan Wilson; © 1994 The New Yorker Magazine, Inc.

Alternative Medicines

Ayurveda

Ayurveda refers to one of the world's oldest medical systems, which has been practiced in India for over 4,000 years. Like other Asian medical practices, **Ayurvedic medicine** embodies a holistic approach to health; it teaches that health results from a balance of mind, body, and spirit, as well as a balance between people and the environment and their relationship to the cosmos. The word *Ayurveda* is from the Sanskrit and is a combination of two words: *ayur*, which means life, and *veda*, which means knowledge. Thus, health is knowledge of life. Ayurveda has been primarily practiced in the past by Buddhists or Hindus, but it is becoming increasingly popular in Western countries.

> To subdue the enemy without fighting is the acme of skill.
>
> SUN TZU

Ayurveda sees nature and people as being made of five elements or properties—earth, water, fire, air, and space; each element consists of both matter and energy. It is the interaction of these basic elements that gives rise to the universe and to human beings, who are viewed as being a microcosm or reflection of the macrocosm. Each element is associated with specific

Terms

alternative medicine: any form of therapy or healing performed by someone other than a physician

integrative medicine: conventional medicine practiced in conjunction with alternative medicine (herbal remedies, acupuncture, massage) to treat sickness

Ayurvedic medicine: a form of medicine that has its roots in the Hindu religion and is practiced widely in India

Wellness Guide

Sources for Information on Alternative Medicines

Chiropractic

Treatment usually involves direct spinal manipulation. Chiropractors contend that the spine is literally the backbone of health, and misalignment sabotages it. Practitioners diagnose with palpation and x-rays.

Information: Foundation for Chiropractic Education and Research, 1701 Clarendon Boulevard, Arlington, VA, 22209; 1-800-637-6244.

Homeopathy

Treatments aim to stimulate the body's defenses with tiny doses of substances that, in larger amounts, would cause the disease's symptoms.

Information: National Center for Homeopathy, 801 North Fairfax Street, Suite 306, Alexandria, VA 22314; 1-703-548-7790.

Aromatherapy

"Essential oils" distilled from plants and herbs are massaged into the skin, inhaled, or placed in baths in an attempt to treat stress, anxiety, and other conditions.

Information: Ann Berwick, Aromatherapy, P.O. Box 4996, Boulder, CO 80306.

Ayurveda

Disease, says this ancient practice from India, is caused by an imbalance of movement, structure, and metabolism. Herbs, diet, meditation, and yoga are treatments.

Herbal Medicine

Plants or plant-based substances are used to treat a wide range of illnesses and enhance physical functions.

Information: American Botanical Council, P.O. Box 201660, Austin, TX 78720; fax 512-331-1924.

Mind-Body Connection

Negative effects of stress are treated with exercise, meditation, and concentration.

Information: Center for Mind-Body Medicine, 5225 Connecticut Avenue, N.W., Suite 414, Washington, DC 20015; 1-202-966-7338.

Chinese Medicine

Ancient healing says an imbalance of vital force, *chi,* causes disease. Diet, herbs, and acupuncture are preventive treatments.

Information: American Foundation of Traditional Chinese Medicine, 505 Beach Street, San Francisco, CA 94133; 1-415-776-0502.

---

properties. For example, the earth element is dense and hard. Solid structures in the body, such as the skeleton, are derived from the earth element. The air element is cold and mobile. In the body, this element governs breathing and movement in the digestive tract. Thought, desire, and the will to do things also are under the control of the air element. The water element is fluid and soft and regulates the blood, secretions, and cerebrospinal fluid. The fire element is hot and light and regulates body temperature and all aspects of digestion. Space plays a unique role in Ayurveda because it permits us to perceive sound and also regulates vibrations that affect the body. Harmony among these five elements in each individual (and in the world) produces health; disharmony in any of the elements produces disease.

The interaction of the body with the environment is further defined by the *doshas,* which mediate the functions of the body tissues and waste products. When the doshas are in balance, people experience health on all levels—physical, emotional, and spiritual. In holistic terms, these individuals are not just free of disease but experience optimal health. They have an abundance of energy and are intelligent and competent in all that they do. They enjoy good relations with other people and with the environment,

and they are emotionally stable and happy. Spiritually, they are attuned with the cosmos. Imbalance in any of the doshas can produce mental, emotional, or physical illness. The goal of Ayurvedic medicine is to restore the balance of the doshas that is correct for each person.

An Ayurvedic physician diagnoses the patient by a technique called pulse diagnosis, which is a highly developed skill in taking a pulse. Also, signs of illness are found by examination of the tongue, urine, and aspects of the body such as the condition of the nails, skin, and lips. Once the nature of the imbalance is determined, the physician provides various remedies. As with modern medicine, nutrition and exercise are among the primary recommendations. Ayurvedic medicine, however, does not define nutrition in terms of fats, proteins, vitamins, minerals, or food groups. Ayurveda recognizes six "tastes": salty, sweet, sour, pungent, bitter, and astringent. These tastes not only are sensations on the tongue but also effects on the body. Each taste is associated with a physiological function, such as elimination, condition of mucus membranes, amount of stress, and so on. The diet is adjusted to restore a balance of the tastes. Exercises such as yoga and t'ai chi are recommended; today, jogging may be included. Other techniques employed by Ayurvedic practitioners include massage, meditation, and herbal remedies. The success of Ayurvedic medicine is attested to by its long history and the increasing number of people who embrace its principles.

Homeopathy

Of all the alternative medicines, **homeopathy** is the most widely used in America and around the world. Approximately half of all licensed physicians in the United States use some form of homeopathy in their practice of medicine. Homeopathy also is used by nurse practitioners, dentists, naturopathic doctors, chiropractors, acupuncturists, and veterinarians. Between 2 million and 3 million Americans take homeopathic remedies each year and spend upwards of $200 million on homeopathic preparations. In European countries, homeopathy is widely used by physicians, and, in India, there are more than 100,000 homeopathic practitioners.

Homeopathy is only about 200 years old and was founded by Samuel Hahnemann, a German pharmacologist and physician. The word *homeopathy* derives from two Greek words, *omoios* meaning similar and *pathos* meaning feeling. Homeopathy is primarily a self-healing system that is assisted by very small doses of medicines or remedies. Hahnemann believed that tiny doses of a substance (a medicine) that evoked symptoms *similar* to the disease symptoms could, in some way, stimulate the body's natural defenses and promote healing. According to Hahnemann, homeopathy is based on four principles:

1. Substances that produce the same symptoms as the disease in an individual as the disease will cure that individual (Law of Similars).
2. Substances are tested by giving them to healthy subjects and observing symptoms (Law of Proving).
3. Smaller doses are more potent than undiluted solutions (Law of Potentiation or Law of Infinitesimals).
4. Vital forces must be released in the treated individual, which will result in reestablishing harmony (homeostasis) in the body.

For example, the substance *belladonna*, which is extracted from a poisonous plant, causes flushing and flu-like symptoms when ingested by a healthy person. Thus, a homeopathic practitioner might use diluted doses of belladonna to treat the flu or high fever. The recommended dose of belladonna might be listed as 30X; this refers to the number of times that the original extract has been diluted. Practically, this means that one drop of the original extract is added to nine drops of water; then one drop of this solution is added to nine drops of water (or alcohol) and so on until 30, tenfold dilutions are reached. Statistically, the final solution is unlikely to have any molecules of belladonna in it. This is the primary reason that homeopathy is dismissed today as bogus by conventional medicine and Western science. Nonetheless, 200 years of experience and observation by patients and physicians show that it does help many patients suffering from many kinds of diseases.

Homeopathy began to be practiced extensively around 1830, a time when conventional medicine was particularly ineffective in treating epidemics of infectious diseases such as cholera, typhus, and scarlet fever. During this period, homeopathic doctors were significantly more successful in treating people than conventional doctors because the remedies worked, because people believed that they worked, or a combination of both. By 1890, at least 15% of conventional physicians used homeopathy and there were 22 homeopathic medical schools and more than 100 homeopathic hospitals operating in the United States.

In the 1800s, the American Medical Association (AMA) offered to include homeopaths in its organization. However, homeopaths chose to remain outside mainstream medicine, and the AMA began to harass and threaten physicians who practiced any form of homeopathy. In 1914, the AMA became the exclusive organization for licensing physicians to practice medicine; as a result, homeopathic medicine disappeared from the American scene for more than 50 years. In the 1970s, along with a general resurgence in alternative medicine, homeopathy again emerged as the choice of many sick people, either as a sole therapy or as an adjunct to conventional medical care.

Homeopathic practitioners use their remedies to evoke symptoms so that the body can recognize them and initiate a healing process from within. Homeopathy is used to treat both acute (infections, injuries) and chronic (arthritis, allergies, high blood pressure) conditions. It does not generally treat structural diseases or those stemming from long-term organic damage, such as cirrhosis, diabetes, chronic obstructive lung diseases, inherited diseases, neurological diseases, or cancer.

Homeopathic remedies are derived from plant, animal, and mineral sources. Examples of plant remedies include herbs, spices, foods, fragrances, and extracts from mushrooms and lichens. Mineral remedies include solutions of metals (copper, gold, tin, zinc), dilute solutions of acids, and substances derived from ores and rocks. Remedies derived from animal

Terms

homeopathy: an alternative medicine that administers very dilute solutions of substances that mimic the patient's symptoms

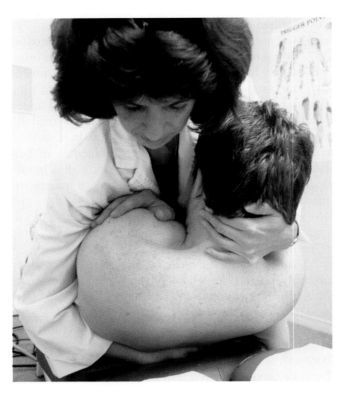

Chiropractic manipulations help many people who suffer from back pain and other musculoskeletal disorders.

substances include venom from insects, spiders, and crustaceans, hormone extracts, and material taken from diseased tissues.

Chiropractic

Chiropractic was founded in the United States around 1900 by Daniel David Palmer, who had no scientific or medical training, but who believed throughout his life that he had a "calling" to heal people. At age 50, Palmer cured Harvey Lillard of deafness by manipulating his spine. Lillard had been deaf for 17 years after working stooped over in a mine. Palmer found a misaligned vertebra, which he manipulated; this allowed Harvey to straighten up for the first time in years and simultaneously restored his hearing. After several other cures by spinal manipulation, Palmer concluded that virtually all diseases are caused by **subluxed** (misaligned) vertebrae.

Palmer coined the name "chiropractic" (from the Greek *cheir* meaning hand and *praktikos* meaning practical; the two words are usually interpreted to mean done by hand. Two years later he opened the Palmer School for Chiropractic in Davenport, Iowa. In 1906, Palmer and his son, Bartlett Joshua (or B. J. Palmer) were arrested for practicing medicine without a license. Palmer was tried, convicted, and jailed. His son's case never came to trial.

B. J. Palmer took over the chiropractic practice and turned it into a multimillion-dollar business. B. J. was a genius at commercializing chiropractic, and he was the first to come up with the idea of mail-order diplomas. B. J.'s philosophy of chiropractic was summed up in his description of the spine: "The principal functions of the spine are to support the head, to support the ribs, and to support the chiropractor." Shortly after B. J. took over, chiropractic split into two distinct schools which still exist today. One group, "the straights," adhere to the original idea that almost all diseases are caused by subluxion of the vertebrae. The other group was founded by John Howard, who believed that other factors also are involved in disease processes. This group became known as the "mixers," and practitioners of this philosophy include nutrition, relaxation, exercise, and other techniques, along with spinal manipulation, in their chiropractic practices.

Although chiropractors treat a wide range of diseases, 90% of patients seeking chiropractic help do so because of back pain, neck pain, or headaches. When the spine is in complete alignment, energy flows freely to all tissues and organs in the body and is the basis for health. Subluxion of vertebrae is the principal cause of disease according to chiropractic theory; subluxion can be caused by genetic disorders, falls, injuries, improper sleeping habits, poor posture, obesity, stress, or occupational hazards.

A number of research studies have demonstrated both short-term and long-term benefits of chiropractic for chronic, disabling lower back pain. Other studies have concluded that chiropractic is cheaper and more effective in treatment of back pain and musculoskeletal disorders than is conventional medicine. However, claims that chiropractic is effective in reducing blood pressure or relieving allergies or ulcers have not been substantiated by research.

There are 18 accredited colleges of chiropractic in the United States and more than 50,000 practicing chiropractors. Until recently, the AMA considered it unethical for physicians to refer patients to chiropractors. However, in 1987, five chiropractors won an antitrust suit against the AMA, and there is no longer any restraint on physicians who refer patients to chiropractors. Most health insurance plans, including

Terms

chiropractic: an alternative medicine that uses manipulation of the spine and joints for healing

subluxation: misalignment of a vertebra from its correct position

osteopathy: an alternative medicine that uses manipulation and medicines for healing; osteopaths receive training comparable to that of physicians and can prescribe drugs

acupuncture: an ancient Chinese alternative medicine that uses thin needles inserted into specific points on the body to produce healing energy

meridians: the channels along the body where energy flows and where acupuncture points are located

Medicare, now cover payments for chiropractic treatments. Chiropractors are licensed to administer any therapy except surgery and prescription drugs.

Osteopathy

Osteopathy, like chiropractic, is basically treatment by manipulation of the spine and other structural parts of the body. Osteopathic physicians, called doctors of osteopathy (D.O.), undergo training that is as rigorous as the education of physicians, and generally osteopaths have the same medical privileges of prescribing drugs and performing surgery as do physicians. However, most practitioners of osteopathy rely primarily on physical manipulation and exercises for their patients' conditions.

Osteopathic medicine was founded in the United States by Andrew Taylor Still, who was born in Virginia in 1828. His father was a preacher-physician, and Andrew grew up observing his father treat patients. He eventually developed his own methods of healing, which depended heavily on manipulation. Today, there are hundreds of osteopathic hospitals in the United States and thousands of doctors of osteopathy.

Acupuncture

Acupuncture is an integral part of traditional Chinese medicine, and the use of acupuncture goes back at least 5,000 years. The accumulated knowledge of acupuncture was passed down over the centuries and recorded in a text called "The Yellow Emperor's Classic of Internal Medicine" written in the second or third century B.C. Although acupuncture has been used in China and other Asian countries for centuries, it became popular in the West only after President Nixon's visit to China in the 1970s. A *New York Times* reporter, James Reston, who was covering Nixon's trip, became ill and underwent an emergency appendectomy. He later wrote an article describing his acupuncture anesthesia, and American physicians began traveling to China to learn more about acupuncture. Today, acupuncture is the most widely used and thoroughly researched alternative medicine.

The underlying principle of acupuncture is the existence of *qi* (pronounced chi)—the vital life force that circulates throughout the body and is carried by channels called **meridians.** There are twelve major meridians that connect all of the major organs, as well as a network of minor meridians. The meridians intersect with the surface of the body at many positions; these are the acupuncture points that are "needled" to restore balance to the qi in order to cure illness or relieve pain. According to Chinese medicine, an organ that is diseased or not functioning properly will manifest symptoms or signs on a corresponding meridian. These may include pain or ache, a change in temperature, sensitivity to touch, or a change in skin texture or color along the affected meridian. Thus, the acupuncturist must first diagnose the cause of the illness by locating the affected meridians; then the correct acupuncture points can be treated.

In acupuncture treatment, very thin metal needles are inserted just under the skin at specific acupuncture points. Usually no more than a dozen or so needles are used (see Figure 20.1). These remain in place for about a half hour, during which they may be twirled or connected to low-voltage generators to increase effectiveness in balancing qi. Sometimes heat is applied to the acupoint in a process called moxibustion. A small piece of an herb, *Artemisia vulgaris* (commonly known as mugwort), is either burned on the tip of the needle or placed on the acupoint.

> *The secret of the care of the patient is caring for the patient.*
> FRANCIS PEABODY, M.D.

In 1997, a scientific panel at the National Institute of Health concluded that traditional acupuncture is effective in relieving postoperative dental pain and in controlling nausea due to surgery, chemotherapy, or pregnancy. Other conditions listed for which acupuncture may be effective include drug and smoking addiction, lower back pain, stroke rehabilitation, menstrual cramps, tennis elbow, headache, and carpal tunnel syndrome (Acupuncture—NIH Consensus Conference,

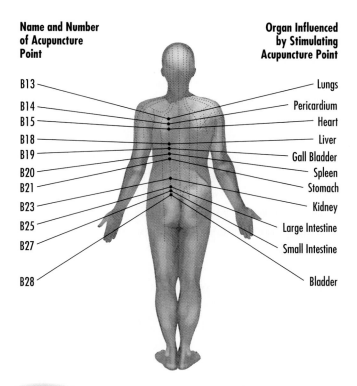

Name and Number of Acupuncture Point	Organ Influenced by Stimulating Acupuncture Point
B13	Lungs
B14	Pericardium
B15	Heart
B18	Liver
B19	Gall Bladder
B20	Spleen
B21	Stomach
B23	Kidney
B25	Large Intestine
B27	Small Intestine
B28	Bladder

FIGURE 20.1 Acupuncture points supposedly influence the functions of internal organs.

1998). Although there is no research to substantiate claims of effectiveness, acupuncture also is used to treat neurological disorders (Ménière's disease, trigeminal neuralgia), gastrointestinal disorders (ulcers, colitis, diarrhea), respiratory disorders (asthma, rhinitus, sinusitis, bronchitis), as well as arthritic conditions.

In the United States, 10 to 15 million acupuncture treatments are performed each year (see Table 20.2). Many physicians have been trained in acupuncture and offer it in addition to conventional medical treatments. Licensing of acupuncturists who are not physicians varies from state to state; however, most states require a licensing exam and some permit acupuncture only when it is performed under medical supervision. As with other alternative medicines, the biological mechanisms that underlie the curative power of acupuncture are unclear.

Herbal Medicine

Herbs in various forms have been used as medicines for centuries to treat every conceivable form of ailment. Ancient Chinese, Greek, and Roman societies compiled extensive *Pharmacopoeia* describing the uses and preparation of herbal remedies. One herbal compilation published by Nicholas Culpepper in the seventeenth century has gone through countless printings and lists over 3,000 herbal remedies.

TABLE 20.2   Conditions Treated with Acupuncture

Allergies	Coughs	Premenstrual syndrome
Arthritis	Diarrhea	Sexual problems
Asthma	Drug abuse	Shoulder/knee pain
Back pain	Fatigue	Smoking
Bladder/kidney problems	Headaches	Stress
Colds	High blood pressure	Vision problems
Constipation		

Herbal medicines consist of materials derived from plants and can be prepared in the form of pills, teas, extracts, tinctures, salves, and other forms. In the 1780s, an English physician noted that one of his patients was cured of dropsy by drinking tea made from dried, powdered foxglove leaves. The physician, William Withering, made the connection between dropsy and heart disease. Subsequently, the chemical digitoxin in foxglove leaves was identified as the ingredient that helps heart functions.

Herbs and other plants have been the source for extracting and purifying modern drugs such as ephedrine, digitalis, atropine, reserpine, quinine, and most recently taxol, used to treat cancer. Herbal medicines often contain a mixture of herbs, so it is diffi-

Wellness Guide

Healing a Headache with Acupressure

Acupuncture is an ancient Chinese healing technique based on balancing the flow of energy through channels (meridians) in the body by inserting needles at acupuncture points on the skin. The acupuncture points for the needles are also "acupressure" points; that is, instead of inserting needles, pressure can be applied to these points to facilitate healing. You might want to experiment by using acupressure to relieve two common conditions.

Many people experience headaches caused by tension in the muscles of the neck and head. Often the tension alters blood supply to the brain, which causes a headache. Pressing acupressure points at two different locations may relieve the headache pain. The points are located just below the base of the skull, at the back of the head, just to the right and left of center.

Cup the back of your head with your fingers and use your two thumbs to press quite firmly just under the skull on either side of center. The thumbs should be an inch or so apart and away from the centerline of the skull. Press hard for up to a minute or until your thumbs become tired. Repeat the pressure two or three times. Breathe deeply while pressing. Notice if the pain has lessened or disappeared.

Two other acupressure points for headache relief are located on the back of each hand in the soft part between thumb and index finger. Using the thumb and index finger (or middle finger) of the opposite hand, press firmly on the acupressure point. This point may be sensitive, so press only as hard as is comfortable. Repeat on the opposite hand. Press these points for up to a minute and

repeat several times. Notice if the headache pain has lessened.

Acupressure also may be useful in helping to stop smoking cigarettes. The earlobes contain acupressure points that reduce the craving for nicotine. Again, using the thumb and index finger of one hand, grab the earlobe and press hard only until it begins to hurt. You can try different locations on the earlobe to find what seems to you to be the most sensitive pressure point. Alternate pressing each earlobe for up to a minute, and repeat the pressure several times. Perform this acupressure treatment each time you have a craving for a cigarette. Notice if the craving decreases.

The best part of self-administered acupressure therapy is that it is free—and it often works.

TABLE 20.3 Herbs and Their Use in Common Ailments

Herb	Use
Aloe	Burns, skin irritations
Black cohosh	Menstrual cramps, PMS, menopause
Chamomile	Digestion
Echinacea	Immune system stimulant
Feverfew	Reduces fever, helps migraine
Foxglove	Control heart rhythm, angina
Garlic	Digestion, protects against high blood pressure
Ginger root	Motion sickness, cough
Ginkgo biloba	Dilates blood vessels, dementia
Ginseng	Reduces stress
Hawthorn	Lowers blood pressure, dilates blood vessels
Milk thistle	Protects damaged liver, prevents toxins from entering liver
Peppermint	Indigestion
Saw palmetto	Enlarged prostate, improves urinary flow, anti-inflammatory agent
Senna	Strong laxative
Tea-tree oil	Skin and vaginal infections, acne
Valerian root	Mild sedative
Willow bark	Headache

Herbal remedies possess the same potential for side effects and harm as with prescription drugs. Many plants contain toxic chemicals that may vary from plant to plant and from season to season; therefore, an herbal remedy that proved safe and effective once may cause harm the next time it is taken. Some herbal remedies that are known to be dangerous include *comfrey* (causes lung, kidney, or liver damage); *ephedra,* or *ma huang* (causes palpitations, raises blood pressure, nerve and muscle damage, stroke, psychosis); *lobelia* (causes drops in blood pressure, rapid heart beat, coma); and *yohimbe* (causes fatigue, paralysis, stomach upset, death). Herbal remedies also may cause allergic reactions and drug interactions and may exert mutagenic effects (Ernst, 1998).

> *The fragrance always stays in the hand that gives the rose.*
> HADA BEJAR

Like other alternative medicines, herbal medicine is widely used in many countries of the world, especially among people who cannot afford expensive drugs. And even in Western industrialized countries including the United States, more and more people

cult to know what component is involved in alleviating symptoms or in healing. Only with the advent of modern chemistry could plant materials be broken down into individual chemical components that can be tested for medicinal properties.

Many herbal remedies have been shown to be beneficial for a variety of ailments and conditions (Table 20.3). However, there are some drawbacks to the use of herbs. For example, many herbal teas concocted by herbalists in China have tastes that are unacceptable to most American palates and, hence, are not often used. Also herbal remedies made in China and in the U.S. usually vary from batch to batch or from one herbalist to another. A recent analysis of certain herbal balls made in China indicated that many of them contained dangerous amounts of arsenic and mercury as well as other toxic substances (Espinoza et al., 1995). Thus, the consumer really does not know how useful or dangerous any particular batch of herbs may be; what worked one time may not work again or might even be harmful.

Terms

herbal medicines: materials derived from plants and other organisms that are made into teas, powders, and salves to treat diseases and injuries

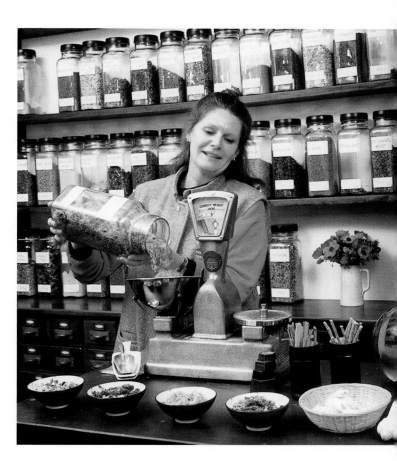

Herbal remedies are continuing to increase in popularity among Americans with a variety of ailments.

consult herbalists for their aches and illnesses. More research is being conducted to test the efficacy of herbal medicines, and some studies show that they do help patients with specific conditions (Wu, 1995).

Naturopathy

Naturopathy is a uniquely American approach to health that arose in the late 19th century. The term was introduced by Dr. John Sheel in 1895; the principles of naturopathy as a system of healing and way of living were formulated by Benedict Lust in 1902. In the early 1900s, more than 20 naturopathic schools of medicine trained naturopathic doctors (ND). But with the rise of conventional medicine, naturopathy all but disappeared from the American health scene. However, it experienced a revival in the 1970s, along with other alternative medicines.

Naturopathy's approach to health emphasizes the prevention of disease and the individual's responsibility for a healthy lifestyle. Naturopathy draws on all available alternative medicines, as well as aspects of conventional medicine. However, it does reject the use of surgery and drugs. If there is a single unifying concept to naturopathy, it is that the body possesses the "energy" or "intelligence" to heal itself. In that sense it is similar in philosophy to Ayurvedic and Chinese medicine.

The eight basic principles of naturopathy are:

- The human body possesses an innate ability to heal itself.
- It is the duty of the naturopathic practitioner to find and treat the underlying cause of illness, not simply the symptoms.
- The naturopathic practitioner is first and foremost a teacher who must educate the patient on how to prevent illness and restore health.
- The naturopathic practitioner must employ therapies that "do no harm." Surgery and drugs are not recommended.
- The focus is mainly on prevention of illness. The patient's lifestyle is examined in detail, and recommendations are made to reduce health risks and to foster health.

Dollars and Health Sense

Beware of Health Fraud

The media are full of advertisements for products that promise to cure cancer, help you lose weight effortlessly, improve sexual vigor, and prevent aging. Anything that sounds "too good to be true" invariably is not true. Do not let your vanity or your hopes for health lure you into trying unproved therapies by unlicensed practitioners. Do not waste money by purchasing products with "secret formulas" or the promise of "miracle" cures for cancer, arthritis, allergies, or a host of other conditions (see table).

In the broadest sense, the attempt to treat illness with any medicine, therapy, or machine that has not been scientifically tested and proven to be safe and effective is called quackery. People who sell useless products are guilty of fraud. Various federal agencies such as the Food and Drug Administration, the Federal Trade Commission, and the Postal Service try to protect consumers by exposing false claims and useless products. However, their efforts usually are too late to prevent millions of people from losing money on useless products. Deceptive advertising still entices millions of people to buy products or services that are completely worthless and sometimes dangerous. Generally, advertisements for worthless products promise "complete satisfaction" and a money-back guarantee. However, customers generally do not receive the refund and eventually quit trying. Do not be the next victim of quackery!

Common Conditions that Attract Health Fraud

Claims for	Fraudulent Schemes
Arthritis	Arthritis affects about 40 million Americans, many of whom seek help from alternative medicine. Arthritis often goes into remission, so what seems like a cure is actually a temporary, natural reduction of symptoms.
Overweight	One out of four Americans is overweight, and some may be searching for magic weight-loss therapy. Weight-loss gimmicks include patches, elastic belts, herbs, and "wonder" diets. There is no easy way to lose weight except by reducing eating and increasing exercise.
Sexual problems	Products to increase breast and penis size and to enhance sexual prowess are worthless. Some chemicals and herbs are sold as aphrodisiacs. Most are only useless, but some can be harmful to health.
Circulatory problems	Promoters of chelation therapy claim that a chemical substance called EDTA can help purify the blood and clear arteries of fatty deposits. No scientific evidence for these claims exists, and EDTA can harm the kidneys and cause other health problems.

- Good nutrition is an essential goal of naturopathy. Without a healthy diet, the body invites illness.
- The treatment must involve the whole person, not just an organ or part of the body. A person's physical, mental, emotional, and spiritual states must be evaluated and altered as necessary to promote health.
- The ultimate goal of naturopathy is optimal health, not just the absence of disease.

These principles of naturopathy are essentially those of modern holistic medicine. The emphasis of the medicine of the future should be to prevent disease by educating patients in the health benefits of good nutrition and in helping them reduce destructive health behaviors such as smoking, drinking, or using recreational drugs. Also, people must find ways to reduce stress, anxiety, and emotional turmoil if they are to enjoy optimal health. In the modern world, these are difficult tasks even for a motivated individual.

Naturopathic doctors receive training that is as complete as a medical school that awards the M.D. degree. A naturopathic doctor who has graduated from one of the half dozen schools offering degrees in naturopathy is well equipped to diagnose and treat a wide range of diseases. It is the approach to healing that distinguishes the ND from the M.D., although many physicians with an M.D. practice naturopathic medicine even though they also can prescribe drugs and recommend surgery. Because naturopathy eschews the use of surgery and drugs, naturopathic doctors do not treat acute illness or conditions that require emergency care. People usually consult a naturopathic doctor in order to construct a lifestyle that will prevent illness and promote overall optimum health.

Therapeutic Massage

Therapeutic massage is a hands-on therapy in which touch is used to heal. Cave paintings dating back approximately 15,000 years depict injured people being treated with what looks like massage. The use of massage to heal is described in ancient Chinese, Greek, and Roman texts. Seemingly miraculous cures have been reported over the centuries by the "laying on of hands" by people believed to have divine powers, such as priests, shamans, and holy persons. Despite its effectiveness as an alternative medicine, some people still regard massage as a guise for sexual stimulation. However, therapeutic massage administered by a trained and licensed professional is a highly effective form of therapy for many conditions.

Human touch is essential to normal development of infants and children and to health in general. Americans tend to touch one another much less than people in other cultures. Psychologists who observe the number of times people touch one another in cafes or other public places report that, on average, Americans touch one another less frequently than almost any other culture in the world. In similar situations, Parisians touch one another more than 100 times per hour and Puerto Ricans almost 200 times per hour! Cultural anthropologists report that cultures that are more physically affectionate toward infants and children have lower rates of adult violence such as domestic and sexual abuse.

The most immediate effect of therapeutic massage is improved blood circulation. As the skin is stretched and the muscles are kneaded, the amount of blood returning to the heart is increased, and toxins released into the blood can be excreted more readily. Enhanced circulation also supplies more oxygen to tissues and to the brain. Massage benefits digestion and elimination, and it hastens wound healing. Massage also eases muscle pain caused by strain or injury; it may stimulate the release of endorphins and enkephalins, pain-relieving chemicals synthesized in the body.

There are certain conditions and diseases in which therapeutic massage should *not* be used because of the possibility of causing further damage to tissues or organs. These are:

- Recent bone fractures or severe sprains
- Herniated disc in the spine
- Excessive blood pressure
- Areas of the body in which hemorrhage has occurred
- Any acute inflammation of the skin or joints
- Blood conditions such as phlebitis and thrombosis
- Severe varicose veins
- Certain kinds of cancer

Therapeutic massage involves five basic kinds of manipulation of a person's skin and muscles. The first is an extended gliding stroke with the whole hand or thumb. This warms the skin and relaxes muscle tension. The next is a kneading motion in which muscles are grabbed and lifted. This relieves soreness and improves circulation. Friction manipulation is used around joints and thick muscles. Repeated circular movement of the hands can help

Terms

naturopathy: an alternative medicine that uses nutrition, herbs, massage, and other techniques to promote healing

therapeutic massage: promotes relaxation and healing by massage of the skin and muscles.

break up adhesions. The hands also can be used in a chopping or tapping motion to stimulate the skin and muscles; this chopping is used when muscles are spastic or cramped. Finally, the fingers or flattened hands are pressed into muscles and "vibrated" for a few seconds. This vibration stimulates nerves and circulation in the area.

Massage therapists are required to pass a licensing exam in most states. Many people claim to be massage therapists who are not licensed or who have limited training. Making sure a therapist is licensed and talking to people who have benefited from that therapist are good ways to ensure that your experience will be helpful. Even if you do not have a specific medical condition that needs massage therapy, getting a massage is relaxing and refreshing.

Aromatherapy

Aromatherapy is a centuries-old alternative medicine in which the essential oils of plants (many of which are fragrant) are administered so that chemicals contained in the oils are absorbed into the body and act as drugs. In that sense, aromatherapy is similar to herbal medicine or to conventional drug therapy. Since the 1980s, aromatherapy has increased in popularity among Americans seeking alternative medicines, and now is a more than $300 million annual business.

Priests and healers in the ancient world used oils and perfumes to treat illnesses and as a prevention against disease. In the Egyptian Ebers Papyrus, which dates to about 1500 B.C., there are descriptions of more than 800 plant and herbal remedies, many of which are fragrant oil extracts. The modern medicinal use of plant oils and fragrances, as well as the term *aromatherapy*, derives from a French chemist who began to study the healing power of plant oils in the 1930s. He became interested after burning his hand in his family's perfume factory. He plunged his burned hand into a vat of lavender oil for relief and discovered that the burn healed rapidly and without scarring.

Some of the most popular aromatherapy oil extracts are derived from:

- The leaves of eucalyptus and peppermint
- The fruits and blossoms of oranges and lemons
- The flowers of lavender and roses
- Woods such as camphor and sandalwood
- Cinnamon bark, lemongrass, fennel, and rosemary
- Dried spices such as clove and fresh garlic bulbs

Essential oils made from plant extracts are very concentrated and contain hundreds of chemicals that can act as drugs. Thus, only minute amounts of oils are used, and a person practicing aromatherapy needs to be knowledgeable about the kinds of chemicals present in different extracts and their effects on the body. Aromatherapists treat people by prescribing oils that can be inhaled directly, applied to the skin as part of a massage, or added to a hot bath, in which case the oils are both absorbed and inhaled. Aromatherapy is used to treat infections, pain, arthritis, skin disorders, headaches, digestive disorders, and other conditions.

Although aromatherapy has been used for thousands of years, there is no scientific evidence that it cures any disease. It is critical that patients using aromatherapy (or other alternative medicine) inform their physicians as to what oils, herbs, or supplements they are using to avoid serious complications from drug-drug or drug-herb interactions. For example, it has recently been discovered that St. John's wort, one of today's more popular herbal supplements, makes birth control pills much less effective, and a number of so-called "miracle" babies have been born to women taking both substances. St. John's wort also interferes with some blood pressure medications and other prescription drugs.

Choosing an Alternative Medicine

Many people are satisfied with the care they receive from modern medicine and the physicians who treat them. However, many Americans also seek alternative medicines to supplement conventional treatments. And some persons choose to rely on alternative medicines exclusively. For many kinds of sickness, alternative medicines may provide relief and healing.

It often is wise to begin with the least invasive form of treatment before undergoing surgery or taking drugs that can also do harm. Our society is gradually coming to the view that healing can be accomplished by both conventional and alternative medicine. And, as we have pointed out repeatedly, the belief of the patient in a particular treatment, physician, acupuncturist, or chiropractor may be what heals.

Terms

aromatherapy: use of fragrant extracts of plants to promote healing

Critical Thinking About Health

1. Suppose that you have been in an auto accident and have a whiplash injury to your neck. It is some months since the accident and your doctor says that your neck has healed and that she cannot find anything wrong. However, you still have pain and difficulty moving your head. What alternative medicines would you now consider to relieve your symptoms? Discuss the rationale behind your choice of alternative medicine(s). If you have actually experienced such an accident, describe the healing process that you went through.

2. Describe any herbal remedy that you are now taking and the condition for which it is being used. Answer each of the questions below and discuss your reasons for taking this remedy and how you think it has helped you (if it has).
   a. Have you investigated whether this herbal remedy has been studied in clinical trials and found to be effective?
   b. Have you investigated whether there are any dangers associated with taking this herb?
   c. Have you discussed taking this herbal remedy with a physician?

3. Therapeutic touch (TT) is a technique widely used by nurses to alleviate suffering and promote healing in patients with a wide variety of ailments, including cancer. TT claims that nurses achieve healing and relief by sensing and manipulating a "human energy field" that is felt above the patient's body. A recent scientific study of TT found that, under controlled laboratory conditions in which nurses had to sense the presence of the experimenter's hand over one of their own without being able to see the person on the other side of a screen, nurses were unable to score significantly above chance (i.e., they had a 50% chance of being correct). The scientists concluded that nurses who practice TT are unable to detect a human energy field, that TT is bogus, and that further professional use of TT is unjustified.
   a. Do you agree with the scientists' conclusions?
   b. Think of reasons why the experiment might not be a valid test of TT and explain your criticisms in detail.
   c. Can you devise an experiment that you think would be better in proving or disproving that TT had beneficial effects on patients?

4. Studies of acupuncture have consistently shown that it is more effective when used on Chinese patients in China than when it is used on patients in the U.S. In addition to being more effective on individual patients, more diseases respond to acupuncture treatments in China than when the same diseases are treated with acupuncture in the U.S.
   a. Make a list of as many reasons that you can think of that would explain these observations (e.g., American acupuncturists are not as proficient as Chinese acupuncturists).
   b. Discuss each of the items on your list and describe how it would explain the observed difference.
   c. Pick one of the items that you have identified and design a scientific experiment that would prove whether your hypothesis was correct or not.

Health in Review

- Alternative medicine consists of hundreds of methods for dealing with sickness and disease in ways that are different from modern medical care performed by physicians.
- The broad categories of alternative medicine include spiritual and mental therapies, nutritional therapies, herbal remedies, and physical therapies.
- Homeopathy administers very dilute solutions of substances that are supposed to mimic the symptoms of sick persons and help the body cure itself of the disease.
- Chiropractic and osteopathy use manipulation of the spine and joints to treat musculoskeletal disorders and other diseases.
- Ayurveda and aromatherapy are ancient healing techniques.
- Acupuncture involves inserting very thin needles into specific points on the body to restore harmony to the functioning of tissues and organs.
- Herbal medicine uses mixtures of herbs in the form of pills, powders, teas, and tinctures to help the healing process.
- Consumers of alternative medicine need to guard against fraudulent claims and unscrupulous persons who advertise therapies of unproved safety and of dubious value.

Health and Wellness Online

The World Wide Web contains a wealth of information about health and wellness. By accessing the Internet using Web browser software, such as Netscape Navigator or Microsoft's Internet Explorer, you can gain a new perspective on many topics presented in *Health and Wellness, Seventh Edition.* Access the Jones and Bartlett Publishers Web site at http://www.jbpub.com/hwonline.

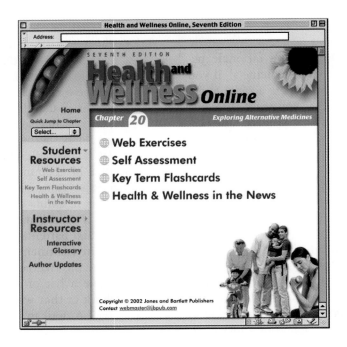

References

Acupuncture—NIH Consensus Conference. (1998). *Journal of the American Medical Association, 280,* 1518–1524.

Angell, M., and Kassirer, J. P. (1998). Alternative medicine—The risks of untested and unregulated remedies. *New England Journal of Medicine, 339.* 839–843.

Eisenberg, D. M., Davis, R. B., Ettner, S. L., et al. (1998). Trends in alternative medicine use in the United States, 1990–1997. *Journal of the American Medical Association, 280,* 1569–1575.

Ernst, E. (1998). Harmless herbs? A review of the recent literature. *American Journal of Medicine, 104,* 170–178.

Espinoza, E. O. et al. (1995). Arsenic and mercury in traditional Chinese herbal balls. *New England Journal of Medicine, 333,* 803–804.

Stokstadt, E. (2000). Stephen Straus' impossible job. *Science, 288,* 1568–1570.

Vandenbroucke, J. P. (1997). Homeopathy trials: Going nowhere. *The Lancet, 350,* 824.

Wu, C. (1995). Yin and yang—Western medicine makes room for Chinese herbal medicine. *Science News, 148,* 172–173.

Suggested Readings

Cassileth, B. R. (1999). *The alternative medicine handbook*. New York: W. W. Norton. A longtime practitioner of alternative medicine discusses all the available therapies and their effectiveness.

Collinge, W. (1996). *American holistic health association's complete guide to alternative medicine*. New York: Warner Books. Describes more than one hundred of the available alternative medicines and how they are used in different conditions.

Dossey. L. (1999). *Reinventing medicine: Beyond mind-body to a new era of healing*. San Francisco: HarperCollins. Discusses the research supporting alternative medicine and ways that it can be incorporated into the medicine of the future.

Is integrative medicine the medicine of the future? Debate between Arnold S. Relman and Andrew Weil. (1999). *Archives of Internal Medicine, 159,* 2122–2126. A very interesting debate between a strong advocate of alternative medicine (Dr. Weil) and an equally strong opponent (Dr. Relman).

Shealy, C. N. (Ed.). (1998). *The illustrated encyclopedia of healing remedies*. Boston: Element Books. A comprehensive reference book, if you need to find out about an alternative medicine and related disorders.

Tyler, V. E. (1997). *The honest herbal: A sensible guide to the use of herbs and related remedies*. New York: Pharmaceutical Products Press. A good source to check out the benefits and dangers of an herb if you are planning to use an herbal remedy.

Study Guide and Self Assessment

Prevention of Unintentional Injury
Prevention of Intentional Injury

Health and Wellness Online

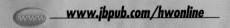 **www.jbpub.com/hwonline**

Chapter 21

Preventing Unintentional Injuries and Accidents: What You Can Do

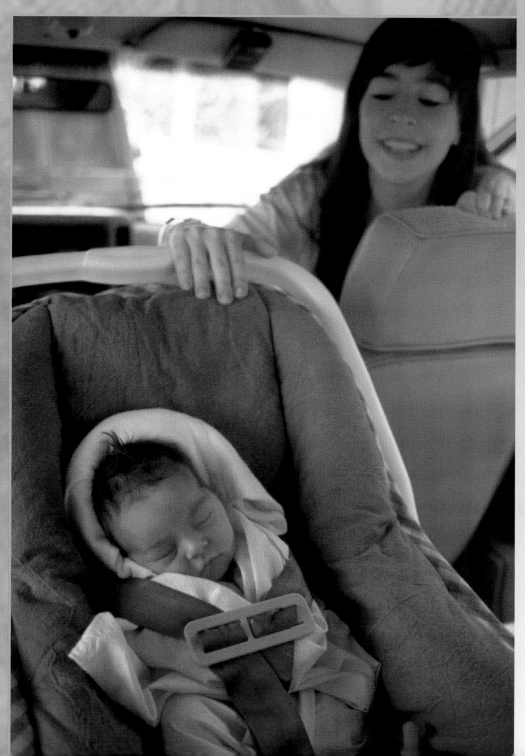

Injuries affect the health and well-being of millions of Americans every year. Unintentional injuries and accidents of various kinds are a far greater source of ill health and death than most people realize. Safety warnings and increased public awareness measures have reduced the number of unintentional deaths significantly in the past thirty years (Figure 21.1). In 1999, the number of unintentional injury deaths from all causes in the United States was 96,900. Over the past 50 years, deaths from unintentional injuries in the United States have ranged from a high of 116,385 in 1962 to a low of 86,777 in 1992. However, because the U.S. population has been increasing steadily, the overall rate of deaths from unintentional injuries has been declining, except for a period in the 1960s and early 1970s. The increased death rate in this period prompted Congress to pass legislation designed to improve safety with safety equipment for automobiles and the use of seat belts. Despite the encouraging reduction in unintentional injury deaths, the adverse health consequences of unintentional injuries are still serious and should be be reduced further.

> *There is no such thing as an accident; what we call by that name is the effect of some cause which we do not see.*
>
> VOLTAIRE

In the United States, unintentional injuries are the leading cause of death among all persons aged 1 to 34 and the fifth leading cause of death among all people of all ages. Unintentional injuries and accidents are responsible for nearly 500 billion dollars in overall costs each year.

Many people believe accidents are ill-fated occurrences over which people have no control. Whereas it

TABLE 21.1   Leading Causes of Unintentional Deaths in the U.S. in 1999
Cause of death is ascribed to a single category, although many factors contribute to all kinds of accidents.

Cause of death	Number of deaths
Motor vehicle crashes	41,300
Falls	17,100
Poisoning by solids and liquids	10,500
Drowning	4,000
Suffocation by ingested object	3,200
Fires, burns, and deaths associated with fires	3,100
Firearm	700
Poisoning by gases and vapors	500
All others (air, water, and land transport, machinery, falling object, etc.)	16,500

Source: National Safety Council, *Accident Facts*, 2000 Edition.

is true that some accidents are the result of bad luck, a vast number of accidents and the injuries resulting from them are caused by social and economic conditions that make the environment hazardous, poor judgment, lapses in attention, recklessness, loss of emotional control, and mental states that are imbalanced by alcohol and drugs. Insofar as the environment can be made safe and individuals made aware and cautious, the degree of unintentional injuries from accidents can be reduced.

Unintentional Injuries and Accidents

What is **safety?** The word "safety" is used in a wide context with various meanings to different individuals. Few individuals or agencies can agree on one universal definition. "Is this a safe part of town to be this late at night?" "He is not a very safe motorcycle driver." "My daughter's safety has been a concern of mine since she obtained her driver's license." "Is that old

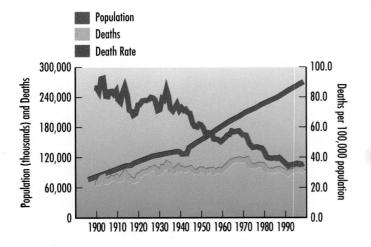

FIGURE 21.1   Deaths Due to Unintentional Injury, Population Increase, and Death Rates in the United States, 1900–1999 The total number of deaths from unintentional injuries has remained relatively constant over the past century. However, because the population has increased dramatically, the death rate has declined significantly.
Source: National Safety Council, *Injury Facts*, 2000.

Terms

safety: an ever-changing condition in which one attempts to minimize the risk of injury, illness, or property damage from the hazards to which one may be exposed

accident: sequence of events that produces unintended injury, death, or property damage; refers to the event, **not** the result of the event

unintentional injury: preferred term for accidental injury; result of an accident

accident mitigation: methods to reduce damage caused by unplanned events

accident prevention: ways to eliminate the occurrence of unintended injuries

ladder safe to use?" As you can see, the word "safe" or "safety" may be used in a variety of situations.

One common tie to all these different scenarios is the word **accident.** As defined by the National Safety Council, an accident "is that occurrence in a sequence of events which produces unintended injury, death, or property damage. Accident refers to the event, not the result of the event."

Each year one in four individuals will sustain some type of serious injury that requires medical attention and that is a result of an accident. Injuries are a serious problem, but many individuals lack the necessary knowledge and skills to provide assistance if an emergency does occur. Injuries are the leading cause of disability in young people today and cause more deaths in children than all the infectious diseases combined.

Unintentional injury is a term often used interchangeably with the term "accident," and we also will use both terms. Unintentional injury is the term preferred by public health officials and refers to the result of an accident or the health consequence of an accident. Deaths due to unintentional injuries result from motor vehicle accidents, home accidents (falls, fires, poisonings), workplace accidents, firearm accidents, and from other causes (see Table 21.1). The greatest number of deaths occur as a result of motor vehicle crashes, falls, and poisonings. However, the age groups that are most likely to die in these kinds of accidents differ significantly. Teenagers and young adults are most likely to die in motor vehicle crashes, middle-aged persons by poisoning, and the elderly by falls (see Figure 21.2).

Unintentional injuries are the fifth leading cause of death overall, exceeded only by heart disease, cancer, stroke, and chronic obstructive pulmonary disease. The five leading causes of death from unintentional

injury are motor vehicles; falls; poisoning by solids and liquids; fires and burns; and drowning: these have been the same since 1970. For most of the twentieth century, the rate of death from accidents has steadily dropped because of increased safety and health efforts. However, in the last 4 years, there has been an increase in total deaths from unintentional injury, which should be a warning that greater attention to increased health and safety efforts is needed to reverse this trend.

The causes of death from unintentional injury change with age. Poor diet, sedentary lifestyle, arthritis, decreased mobility, poverty, chronic diseases, or lack of access to primary medical care may contribute to injuries and accidental death as people get older.

Reducing the Risk of Accidents

When considering accidents, their prevention, and their consequences, public health professionals focus on **accident mitigation**—methods to reduce damage caused by unplanned events—and **accident prevention**—ways to eliminate the occurrence of unintended injuries. Accident mitigation and prevention can be viewed in two contexts: (1) individual or personal and (2) environmental or community.

Many factors are involved in unintentional injury: knowledge, attitudes, beliefs, and behaviors; economic and social conditions; ability level of the performer of tasks; conditions of the environment; and alcohol and other drug use. Positive changes in these factors will reduce injuries, but more attention should be directed to prevention strategies. Even though unintentional injuries have decreased by more than half over the past century, the cost is still staggering (Figure 21.3).

Attitudes and beliefs may be the greatest factor involved in unintentional injuries. Your individual

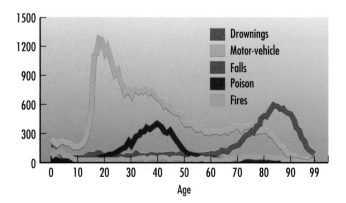

FIGURE 21.2 **Leading Causes of Death by Unintentional Injury According To Age in the United States, 1997** People of different ages have very different risks of accidental death from different causes.
Source: National Safety Council, *Injury Facts,* 2000.

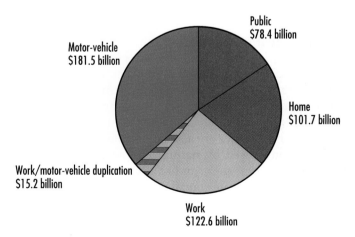

FIGURE 21.3 **Costs of Unintentional Injuries by Classification, 1999** Total cost of unintentional injuries was over $469 billion; the greatest cost is from motor-vehicle injuries and property damage
Source: National Safety Council, *Injury Facts,* 2000.

attitude toward safety precautions greatly influences the likelihood of an injury. You may believe that safety precautions are a waste of time, that you have no control over the situation (what will happen, will happen), or you may have a reckless attitude (you like to take risks).

Lack of knowledge and skills also play a role in unintentional injury. In special circumstances, especially when performing a new procedure or task, lacking the proper knowledge or skills could result in unintentional injury (e.g., operating a new power tool before reading the instructions, operating a motorcycle the first time, or using a new kitchen appliance).

Socioeconomic factors also play a role in unintentional injury. Some individuals may lack the necessary funds to replace unsafe or old equipment. Some may even lack the necessary funds to obtain proper training in safety-related matters. Safety training can be received through a local National Safety Council office on such topics as proper storage of household cleaning items, tool safety, and safety tips for the babysitter. Local health departments may also provide educational workshops on safety issues.

Some social settings may lend themselves to accidents. Attitudes and beliefs as well as the social setting can raise or lower the probability of an unintentional injury. For example, alcohol and drug use and abuse definitely affect the frequency of unintentional injuries. Prescribed medications, especially ones with a sedative effect, can increase the likelihood of an accident while operating a motor vehicle, motorcycle, or power tool.

The ability of the individual performing a task or activity may affect the probability of an unintentional injury. The person may be a child who is too young to perform a task competently. At the other end of the spectrum, an elderly individual may not be strong enough or steady enough to perform a simple task like carving Thanksgiving turkey with an electric knife.

The environment can be the most unpredictable risk factor in unintentional injuries. Environmental risks include appropriate maintenance of streets, safe power transmission and sewage treatment, and laws that regulate the hazard risk of appliances and tools. Natural disasters such as floods, hurricanes, earthquakes, or tornadoes are also environmental risks. The devastation caused by natural disasters affects every one of us at some point in our lifetime.

Stress and fatigue contribute greatly to higher rates of unintentional injuries. Stress may interfere with your concentration when performing even a simple task or may distract you while you are engaged in an activity. Fatigue causes you to be less alert or have slower reaction times; affects your coordination; and, at worst, can cause you to fall asleep. It is not wise to attempt difficult tasks while you are fatigued or under stress.

Analysis of Unintentional Injury

Scientific study of unintentional injury tries to uncover why injuries occur, what factors play a role, and who or what age group is most at risk. Analysis of unintentional injury provides us with data that are necessary before effective educational, preventive, or enforcement strategies can be implemented.

Injury epidemiology, used to investigate risk factors that cause unintentional injuries, is analogous to the epidemiologic model for disease. For injuries to result, three factors are involved: (1) the agent or source of energy exchange, i.e., mechanical, chemical, electrical, or thermal; (2) the vehicle for the transmission of mechanical energy, i.e., a car, truck, motorcycle, powerline, or poison; and (3) a host or object, i.e., a person, school building, or house (Figure 21.4).

Most unintentional injuries involve many factors; interactions among risk factors affect the likelihood of an accident. For example, cutting trees with a chain

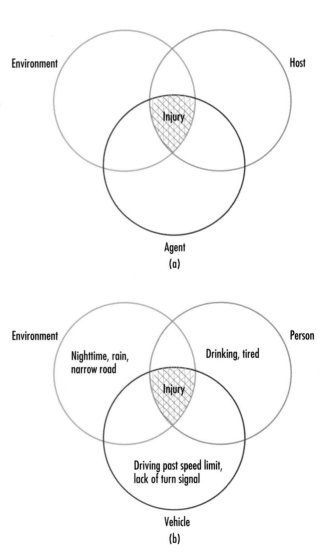

FIGURE 21.4 **Epidemiologic Model for Unintentional Injuries**

saw on a windy or rainy day may increase the risk of accident, whereas choosing a dry, calm day might reduce the chance of an accident.

The Haddon matrix is one of the scientific models used in unintentional injury analysis. Developed by William Haddon, Jr., in the 1960s, this model was used originally to investigate motor vehicle risk factors and to develop and implement programs to prevent or reduce the occurrence of car accidents.

According to some estimates "every two miles, the average driver makes 400 observations, 40 decisions, and one mistake. Once in every 500 miles, one of these mistakes leads to a near collision, and once in every 61,000 miles, one of these mistakes leads to a car crash" (Gladwell, 2001). The Haddon matrix analyzed accidents in three phases:

- *Phase 1: Pre-event phase.* Includes factors that may determine if an accident will happen; lack of knowledge or skills or alcohol use are the most significant factors.
- *Phase 2: Event phase.* Occurs when the host comes into contact with forces of energy. Many preventive measures, such as the use of helmets, safety belts, or protective goggles, are associated with this phase.
- *Phase 3: Post-event phase.* Includes emergency procedures provided after the injury has occurred. Preventive signaling devices, smoke and carbon

monoxide detectors, or fire alarms will increase the speed with which help reaches an injured person. Emergency transportation and care of an injured or sick person occurs in this phase.

All approaches to unintentional injury reduction include: (a) educational and prevention strategies; (b) stricter laws and regulations (e.g., mandates to enforce safety belt and helmet compliance); and (c) better product design and automatic protection devices (e.g., air bags, child-proof car door locks, child-proof safety caps on medicines).

Motor Vehicle Safety

Even though motor vehicle death rates have been declining since 1962, the number of deaths is still a major concern. Motor vehicle travel is the primary means of transportation in the United States, and it provides an unprecedented degree of mobility. Yet, for all its advantages, injuries resulting from motor vehicle crashes are the leading cause of death from age 6 to 27. In 1999, an estimated 41,300 people were killed in motor vehicle traffic crashes and approximately 2,000,000 were injured.

The National Highway Traffic Safety Administration (NHTSA) estimates that alcohol was involved in 39% of fatal crashes and 7% of all traffic accidents, fatal and nonfatal. Approximately three in every ten Americans will be involved in an alcohol-related traffic accident some time in their lives. Alcohol involvement in fatal crashes during the day is 17% but rises to 60% at night. Heed the warning: *Do not drink and drive.*

Terms

injury epidemiology: the study of the occurrence, causes, and prevention of injury

Wellness Guide

Driving Defensively

Driving defensively means not only taking responsibility for yourself and your actions but also keeping an eye on "the other guy." The National Safety Council offers the following guidelines to help reduce your risks on the road:

- Don't leave the driveway without securing each passenger in the car, including children and pets. Safety belts save thousands of lives each year!
- Remember that driving too fast or too slow can increase the likelihood of collisions.

- Don't kid yourself. If you plan to drink, designate a driver who won't drink. Alcohol is a factor in almost half of all fatal motor vehicle accidents.
- Be alert! If you notice that a car is straddling the center line, weaving, making wide turns, stopping abruptly, or responding slowly to traffic signals, the driver may be impaired.
- Avoid an impaired driver by slowing down, letting the driver pass, pulling onto the shoulder, or turning right at the nearest corner. If it appears

that an oncoming car is crossing into your lane, pull over to the roadside, sound the horn, and flash your lights.

- Notify the police immediately after seeing a motorist who is driving suspiciously.
- Follow the rules of the road. Don't contest the "right of way" or try to race another car during a merge. Be respectful of other motorists.
- While driving, be cautious, aware, and responsible.

Many accidents involving young persons occur after dark, after parties, and after drinking. Alcohol in the blood and brain impairs a driver's judgment, coordination, and reaction time. The effects of alcohol vary considerably from one person to another, so even small amounts of alcohol may impair driving skills and cause an accident. New laws have been proposed that set a zero tolerance for blood alcohol for persons under age 21.

Many factors other than alcohol use contribute to motor vehicle fatalities and injuries, e.g., road conditions and speed at which the vehicle travels. The interaction between these two factors is particularly risky. In all severe accidents, rural and urban, exceeding the posted speed limit was the most common factor. Defects in a vehicle, such as faulty tires, brakes, headlights, steering system, body, door, and hood, also contribute to the risk of motor vehicle accidents.

Driving can be difficult even when you are concentrating on the road and your surroundings. But driving while you dial or talk on a cellular phone can be distracting and potentially dangerous. Cell phones may be convenient, but if not used properly, they are a danger to the user and everyone on the road. At 55 miles per hour, a vehicle travels the length of a football field in 3.7 seconds, less time than it takes to dial a phone number. Anything that takes a driver's concentration off the road increases the possibility of an accident. America's growing enchantment with cellular phones in automobiles brings with it the need for renewed emphasis on safe driving practices.

Some countries already have banned the use of cell phones while driving, and some states also are considering restricting their use. Studies show that carrying on a conversation over a cell phone is much more distracting than having a conversation with someone in the car or listening to the radio. Doing business or having an argument with someone in a cell phone conversation increases the risk of an accident. The National Safety Council has recommended that "the best practice is to not use electronic devices, including cell phones, while driving. When on the road, drivers shall concentrate on safe and defensive driving and not on making or receiving phone calls, delivery of faxes, using computers, navigation systems, or other distracting influences."

Lap/shoulder seat belts are still the best protection against fatal injury in a crash. Seat belts are estimated to reduce the risk of fatal injury to front seat occupants by 45%; between 1975 and 1999, it is estimated that 112,086 lives were saved by the use of seat belts. Air bags provide additional protection, but are not very effective by themselves except in a head-on collision; they should always be used in conjunction with a lap/shoulder seat belt.

All states (except for New Hampshire) and the District of Columbia have mandatory seat belt safety laws. However, the degree of seat belt use varies widely from state to state because of differences in public attitudes, enforcement, and education programs. Government regulations, use of lap/shoulder seat belts and child safety seats, and installation of air bags have markedly reduced the number of motor vehicle fatalities and injuries.

When driving, observe the following safety ABCs:

- **A**lways slide the seat back as far as possible and sit back.
- **B**uckle everyone up.
- **C**hildren aged 12 and under should ride properly restrained in the back seat.

Motorcycle Safety

Motorcycles appeal to many individuals for various reasons: low cost to purchase, repair, and operate; the exciting feeling of open-air riding; and association with fellow motorcycle riders. However, higher risks include less crash protection than an automobile, and less visibility by other drivers. Motorcycle operators can ensure a safer ride by securing proper training in operational procedures and by using a helmet and proper protective clothing. Less than 10% of all

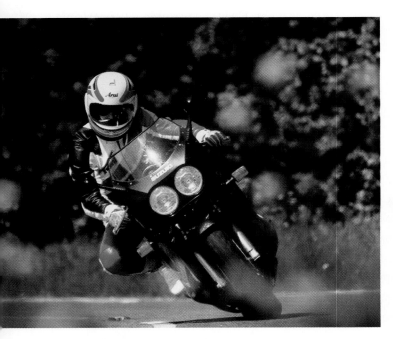

A helmet and protective clothing are essential to motorcycle safety.

motorcycle operators receive any formal training. Wearing a motorcycle helmet reduces the likelihood of fatal injuries in an accident. Protective clothing, such as long sleeves and pants, jackets, and boots, may lessen the chance for abrasions should an accident occur or protect from bad weather.

In 1966, Congress mandated that motorcycle riders and passengers use helmets in all states. If states did not enforce this mandate, they would lose federal highway funds, but only three states at first adopted helmet laws. However by 1975, 47 states had helmet laws in force. During this ten-year period (1966–1975), fatal motorcycle accidents declined from 12.8 to 6.5 deaths per 100,000. All motorcycle helmets sold in the United States are required to meet federal guidelines, which establish the minimum level of protection helmets must afford each user.

Pedestrian Safety

In 1999, traffic accidents injured 95,000 pedestrians and killed 5,800 pedestrians in the United States. About half of all pedestrian deaths and injuries involve children aged 5 to 9 who are either crossing or entering a street. Among young children, implementation of preventive strategies and educational efforts addressing safety procedures in traffic areas may reduce accidents. Many young children don't know what traffic signals or signs mean. Young children are also unable to judge the distance and speed of vehicles, which puts them in danger when trying to cross a busy intersection. Close supervision by adults helps prevent accidents; education of childcare workers is another preventive strategy.

The elderly are especially at risk for pedestrian injuries, as a result of failing eyesight, hearing, and mobility problems. Some pedestrian injuries occur when individuals dart into a busy street or are unable to see oncoming traffic because their view is blocked by a parked vehicle. Many pedestrian injuries involve joggers, runners, and walkers. Bright-colored clothes, especially reflective clothes, offer protection for pedestrians during both day and night. Also, just as alcohol impairs the judgment of motor vehicle operators, it also impairs the judgment of pedestrians.

Other preventive strategies can also help reduce the number of pedestrian injuries and deaths. Underpasses and overpasses in high traffic areas, well-marked crosswalks, and pedestrian guardrails all offer

Managing Stress

Mindful Meditation

Ninety percent of all accidents are the result of human error. This fact suggests what those in the field of stress management already know: the mind can focus on only one thing at a time. When the mind is overwhelmed with thoughts, attention drops. When you are sitting at your desk studying for an exam and your mind wanders, your life isn't in jeopardy. But when you are engaged in driving your car, and you are talking on your cell phone, and also listening to the news, an accident is waiting to happen.

Most accidents occur because your mind is somewhere other than where it is supposed to be. Drifting attention, unfocused thoughts, and mental distractions are normal in the course of a typical day, but the mind *can* be trained to stay focused. Training the mind in this fashion is called "mindful meditation," a type of meditation used to focus your thoughts and increase awareness. Athletes, surgeons, and actors practice this technique to improve their performance. It is a technique that everyone should master, especially to reduce the risk of accidents.

Mindful meditation can take many forms and with repeated practice, the effects of one experience (like eating an apple) can transfer to virtually any activity. Mindful meditation is a way to keep focused on whatever task you are engaged in. Try this exercise.

1. Take an apple and hold it in your hand.

2. Sit comfortably with your back straight. You may choose to sit against a wall for support.

3. Hold the apple and feel its weight in your hand. Feel the apple. Feel the texture of the apple's skin. Feel the curves. Feel the stem if there is one. Notice all the nuances of the apple with your fingers.

4. Look at the apple. What color is it? Look at it carefully. Study it. Know this apple so well, that if it was put back in a barrel of apples, you could easily find it.

5. Now smell the apple. Close your eyes and focus your sense of smell on the apple. What does it smell like?

6. Bite into the apple. Savor its taste, flavor, and texture. Feel your tongue and jaws move as you chew.

Now, sensing and eating an apple may seem far removed from preventing an accident, but the truth is that the skills of concentration and focusing are important in every activity. Practice mindful meditation and use it when driving.

protection for the pedestrian. Limiting traffic during peak hours of pedestrian traffic—for instance, before and after school or church—is also beneficial.

Bicycle Safety
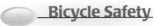

Safety concerns have been increasing as more bicycles are used for exercise and recreation. Few bicyclists wear a protective helmet every time they ride their bike yet the single most important factor in reducing bicycle deaths is the use of protective helmets. A total of 70,000 bicyclists were injured and 900 were killed in collisions with motor vehicles in 1999.

Bicycle riders are required to follow the same rules of the road as automobile operators. But many bicycle riders lack knowledge of these rules, do not use proper hand signals, or ride on the wrong side of

---

Wellness Guide

Protect Your Kids in the Car

The type of child safety seat to buy and how you position it depend on the child's age, weight, and size. Every state and the District of Columbia have child protection laws. The safest place for any child aged 12 and under is in the back seat. Every child should be buckled into a child safety seat or a booster seat or a lap-shoulder belt, if it fits. A few pointers:

Riding with Babies

- Infants up to about 20 pounds and up to age 1 should ride in a rear-facing child seat. The child seat must be in the BACK seat and face the rear of the car, van, or truck.

- Babies riding in a car must never face front. In a crash or sudden stop, the baby's neck can be hurt badly.

- Infants in car seats must never ride in the front seat of a car with air bags. In a crash, the air bag can hit the car seat and hurt or kill the baby.

- Never hold your baby in your lap when you are riding in the car. In a crash or sudden stop, your child can be hurt badly or killed.

Riding with Young Kids

- Kids over 20 pounds and older than 1 year should ride in a car seat that faces the front of the car, van, or truck.

- It is best to keep kids in the foreward-facing car seat for as long as they fit comfortably in it.

- Older kids over 40 pounds should ride in a booster seat until the car's lap and shoulder belts fit them correctly. The lap belt must fit low and

snug on their hips. The shoulder belt must not cross their face or neck.

- Never put a shoulder belt behind a child's back or under a child's arm.

Remember . . .

- All kids are safest in the back seat, in a safety seat or seatbelt.

- Always read the child seat instructions and the car owner's manual. Test the child seat to ensure a snug fit by pulling the base to either side or toward the front of the car.

Source: National Highway Traffic Safety Administration, U.S. Department of Transportation, *Protect Your Kids in the Car*, August 1997.

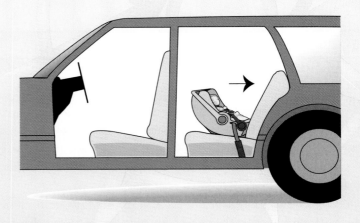

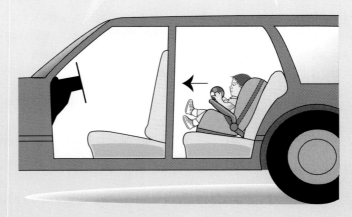

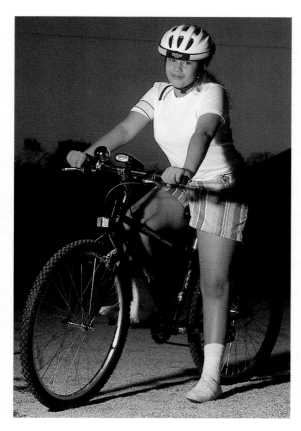

Appropriate helmet and reflector use are crucial to bicycle safety.

the street, contributing to bicycle injuries and fatalities. Also, lack of skill in handling a bicycle increases the risk of an accident. Individuals who purchase a new bicycle should be familiar with all its devices before riding it. Also, many young bicycle riders are unaware of the rules of the road or are too small to see over motor vehicles.

Bicycle riders need to wear bright, reflective clothing, and the bicycle itself should be properly equipped with reflectors and lights. A recent and dangerous phenomenon is wearing headphones while riding. Inability to hear the sounds of traffic, the honk of a horn, or a shout of warning may contribute to an accident. Construction of more bicycle paths, underpasses, overpasses, and guardrails along with defensive riding skills can reduce bicycle injuries and deaths.

Home Safety

Accidental deaths in the home are gradually declining but are still a major source of concern. Accidents in the home take a special toll on both young and elderly persons. As the elderly population continues to grow, accidents in the home will increase. The main categories of home accidents include falls, poisonings, drowning, choking and suffocation, and fires and burns. Although

not all falls, drownings, or poisonings occur in the home, they are classified as home accidents.

Between 1912 and 1999, deaths from unintentional home injury per 100,000 population were reduced 61%. One person in 75 in the United States was disabled half a day or more by unintentional injuries received in the home. Disabling injuries are more numerous in the home than they are in the workplace and in motor vehicle accidents combined. In 1999, various home injuries totaled almost 7 million—28,800 of which were fatal (see Figure 21.5).

> *Experience is something you don't get until just after you need it.*
> ANONYMOUS

Falls

People of all ages fall, but most fatal injuries occur among elderly persons. Falls are the leading cause of deaths from unintentional injuries in the home. Children often fall because of their strenuous activities, but usually the injuries are minor and heal rapidly. However, children also fall down stairs, out of trees, from open windows, and from the backs of trucks. They fall while climbing, jumping, or running. People responsible for watching children at play must be alert to the danger of a fall.

Falls are a more serious problem for older persons, who often fracture hip or head bones. For people over age 79, falls were the leading cause of death from unintentional injury. Bone breaks in elderly persons heal slowly and often lead to complications and death. If hospitalized, an elderly person may contract nosocomial infections (see Chapter 9) and die. Being careful

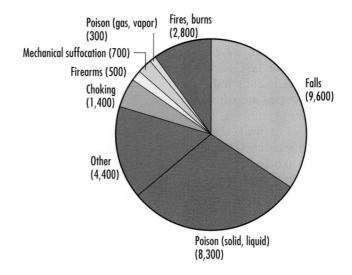

FIGURE 21.5   **Unintentional Injury Deaths at Home, United States, 1999**
Choking includes inhalation or ingestion of food or other object.
Source: National Safety Council, Injury Facts, 2000.

and in good physical condition are the best deterrents to being seriously injured in a fall.

Certain areas in the home are hazardous for falls. The kitchen, bathroom, and laundry room are dangerous because they often have wet floors. Stairs are also hazardous; a person may stumble while walking up or down, particularly if he or she is distracted or if the stairs are not well lit. Bumping into furniture or tripping over the legs of tables, chairs, or loose rugs are also common causes of falls. Climbing ladders may be an invitation for a fall if a person is careless or the ladder is weak or unstable. When performing any activity in which a fall is possible, take extra safety measures, such as having someone hold the ladder that you are climbing. After motor vehicle accidents, falls cause the greatest number of unintentional injury deaths.

Poisonings

A **poison** is any chemical substance that causes illness, injury, or death. Poisons enter the body by being ingested (medicines, drugs, mushrooms, shellfish, chemicals), inhaled (carbon monoxide, hydrogen sulfide), injected (bee sting, snake bite), or by contact with the skin (poison ivy, solutions that burn). Poisonings from spoiled foods, i.e., salmonella, are excluded here and are classified as disease deaths. Chemical poisons such as pesticides disturb essential biological reactions in the body and cause a variety of symptoms and may cause death. Some poisons cause only transitory symptoms; the body returns to normal once the poison is eliminated. However, some poisons that do not kill can cause permanent and irreversible damage to body functions.

Many cultivated and wild plants, trees, and bushes contain poisonous compounds. Eating the berries, seeds, roots, or leaves of many plants can produce mild or severe symptoms or death. Many common household plants are also poisonous, even the Christmas poinsettia. Collecting and eating wild mushrooms can be dangerous unless you are knowledgeable about what species are edible.

Young children, especially once they have learned to crawl or walk, are particularly susceptible to poisoning accidents. Children are curious, active, and adventurous, and it is natural for young children to put things in their mouths, including nonfood items such as paint chips, dirt, marbles—almost any small object. When children are hungry, thirsty, or just curious, they are likely to ingest whatever is closest to hand—medicines, pills, household products, pesticides. Children between ages 1 and 5 suffer the greatest number of accidental poisonings.

Precautions by manufacturers of drugs, solvents, paints, and other products have markedly reduced the number of accidental childhood poisonings. Child-resistant lids, tamper-proof caps, and internal seals help to prevent children from ingesting harmful substances. Precautions by parents and other child caregivers are essential to reduce the risk further. All household products and medicines should be kept out of reach of small children. Dangerous substances should be kept in locked cabinets. Small children should not be left unsupervised in areas like bathrooms, kitchens, and garages, where dangerous household products are stored.

There are several hundred poison control centers across the country. Should a poisoning accident occur, someone at a poison control center can give you immediate expert advice. Keep the number of a poison control center near the phone in case of emergency.

Poisoning by gases and vapors is mainly caused by carbon monoxide. Carbon monoxide results from incomplete combustion in cooking stoves, heating equipment, and standing running motor vehicles. Most deaths are the result of suicide, but many are accidental. The largest number of carbon monoxide fatalities occurred in the group aged 15 to 24; males commit suicide with carbon monoxide three times as often as females. Most carbon monoxide deaths occurred in stationary motor vehicles, although fireplaces, stoves, and appliances using natural or liquid propane gas were responsible for 10% of all unintentional carbon monoxide fatalities. Regulations that have lowered carbon monoxide emissions have contributed significantly to reducing the rates of unintentional carbon monoxide fatalities.

Drowning

Drowning accounts for many unintentional injuries and fatalities in the home; young children are especially vulnerable. Young children can drown in five-gallon buckets or in toilet bowls. About half of all drownings occur during June, July, and August when many people are engaged in summer water activities. Recreation in large bodies of water, rivers, and streams provides the opportunities for accidental drowning.

When a person is under water and inhales water instead of air, an automatic muscular contraction of the larynx occurs that is called **laryngospasm.** This muscular reflex closes the body's main airway in an attempt to keep water from entering the lungs. The spasm continues as long as the person is under water and within a few minutes can lead to death by suffocation. Once the laryngospasm relaxes, water enters the lungs. Only about 10% of people survive not breathing under water for as long as 6 minutes and these victims will survive only if artificial respiration is applied immediately. Few people recover if breathing has stopped for as long as 10 minutes.

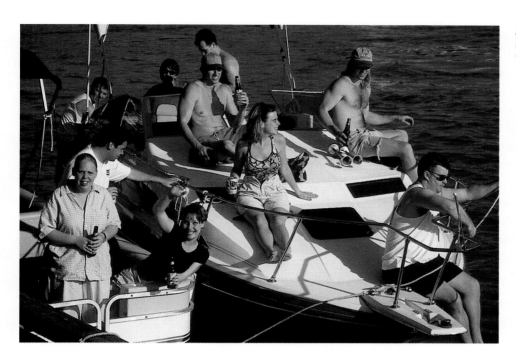

Many boating accidents are associated with drinking alcohol while having fun on the water.

Scientific evidence does not support the widely held belief that swimming shortly after eating induces stomach cramps, thereby increasing the risk of drowning. However, it is true that after eating, blood is diverted to the stomach to assist digestion and consequently less oxygen may be available for muscles, which can lead to muscle spasms. This sequence poses no problem for a healthy person, but if a person is in poor health, is overweight, or has existing heart disease, the risk of drowning may be increased.

Knowing your swimming ability and avoiding swimming in dangerous waters are ways to reduce the risk of accidental drowning. Using a personal flotation device (commonly called a life jacket) while you engage in water sports can also reduce the risk of drowning.

Alcohol and other drugs may be the biggest predisposing factor in drowning for individuals aged 15 or older. Impairment of the individual's judgment may lead to the death of others as well, for example, operating a boat with passengers while intoxicated or supervising children who are in or near the water while drinking.

Choking and Suffocation

Choking to death as a result of an object lodged in the airway passage occurs more often than one might expect. Each year in the United States more than a thousand people die because a piece of food or a foreign object became stuck in their throats and caused them to stop breathing. Food that is swallowed without being chewed sufficiently is a common cause of choking and blockage of the air passage. Small bones from fish or chicken also can be swallowed inadvertently and become stuck in the airway. Sometimes dentures, fillings, or crowns become loose, are accidentally swallowed, and may cause the person to choke. Being intoxicated also increases the risk of swallowing improperly.

When the airway is completely blocked, a choking victim is unable to speak, breathe, or cough. A choking person often clutches his or her throat. If the object is not removed quickly, the victim may become unconscious and death may follow rapidly from lack of oxygen.

Mechanical suffocation is another type of unintentional injury, occurring most frequently in young children up to 4 years old. A small child can get into tight spaces and become trapped or wedged, resulting in suffocation. As infants become more mobile and inquisitive, the risk of entrapment and suffocation increases. Long cords dangling from appliances, draperies, or blinds should be placed well out of the way of a curious infant or toddler. Bulky bedding materials have been responsible for the suffocation of young children, especially fluffy comforters or infant bean bag cushions, and some household items, such as the bean bag cushion, have been recalled because of suffocation risks.

Prevention and education strategies reduce the risk of suffocation of young children. Eliminate dangerous products and access to dangerous areas in the house by

Terms

poison: any chemical substance that causes illness, injury, or death

laryngospasm: spasm of the larynx due to inhaling water

Wellness Guide

Smoke Detectors Give You a Chance

Most deaths and injuries in fires result from inhalation of smoke and toxic gases that reach victims before the flames do. Survival depends on an early warning system that gives you time to vacate the premises at once. The best warning system available is a smoke detector that cuts your risk of dying in a fire in half. The U.S. Consumer Product Safety Commission offers these suggestions about smoke detectors:

- Many localities require that you have a smoke detector in your home, so buy one—at least one. They're inexpensive and are available at most hardware stores and supermarkets. Check your local codes and regulations; they may require you to purchase a specific kind.

- Read the instructions that come with the detector for advice on where to install it. You should purchase at least one for every floor in your house. Preferably you should place one outside every bedroom.

- Manufacturers know what is best for their products and tell you how to care for them. Follow their instructions. Detectors can save lives, but only if you install and maintain them properly.

- Never disconnect a fire detector. If it goes off at wrong times because of heat from a stove or steam from a bathroom, move it to another location.

- Replace the battery annually (January 1 is an easy day to remember) or when you hear a "chirping" sound. And press the test button regularly to be sure the batteries work.

- Keep your detector clean. Dust, grease, or other materials can interfere with efficient operation. You may want to vacuum the grill work on the detector.

using a safety gate or closing doors. Child-care providers should know what steps to take to prevent unintentional injuries of young children in the home.

Fires

House fires cause more than 3,000 deaths and 17,000 injuries each year in the United States. Those at highest risk include the elderly, minority, and low-income populations (Istre, McCoy, Osborn et al., 2001). Fires in the home may be attributed to many factors: fireplaces, wood stoves, kerosene or space heaters, improper placement of appliances, faulty wiring of the house or appliances, grease fires in the kitchen (loose sleeves dangling over open flames), improper storage of combustible materials, or a careless smoker in the house.

Death rates from fires or burns have markedly decreased since the 1950s. Smoke detectors, portable ladders, and fire extinguishers have helped reduce fatalities. Also, many elementary school students are receiving annual training from local fire departments concerning fire safety. Prevention and education are, once again, the best strategies to eliminate unintentional injuries from fires and burns. Each household should have a planned escape route, smoke detectors placed at key locations throughout the home, and posted emergency phone numbers. Everyone should know how to operate a fire extinguisher and know exactly where it is kept, and in two-story houses, a portable ladder should be readily accessible.

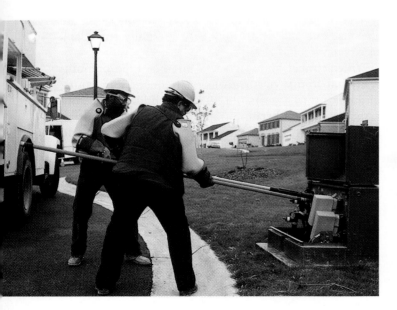

Workers should always wear the appropriate safety equipment while on the job.

 ### Work Safety

Between 1912 and 1999, unintentional injury deaths in the workplace were reduced by 90%. However, there still were almost 4 million disabling injuries and 5,100 deaths in 1999. Occupational illnesses also occur with high frequency, and together with nonfatal injuries account for many lost days at work (see Figure 21.6).

Occupational illnesses occur most often in manufacturing industries. Agriculture has the highest incidence of skin diseases and disorders, which may be attributed to agricultural workers' close contact with

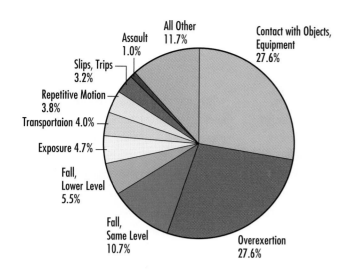

FIGURE 21.6 **Nonfatal Occupational Injuries and Illnesses Involving Days Away from Work, 1998** According to the Bureau of Labor Statistics, more than half of the 1,730,500 nonfatal injuries and illnesses in private industry were due to overexertion or to contact with equipment and other objects.

Source: National Safety Council, *Injury Facts* 2000

Cumulative motion disorders

Cervical radiculopathy: People who look up to a computer screen or who balance a phone on their shoulder are at risk.

Pronator syndrome: Mechanics, baseball pitchers, and barbers are at risk.

Carpal tunnel syndrome: Typists, computer programmers, and potters are at risk.

Thoracic outlet syndrome: Violinists and other musicians are at risk.

Cubital tunnel syndrome: Truck drivers or other persons who keep their arms in fixed, flexed positions are at risk.

Distal ulnar neuropathy: Meat packers, assembly-line workers, and machine operators are at risk.

FIGURE 21.7 **Cumulative Motion Disorders** These injuries affect muscles, tendons, and nerves.

hazardous chemicals. Common occupational illnesses include skin disorders, respiratory conditions caused by inhalation of toxic substances, disorders associated with repeated trauma, poisonings, and dust-related diseases of the lungs. The incidence is suspected to be higher than reported, because many workers do not seek medical attention for their illnesses or injuries.

Carpal tunnel syndrome is one of a group of injuries known as **cumulative motion disorders,** caused by repeated stress of a body part, resulting from repetitive motion for long periods (Figure 21.7). Symptoms of carpal tunnel syndrome are burning, numbness, tingling, and stiffness of the hand, fingers, or wrist. Dentists, dental hygienists, supermarket cashiers, seamstresses, musicians, factory workers, computer keyboard operators, and surgeons are at risk for carpal tunnel syndrome. Better product design, correct positioning of the operator and the tool, and limiting time spent at the same task are being investigated as possible solutions to the rising incidence of cumulative trauma disorders.

A recent phenomenon of work-related injury and illness is **sick building syndrome,** a variety of symptoms reported by workers in modern office buildings. Recent investigations have found a correlation between pollutants in or near the building or a poor ventilation system and sick building syndrome. Much of the evidence of these symptoms is self-reported by the workers or documented by physicians. Symptoms include asthma, lung infections, dizziness, nausea, throat and eye irritations, fatigue, cough, and shortness of breath. Based on limited research to date on sick building syndrome, ventilation alone was not a significant factor.

Possibly the combination of the ventilation system and volatile organic substances used in many new building products may be the determinants.

First Aid and Emergencies

First aid and medical emergencies can be handled appropriately if you take a deep breath and tell yourself you can handle the situation until a qualified medical professional arrives to take over. First aid is defined as the immediate care given to an injured or ill person. First aid is temporary assistance given until a person has recovered or until a qualified medical person can provide assistance.

Knowledge about first aid and medical emergencies can literally mean the difference between life and death and can help prevent disability or permanent injury. Knowledge of first aid skills will increase your confidence in dealing with both minor and major emergencies and will be reassuring to an injured person.

Taking Risks and Preventing Accidents

Risks cannot be avoided in life; accidents and unintentional injuries are a consequence of the risks we

Terms

cumulative motion disorders: disorders caused by repeated stress to a body part; carpal tunnel syndrome is a cumulative motion disorder

sick building syndrome: collection of symptoms reported by workers in some modern buildings

Dollars and Health Sense

Workplace Injuries and Government Policy

According to the Bureau of Labor Statistics, about 4% of workplace injuries are classified as repetitive motion disorders; 582,300 such injuries were reported in 1999 and resulted in an average of 17 days off from work. Carpal tunnel syndrome, the most common form of repetitive motion disorder, caused an average of 27 days off the job. The workers most affected by this disorder are truck drivers, manual laborers, and nursing aides and orderlies. The Office of Safety and Health Administration (OSHA), which oversees health and safety concerns in the workplace, conducted an intensive study of repetitive motion disorders and developed ergonomic workplace rules that would have markedly reduced these kinds of injuries and saved million of dollars in health costs. Just before leaving office, former President Bill Clinton implemented the OSHA rules by executive order.

The new rules proved to be highly controversial. Labor unions and workers favored them; business groups did not. Although the new rules were expected to reduce injures, lost work time, and overall health costs, the rules also would have increased costs for some businesses by limiting the time workers could perform repetitive manual tasks such as working at a computer keyboard, slicing meats, grasping tools, or operating a grocery scanner. Shortly after taking office, President George W. Bush, under pressure from business interests, signed a law repealing the new OSHA rules.

Carpal tunnel syndrome is treated traditionally with wrist splints, anti-inflammatory drugs, injection therapy, and surgery. Many victims are forced to change careers. A recent study of 400 volunteers suffering from carpal tunnel syndrome showed that a specific set of yoga and relaxation exercises was more effective than wrist splints in relieving symptoms (Garfinkel, Singhai, Katz et al., 1998). The yoga exercises strengthened the upper body and hand grip and reduced pain.

Individuals who are susceptible to repetitive motion injuries at their jobs should try to learn what ergonomic measures can be taken to ward off injuries. Ergonomic chairs and desks that impose better posture can be of significant benefit in many jobs. If the employer allows it, taking frequent breaks and using stretching and relaxation exercises also can help. As with most aspects of health and safety, self responsibility can ward off the pain, suffering, and possible permanent damage resulting from a repetitive motion disorder.

---

take. As soon as a child learns to crawl, he or she begins to take risks to explore and understand the environment. At each stage of life we take risks to learn and to expand our capabilities and experiences. We take a risk when we cross the street in traffic, run to catch a bus, or swing from the branch of a tree. When we go hiking or climbing or engage in sports, we are taking risks.

The important question YOU need to ask is: "What risks are necessary and acceptable for me to live the way I want to?" The answer will also, to some extent, determine your risk of unintentional injury. People differ enormously in their need for risk-taking behaviors. Some people thrive on high-risk endeavors, such as playing polo, racing cars, or climbing mountains. However, even people who live more sedate lives may be at risk for unintentional injuries because of destructive behaviors or unhealthy mental attitudes.

> If at first you don't succeed, skydiving is not for you.
>
> ANONYMOUS

Whatever your personal beliefs, a commitment to safe living can be made at any time. Why not make the commitment now? Eliminating or reducing the use of alcohol can reduce the risk of many kinds of injuries, especially motor vehicle accidents. Lowering your stress level will also contribute significantly to reducing unintentional injuries. Not keeping a loaded firearm in the house can eliminate the risk of an unintentional firearm injury. Reading and following the manufacturer's instructions and warnings before operating a new product will also help to reduce the risk of unintentional injury. Before undertaking any sport activity, climbing a ladder, or riding a bike, take a moment to consider essential safety measures. Observe posted safety rules and warning signs. Keep in good physical condition and have a positive mental attitude when undertaking a potentially dangerous activity.

Although unintentional injuries are usually not a laughing matter, one accident statistic does sound a humorous note. Saturday and Sunday are the two most dangerous days of the week for fatal accidents. Going out on the weekends just to have fun increases the risks of serious injuries. Maybe studying or reading on weekends is a good idea after all.

Critical Thinking About Health

1. Briefly explain a recent injury that occurred to you, a friend, or family member using the epidemiological triad presented in Figure 21.4.
   a. What were the human factors involved in the injury?
   b. What were the environmental factors (physical as well as social) involved in the injury?
   c. What were the vehicle (or agent) factors involved in the injury?
   Which factor(s) could have been modified in such a way that may have prevented the injury from occurring?
2. Alcohol is a contributing factor in about 40% of traffic fatalities. What are your campus and community doing to help prevent people, both young and old, from driving while intoxicated? Some questions to consider:
   a. Are there educational programs? If so, what are they and who do they target?
   b. How would you design an educational program to keep your peers from drinking and driving?
   c. Are there seasonal programs that increase awareness about the dangers of drinking and driving (e.g., high school prom, Fourth of July)?
   d. What is the role of local law enforcement, both on and off campus, with regards to decreasing drinking and driving accidents and fatalities?
3. Federal, state, and local governments have written and passed laws and regulations that enforce certain safety behaviors that have an impact on the individual and/or community. Such laws regulate using a seatbelt, restraining your child in a car seat, and wearing a helmet while riding a motorcycle or bicycle. Some people believe that the government (at any level) should not mandate laws regarding individual safety and injury prevention. Others believe that the government has a right to demand certain safe behaviors among its citizens for the public good. What's your opinion? Should the government be allowed to regulate individual safety behaviors? Explain why or why not.

Health in Review

- Unintentional injuries and deaths cost Americans billions of dollars in medical costs as well as costs due to loss of work each year. Unintentional injuries and deaths are preventable!
- Many factors contribute to unintentional injuries: knowledge, attitudes, beliefs, and behaviors; economic and social factors; competence; environmental conditions; and use of alcohol and other drugs.
- The Haddon matrix was developed to assess motor vehicle risk factors and is used to develop prevention programs.
- A multidimensional approach to injury prevention includes education, prevention strategies, stricter laws and regulations, and better product design.
- Motor vehicle deaths are decreasing; however, in 1999 about 41,300 people were killed in motor vehicle crashes. Approximately one alcohol-related fatality occurs every 32 minutes.
- Pedestrian and bicycle safety rules and equipment are keys to preventing accidents. Wear reflective clothing and obey the rules of the road.
- Safety in the home includes preventing falls, poisonings, drownings, choking, and fires.
- Work-related injuries have decreased since 1984; however, they still cost employers and employees large amounts of time and money. Injuries to the back are most frequent, followed by legs, arms, and trunk. Proper work safety procedures can prevent the majority of work-related injuries.
- Accidents and injuries are a consequence of the many risks we take. Although most of what we do has some degree of risk, we can decrease that risk by increasing safety knowledge and taking the necessary precautions.

Health and Wellness Online

The World Wide Web contains a wealth of information about health and wellness. By accessing the Internet using Web browser software, such as Netscape Navigator or Microsoft's Internet Explorer, you can gain a new perspective on many topics presented in *Health and Wellness, Seventh Edition.* Access the Jones and Bartlett Publishers Web site at http://www.jbpub.com/hwonline.

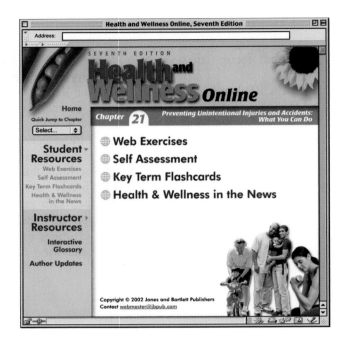

References

Garfinkel, M. S., Singhai, A., Katz, W. A., et al. (1998). Yoga-based intervention for carpal tunnel syndrome. *Journal of the American Medical Association, 380,* 1601–1603.

Gladwell, M. (2001, June 11). Wrong turn. *The New Yorker,* 50–61.

Istre, G. R., McCoy, M. A., Osborn, L. et al. (2001). Deaths and injuries from house fires. *New England Journal of Medicine, 344,* 1911–1916.

National Safety Council, *Injury facts,* 2000 edition. Itasca, IL.

Suggested Readings

Barss, P., Smith, G., Baker, S., and Mohan, D. (1998). *Injury prevention: An international perspective.* Cary, NC: Oxford University Press. Injuries are rapidly assuming epidemic proportions throughout the world. This book provides a worldwide overview of injury problems, including the epidemiology of injury, surveillance, and policy.

Gladwell, M. (2001, June 11). Wrong turn. *The New Yorker,* 50–61. An interesting look at why automobile safety measures may not be working as originally expected.

Injuries in the school environment: A resource guide. (1997). Children's Safety Network, 55 Chapel Street, Newton, MA 02158-1060 (free). The Children's Safety Network designed this packet of information to inform school personnel and other professionals about the extent of the problem of injury and to stimulate discussion.

Turkington, C. (1994). *Poisons and antidotes.* New York: Facts on File. Describes more than 600 toxic substances, symptoms, and treatments for poisoning.

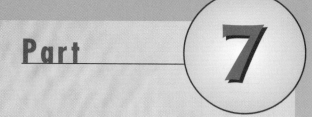

Part 7

Overcoming Obstacles

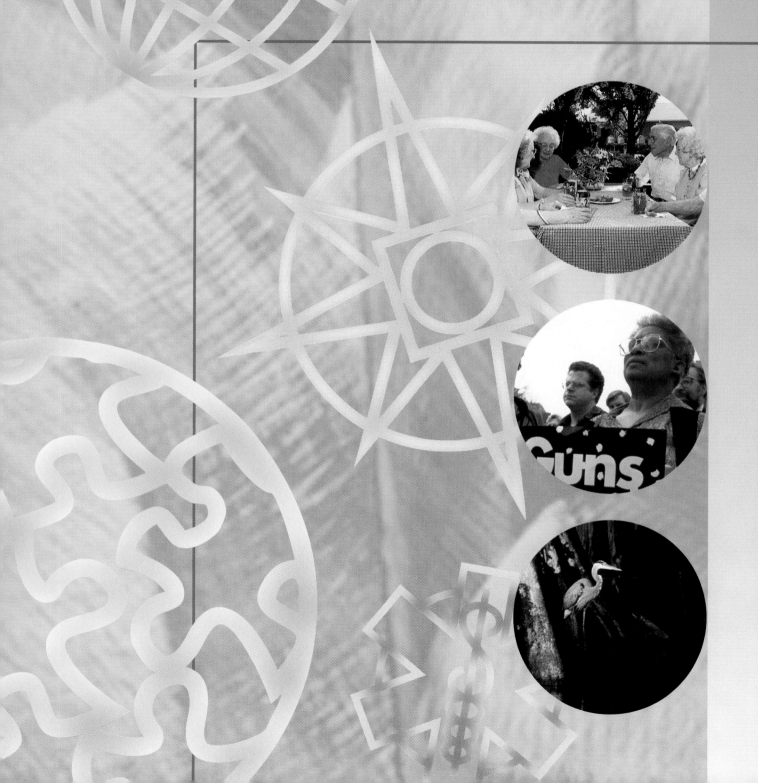

Learning Objectives

1. Describe some of the biological changes that occur with aging.
2. Define aging, maximum life span, average life span, life expectancy, ageism, and gerontology.
3. Discuss some of the health-related and social implications of the average increase in age of the U.S. population.
4. Briefly explain two theories of aging.
5. Explain how undernutrition affects the aging process.
6. Discuss Alzheimer's disease and senile dementia.
7. Describe several ways to prevent osteoporosis.
8. Identify the stages of dying as defined by Elizabeth Kubler-Ross.
9. Explain differences between euthanasia and physician-assisted suicide.
10. Compare palliative care with physician-assisted suicide.
11. Describe factors involved in healthy aging.

Study Guide and Self Assessment

A Simple Test for Loss of Cognitive Function

Health and Wellness Online

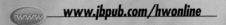 **www.jbpub.com/hwonline**

Chapter 22

Understanding Aging and Dying

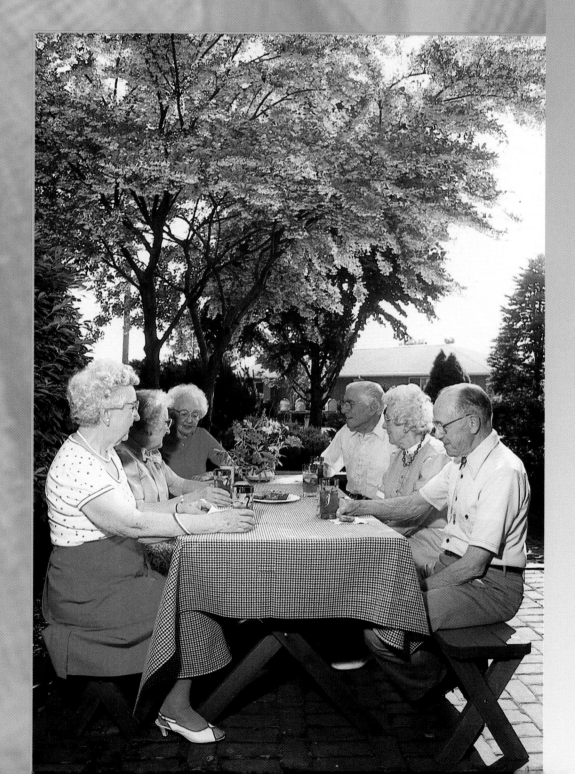

Everything in the universe—plants, animals, mountains, planets, and stars—changes over time and eventually dies (plants and animals) or disintegrates and disappears (planets and stars). Our planet is aging in the sense that its resources are being used up and the environment is changing. The nuclear reactions that fuel the sun will eventually slow down, and the sun is expected to explode about five billion years from now.

> It is silliness to live when
>   to live is torment;
> and then have we
>   a prescription to die
> when death is
>   our physician?
>
>   SHAKESPEARE
>   OTHELLO

Many people associate aging with sickness, disability, loneliness, and increased inactivity. However, such negative views of aging are exaggerated; many older persons today are sexually and physically active and continue to work well into their 80s or even 90s. George Burns, comedian and movie star, performed on stage and in movies until he was nearly 100 years old.

In America, negative views about aging are still prominent in movies, television, and, especially, advertising. The ideal American is portrayed as eternally young, active, attractive, and wrinkle-free. Advertisements exhort people to retard the noticeable signs of aging by using face and body creams that restore youth, dyes for graying hair, and special herbs or vitamins that stop aging or by resorting to various kinds of cosmetic surgery.

The normal processes of aging are not caused by disease, so aging cannot be cured. The noticeable effects of aging result from wear and tear on organs, bones, and tissues in the body that change and become less efficient over the years—muscles weaken, immune system functions decrease, and sex drive is reduced. Even the healthiest body wears out slowly. However, by developing healthy habits while young and by understanding aging processes, one can remain vigorous and healthy until the very end of life.

Today, many people in this country can look forward to an "old age," but this was not always the case. According to an expert on aging:

> For more than 99.9% of the time that human beings have inhabited this planet, life expectancy at birth has been no more than 30 or 40 years. It is only after we learned how to avoid animal predators, massive homicides, starvation, most causes of accidents, and infectious diseases that it has been possible for a substantial portion of the population of developed nations to grow old. (Hayflick, 1997).

Life expectancy for newborns in the U.S. is close to 80 years. To attain that, however, requires implementing the healthy lifestyles that we have been describing while you are still young.

Wellness Guide

Will Hormones Keep You Young?

Many women use estrogens (called hormone replacement therapy, or HRT) to alleviate the symptoms of menopause, to reduce the risks of osteoporosis and heart disease, and for other health benefits. Now many men are trying hormone therapy to counteract the effects of aging—reduced physical vigor, lowered levels of testosterone and sex drive, difficulty sleeping, and other symptoms that begin to appear after age 50.

An over-the-counter hormone, called dehydroepiandrosterone (DHEA), is believed to be used by millions of men in this country to slow down the effects of aging and to increase physical and sexual vigor. DHEA is normally produced in the adrenal glands and is used in the body to manufacture other hormones, such as testosterone. After age 35, the production of DHEA declines and eventually falls to about 20% of the level measured in early adulthood (Eweksler, 1996).

The Food and Drug Administration, which regulates the sales of prescription drugs, does not regulate substances that are marketed as food supplements. Vitamins, herbs, amino acids, and hormones come under this category and, consequently, can be sold without federal regulation.

There is no question that DHEA raises testosterone levels, and many men are convinced that they feel and act younger in many ways after taking it. In fact, at a scientific research meeting on DHEA, about 25% of the investigators acknowledged that they were using it.

Hormones are substances that exert many effects on the body, some of which are not always healthy. Reported side effects of DHEA in men include acne and increased risk of prostate cancer; women who take DHEA may experience increased growth of facial hair and have an increased risk of breast cancer. At present, the official position of the National Institute on Aging and most physicians is that not enough is known about DHEA to justify recommending it as a safe and effective anti-aging medication.

America's Aging Population

Aging refers to the normal changes in body functions that occur after sexual maturity and continue until death. In an idealized situation, everyone would survive close to the **maximum life span** for the species; for human beings, maximum life span is about 120 years (Figure 22.1). The oldest person whose age has been reliably documented is Jeanne Calment, who died in Arles, France on August 4, 1997 (Robine & Allard, 1998). At the time of her death she was 122 years and 164 days old. She also had a brother who lived to 97 and other long-lived relatives, which suggests that her genetic makeup played a role in her longevity. The **average life span** is defined as the age at which half of the members of a population have died. Insurance companies use data based on actual populations to determine what insurance premiums are necessary to pay survivor benefits. **Life expectancy** is the average length of time that members of a population can expect to live. The average life expectancy at birth in the U.S. has increased by almost 30 years since 1900 and now averages about 76 years. However, not all countries have been as fortunate. Life expectancy for men in Russia declined from 63.8 years to 57.7 years between 1990 and 1994 (Notzon, Komarov, Sergei et al., 1998). This sharp decline is attributed to the collapse of the economy and a deteriorating health care system following the collapse of the communist Soviet Union. Life expectancy in many African countries with serious AIDS epidemics also is declining rapidly.

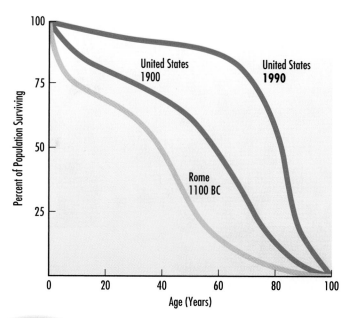

FIGURE 22.2   **Approximate Survival Curves for Various Populations**   The U.S. population is beginning to approximate the idealized curve.

Because of disease, accidents, and other factors, populations in the real world do not survive according to the idealized situation but have followed various curves throughout history (Figure 22.2). The average U.S. life span has increased dramatically in the last century. Because of this increase in the average life span, the U.S. population is becoming increasingly older.

Although genes certainly play a significant role in aging and the life span of human beings, studies show that genes account for much less than half of the differences in life span between different persons. If genes were the dominant factor in life span, identical twins should age and die at more or less the same age, but they do not. From identical and fraternal twin studies, genes are estimated to account for no more than 35% of individual differences in life spans (Finch and Tanzi, 1997).

The "graying" of America will create a broad range of social, medical, and economic problems. First and most important is the ability of the federal gov-

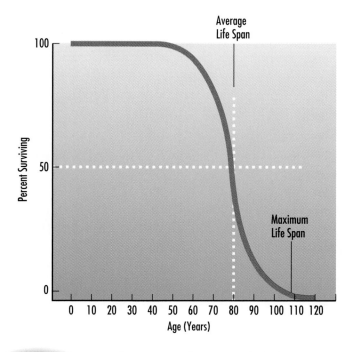

FIGURE 22.1   **Survival as a Function of Years in an Idealized Human Population**

Terms

aging: normal changes in body functions that begin after sexual maturity and continue until death

maximum life span: the theoretical maximum number of years that individuals of a species can live

average life span: the age at which half the members of a population have died

life expectancy: average number of years a person can expect to live

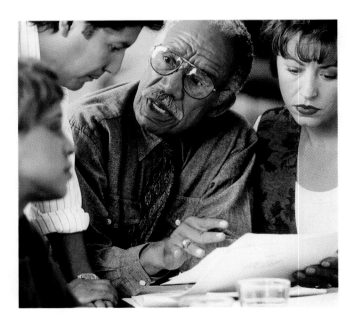

Many elderly people continue to enjoy work long after the "normal" retirement age.

ernment to sustain Social Security payments. At the present rate, the government has estimated that the Social Security system will run out of money within 10 to 20 years. To avoid this, Congress has begun to discuss ways to reform Social Security so that future retirees still will receive benefits. Another problem is the extra medical care required by this group of older people. Although many older people are vigorous and healthy, a large number of people over age 65 have chronic illnesses and disabilities that require ongoing medical care and some need expensive, long-term care. The costs of health care for the elderly are rising rapidly and will be a burden to the government and the general public, which is why there is an urgent need for health care reform (see chapter 19).

How Long Can Human Beings Live?

Some experts in **gerontology** (the science that studies the causes and mechanisms of aging) believe that populations in many countries are approaching the current maximum average life span, estimated at 85 to 90 years, although, as noted above, a few exceptional individuals may live longer. One bit of evidence for a maximum average life span of 85 to 90 years comes from government estimates that show differences in the life expectancies of people in their countries (Table 22.1). Australia, Japan, and Iceland top the list with average life expectancies of 80.6 years. At the bottom of the list are countries where life expectancy is still less than 50 years.

The average life expectancy at birth for all Americans is now 77.6 years, but there are significant differences between the sexes and races. These differences probably result from socioeconomic factors, education, and access to health care.

Other evidence also suggests that the maximum average life span cannot be increased significantly above 85 to 90 years. Statistical studies can estimate how much average human life expectancy would increase if major diseases were eliminated. For example, if *all* cancers could be cured or prevented, only about 3 years of life would be added to the average lifespan of a baby born today. If *all* heart disease was eliminated, average life expectancy at birth would increase by about 14 years (Hayflick, 1994). So, even with remarkable (and unexpected) breakthroughs in medical care, most people still would die before age 100.

A slightly different picture of aging emerges from studies of people between the ages of 85 and 100—a

TABLE 22.1   Life Expectancy in Various Countries
Countries at the top of the list have populations that are approaching the maximum average life expectancy. Note that countries at the bottom of the list have populations with life expectancies that are 40 to 50 years less, and in developed countries, women live an average of six years longer than men. Rank of the countries is based on the sum of male and female life expectancies.

Country	Life expectancy at birth	
	Female	Male
Australia	83.5	77.5
Japan	83.5	77.1
Iceland	81.3	76.9
France	82.8	74.9
Spain	81.8	74.2
United Kingdom	80.3	74.9
United States	79.8	73.4
Mexico	75.6	69.3
China	71.9	68.8
Russia	71.0	59.1
Brazil	68.4	59.3
Bangladesh	61.1	61.2
South Africa	56.0	51.8
Haiti	54.1	49.7
Afghanistan	47.4	48.3
Botswana	40.0	39.4
Zambia	37.1	36.6

Source: World Almanac, 2000.

group known as the "oldest old." Statistical studies of oldest old Scandinavians suggest that, in the absence of disease, senescent death (death from old age) could occur as late as 110 years. However, whether the maximum life expectancy for most people in the absence of disease is 85, 100, or 110 years, no human being is going to live to be as old as Methuselah, the biblical patriarch who is said to have lived for 967 years.

Theories of Aging

Biological Clocks Regulate Aging

Theories of aging fall into two broad categories. One ascribes aging to biological and genetic mechanisms that are specific for each species of animal and determine its maximum life span and rate of aging. The other theories focus on environmental factors that affect aging, such as nutrition, susceptibility to diseases, and exercise. Evidence for a "biological clock" that determines the maximum life span comes from measuring the amount of energy per gram of body weight consumed per day by mammals of different species. This energy consumption per day, called the **specific metabolic rate,** shows a striking correlation with the maximum life span of different species (Figure 22.3). Mammals that have the highest specific metabolic rate have the shortest life span; human beings have the slowest metabolic rate and the longest life span.

Further evidence for a biological clock that governs aging comes from studying the growth of cells in the laboratory. Conditions have been established in which cells from various tissues of different animals can be grown under fixed laboratory conditions. The surprising result of these experiments is that cells grow and divide in a laboratory medium for a fixed number of generations and then die (Hayflick, 1994). The number of generations of growth is related to the maximum life span of the animal from which the cells were taken. Mouse cells only divide a few times, but human cells divide many times before dying. The inescapable conclusion from these experiments is that built into the cells of every animal is a genetically controlled clock that determines how many times cells can grow and divide before a signal tells them to stop.

A distinguishing feature of cancer cells is that they are immortal when grown under the same laboratory conditions used for growing normal cells. Cancer cells grow and divide indefinitely as long as fresh nutrients are provided; cells taken from human

Terms

gerontology: science that studies the causes and mechanisms of aging

specific metabolic rate: the amount of energy per gram of body weight consumed per day

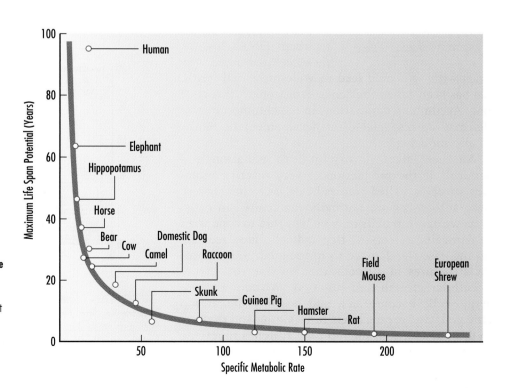

FIGURE 22.3   Correlation between the Rate of Energy Consumed and Maximum Life Span Potential   Rate of energy consumption is calculated as energy per gram of body weight per day. Life span of various mammalian species is shown. The correlation suggests that the maximum human life span is a function of human biology and ultimately of human genes.

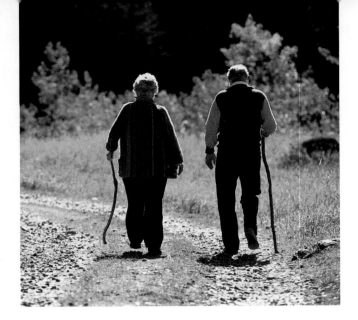

Shared activities are healthful at any age.

tumors more than 30 years ago are still kept growing in the laboratory. Thus, cancer cells have lost the ability to regulate normal growth and aging both in people and in the laboratory (see Chapter 13).

Environmental Factors Affect Aging

Although genetic factors contribute to aging, environmental factors play an even greater role. The longer we live, the more we are exposed to radiation and chemicals that can damage DNA in cells and, over time, may cause the death of essential cells in the body. For example, most cells possess enzymes that repair damage to their DNA; loss of these cellular repair enzymes with age could lead to widespread cell death. This has been called the "error catastrophe" theory of aging. Accumulated mutations in the chromosomes of cells may be responsible for development of cancer and also for aging.

> *If I'd known I was going to live this long, I'd have taken better care of myself.*
> EUBIE BLAKE

Another effect of exposure to radiation and chemicals is the production of very reactive molecules in cells, called free radicals (see chapter 14). These substances are normally inactivated in cells, but as we age, our cells may be less able to cope with the damaging effects of free radicals. Free radicals also increase the damage to mitochondria, the complex structures in all cells that provide the energy for cellular growth and function. Without enough energy, cells become sick and possibly die; if too many cells die, organs cease functioning and the person dies. In addition, the immune system's functions become less efficient with age so that we become more susceptible to infections and autoimmune

diseases. Overall, aging is a complicated process brought on by a combination of genetic and environmental factors.

Undernutrition Slows Aging

A large body of evidence from ongoing studies of animals shows that **undernutrition** does allow them to live longer (Campisi, 2000). For example, a laboratory rat usually has a maximum life span of about 40 months; rats whose caloric intake is restricted have a maximum life span of about 57 months (Figure 22.4). Moreover, the older rats in the calorie-restricted group are healthier and act younger than old rats in the control group who have been well fed (Weindruch, 1996).

Undernutrition does not mean malnutrition; the laboratory animals that live longer are not starved or deprived of any essential nutrients. Only the total amount of food that they are allowed to eat each day is restricted. Calorie restriction studies similar to those performed with rats also extend life in other animal species.

One problem with caloric restriction is knowing when to begin restricting the amount of food. Young animals (including young children) require abundant nutrition for physical growth and for brain development. In the rat studies, it was shown that caloric restriction is of no value in prolonging life if it is begun too late in the animal's life. At present not enough is known about undernutrition and life span to make any recommendations to people, except that everyone should consume a varied and healthy diet and not become overweight.

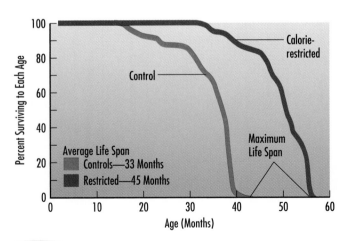

FIGURE 22.4   Survival of Mice Fed Either an Unrestricted Diet or a Calorie-Restricted Diet. The rats whose diets are restricted in amount live, on average, 45 months compared with 33 months for rats that are allowed to eat as much as they want. The maximum life span of the calorie-restricted rats also is markedly increased.

Source: "Caloric Restriction and Aging," Richard Weindruch. Copyright © 1996 by Scientific American, Inc. All rights reserved.

Alzheimer's Disease and Senile Dementia

In the absence of disease, normal mental functions can be maintained to age 100 or longer. However, approximately 20% of people over age 85 have loss of normal cognitive functions that is readily determined by a few simple questions. The medical term for impairment or loss of mental functions in elderly persons is **senile dementia.** More than 2 million Americans currently suffer from some form of dementia (Fago, 2000). Many diseases and conditions can result in senile dementia, but the most common cause is **Alzheimer's disease,** which is characterized by memory loss, reduced ability to use language, losses in perception and problem-solving abilities, and reduced mobility.

More than 4 million Americans suffer from Alzheimer's disease now, and the number will rise dramatically in the next century as the population continues to age (St. George-Hyslop, 2000). The prevalence of Alzheimer's disease increases linearly with advancing age; more than half of the population at age 90 have symptoms of Alzheimer's disease. Even if Alzheimer's disease cannot be cured, any treatment that delays or prevents symptoms from progressing is of great benefit to society in terms of the number of Alzheimer's patients who need care (Figure 22.5).

The disease is named for Alois Alzheimer, a German physician who, in 1907, described the abnormal brain structures he observed under the microscope in tissues obtained from patients who died from senile dementia. Alzheimer's findings at autopsy revealed what are still the diagnostic criteria for the disease: (a) the presence of bundles of tangled nerve fibrils in certain areas of the brain; and (b) the presence of a specific protein called **amyloid protein,** which is localized in certain areas and blood vessels of the brain. How these changes affect the brain to produce loss of cognitive functions is still not understood.

No definitive cause for Alzheimer's disease is known, although it seems to develop as a result of both genetic and environmental factors. In some families, Alzheimer's disease occurs over several generations and family members often die at an early age. In these families, inherited genes must contribute to disease susceptibility. However, Alzheimer's disease also occurs in individuals whose families have never had a previous case. Most cases of Alzheimer's disease fall into this category and result from unknown environmental factors.

Researchers have discovered genes that increase a person's susceptibility to Alzheimer's disease. Three genes *(APP, PS1,* and *PS2)* occur in rare families (only a hundred or so, worldwide), in which many members suffer from Alzheimer's disease, some as young as age 40. The presence of one of these genes makes it virtually certain that the carrier eventually will develop Alzheimer's disease. The other susceptibility gene (APOEϵ4) is associated with increased risk of developing Alzheimer's disease but does not cause it (Roses, 1997).

The presence of the APOEϵ4 gene can be determined by genetic tests, but people need to carefully weigh the benefits and disadvantages of finding out about their Alzheimer's risk status. Although the presence of this gene increases the risk of developing Alzheimer's disease late in life, many people with this gene still will never develop the disease. Is it useful

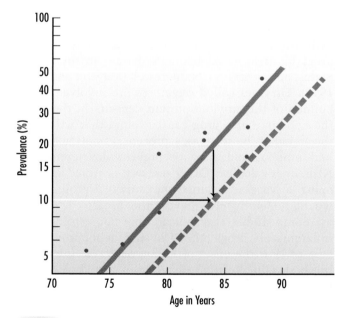

FIGURE 22.5   Benefits of Slowing Onset of Alzheimer's Disease   Approximately 5% of the U.S. population will have Alzheimer's disease by age 75; this increases to 10% by age 80 and to almost 50% by age 90, which shows a linear increase in the disease with increasing age. If the onset of symptoms could be delayed by only 5 years, the prevalence of the disease would be only half as great, about 10% of the population affected at age 85 instead of 20%, which is the current estimate. This marked reduction in the number of persons with symptoms of dementia would be of enormous benefit to society and save a substantial amount of health dollars.

Source: Courtesy Robert Katzman, University of California, San Diego.

Terms

undernutrition: restricting the daily caloric intake of an animal or person without causing malnutrition

senile dementia: loss of cognitive functions in elderly people

Alzheimer's disease: a common cause of senile dementia and other symptoms, eventually leading to death

amyloid protein: an abnormal protein in the brain of patients with Alzheimer's disease

Wellness Guide

Extracts of *Ginkgo Biloba* Slow Alzheimer's Dementia

Ginkgo biloba (maidenhair tree) extracts have been used for centuries in China and Asia to treat a variety of diseases. The dried leaves of the ginkgo tree are used to make teas that are consumed to alleviate symptoms of numerous ailments, particularly ones associated with aging. The main use of ginkgo extracts in western countries is for conditions related to "cerebral insufficiency," which includes conditions such as difficulty concentrating, poor memory, confusion, and absentmindedness. These symptoms often are associated with early stages of dementia that are characteristic of Alzheimer's disease. In 1998, *Ginkgo biloba* was the top-selling herbal remedy in the United States.

In countries such as France and Germany, where *Ginkgo biloba* is one of the most commonly prescribed drugs, extract procedures have been standardized. EGB 761 is a particular extract of *Ginkgo biloba* leaves that has been tested in clinical trials on patients with cognitive disorders. In a one-year, placebo-controlled, double-blind study of more than 200 patients suffering from dementia, EGB 761 was able to stabilize the mental deterioration in a significant number of patients, including some with Alzheimer's disease. EGB 761 does not cure dementia or Alzheimer's disease, but may delay or improve mental functions in people who are losing cognitive abilities because of disease.

---

for people to find out while young that they are at increased risk for Alzheimers's disease many years down the road, even when they may never contract the disease? Knowing that one is destined to lose mental function eventually may be more than many people can handle, even with counseling.

A number of drugs that may slow the progression of Alzheimer's disease have been developed. However, all of these drugs are only marginally effective in slowing progression of symptoms. Tacrine, donepezil (Aricept), and rivastigmine (Exelon) are FDA-approved drugs for treating Alzheimer's disease in the United States, and others are being tested (Mayeux and Sano, 1999). Enzymes called *secretases* are involved in the buildup of the amyloid protein deposits in the brain; the hope is that a drug can be found that will block the action of the secretases, prevent formation of amyloid protein, and slow or prevent development of Alzheimer's disease. Other research is aimed at developing a vaccine against the amyloid protein that would, hopefully, also prevent the disease.

Some studies also indicate that nonsteroidal anti-inflammatory drugs (NSAIDs) such as ibuprofen may help to slow the onset of Alzheimer's. Vitamin E and the herb *Ginkgo biloba* have been tested in clinical trials and some patients have shown a very slight improvement, about equivalent to that observed with the prescription drugs (Rae, 2000).

Despite the current research emphasis on finding defective genes linked to Alzheimer's disease risk, environmental factors also are very important. Epidemiological studies show that people with more education (college graduates) are much less likely to develop Alzheimer's disease than are people with little or no education (Mortimer and Graves, 1993). A study of Catholic nuns who died between ages 76 and 100 has confirmed the importance of education. All of these Catholic nuns were college-educated and had a much lower prevalence of Alzheimer's disease than the general population. And among the few who did develop the disease, it could be shown by studying their brains after death that stroke was a primary trigger of the clinical symptoms of Alzheimer's disease (Snowden et al., 1997).

It is not simply the level of education that helps to prevent the development of Alzheimer's disease. The key is to use the brain throughout life. Keep learning new things, explore new ventures—even doing crossword puzzles may help. It is now clear that brain cells continue to grow and establish new connections throughout life and that brain growth and health is dependent on mental stimulation. Just as exercise is necessary to maintain the body's fitness at all ages, exercising the brain is necessary to maintain mental functions.

If you were thinking of dropping out of school, remember how education helps protect your brain's health. Take more challenging courses. Take night classes if you have a job all day. And remember that watching TV is *not* a useful form of physical or mental exercise!

Parkinson's Disease

Parkinson's disease (PD) is the second most common cause of neurodegenerative disease (after Alzheimer's disease) among older persons (Nussbaum, 1998). About 1 million Americans suffer from PD, and about 50,000 new cases are diagnosed every year. Like other major neurological diseases such as Alzheimer's or Lou Gehrig's disease (ALS), Parkinson's disease is chronic and progressively worsens despite treatments that alleviate symptoms. PD was first described in 1817 by an English physician, James Parkinson, who described the symptoms as "the shaking palsy."

The four defining symptoms of PD are:

Tremor: The tremor of a person suffering from PD involves a rhythmic back-and-forth motion of the thumb and forefinger that appears as if the patient is rolling a pill between the fingers. Although the tremor usually is observed in a hand, it can also arise in a foot or in the jaw.

Rigidity: A basic principle of all movements of the body is that all muscles have opposing muscles. Movement occurs when one set of muscles contract and the opposite set relaxes. The signals that tighten or relax muscles originate in the brain and are transmitted automatically to the muscles so that we make the movement that we desire. In PD patients, the signals from the brain are not coordinated, and the delicate balance between muscle tension and muscle relaxation is lost. In PD, the muscles stay constantly tensed and contracted, and the patient feels stiff and achy.

Bradykinesia: This is probably the most distressing symptom of PD. Bradykinesia refers to the slowing down and loss of spontaneous movement. One moment, a person with PD is moving normally—crossing a street, for example—the next moment, the patient is frozen and cannot move, possibly in the middle of the crosswalk. Daily activities such as washing or putting on clothes may take hours because routine movements cannot be performed rapidly or continuously.

Postural instability: Because PD patients have impaired balance and coordination of movements, they develop a tendency to lean forward or backward and to fall easily. As the disease progresses, walking becomes increasingly difficult; a patient may freeze in midstep and topple over if someone is not there for support.

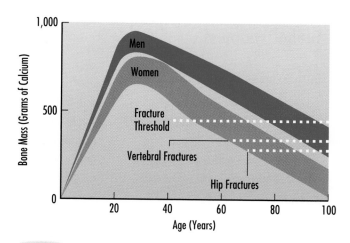

FIGURE 22.6 **Changes in Bone Mass in Aging Men and Women** The risk of bone fracture from osteoporosis occurs when bone mass falls below a theoretical threshold and even a slight strain can cause a fracture.

The most effective drug used to treat PD is L-dopa (L-3,4-dihydroxyphenylalanine). Discovered in the 1960s, L-dopa delays the onset of the symptoms described and gives patients a period of time during which they can function more or less normally. Not all patients with PD are helped to the same degree by L-dopa and not all symptoms of PD improve to the same degree. Today, L-dopa usually is taken with another drug, carbidopa; this reduces the dose of L-dopa needed and increases its effectiveness. Although L-dopa therapy, in combination with other drugs, is effective for some time, eventually the drugs' effectiveness diminishes as the disease progresses. The hope for PD patients lies in new drugs that may be able to halt the loss of dopamine neurons in the brain or in direct replacement of neurons by transplantation of healthy tissues (Olson, 2000).

Osteoporosis

The skeleton provides a means of locomotion, protection of vital organs, and a readily available store of calcium and phosphorus. Only recently has it been recognized that the skeleton is a delicately balanced regenerating tissue, regulated as precisely as the destruction and synthesis of blood cells (Travis, 2000). The most common metabolic bone disease is **osteoporosis,** which results from many environmental factors such as

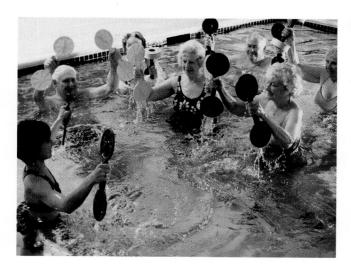

Regular exercise is important for reducing the risk of osteoporosis.

Terms

Parkinson's disease: a neurodegenerative disease in which brain functions that control movements of the body are gradually lost

osteoporosis: a condition in older people, particularly women, in which bones lose density and become porous and brittle

Global Wellness

Can Beliefs Influence Life Span?

Just how powerful are thoughts and feelings in influencing health? Can beliefs affect the duration of a person's life? A recent survey of the causes and ages of death among Chinese-Americans shows that strongly held beliefs can affect the cause of death and how long a person lives (Phillips et al., 1993).

In Chinese astrology, a particular phase—metal, water, wood, fire, or earth—is associated with the year of a person's birth. Also associated with each phase is susceptibility to particular diseases (see table). According to Chinese astrology and medicine, being born in a particular year makes a person more likely than usual to succumb to

diseases associated with the phase of their birth year. An analysis of almost 30,000 death certificates of Chinese-Americans showed that people with the predicted combination of birth year and disease susceptibility died 2 to 5 years before white Americans with the same diseases and phases.

The more traditional the Chinese lifestyle of the person, the shorter their life was once they contracted the disease associated with their birth year. The most plausible explanation of the findings is that Chinese-Americans who believe in the predictions of Chinese astrology are the most likely

Birth year ends in	Phase	Susceptibility to
0 or 1	Metal	Pulmonary diseases
2 or 3	Water	Kidney disease
4 or 5	Wood	Cirrhosis of liver
6 or 7	Fire	Heart attack
8 or 9	Earth	Cancer, diabetes, ulcers

to succumb to the disease that they expect will kill them. It appears that beliefs not only affect health through the onset of disease but also affect life span.

---

poor diet, smoking, alcohol consumption, and lack of exercise. Genetic variation among individuals also may be an important factor in the development of osteoporosis in some individuals but not others. In osteoporosis, the breakdown of bone exceeds the rate of bone renewal.

Osteoporosis affects 25 million women in the United States and is responsible for 250,000 hip fractures each year (Barzel 1996). Medical costs of caring for people with bone fractures from osteoporosis are $10 billion each year and will rise sharply as the American population ages.

Osteoporosis occurs because the rate of bone breakdown exceeds the rate of bone renewal; many factors contribute to this. In older women, estrogen loss following menopause contributes to loss of bone material. In both older men and women, aging results in bone loss and increases the risk of fracture, depending on how much bone mass is reduced (Figure 22.6). Generally, the bone loss in women caused by low estrogen levels is significantly greater than the bone loss caused by normal aging processes.

The risk of osteoporosis in older women can be lessened by replacing the lost estrogen with **hormone replacement therapy (HRT).** For most women HRT is beneficial because it reduces the risk of osteoporosis (and heart disease, to some degree) but for other women HRT may increase the risk of breast and uterine cancer. Another benefit of HRT is that women who take estrogen for even a limited time during menopause have about half the risk of developing Alzheimer's disease compared with women who do not take the hormone. Thus, the use of HRT must be carefully weighed by each postmenopausal woman.

Women whose families have a history of breast cancer or blood clotting problems are not good risks for estrogen supplementation, although this recommendation also is controversial (Shoupe, 1999).

The best way to avoid osteoporosis is to build up as much bone mass as possible while young through a healthy diet with sufficient calcium and exercise. Although widely regarded as a disease of the elderly, osteoporosis begins in childhood. Only 10% of American children get enough calcium or vitamin D or exercise enough to prevent osteoporosis later in life. Even children can be diagnosed with low bone mass that will only worsen as time goes on. After maturity, calcium and vitamin D still are needed to maintain bone mass. Consuming at least a gram of calcium daily is recommended, but nutritional surveys indicate that half of all Americans do not consume that amount. Vitamin D is essential because it assists in the absorption of calcium and in bone formation.

Scientists hope to develop drugs such as osteoprotegerin (OPG) that may protect the integrity of bone or stimulate new growth. In mice, injections of OPG prevented bone and cartilage destruction. Other drugs called "statins" have been used for years to lower high cholesterol levels and reduce the risk of a heart attack. Recently, it has been discovered that these drugs stimulate bone formation; it may be possible to redesign these drugs so that they stimulate bone formation without affecting cholesterol in people with osteoporosis and normal cholesterol levels.

Because many Americans live sedentary lives, especially as they age, osteoporosis is a growing problem among the elderly. Exercise, especially weightlifting, running, hiking, and walking briskly, reduces the risk of osteoporosis because bone is renewed with exercise. In addition, not smoking and not consuming alcohol in excessive amounts help prevent osteoporosis.

Fear of Aging and Dying

Nobody wants to grow old or die. When we are young, we never think about becoming old nor can we imagine what it is like not to be strong, vigorous, and active. With few exceptions, the media portray aging as a time of life beset with sickness, inactivity, and deterioration of physical, sexual and mental functions. These negative views of aging are used to sell products and do not truthfully portray the experiences of most older Americans.

Of all human fears none is greater than the fear of death. When we are young, thoughts of death and dying are rare. Instead we are occupied with living, learning, and daily activities. We can't imagine that someday we will die. As we grow older and see parents, relatives, and friends die, we become more aware of our own mortality. We may begin to ponder our own death.

Fear of aging and death may lead to anxiety and stress that may hasten aging processes. A few of the many fears that people associate with aging are illness, poverty, being attacked or victimized, falling and being injured while alone, loss of responsibility for one's life, memory loss, and sexual inadequacy. Most of these fears are unfounded, but they may turn out to be self-fulfilling prophesies. However, chronological age often does not correlate with biological age. Some people feel and act young even in old age.

Death with Dignity

Death can strike without warning in the form of an accident or an unexpected heart attack. However, for most people, thoughts of death do not occupy their daily lives until old age. People in their 20s are too busy living to think about dying. But people in their 70s and 80s realize the inevitability of death and may modify their lives and affairs accordingly. Younger people who acquire a life-threatening disease such as cancer also are forced to face the reality of death.

Most people would prefer to die peacefully in their sleep after living a full, satisfying life. Some may be fortunate to die like this, but others may have to endure considerable pain and suffering for years. In addition to wondering how they are going to die, people usually wonder what will happen to them after death. Christianity provides a heaven where one's "soul" can exist in the grace of God for all eternity. Buddhism embraces a belief in reincarnation; after a series of deaths and rebirths a person can attain "Buddhahood," a perpetual state of enlightenment.

In our society, death is not discussed openly, although this is beginning to change. (In 1997, public radio ran a series of programs on death and dying that included interviews with people who had been diagnosed with a terminal illness and were facing death within weeks or months.) Dying people are often isolated in hospitals and their care is left to physicians who may perform unwanted or unnecessary treatments. Sterile, impersonal death in a hospital or nursing home has increased many people's fears of death and the process of dying.

Fear is a crippling emotion; it paralyzes thoughts and actions and stifles spiritual growth. Here are some suggestions to help you overcome fears associated with death.

- Become a volunteer with the American Cancer Society or American Hospice Centers. Spend time with cancer or AIDS patients who are dying and who may be willing to share their thoughts with you.
- Write down your feelings about death and dying. Record any experiences you have had at funerals or with someone who was dying. Write down how you felt and how you coped with your feelings and fears.
- A powerful technique for dealing with fear is humor. Humor associated with death and dying is called "black humor" because it deals with the dark side of thoughts and feelings. Black humor was used to cope with issues of death in the long-running TV show M*A*S*H. Many movies also portray death in a humorous way in order to make audiences comfortable. Many cartoons by Gary Larson *(The Far Side)* and John Callahan (who has quadriplegia) portray death and dying in humorous ways. Confront your fears by drawing cartoons or writing a humorous story about dying.

Stages of Dying

People have different attitudes toward death and dying. In conversations with many persons who were facing death, Elisabeth Kubler-Ross (1975) identified

Terms

hormone replacement therapy (HRT): administration of estrogen to menopausal and postmenopausal women to help prevent symptoms of menopause, osteoporosis, and heart disease

five distinct stages in the process of dying. Not all persons experienced all stages, but most experienced some of them. These stages of dying are: (1) denial and isolation, (2) anger, (3) bargaining, (4) depression, and (5) acceptance.

The work of Kubler-Ross has found widespread acceptance, especially among counselors and those who help dying patients, but it has also received criticism. The main objection is that the studies were not conducted scientifically but were based on personal observation and interpretation. Another criticism is that because the stages of dying that Kubler-Ross proposed have been widely accepted and publicized, some dying patients may feel obliged to follow the stages she described.

More and more it is recognized that dying, like living, is an individual, personal matter. People can do as poet Dylan Thomas recommended and "Rage, rage against the dying of the light." Or they can embrace the idea that " . . . with a better understanding of aging, it will become easier to accept the fact that life ends" (Campion, 1998).

Living Wills

Some people are more concerned about the quality of life than about its duration. For them, the issue is not how long they live but the quality of life. These people do not want to lose control of their life because of serious accident or unforeseen serious illness. They do not want to delegate to their physicians or others the right to make decisions about treatments if they are unable to make the decisions themselves.

One physician describes the need for a living will as follows:

> For many, the "golden years" are a euphemism. There comes a time when even the most buoyant of personalities cannot find enough quality of life to enjoy it. We sometimes find more suffering at its end than we want to endure. While vigorously preserving our right to live, however, we can still choose to reject in advance overaggressive, inappropriate medical interventions under future circumstances when we may no longer consider them desirable (Stollerman, 1997).

A **living will** or a similar document can spell out what your wishes are with respect to medical care if you are incapacitated (Figure 22.7). A living will should be given to your primary physician and close relatives so that they can follow your wishes if the occasion arises.

Euthanasia

Almost everyone would like to live a full, active, satisfying life right up to the moment of death. But some people will experience illnesses that bring on a prolonged period of disability, suffering, and pain that cannot be relieved by medical care. Modern medical technology often has the means to prolong life beyond the point where the dying person wishes to live. Given the choice, some terminally ill patients would elect **euthanasia,** which is defined as the act of helping a person experience a peaceful, painless death. In recent years **physician-assisted suicide** has become an alternative to active euthanasia.

Dollars and Health Sense

What Price Immortality?

> I don't want to achieve immortality through my work.
> I want to achieve immortality by not dying.
> > Woody Allen

People worry about dying and wonder what happens to them after death. Most people comfort themselves with the thought that their "soul" will persist forever and is the basis for their immortality even if their physical body is gone. However, a few people believe that immortality can be achieved by preserving their entire body immediately after death. They believe that their body can be revived at some time in the future when aging and diseases

have been conquered, and then their preserved bodies can be restored to life. Cryonic (freezing) suspension provides a means of preserving a body until such time in the future that science has progressed to the point that death and disease can be overcome (as depicted in Steven Spielberg's film, *A.I. Artificial Intelligence*).

If you believe in cryopreservation (and have sufficient money), you can have your body frozen immediately after death and maintained in a deeply frozen state by Alcor Life Extension Foundation, an organization that has been cryopreserving bodies for more than 30 years. For about $120,000, Alcor

personnel will stand by to freeze your body after death and transport it to their headquarters in Arizona, where it will be kept in a frozen state until you can be revived. For $50,000, you can have only your brain frozen if you are comfortable with the idea of being hooked up to a new body in the future. Presumably, your mind, memories, and personality will be preserved by freezing your brain.

Alcor argues that becoming immortal through cryopreservation will become a reality in the not-too-distant future when advanced biotechnologies will be able to repair damaged tissues and even construct new organs and physical bodies.

FIGURE 22.7   **Example of a Living Will**   A copy should be given to your physician and relatives so that they will understand your wishes. Many states have passed laws upholding the legality of living wills.

A LIVING WILL

TO MY FAMILY, MY PHYSICIAN, MY LAWYER, MY CLERGYMAN
TO ANY MEDICAL FACILITY IN WHOSE CARE I HAPPEN TO BE
TO ANY INDIVIDUAL WHO MAY BECOME RESPONSIBLE FOR MY HEALTH, WELFARE
OR AFFAIRS

Death is as much a reality as birth, growth, maturity and old age—it is the one certainty of life. If the time comes when I, _____, can no longer take part in decisions for my own future, let this statement stand as an expression of my wishes, while I am still of sound mind.

If the situation should arise in which there is no reasonable expectation of my recovery from physical or mental disability, I request that I be allowed to die and not be kept alive by artificial means or "heroic measures." I do not fear death itself as much as the indignities of deterioration, dependence, and hopeless pain. I, therefore, ask that medication be mercifully administered to me to alleviate suffering even though this may hasten the moment of death.

This request is made after careful consideration. I hope you who care for me will be morally bound to follow its mandate. I recognize that this appears to place a heavy responsibility on you, but it is with the intention of relieving you of such responsibility and of placing it upon myself in accordance with my strong convictions, that this statement is made.

Date_____   Signed_____
Witness_____   Witness_____

Copies of this request have been given to:

_____   _____
_____   _____

In physician-assisted suicide, a terminally ill patient who is mentally competent must express a desire to die on a number of occasions. Then a second physician would be consulted. Finally, if both physicians agree that the patient is mentally competent and has an incurable, painful disease, one physician would supply the patient with the drugs needed to commit suicide or otherwise help the patient end his or her life.

Thousands of people in the United States are kept alive in hospitals in a permanent vegetative state. They are fed artificially and maintained by machines and medical technology. There is no hope of recovery for these persons and most would die if they were unhooked from the machines that keep them alive. There is intense legal and ethical controversy about proper choices regarding comatose and terminally ill patients who want the option of physician-assisted suicide.

In 1997, Oregon passed the Death with Dignity Act, which legalized physician-assisted suicide in that state. In the first year after the bill passed, 23 persons received prescriptions for lethal medications, and 15 actually took the medicine and died. In 1999, physicians prescribed lethal medications to another 33 patients, but some died before they could take the drugs (Sullivan, Hedberg, and Fleming, 2000). It is clear from these numbers that, so far, there has not been a rush among terminally ill patients in Oregon to end their lives.

Physician-assisted suicide also has been practiced in the Netherlands for a number of years, even though it was officially illegal. In the Netherlands, several thousand seriously ill patients die each year with the help of their physicians; the criteria for physician-assisted suicide in that country include:

- The patient must repeatedly and explicitly request the desire to die.
- The patient's decision must be well informed and free.
- The patient must be suffering from severe physical or mental pain with no prospect of relief.
- All other options for therapy must have been exhausted.
- The physician must consult at least one other physician.

Despite growing public support for physician-assisted suicide in the United States, there is still great resistance to its use among physicians, clergy, and members of right-to-life activist movements.

There is general agreement that end-of-life care needs to be improved substantially. Studies show that of the more than 2 million people that die each year in the United States, almost half of hospitalized patients suffer serious pain in the days preceding death. And only about one third of patients in nursing homes receive adequate pain relief. Two national health care organizations have proposed that every physician attending to a dying patient should make the following six promises (Mitka, 2000):

- You will have the best of medical treatment, aiming to prevent exacerbation, improve function and survival, and ensure comfort.
- Your care will be continuous, comprehensive, and coordinated.
- You and your family will be prepared for everything that is likely to happen in the course of your illness.
- Your wishes will be sought and respected, and they will be followed whenever possible.

Terms

living will: a legal document that expresses your wishes regarding treatment if you become unable to make your own medical decisions

euthanasia: helping someone who is on the verge of death or in a coma to die without suffering

physician-assisted suicide: a form of active euthanasia in which a physician helps a patient who no longer desires to live because of pain or an incurable illness to commit suicide

- We will help you consider your personal and financial resources and we will respect your choices about their use.
- We will do all we can to see that you and your family will have the opportunity to make the best of every day.

The public discussion over end-of-life treatments and legal options and problems has been active in the United States for more than a quarter of a century and is still far from being resolved to everyone's satisfaction. In 1990, the U.S. Supreme Court did rule that withholding or withdrawal of life support to dying patients who can no longer be helped medically is legal. However, physician-assisted suicide is still illegal in most states.

Palliative Care

Palliative care is a newly recognized branch of medicine that focuses on noncurative treatments for the dying (Goodlin, 1997). The World Health Organization (WHO) defines palliative care as follows:

- Affirms life and regards dying as a normal process
- Neither hastens nor postpones death
- Provides relief from pain and other distressing symptoms
- Integrates the psychological and spiritual aspects of patient care
- Offers a support system to help patients live as actively as possible until death
- Offers a support system to help families cope with the patient's illness and death

When a person elects palliative care, the emphasis of treatment shifts from prolonging life to enhancing the quality of life that remains, preserving a person's dignity, and relieving suffering. Usually a team of health professionals, in consultation with the patient and family, will decide if palliative care is appropriate.

> *The true traveler is without goal, it is the absence of goals which creates the ultimate traveler.*
> GAO XINGJIAN
> SOUL MOUNTAIN

Many opponents of physician-assisted suicide embrace the concept of palliative care and believe that it is more in accord with the ethics of medical

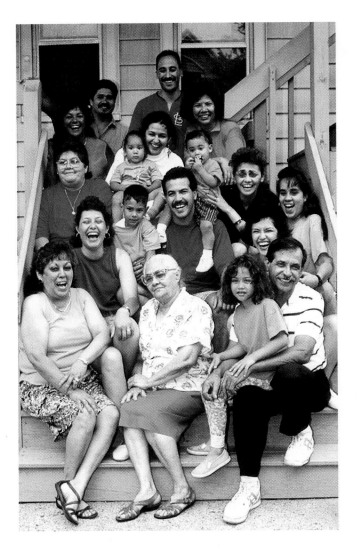

Strong family ties are healthy for young and old alike.

practice. Now that palliative care is seen as a a reimbursable form of therapy by many health insurance programs, eventually all terminally ill patients may have access to such care and no longer have to fear prolonged pain and suffering.

The Hospice

The term **hospice** originally applied to medieval Christian hospitals caring for the poor, the aged, and the sick. Hospices also provided refuge for people on religious pilgrimages. Providing physical necessities, medical care, and spiritual comfort was the primary purpose of the early religious hospices. In the United States today there are over 2,000 hospices offering comprehensive care for terminally ill patients. The goal of a hospice is to meet the total health needs—physical, psychological, and spiritual—of patients who have weeks or months to live. Medications are given to ease pain, but heroic treatments are not attempted. Family and friends are free to visit with

Terms

hospice: a place for terminally ill patients to spend the time before death in an environment that attends to their physical, emotional, and spiritual needs but does not administer any further treaments; hospice care also can be given in a patient's home

the patient in a comfortable setting, whether it is in a patient's home or a hospital with a hospice attached.

The hospice philosophy is that dying is part of living and should not be resisted with every weapon in the modern medical arsenal. Hospice care is designed to control pain and make patients comfortable, but staff also are trained to discuss emotional and spiritual issues relevant to death. Counseling and social services are available in hospices and close family members are encouraged to participate in daily activities. About two-thirds of hospices in the United States are certified for Medicare reimbursement.

More than 200,000 patients each year in the United States elect to spend their final weeks or months in hospice care. As the population in this country becomes older, more and more families and individuals will have to face the issues raised by terminal illness and death. Although hospices do everything possible to make patients comfortable, they do not permit active euthanasia.

 ## Healthy Aging

With the dramatic upward shift in average life expectancy in the U.S. and other countries, finding ways to improve health in elderly people has become a major challenge. Generally, increasing age is associated with increasing disability and functional impairments, such as loss of mobility, sight, or hearing. One goal of gerontology is to find ways to minimize or postpone the disabilities that accompany aging so that quality of life extends to, or close to, the end of life.

The scientific evidence is now quite overwhelming that most of the disability and long-term medical care in elderly persons results from major chronic diseases that were already present in mid-life (Reed et al., 1998). The most significant predictors of a healthy old age are low blood pressure and low serum glucose levels, not being obese, and not smoking cigarettes while young. These factors are also important in predicting such diseases as cardiovascular disease, cancer, and diabetes. Thus, the evidence points to the importance of developing healthy habits while young if the "golden years" are going to be enjoyed with one's physical and mental abilities intact.

Persons surviving to age 55 today can expect to live, on average, another 25 years; those surviving to age 75 can expect to live another 10 to 12 years. Many of these older people are relatively healthy and the length of time that they will be disabled before death is short. In general, people who live to the oldest ages without disabilities are those who have practiced good nutrition, were physically and mentally active, and did not use tobacco or drink alcohol excessively. (George Burns may have been an exception to the rule, or maybe he didn't inhale his ever-present cigar.)

TABLE 22.2   Anti-Aging Supplements and Recommended Maximum Daily Doses
If you take a multivitamin and mineral supplement, you may want to reduce the recommended amounts shown below.

Supplement	Recommended amount
Vitamin E	400 IU
Vitamin C	1,000 milligrams (1 gram)
Beta carotene (vitamin A)	10 milligrams*
Chromium	200 micrograms
Selenium	200 micrograms
Calcium	1,000–1,500 milligrams (1 to 1.5 grams)
Zinc	15 milligrams
Magnesium	200–300 milligrams
Coenzyme Q	30 milligrams (probably not worth the money)

*may increase risk of lung cancer in smokers

More and more attention is being paid to the role of nutrition in healthy aging. Increased consumption of fresh fruits and vegetables are thought to slow the aging processes; those containing antioxidant chemicals are regarded as particularly potent anti-aging foods. These include avocado, berries, broccoli, cabbage, carrots, citrus, grapes, onions, tomatoes, and spinach. But according to believers in the antioxidant theory of aging, supplements still are needed to ensure that you are getting sufficient amounts of antioxidant vitamins and minerals (Table 22.2). Taking vitamin and mineral supplements from early adulthood on may contribute to a healthier old age (Carper, 1995).

There is no way of knowing how or when we are going to die or what we will do or think when confronted with death. Most of us only think about death when someone close to us dies or if we ourselves become seriously sick or injured. However, if thoughts of death do arise often, or if you feel that you are unreasonably afraid of death, then it is advisable to seek help to overcome fears.

Every age of life provides opportunities for growth and satisfaction. Even though we have no way of knowing when serious illness or death will confront us, we do have control of how we live each day and the satisfactions we find in life. The way we choose to live when we are young will greatly affect our health later. For example, smoking while young increases the likelihood of developing cancer and heart disease later. Drinking alcohol to excess and taking unnecessary chances invite accidents that can cause death or permanent disability. While each person's life span is partly determined by genes, environmental factors, such as nutrition, exercise, and lifestyle, are also important not only in determining how long we live, but how well we live.

Critical Thinking About Health

1. Since the breakup of the former Soviet Union, the life expectancy of people in Russia has been declining dramatically. Make a list of all the factors you can think of that would contribute to a shorter life expectancy in Russia now compared with previously. Discuss each factor and how important you think it is in contributing to the decline. Also indicate if any of the factors you have discussed for the decline of life expectancy in Russia are important in explaining the difference in life expectancy between black and white Americans discussed in this chapter.

2. Imagine that you have just learned that your mother is suffering from terminal cancer that cannot be treated. The physician estimates that death can occur at any time within a few months and that your mother's pain will be considerable. While drugs can alleviate some of the pain, the doctor honestly does not know how effective the pain relief will be. Your mother is 75 years old and is aware of her condition. When you and she discuss her condition, she expresses a strong desire not to suffer in order to survive a few weeks or months. She asks you to help her obtain drugs that she can use to end her life peacefully whenever she chooses.

   Describe how you would feel in such a situation and what actions you would take. Would you discuss the problem with her physician, with a religious counselor, or with someone else? Would you be concerned about legal problems if you did obtain the lethal drugs and give them to your mother? Would you tell your mother that you want to keep her alive at all costs and you will do all that you can to reduce her suffering? Make a list of all the steps you would take in this situation, and explain your reasons for each action.

3. Make a list of all the health-related factors in your life that you think might play a role in how healthy you will be at age 70 (e.g., you smoke cigarettes, you are significantly overweight). After thinking about the list you have made, ask yourself if some behaviors or lifestyle factors are worth changing to help ensure that you will enjoy a healthy old age. Or perhaps you feel that it is not worth worrying about old age now and that the important thing is how to enjoy life at the present time. Discuss these different views and try to develop a personal philosophy of aging that is right for you.

4. Because both of your grandmothers have Alzheimer's disease, the other members of your family are very concerned over their own future mental health, even though both of your parents are only in their 50s. Having read that a particular gene contributes to the risk of Alzheimer's disease and that doctors can test for the presense of this gene, your mother and father have been discussing the advisability of getting the test. They also have asked if you would like to be tested for the Alzheimer's gene. What advice would you give them? Would you want to be tested for the Alzheimer's susceptibility gene? Discuss in detail the reasons for your advice to them and the decision you would make for yourself.

Health in Review

- Aging and dying are natural stages of life. People should strive to remain physically, emotionally, mentally, and spiritually active at all stages of life regardless of chronological age.
- The maximum human life span is approximately 115 years; the average life span in many countries is 80+ years, which means that a majority of people in those countries will live to be 80 years of age or older.
- The average age of the population in the United States is increasing, causing increasing health care costs and financing problems for the Social Security system.

- Aging is partly determined by genes and partly by environmental factors that cause cellular changes with age. Undernutrition slows aging in laboratory animals and may slow down aging processes in people.
- Loss of cognitive mental functions in older people is called senile dementia; the most common cause of this is Alzheimer's disease. Bone loss with age is called osteoporosis and occurs most often in postmenopausal women. Parkinson disease affects movement.

- Active euthanasia refers to helping someone die without pain or suffering. Physician-assisted suicide is a form of active euthanasia that is presently illegal in the United States, although some states have attempted to enact laws legalizing it.

- Palliative care is treatment that does not cure but relieves pain and suffering of dying patients and deals with the distress of family members.
- Hospice care provides terminally ill patients with medical, emotional, and spiritual support during the final weeks or months of their lives.

Health and Wellness Online

The World Wide Web contains a wealth of information about health and wellness. By accessing the Internet using Web browser software, such as Netscape Navigator or Microsoft's Internet Explorer, you can gain a new perspective on many topics presented in *Health and Wellness, Seventh Edition*. Access the Jones and Bartlett Publishers Web site at http://www.jbpub.com/hwonline.

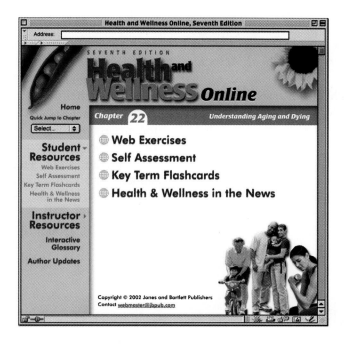

References

Angell, M. (1997). The Supreme Court and physician-assisted suicide—The ultimate right. *New England Journal of Medicine, 336*, 50–53.

Campion, E. W. (1998). Aging better. *New England Journal of Medicine, 338*, 1064–1066.

Campisi, J. (2000). Aging, chromatin, and food restriction—connecting the dots. *Science, 289*, 2962–2964.

Carper, J. (1995). *Stop aging now!* New York: HarperCollins.

Dawson-Hughes, B., Harris, S. S., Krall, E. A., and Dallal, G. E. (1997). Effect of calcium and vitamin D supplementation on bone density in men and women 65 years of age or older. *New England Journal of Medicine, 337*, 670–676.

Eweksler, M. (1996). Hormone replacement for men. *British Medical Journal, 312*, 859–860.

Fago, J. P. (2001, January 15). Dementia: Causes, evaluation, and management. *Hospital Practice*, 59–69.

Finch, C. E., and Tanzi, R. E. (1997). Genetics of aging. *Science, 278*, 407–411.

Goodlin, S. J. (1997, February 15). What is palliative care? *Hospital Practice*, 13–16.

Hayflick, L. (1994). *How and why we age*. New York: Ballantine.

Hayflick, L. (1997, January). Myths of aging. *Scientific American*, 110–113.

Kubler-Ross, E. (1975). *Death: The final stage of growth.* New York: Prentice-Hall.

Leon, D. A. (1998). Social stress and the Russian mortality crisis. *Journal of the American Medical Association, 279*, 790–791.

Mayeux, R., and Sano, M. (1999). Treatment of Alzheimer's disease. *New England Journal of Medicine, 341*, 1670–1680.

Mitka, M. (2000). Suggestions for help when the end is near. *Journal of the American Medical Association, 284*, 2441–2442.

Mortimer, J. A., and Graves, A. B. (1993). Education and other socioeconomic determinants of dementia and Alzheimer's disease. *Neurology, 43* (Suppl 4), S39–S44.

Notzon, F. C., Komarov, Y. M., Ermakov, S. P. et al., (1998). Causes of declining life expectancy in Russia. *Journal of the American Medical Association, 279*, 793–800.

Nuland, S. R. (2000). Physician-assisted suicide and euthanasia in practice. *New England Journal of Medicine, 342*, 583–584.

Nussbaum, R. L. (1998). Putting the Parkin into Parkinson's. *Nature, 392*, 544–545.

Olson, L. (2000). Combating Parkinson's disease—step three. *Science, 290*, 721–724.

Orentlicher, D. (1996). The legalization of physician-assisted suicide. *New England Journal of Medicine, 335*, 663–667.

Phillips, D. P., Ruth, T. E., and Wagner, L. M. (1993, November 6). Psychology and survival. *The Lancet, 342*, 142–145.

Rae, S. Vanishing act. (2000, November-December). *Modern Maturity*, 34–37.

Reed, D. M. et al. (1998). Predictors of healthy aging in men with long lives. *American Journal of Public Health, 88*, 1463–1468.

Robine, J. M., and Allard, M. (1998). The oldest human. *Science, 279*, 1834–1835.

Roses, A. D. (1997, July 15). Alzheimer's disease: The genetic risk. *Hospital Practice*, 51–69.

Shoupe, D. (1999, August 15). Hormone replacement therapy: Reassessing the risks and benefits. *Hospital Practice*, 97–114.

Snowden, D. A. et al. (1997). Brain infarction and the clinical expression of Alzheimer's disease—The nun study. *Journal of the American Medical Association, 277*, 813–817.

St. George-Hyslop, P. H. (2000, December). Piecing together Alzheimer's. *Scientific American*, 76–83.

Stollerman, G. H. (1997, March 15). Seven rules for successful aging: A physician's advice to elderly patients. *Hospital Practice*, 235–238.

Sullivan, A. D., Hedberg, K., and Fleming, D. W. (2000). Legalized physician-assisted suicide in Oregon—the second year. *New England Journal of Medicine, 342*, 598–604.

Travis, J. (2000). Boning up. *Science News, 157*, 41–43.

Suggested Readings

Callahan, D. (2000). Death and the research imperative. *New England Journal of Medicine, 342*, 654–656. The author of this article argues that built into modern medicine is the goal of preserving life at any cost. This goal puts medical care at odds with patients who want to accept "death with dignity."

Goodwin, J. S. (1999). Geriatrics and the limits of modern medicine. *New England Journal of Medicine, 340*, 1283–1285. A thoughtful article about how we have "medicalized" many of the problems of old age and should be less aggressive in treating people in their 80s and 90s.

Humphry, D., and Clement, M. (1998). *Freedom to Die—People, politics, and the right-to-die movement.* New York: St. Martin's Press. Presents arguments supporting the idea that physician-assisted suicide should be an option for terminally ill patients.

Olshansky, S. J., and Carnes, B. A. (2001). *The quest for immortality: Science at the frontiers of aging.* New York: W. W. Norton. Discusses the reasearch that attempts to uncover the biological basis for aging and ways to slow the aging processes.

Weindruch, R. (1996, January). Caloric restriction and aging. *Scientific American*, 46–52. Discusses how restriction of food intake in rats prolongs their lives by almost one third. Speculates on the usefulness of caloric restriction in human beings to prolong life.

Winters, P. A. ed. (1998). *Death and dying—Opposing viewpoints.* San Diego: Greenhaven Press. A collection of articles on such controversial issues as individuals' right to die, coping with death, life after death, and at what point treatment for terminally ill patients can be stopped. Articles present both sides of these issues.

Learning Objectives

1. Describe the different kinds of interpersonal violence.
2. Explain ways that violence affects health.
3. Discuss the symptoms and long-term effects of post-traumatic stress disorder.
4. Describe the different forms of child abuse and why the incidence is different in different cultures.
5. Define sexual assault, forcible rape, and acquaintance rape.
6. Discuss the reasons that underlie forcible rape and acquaintance rape.
7. Define elder abuse and the factors that contribute to it.
8. Discuss the ways in which firearm abuse affects the health of individuals and disrupts society.

Study Guide
and
Self Assessment

Crime Prevention Tips

Health
and Wellness
Online

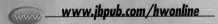 **www.jbpub.com/hwonline**

Chapter 23

Violence in Our Society

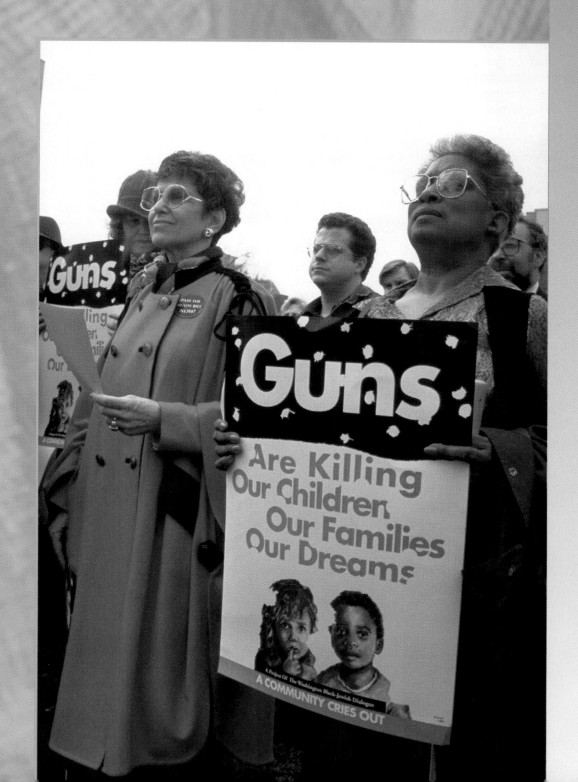

Violence is an integral part of the animal kingdom, as the expression "eat or be eaten" implies. Predator animals practice offensive violence, while their victims practice defensive violence. Animals invariably engage in these kinds of violent behavior to gain access to food and water and to reproduce. Human beings, however, are far ahead of all other animal species in the degree and occasions for practicing violence. In peace, as well as in war, people attack, injure, and kill other people for a multitude of reasons.

Violence is a physical or verbal behavior in which the intent is to harm, injure, or destroy someone or something. Human beings are unique in understanding the future possibility of injury and death and so will fight for many reasons, including being threatened by loss of personal freedom. People also have many intangible things to fear—fear of being hungry, fear of being poor, fear of being attacked, and fear of being unwanted or unloved are examples. All of these fears can provoke violent behavior.

Some people use violence as a means of gaining power over others. In its simplest form, power is the ability to satisfy one's needs. Power and its accompanying violence manifest in society in a variety of ways—as rape, domestic violence, child abuse, elder abuse, homicide, suicide, terrorist attacks, gang fights, and wars between nations.

More than 20,000 persons die in the U.S. every year from homicide, and over 2 million persons are injured in violent attacks. Homicide is the second leading cause of death among persons aged 15 to 24, and suicide is the third in the same age group. The consequences of violence in society are broken families, battered women, maimed and handicapped children, and countless unnecessary injuries and deaths.

To repair the effects of violence on the minds and bodies of people is expensive, difficult, and often unsuccessful. The *only* solution to violent human behavior, as with other serious diseases, is prevention (Gellert, 1997). While some people believe that violence in human societies is inevitable, many others do not and choose to live nonviolent lives.

Interpersonal Violence

Historically, violence in the family was ignored for centuries both in the United States and in other developed countries. Until the 1960s, most people considered family violence a rare event. Since then, awareness of interpersonal violence as a major health problem has increased partly as a result of required reporting of suspected cases of domestic violence and child abuse

You never know when you're making a memory.
RICKIE LEE JONES

by hospitals, physicians, and police departments and partly to increased research (Kantor and Jasinski, 1998). In the 1990s, publicity about child abuse, sexual abuse, spousal abuse (primarily by men), and elder abuse has greatly increased public awareness.

The killings of Nicole Brown Simpson and Ronald Goldman focused public attention on interpersonal violence as never before in the 1990s. (Gelles, 1997). The three most widely quoted facts about interpersonal violence are:

- More women are treated in hospital emergency rooms for battering injuries each year in the U.S. than for muggings, rapes, and traffic accidents combined.
- Interpersonal violence has killed more women in the past 5 years in the United States than the total number of Americans killed in Vietnam.
- Battering during pregnancy is the leading cause of birth defects and infant mortality.

The FBI estimates that a woman is beaten by her husband or boyfriend every 15 seconds in this country. Clearly, interpersonal violence is an epidemic. Recognizing that domestic violence is as serious a health problem as communicable diseases, the federal government has declared every October as National Domestic Violence Month. During this month, extra efforts are made to increase public awareness and to educate people on how to prevent and avoid violence in the family.

Domestic Violence

Women who experience battering or rape by a partner or acquaintance not only have medical problems but also may suffer from anxiety, depression, chronic pelvic pain, gastrointestinal upset, substance abuse, obesity, or headaches. Assaulted women may also develop symptoms of **post-traumatic stress disorder (PTSD)** and its variants, which are battered women's syndrome or rape trauma syndrome. Many long-term health consequences of battering, rape, and sexual abuse are associated with PTSD. For example, traumatized individuals tend to be more susceptible to arousal by stimuli that makes it difficult for them to differentiate normal aches, pains, and sensations from signals of disease, leading to increased incidence of seeking help from health professionals.

Terms

violence: a physical or verbal behavior, in which the intent is to harm, injure, or destroy someone or something

post-traumatic stress disorder (PTSD): reactions after an event that is outside the range of usual human experience and would be distressing to almost anyone

Also, emotional tension and guardedness can produce painful muscle tension and skeletal misalignment. Chronic anxiety can lead to gastrointestinal upsets. Alcohol, nicotine, and other drugs may be used to block out memories of abuse and to alleviate uncomfortable emotions and physical sensations that accompany memories of the assault or abuse.

Recovering from the trauma of relationship violence requires patience and support. Victims are encouraged to seek psychological counseling from professionals who specialize in helping victims of relationship violence and to join support groups of other assaulted individuals. Support can hasten healing and recovery and help restore the trust that is shattered by assault. Support groups can also provide a place to stay if the victim needs to escape the abuser, or the group can offer companionship if the victim is afraid to be alone.

Symptoms of PTSD include:

- Re-experiencing the traumatic event(s) via recurrent intrusive images, thoughts, dreams of the trauma, and "flashbacks"—having a sense of reliving the trauma, including re-experiencing the disturbing accompanying emotions.

- Intense reactions to things that symbolize the traumatic experience. For example, in recovering from a rape, victims may intensely fear being in locales that resemble the scene of the assault.

- Some may experience nausea when thinking of the rape, and some may have difficulties with sexual relations.

- Being unable to recall the trauma (denial), or being able to "make the mind go somewhere else" to avoid the pain associated with the memory of the trauma (dissociation). They may feel detached or estranged.

- Manipulation of others and the environment as a way to keep things calm and under control. They may become compliant as a way to avoid real or imagined abuse.

- Persistent arousal symptoms, such as difficulty falling or staying asleep, being edgy, jumpy, irritable, and sometimes irrationally angry. Victims may have difficulty concentrating, be hypervigilant to their surroundings, and have an exaggerated startle response.

Causes of Domestic Violence

There is no single cause of domestic violence, but contributing factors include:

- A high level of conflict and stress in the family
- Male dominance and the view that women and children are men's property

- Cultural norms that permit family violence
- Displays of violence on TV and other media
- Being raised in a violent family
- Alcohol and drug abuse
- Victim-blaming ("people get what they deserve")
- Denying the existence of physical violence or sexual abuse

Women who are at the greatest risk for serious injury from domestic violence include those with male partners who abuse alcohol or drugs, are unemployed or intermittently employed, have less than a high-school education, and are former husbands or boyfriends of the women (Kyriacau et al., 1999).

Ways to prevent domestic violence include providing shelters, safe houses, and other protective environments for abused women; reducing contributing social and economic factors (unemployment, poverty, and racism); holding the abusers accountable for their actions; training law enforcement and health care professionals to recognize and intervene in cases of domestic violence; training everyone in nonviolent conflict resolution; and reducing the amount of violent imagery on TV, in films, and in popular music. Physicians also are receiving more training in recognizing, treating, and helping victims of domestic violence, most of whom are women, find shelter and support (Eisenstat & Bancroft, 1999).

Domestic violence not only affects adults who are in an abusive relationship; children who share the abusive environment also suffer (Table 23.1). Resolution of

> *I have learned that a man has the right to look down on another man only when he has to help the other get to his feet.*
> GABRIEL GARCIA MARQUEZ

TABLE 23.1   Symptoms of Parental Violence in Children
Children who are exposed to parental violence are subject to a variety of symptoms.

Behavioral symptoms			
Aggression	Tantrums	Immaturity	Delinquency
Emotional symptoms			
Anxiety and depression	Low self-esteem	Anger	Withdrawal
Cognitive symptoms			
Poor performance in school	Poor language skills		
Physical symptoms			
Eating disorders	Poor motor skills	Sleep problems	Retarded growth
Psychosomatic disorders			

conflicts between parents or partners is essential to the long-term health of children. And children who grow up in physically or sexually abusive environments are much more likely to find themselves in abusive relationships as adults.

The Brain Controls Violent Behavior

While personal experiences, social environment, and cultural norms all contribute to the expression of violent behavior, it is also a fact that there are specific areas of the brain that govern violent, antisocial behaviors. Neurological and biological factors, as well as environmental influences, contribute to the development of what is regarded as acceptable personality and behavioral traits. The brain's intimate control of behavior was demonstrated by a bizarre accident that occurred more than a century ago.

On September 13, 1848, a 25-year-old railroad construction foreman named Phineas P. Gage was setting blasting charges in rock to level terrain for the laying of railroad ties. Holes were drilled in the rocks, a powder charge was inserted and tamped down with an iron rod. On this day, Gage was tamping down a charge when it went off prematurely. The steel tamping rod, one inch thick and a yard long, shot through his face, through his brain, and emerged from his skull and landed yards away. Remarkably, within moments after the accident, Gage regained consciousness, was able to talk, and able to walk away with the help of his men (Damasio, Grabowski, Frank, et al., 1994).

Gage survived the catastrophic injury with all his intelligence and physical abilities intact. His speech was unaffected. His memory was complete and accurate. However, Gage was a different man. Before the injury he had been responsible, socially well adjusted, and popular with his peers and bosses. After the accident he became profane, argumentative, and irreverent. He lost all respect for social conventions. He could not be trusted or relied on in any assignment. His employers, who had called him "the most efficient and capable" man in their employ, had to dismiss him. Gage spent the remaining 15 years of his life wandering around, largely unemployed, and unaccepted in any company. His family wound up caring for him until his death.

Managing Stress

Coping with Anger

Anger. The word itself brings to mind images of pounding fists, yelling, and violent behavior. But anger is as natural a human emotion as love. Anger is a survival emotion; it's the fight component of the fight or flight response. We use anger to communicate our feelings, from impatience to rage. We employ anger to communicate boundaries and defend values. Although feeling angry is within the normal limits of human emotions, anger is often mismanaged and misdirected. Unfortunately, we have been socialized to suppress our feelings of anger. As a result, it either tears us apart from the inside or promotes intermittent eruptions of verbal or physical violence, which can be seen played out in local and national headlines. In most cases, we do not deal with our anger wisely.

Research reveals four very distinct ways in which people mismanage their anger. They include:

1. **Somatizers:** People who never show any signs of anger and internalize their feelings until eventually there is major bodily damage (i.e., temporomandibular joint syndrome, colitis, migraine headaches).

2. **Exploders:** Individuals who erupt like a volcano and spread their temper like hot lava, destroying anyone and anything in their path with either verbal or physical abuse. This type of mismanaged anger style is what makes the news headlines.

3. **Self-Punishers:** People who neither repress their anger nor explode, but rather deny themselves a proper outlet of anger because of feelings of guilt. Examples of their behavior include excessive sleeping, eating, and shopping.

4. **Underhanders:** Individuals who sabotage or seek revenge against someone through barely socially acceptable behavior (e.g., sarcasm, tardiness, not returning phone calls).

When anger is mismanaged and left unresolved it becomes a control issue, if not a control drama.

Here are some ways to deal with anger sensibly or creatively:

1. Take "time-out" from the situation, followed by a "time-in" to resolve the issue.

2. Communicate your feelings diplomatically.

3. Think of the consequences of your anger.

4. Plan several options to a situation.

5. Lower personal expectations.

6. Most important, learn to forgive—"make past anger pass."

Although anger is an emotion we all experience and should recognize when it arises, it is crucial to manage anger. Sometimes just writing down what frustrates you can be the beginning of the resolution process. Above all, make a habit of resolving your angry feelings once they arise. Learn to let go of your feelings of anger before they become toxic to your mind, body, and spirit.

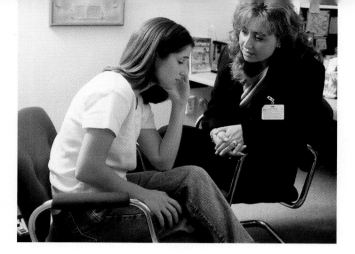

Being able to tell an understanding person what happened helps.

Twenty years after the accident, a scientist named John Harlow postulated that the behavioral and personality changes observed in Gage after the accident resulted from damage to a particular area of the brain. This was the first scientific insight that acceptable personal and social behavior, what we commonly refer to as rationality, is controlled by the brain. In effect, there is a neural basis not only for intelligence, but for ethical, moral, and social behaviors as well.

Modern neurological experiments have confirmed Harlow's insight. Other patients have also been identified who have suffered damage to their frontal lobes and who exhibit deficits in rational behaviors and in the processing of emotions. Future research may elucidate how neurons in the frontal lobe function to generate socially acceptable behaviors—or their opposite.

Child Abuse

Children have been abused for centuries in all cultures and countries. A definition of **child abuse,** which applies to all cultures, is: Child abuse is the portion of harm to children that results from human action that is proscribed, proximate, and preventable (Finkelhor and Korbin, 1988). In plain English, child abuse is any human action that causes injury to children and is preventable.

About 16 million American children are taken to hospital emergency rooms each year for treatment of injuries caused by child abuse (Peterson and Gable, 1998). Several hundred thousand of these children require hospitalization, and at least 30,000 of them suffer permanent disabilities. Child abuse assumes several forms, all of which invariably lead to serious harm.

Physical Abuse When intentional force of any kind that results in injury is used on a child, the child has suffered physical abuse. Injuries can also result from accidents, which are not the result of physical abuse. For example, a child may fall and be bruised while running during play. This is understood by the child to be an accident and may lead to more careful behavior. It may also be something the child is proud of and can be "brave" about.

However, physical force that is used to discipline or control a child or adolescent can cause serious physical and psychological injury. Often a parent is venting anger over some other issue that is irrelevant to the child's behavior; the child is the unwitting victim of the anger and knows that the punishment is unjust. The younger the child, the more likely a serious injury will result from the use of physical force. Shaking a baby repeatedly to get it to stop crying, or for any other reason, can cause death.

Emotional abuse Psychological abuse can cause severe emotional distress and can produce illness and violent behavior that may lead to suicide or homicide. Being screamed at repeatedly, and told that one is worthless, stupid, or defective can permanently damage psychological and social development.

Sexual abuse This is another form of maltreatment of children. Sexual contact between adults and children is forbidden by both cultural taboos and by criminal law. Although it is difficult to determine with accuracy the prevalence of child sexual abuse in this country, some surveys find that as many as 15% of women and 6% of men have experienced sexual abuse as children (Swenson and Hanson, 1998). Because this subject is not one that most people are willing to discuss, the prevalence of child sexual abuse may be higher than reported. Sexual abuse of children may result in depression, anxiety, and general dysfunction later in their lives.

Neglect This is probably the most common form of maltreatment of children. Neglect includes failure to provide a child with adequate nourishment, proper clothing, prescribed medications, or to oversee a child's hygiene. Neglected children are left to their own devices for long periods without adult supervision, and many neglected children engage in self-destructive behaviors.

While it is true that males are the usual perpetrators of violence on children, especially female children,

Terms

child abuse: physical or mental injury, sexual abuse or exploitation, maltreatment, or neglect of a child by a person who is responsible for the child's welfare; circumstances in which a child's health or welfare is harmed or threatened

mothers also abuse their children both physically and sexually. Women who inflict serious injury on their children are often mentally ill and may suffer from dissociative identity disorder, formerly known as multiple personality disorder (Mitchell and Morse, 1998).

Child abuse affects children not only physically (e.g., broken bones, burns, or even death), but emotionally as well (e.g., they may become abusive themselves, suicidal, or withdrawn). Effects are both short- and long-term and invariably devastating to all victims. As the abused child reaches age 10 and older and becomes more independent, he or she may feel in a hopeless situation and may run away from home. The consequences for many runaways are dismal: teenage prostitution, illicit drug and alcohol use, higher rates of juvenile crimes, and higher school dropout rates. Child abuse is costly to society and directly or indirectly affects everyone.

Social Aspects of Child Abuse

Because many cases of child abuse go unreported, reliable data are difficult to obtain; also, abusers and the abused usually do not offer information freely. As a result, much information on child abuse has been incorrect or misleading (Allen and Epperson, 1993).

As more women enter the work force, more males assume greater responsibility for child care. For whatever reasons, males tend to abuse their children at a higher rate than females. However, no unique factors have been found that distinguish male abusers of children from female abusers. Male children are abused more frequently and seen by parents as more deserving of harsh treatment than female children. Male children even blame themselves more than female children do for their own maltreatment.

Two-thirds of all abused children are between the ages of 5 and 17. Younger children are abused more frequently because they lack both physical strength to resist child abuse and knowledge about what is normal and abnormal behavior. Infants are attacked less frequently than older children by abusive parents, but are at greater risk of death than older children, especially when shaken. As children pass the age of 15, they are more likely to be abused by peers than by family members.

Children with physical or mental handicaps such as blindness, deafness, mental retardation, or cerebral palsy are at a greater risk for child abuse than others. It is unclear if the physical handicap itself provokes the abuse or if stress created by caring for such a child is the underlying cause of the abuse. Children who are temperamental, impulsive, aggressive, depressed, or hyperactive are also at a higher risk for being abused. These behaviors create parental stress that may contribute to child abuse.

Cultural Aspects of Child Abuse

Different cultural beliefs play a role in the risk of child abuse. Latino men tend to regard themselves as *macho* (masculine), which may be used to justify abusive behavior towards their families and children. Their society accepts macho behavior as the social norm, although as Latino families become acculturated to the value system of middle-class Americans, child abuse declines. *Machismo* (the need for males to appear powerful) is observed in all ethnic groups and child abuse occurs among all socioeconomic classes.

Lack of knowledge and skills about child care may predispose parents to child abuse, possibly because of frustration and stress created by the needs of a child and its apparent lack of cooperation. Males who are primary care givers usually have received little or no training regarding child care.

The same holds true for adolescent mothers and mothers with low levels of education, for example, high school dropouts. They, too, lack the knowledge and skills necessary for adequate child care. This lack places them in a stressful situation in which abuse is more likely to occur. These mothers feel they have no one to turn to for help, and they may not even know where to obtain help. In frustration, they abuse their children.

If the family lives in an unsafe neighborhood, family members may feel afraid to venture out to seek help for their problems. This fear results in even more isolation and may exacerbate family conflicts and abuse. If the family lives in an area of limited public transportation or owns no car, these factors also contribute to the risk of child abuse. Contributing reasons for child abuse seem to be social isolation, lack of friends, dangerous neighborhoods, or lack of access to transportation (Finkelhor and Dziuba-Leatherman, 1994).

Child Abuse Prevention

There are child abuse prevention programs that can help parents reduce the stress that is a risk factor in child abuse. These programs emphasize educating parents on how to care for their children and how to avoid abuse. Different stress reduction programs have been developed for adolescent mothers, young parents, fathers who have never been in charge of child care before, working mothers, single parents, step parents, and siblings who are in charge of child care. Stress management programs are particularly important in communities where unemployment rates are high.

Conflict resolution programs can also help prevent child abuse. If people are able to manage conflict without using physical force, the risk of child abuse is lower. Both anger mediation programs and conflict resolution programs have been shown to help lower rates of child abuse. Training in life and social skills for all individuals involved with child abuse is recommended.

Training in parenting skills for both males and females of all ages is also strongly suggested. This training also educates them about resources for assistance.

Sexual Assault

Rape, incest, attempted rape, and unwanted sexual touching are called **sexual assault.** There has been a significant increase recently in public recognition of sexual crimes against women, including intense media scrutiny of rape issues in high profile rape trials. The legal definition of **forcible rape** varies from state to state. However, rape is generally viewed as penetration by force or threat of force of a body orifice, including the mouth, rectum, or vagina. Penetration includes the use of objects or other body parts, such as fingers. Forced sexual activity can occur between men and women,

Terms

sexual assault: violent actions that include rape, incest, attempted rape, and unwanted sexual touching

forcible rape: sexual assault using force or threat of force and involving sexual penetration of the victim's vagina, mouth, or rectum

men and men, women and women, and married and unmarried people. Regardless of the identity of the victims and perpetrators, sexual assault is a criminal activity; it is not sex and has nothing to do with sex. Sexual assault is an act of power, an attempt to humiliate a victim. Whether the term is sexual assault or forcible rape, the end result is physical violence to the victim.

Some men try to deny the fact of sexual assault with statements such as "women enjoy being raped," "she asked for it," and "I didn't think she meant no." These kinds of statements are heard repeatedly; however, the facts of sexual assault are plain:

- Sexual assault is an act of power and control—*not* an act of sex or passion.
- Most sexual assaults go unreported.
- Most sexual assaults do not occur on impulse or in remote areas.
- In 80% of all sexual assaults, according to some estimates, the assailant was a casual acquaintance, friend, or relative of the victim.
- Sexual assailants come from *all* socioeconomic and ethnic backgrounds.
- Rapists are not sexually deprived people.
- Women do not secretly want to be raped.
- Forced intimacy in a dating situation is sexual assault.

Managing Stress

"Road Rage" on the Rise

A report by the American Automobile Association observed that "motorists . . . are increasingly being shot, stabbed, beaten, and run over for inane reasons." The reasons that provoke rage among today's drivers include being cut off by a car pulling into your lane, aggressive tailgating, headlight flashing, and verbal abuse (Adler, 1997).

All of us have been irritated at one time or another while driving; most of us also have driven in a manner that was irritating to another driver. There is something about getting behind the wheel of a two-ton automobile that seems to raise the level of aggression in many people and causes them to ignore the safety of others. It is no coincidence that sport utility vehicles, large vans, and pickup trucks are called "suburban assault vehicles."

Whenever you get into a car to drive somewhere, remind yourself that being courteous

(even if the other driver is not) can save your life. Play a relaxing tape while driving. Your goal should be to get where you are going as safely as possible

and without incident. Your health and survival depend on it. Do not let yourself become a victim of "road rage."

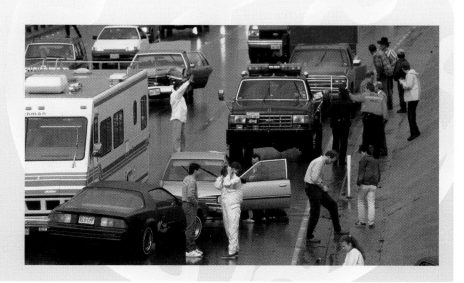

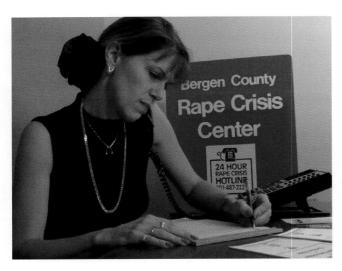

Many communities have crisis centers for rape victims.

Acquaintance Rape

Acquaintance rape, or date rape, occurs when a person known to the victim uses force to coerce the victim into having sex. Warsaw (1988) reports that 84% of all sexual assaults are committed by an acquaintance of the victim, 57% of all sexual assaults occur during a date, and 60% of men raped by other men knew their attacker. Acquaintance rape carries the same legal penalties as sexual assault committed by a stranger.

Women of high school and college age are the most vulnerable to acquaintance rape. A survey of 6,000 students from 32 colleges found that one in six female students had been a victim of rape or attempted rape within the preceding year, and one of fifteen male students reported committing sexual assaults within the preceding year (Koss and Harvey, 1991).

Every year, more than 100,000 forcible rapes are reported in the U.S. This number is probably low, because many rapes are not reported by the victim. In 1960, only about 15,000 forcible rapes were reported, a statistic that provides a sad record of how much this form of violence has increased.

Cultural views on sexual relationships between men and women play a significant role in acquaintance rape. Many young women who are victims of attacks that meet the legal definition of rape do not know that what happened to them was sexual assault. Victims may believe that a sexual assault can only be committed by a stranger or they may blame themselves for the act. A rapist may not realize that the victim's refusal really means NO. Aggressive males mistakenly believe that when women say no, men should insist. In a survey conducted by *MS.* magazine, 84% of men whose actions came under the legal definition of sexual assault believed they had not committed sexual assault.

Consequences of Acquaintance Rape

Victims of acquaintance rape often suffer serious, long-term psychological effects. Compared with victims of stranger rapes, acquaintance rape victims often blame themselves for what happened. They often have difficulty trusting people in later relationships. It may take acquaintance rape victims longer to recover, particularly if the rape involved physical violence. Acquaintance rape victims are less likely than other rape victims to seek crisis services, tell someone, report the incident to the police, or seek counseling. Family and friends may not provide the same support for acquaintance rape victims as they might offer victims of stranger rape. If victims tell friends or family, the severity of the attack may be minimized or the victim may be blamed for the sexual assault.

Terms

acquaintance rape: (also known as "date rape") sexual assault occurring when the victim and the rapist are known to each other and may have previously interacted in some socially appropriate manner

Wellness Guide

How to Prevent Date Rape

Be wary of a relationship that is operating along classic stereotypes of dominant male and submissive, passive female. The dominance in ordinary activities may extend to the sexual arena.

Be wary when a date tries to control behavior or pressure you in any way.

Be explicit with communication. Don't say "no" in a way that could be interpreted in any way as a "maybe" or "yes."

Avoid ambiguous messages with both verbal and nonverbal behavior. Saying "no" and permitting heavy petting implies confusion or ambiguity.

First dates with an unknown companion may be safer in a group.

Avoid remote or isolated spots where help is not available.

TABLE 23.2   Reactions and Feelings of Significant Others of Sexual Assault Victims

Anger	Concern	Guilt	Embarrassment	Vulnerability
• At assailant for committing crime • At system for letting "those kinds of people" run the streets • At victim for engaging in "risky behavior"	• For the victim's well-being and safety • About how the relationship between victim and significant other will change • For the victim's rights	• For not having prevented assault ("I should have been with her" OR "I should have given her a ride home") • For not having been there to protect victim	• Worry about gossip (myth and stigma hold strong effect) • Embarrassed for victim	• Realization that it can happen to me as well • Intensely heightened awareness of environment

Source: Adapted with permission from *Illinois Coalition Against Sexual Assault,* Springfield, Ill.: 1993.

Family members and significant others have also been victimized when someone they know, love, and care for has been sexually assaulted. Significant others may also have expressed or controlled reactions that indicate a state of shock from the incident. Some common feelings felt by the sexual assault victim's family members and significant others are listed in Table 23.2.

Victims usually have two types of behavioral reactions, expressed or controlled. Those who express their feelings usually manifest fear, anger, and anxiety. They may display these emotions through crying, tension, nervousness, restlessness, and hysteria. Those who control their feelings may appear calm or quiet, but either reaction indicates that the victim is in a state of shock (Table 23.3). Expressed or controlled feelings may occur at any time and often come and go more than once after the incident. Acknowledging or recognizing these feelings are a normal part of the healing process.

What to Do after a Sexual Assault

A person who has been sexually assaulted is advised to do the following:

• Contact a rape-crisis hotline.
• DO NOT shower, bathe, douche, change or destroy clothing, or straighten up the area where the sexual assault occurred (if indoors), because these actions would destroy important evidence.
• Go to the nearest hospital emergency room.
• Notify the police.
• Seek professional counseling.

Each person's reaction to being sexually assaulted is different, and it is natural that each victim's pain and needs are unique. All victims of sexual assault should seek counseling from someone they trust.

 ## Elder Abuse

We are an aging society, and with increasing frequency adult children are required to care for disabled or demented elderly parents and grandparents. It is only within the last generation that the problem of elder abuse has been recognized and documented. Studies now indicate that over 1 million elderly persons are victims of abuse each year in the U.S. (Quinn and Tomita, 1997). In addition to abuse by their adult

TABLE 23.3   Feelings Reported by Sexual Assault Victims

Fear	Embarrassment	Shame	Guilt	Anxiety
• Fear of death • Fear of rapist	• Embarrassed to discuss details • Embarrassed about their bodies	• Destruction of self-esteem, self-worth, self-respect • Ashamed at having the medical exam • Ashamed at having to perform a sexual act in order to stay alive	• Feelings of shame and of having provoked the rape • Feeling of blame for the assault	• Shaking • Nightmares • Difficulty sleeping or sleeping all the time • Constantly reminds self what "should or shouldn't have" been done
Stupidity	**Vulnerability**	**Concern**	**Anger**	**Loss of control**
• Feels stupid for engaging in risk-taking behavior(s) • Feels stupid for being too trusting	• General fear of people • Paranoid feelings • Intensely heightened awareness of environment	• Will the rapist get psychiatric help? • What will happen to offender if rape is reported?	• Toward assailant • Toward self • Toward men and women in general, especially if they resemble assailant	• Small decisions seem monumental • Unsure about self or actions

Source: Adapted from *Illinois Coalition Against Sexual Assault,* Springfield, Ill.: 1993.

children, elderly persons also are abused frequently by their spouses. The magnitude of elder abuse in the U.S. is now only slightly less than that of child abuse.

Elder abuse is defined as the physical, sexual, or emotional maltreatment or financial exploitation of an adult, age 60 or older. The abuse or neglect may be by any caregiver—spouse, child, relative, or friend—and occurs in a domestic setting. Self-neglect is also included in the definition, because almost half of the cases of elder abuse involve self-neglect.

Self-neglect may result from physical or mental disability of the elder person. He or she may not be able to obtain essential food, clothing, shelter, or medical care. Quite often the financial affairs of a neglected elder person are in disarray. Despite increased public attention to the problems of elder abuse, much maltreatment of elders still remains hidden to a large extent.

A variety of abusive methods are used by caregivers in the domestic setting to control the elder persons under their care. These include screaming and yelling (the most frequent form of abuse), physical restraint, forced feeding or medicating, blows and slaps, and threats to send the person to a nursing home.

However, the abuse is not all one way. Elder persons who are disabled or immobilized also use abusive methods to control their caregivers. Elder persons scream and yell, pout and withdraw, refuse food and medication, cry or become emotional, throw objects, and threaten to call the police. As with other forms of abuse, the reasons for the abusive behaviors by both persons in the relationship are many. Alcohol plays a role in many situations, and emotional illness contributes, as does mental impairment, on the part of one or both parties.

The reason why much elder abuse remains hidden or undocumented is that many elderly people are concerned about the family's privacy and fear public exposure and embarrassment. The victim also may feel shame at having raised the child who has now become abusive. If the child is stealing money, the elderly parent may fear that the child will be sent to jail if the abuse is reported. And, despite the abusive treatment, the elder person may feel that the situation is preferable to being sent to a nursing home. Elder abuse will become an ever greater problem during the next century, as more and more people live to be age 80 or older and as the number of people with dementia increases (see chapter 22).

Firearm Violence

Year after year, the use of firearms causes thousands of deaths—both deliberately inflicted and accidental—in the United States. In 1994, more than 38,000 deaths were caused by firearms; about half of this number were suicides, slightly less than half were homicides, and the rest were unintentional firearm fatalities. In addition to firearm fatalities, more than 100,000 injuries result each year from guns.

Firearms are the second leading cause of death among young people between the ages of 10 and 24. In 1995, a national survey found that one student in twelve (7.6%) admitted to carrying a firearm within the past month, either for defense or for fighting. People living in homes in which guns are kept have a risk of suicide that is five times greater than for people living in homes without guns. Surveys also show that the vast majority of teenage suicides are accomplished with guns. Numerous studies come to the same conclusion; ready availability of firearms in the United States is associated with an increased risk of suicide and homicide (Sherman, 2000).

Americans have a longstanding love-hate relationship with firearms, and many people believe strongly in the constitutionally guaranteed right to carry and use firearms. Their views are defended with money and lobbying by the National Rifle Association (NRA), which works to prevent passage of laws limiting or regulating the purchase and use of guns by civilians. The NRA is opposed by physicians, health organizations, and law enforcement agencies including the Federal Bureau of Investigation (FBI), which supports stricter gun control laws.

In 1993, in response to the escalating number of homicides, suicides, and assaults, 11 states, including New York, New Jersey, and California, passed gun control laws. In addition, the U.S. Congress passed a gun control law known as the Brady Bill. (Jim Brady was permanently disabled in the assassination attempt on President Ronald Reagan in 1981.) The Brady Bill imposes a five-day waiting period for the purchase of handguns and requires local police agencies to determine if the prospective buyer has a criminal record (Cole, 2001).

Violence and the use of firearms in the United States has become one of society's most pressing concerns. Juveniles under 21 now account for about one-quarter of all arrests for the possession or use of a gun. Black American youths are three times more likely to be arrested for a gun violation than are white American youths, and about half of all homicide victims are black Americans. Most homicides are not racially motivated, however, because 94% of victims are killed by members of their own race and 83% of white American murder victims are killed by other whites.

Terms

elder abuse: physical, sexual, or emotional maltreatment or financial exploitation of an adult age 60 or older

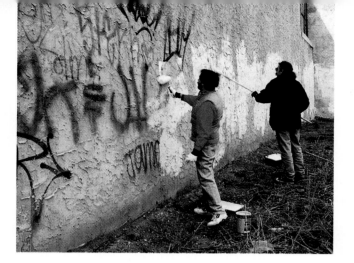

Graffiti is one form youths use to express anger.

The majority of homicides involve juveniles, many of whom are in gangs and involved in selling and using illegal drugs. While law enforcement can be increased in some ways, laws cannot solve the problems of violence and murder. Solutions to the social problems that underlie the violence must come from parents, clergy, teachers, and the youths involved.

Youth Gangs

Youth gangs exist in nearly every major city in the U.S. Recent surveys indicate that more than 200,000 adolescents and young adults are members of almost 4,000 gangs. Previously, gangs were primarily focused in major cities, such as Los Angeles, Chicago, and New York, but they have since spread to most large cities in the midwest, northwest, south, and southwest. The sale of drugs has been a key factor in the movement of gangs to more and more cities. In most cities with gangs, it is not only poor areas that are affected; gang activities have also spread to traditionally safe suburbs and to schools.

A number of factors contribute to a teenager or young adult deciding to join a gang: poverty, failure at school, substance abuse, dysfunctional family life, and family violence. Easy access to illegal drugs and the lure of financial rewards from drug dealing are both powerful at-

> *War is but a spectacular expression of our daily conduct.*
> KRISHNAMURTI

tractants for a young person with no money, no education, no job, and no future. For them, gang life is exciting and rewarding.

Gang recruits often have a poor self-image, low self-esteem, and no adult to provide counseling and support. Some gang members are the children of gang members and are following in their parents' footsteps. Gang members often gain recognition from other gang members and from a society that fears them—in this way they gain attention and respect.

Drugs and guns are an integral part of gang acceptance. Often a recruit is not deemed fit until he or she has obtained a gun—and used it, either on a rival gang member or in committing a crime. About half of the juvenile inmates of prisons report that their gang regularly bought and sold guns and that gun theft was an important gang activity. Thus, the ready accessibility of guns in the U.S. directly contributes to gang activities and the destruction of the lives of thousands of young people.

School Violence

The problem of guns in schools became the focus of national attention in 1998. A series of shootings by teenagers in schools across America brought horror

---

Managing Stress

Check Your Anger Level

Answer the questions below using the following scale:

Almost never . . . . 1 point
Sometimes . . . . 2 points
Often . . . . 3 points
Almost always . . . . 4 points

1. I am quick tempered. _____
2. I would say that I have a fiery temper. _____
3. I am a hotheaded person. _____

4. I get angry at others' mistakes. _____
5. I feel annoyed when my work is not recognized. _____
6. I fly off the handle easily. _____
7. When I get angry, I say nasty things and swear. _____
8. It makes me furious when I am criticized in front of others. _____

9. When I am frustrated, I feel like hitting someone. _____
10. I get angry when I do a good job and get a poor evaluation. _____

A score of 22 points or more indicates a high anger level. To double-check your score, ask one or more friends to take the same test and mark the answers as if they were you. If your anger score remains high, you may want to consider anger counseling. Anger often leads to violence against another person.

Global Wellness

Violence in the U.S. Exceeds That of Any Other Nation

The ultimate measure of violence is homicide, the killing of another person. The U.S. leads all technologically advanced, industrialized nations in the number of homicides per capita (see figure). Compared with Italy, the country with the next highest homicide rate, the U.S. rate is eight times greater. And compared with Japan, it is about 40 times as great. Even compared with Canada, a country that is culturally similar to ours, the U.S. homicide rate is 20 times greater.

If one looks at data on other forms of violence, such as forcible rape, the graph is pretty much the same. In fact, if one looks at the statistical data for any form of interpersonal violence, the U.S. is ahead of every other nation by a factor of 10 or more. A consequence of this violence is that the U.S. also imprisons a higher percentage of its population than any other industrialized nation. Whether a nation can long endure with this level of violence— violence that continues to escalate year after year—is a question that many people ask but are afraid to answer.

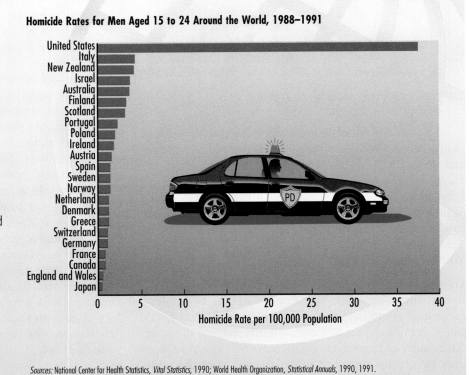

Homicide Rates for Men Aged 15 to 24 Around the World, 1988–1991

Homicide Rate per 100,000 Population

Sources: National Center for Health Statistics, *Vital Statistics*, 1990; World Health Organization, *Statistical Annuals*, 1990, 1991.

and tragedy into the affected families and communities. A partial list of school shootings include:

October 1997, Pearl, Mississippi: A 16-year-old boy shoots and kills his mother, his ex-girlfriend, and a student.

December 1997, West Paducah, Kentucky: A 14-year-old boy shoots and kills three students.

March 1998, Jonesboro, Arkansas: A 13-year-old boy and an 11-year-old boy shoot and kill five students.

April 1998, Edinboro, Pennsylvania: A 14-year-old boy shoots and kills a teacher at a school dance.

May 1998, Fayetteville, Tennessee: An 18-year-old boy shoots and kills a classmate.

May 1998, Springfield, Oregon: A 15-year-old boy shoots and kills his parents and then goes to school and kills two students. Others are critically wounded.

April 1999, Littleton, Colorado: Two teenage boys go on a methodical shooting spree, killing 12 students, a teacher, and themselves.

March 2001, Santee, CA: A disturbed 15-year-old boy shoots and kills two classmates and wounds 13 more.

What prompts such senseless violence by teenage boys all across America? Experts of all kinds offer explanations and social theories, but as a friend of the family whose son was accused of the murders in Springfield, Oregon, remarked, "There's no obvious explanation for it. Young Kip was just a bad seed" (King and Murr, 1998). These school killings occurred in middle-class American communities and received much more media attention than killings in inner city schools in poor neighborhoods. Today, no parent can feel entirely at ease when a child is at school. All unusual behaviors and threats must be taken seriously. The continuing epidemic of violence and murder in America's schools has generated public demands for more money and research to solve the problems of teen violence (Marshall, 2000).

School killings focus on the controversy over the right of citizens to own firearms in this country, a right that many argue is guaranteed by the U.S. Constitution. The NRA persistently argues that ownership of guns has nothing to do with violence and killings. After the killings in Springfield, Oregon, a spokesman for the NRA stated, "Lawful arms ownership has nothing to do with this tragedy." In refuting this, a prominent physician points out that:

> "Children and adolescents are by definition immature and may lack judgment. Life's embarrassments, rejections, and torments may send them into fits of temper, even rage, and may prompt a desire for revenge. Impulsively, some children lash out at others and at themselves. Nonetheless, they are only murderous when they have the means, and a loaded gun is the 'perfect' tool" (Kassirer, 1998).

Almost everyone in America has experienced some form of violence in their lives. In many cities and communities, people are afraid to go out at night or to go walking or jogging alone. Now there is fear among students about going to school. Two critical questions must be addressed by American society. First, what are the factors contributing to the continued rise in all forms of violence—child abuse, spousal abuse, bombings, homicide, and sexual abuse of all kinds—and what can be done to reduce violence? Second, will Americans find the will to disarm private citizens and, thereby, reduce the cause of most violent crimes?

Many studies indicate that social and interpersonal violence stems from inequality—inequality in wealth, inequality in education, inequality in medical care, and inequality in job opportunity (Chasin, 1997). Changing these inequalities in American society may prove to be difficult or impossible. If that is so, then violence, and its many negative effects on health and life, is likely to increase in the years ahead.

Other experts believe that anger and aggression underlie violent acts (Robbins, 2000). Many factors contribute to anger and aggression—culture, violent portrayals in all forms of media, alcohol, illegal drugs, poverty—the list is probably much longer.

Many people believe that violence among people and in societies is inevitable, that is, violence is biologically determined and cannot be changed. At best, society can try to limit the amount of violence and punish offenders. This belief is not substantiated by cultural studies of societies around the world that have little or no violence as long as their traditional life-style is not disrupted. Examples of nonviolent societies include the Semai Senoi people of Malaysia, Mabuti pygmies of Zaire, the Inuit Eskimos of Canada, the Zuni Pueblo Indians of New Mexico, and the Ladakh people of northwestern India (Adler and Denmark, 1995). The Ladakh, in particular, is a Buddhist culture whose doctrines identify greed, hate, aggression, lust, envy, jealousy, and pride as the ultimate sources of human unhappiness. In American society, we have come to accept these human behaviors.

We believe that the point to remember about violence is that it is a personal decision to be violent or not, just as it is a personal decision to exercise or not. The fact that nonviolent societies do exist and that people may choose to live nonviolent lives should encourage everyone who abhors violence to reduce the level of violence in their lives. In so doing, the violence in society is reduced.

World Violence and Bioterrorism

The nature of violence in the United States (and the world) changed forever on September 11, 2001. On that day, four commercial airplanes were hijacked by suicidal terrorists and crashed into the World Trade Center in New York City, the Pentagon in Washington D.C., and a field in Pennsylvania.

> *An eye for an eye leaves both parties blind*
> MARTIN LUTHER KING

Thousands of people in the planes and on the ground were killed. The World Trade Center towers in New York City collapsed, leaving a smouldering ruin in lower Manhattan.

Shortly after the airplane hijackings, lethal anthrax spores were sent in letters to offices in Florida, New York, and Washington, D.C. Several people died from inhalation of the deadly spores, many others became ill, and thousands had to take antibiotics as a precaution against possible infection. Buildings had to be closed and decontaminated. The U.S. postal system was forced to revise the way mail was processed, delivered, and opened. Bioterrorism was used to attack politicians and media personnel, and to disrupt basic American services and business operations. As of this writing, no one can predict whether these acts of bioterrorism (or other forms of terrorism) will continue or escalate with the use of other kinds of deadly bacteria, viruses, or toxins.

The violence that has recently been unleashed in the world has heightened people's stress and fears. Agencies of the U.S. government at both the federal and local levels are struggling to cope with the new threats to public health and safety. In this time of violence, each individual must continue to strive to reduce the level of anger and stress in his or her personal life, and in the world at large. Understanding, compassion, and patience are what we need to live in these troubled times of uncertainty and unrest.

Critical Thinking About Health

1. Imagine that you are in a debate in school over this question: "Should all Americans over 21 years of age be allowed to own (a) a handgun; (b) a rifle; (c) a semiautomatic weapon; or (d) an automatic weapon?"

   Take a position on this issue with respect to owning or not owning guns in general. If you favor the ownership of guns, give your reasons for owning or not owning each of the four categories of guns. If you do not favor the ownership of guns, explain your reasons. Whatever side of the issue you are on, discuss whether or not you believe that ownership and availability of guns contributes to violence and crime in America.

2. You and Jennifer have been close friends for more than 15 years (since you both were in high school). Jennifer has recently divorced and has a 5-year-old son, Timmy, who is a "handful" in your view. You and Jennifer have shared many thoughts and feelings over the years. One day after work you stop by to see how Jennifer is doing. You notice that Timmy is limping and has several bruises on his legs. When you comment on Timmy's limp, Jennifer looks at the boy sharply and says, "You fell out of a tree. Isn't that right, Timmy?" The boy mumbles, "Yes" and limps from the room. Jennifer seems tense and doesn't want to talk. You soon leave but not before you smell alcohol on her breath.

   Do you think that this might be a case of child abuse? If so, what do you think your actions should be? In your discussion, indicate whether you are a male or female. Do you think a male or female friend of Jennifer's would act differently in this situation?

3. Volunteer to help at a retirement or nursing home in your community. Ask the older persons what they enjoy and dislike most about being elderly or infirm. Observe how many of the persons living there are mentally incompetent in your judgment and to what degree. Make a report of your findings and observations. Describe how your views of the elderly have changed as the result of your volunteer work.

4. By all statistical measures, the U.S. is the most violent society among all industrialized countries in the world by a large margin. The U.S. has more forcible rapes, more battered women, more homicides, and more suicides than any other nation on a per capita basis. Discuss why you think our society is so violent and what could be done to change its violent nature.

Health in Review

- Domestic violence includes relationship abuse and child abuse. Violence refers to use of force and power.
- Child abuse encompasses physical abuse, emotional abuse, sexual abuse, and neglect.
- Women who have been assaulted may experience anxiety, depression, substance abuse, headaches, and other medical problems. These are symptoms of post-traumatic stress disorder (PTSD). Many long-term consequences of sexual abuse are associated with PTSD.
- Acquaintance rape or date rape occurs when a person known to the victim uses force or power to coerce the victim into having sex. Women of high school and college age are most vulnerable to acquaintance rape.

- Child abuse is a form of domestic violence that reaches across all social, economic, racial, ethnic, geographic, and educational barriers.
- Education is the key to all forms of violence prevention, including firearm violence, relationship abuse, acquaintance rape, and child abuse.
- The United States exceeds all other developed nations in the per capita rate of rapes, homicides and suicides and in the percentage of its population in prisons.
- Violence and the presence of handguns in schools mirror our communities. Violence is generating fear in our schools, not learning.
- Violence is not an essential part of human behavior, and many societies in the world are nonviolent.

Health and Wellness Online

The World Wide Web contains a wealth of information about health and wellness. By accessing the Internet using Web browser software, such as Netscape Navigator or Microsoft's Internet Explorer, you can gain a new perspective on many topics presented in *Health and Wellness, Seventh Edition*. Access the Jones and Bartlett Publishers Web site at http://www.jbpub.com/hwonline.

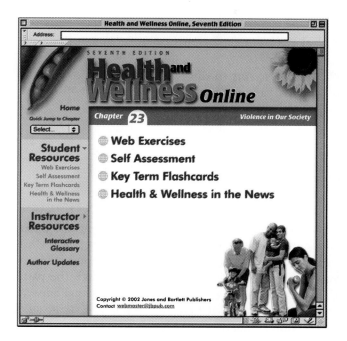

References

Adler, J. (1997, June 2). 'Road rage': We're driven to destruction. *Newsweek,* 70.

Alexander, L. L., and LaRosa, J. H. (1994). *New dimensions in women's health.* Boston: Jones and Bartlett.

Allen, C. M., and Epperson, D. L. (1993). Perpetrator gender and type of child maltreatment: Overcoming limited conceptualizations and obtaining representative samples. *Child Welfare, 72*(6): 543–554.

Chasin, B. H. (1997). *Inequality and violence in the United States.* New Jersey: Humanities Press.

Cole, T. B. (2001). Complementary strategies to prevent firearm injury. *Journal of the American Medical Association, 283,* 1071–1072.

Damasio, H., et al. (1994). The return of Phineas Gage: Clues about the brain from the skull of a famous patient. *Science, 264,* 1102–1105.

Eisenstat, S. A., and Bancroft, L. (1999). Domestic violence. *New England Journal of Medicine, 341,* 886–892.

Finkelhor, D., and Dziuba-Leatherman, J. (1994). Victimization of children. *The American Psychologist, 49*(3): 173–184.

Finkelhor, D., and Korbin, J. (1988). Child abuse as an international issue. *Child Abuse and Neglect, 12,* 3–24.

Geles, R. J. (1997). *Intimate violence in families* (3rd ed.). Thousand Oaks, CA: Sage Publications, pp. 3–4.

Gellert, G. A. (1997). *Confronting violence.* Boulder, CO: Westview Press.

Illinois Coalition against Sexual Assault [ICASA] (1993). Springfield, Ill.

Kantor, G. K., and Jasinski, J. L. (1998). Dynamics and risk factors in partner violence. In Jasinski, J. L., and Williams, L. M. (Eds.), *Partner violence* (pp. 1–43).

Kassirer, J. P. (1998). Private arsenals and public peril. *New England Journal of Medicine, 338,* 1375–1376.

King, P., and Murr, A. (1998, June 1). A son who spun out of control. *Newsweek*, 32–33.

Koss, M. P., and Harvey, M. R. (1991). *The rape victim: Clinical and community interventions*. Newbury Park, Calif.: Sage Library of Social Research, Sage Publications.

Kyriacou, D. N. et al. (1999). Risk factors for injury to women from domestic violence. *New England Journal of Medicine, 341*, 1892–1898.

Marshall, E. (2000). The shots heard round the world. *Science, 289*, 570–574.

Mitchell, J., Morse, J. (1998). *From victims to survivors*. Washington, DC: Taylor and Francis Group, pp. 25–66.

Peterson, L., and Gable, S. (1998). Holistic injury prevention. In J. R. Lutzker (Ed.), *Handbook of child abuse: Research and treatment*. New York: Plenum, pp. 291–318.

Sherman, L. W. (2001). Gun carrying and homocide prevention. *Journal of the American Medical Association, 283*, 1193–1195.

Swenson, C. C., and Hanson, R. F. (1998). Sexual abuse of children. In J. R. Lutzker (Ed.), *Handbook of child abuse research and treatment*. New York: Plenum, pp. 475–500.

Warsaw, R. (1988). *I never called it rape*. New York: Harper and Row.

Suggested Readings

Byers, E. S., O'Sullivan, L. F. (1996). *Sexual coercion in dating relationships*. New York: Haworth. Provides a good overview of the growing problem of "date" rape and steps to take to avoid the problem.

Gellert, G. A. (1997). *Confronting violence: Answers to questions about the epidemic destroying America's homes and communities*. Boulder, CO: Westview Press. A thoughtful and comprehensive discussion of all aspects of violence in America. The best source for persons who want to know more about specific kinds of violence and what to do about them. The author was working two miles from the blast that killed 169 people in Oklahoma City on April 19, 1995.

Munson, L., and Riskin, K. (1995). *In their own words: A sexual abuse workbook for teenage girls*. Washington, DC: Child Welfare League. Two therapists have designed a workbook to help teenage girls work through the pain and emotional damage resulting from sexual abuse.

Robbins, P. E. (2000). *Anger, aggression and violence*. Jefferson, NC.: McFarland Publishers. Explores how anger and aggression lead to violence.

Wissow, L. (1995). Current Concepts: Child abuse and neglect. *New England Journal of Medicine, 332*(21): 1425. Defines the various kinds of child abuse and treatment strategies.

Learning Objectives

1. Discuss the relationship between environment and health.
2. Describe the health effects of air pollution, including smog and the hole in the ozone layer.
3. Explain the greenhouse effect and the predicted consequences of global warming.
4. Describe the effects of lead on children's health and intelligence.
5. Describe substances that pollute water in the United States.
6. Discuss the impact of land pollution on food production and health.
7. Describe sources of pesticide contamination and their effects on health.
8. Identify the potential health problems associated with noise pollution and EMFs.
9. Discuss how human population growth will affect global health and environmental issues.

Study Guide
and
Self Assessment

How Do You Score on Environmental Awareness?

Health
and Wellness
Online

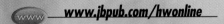 **www.jbpub.com/hwonline**

Chapter 24

Working Toward a Healthy Environment

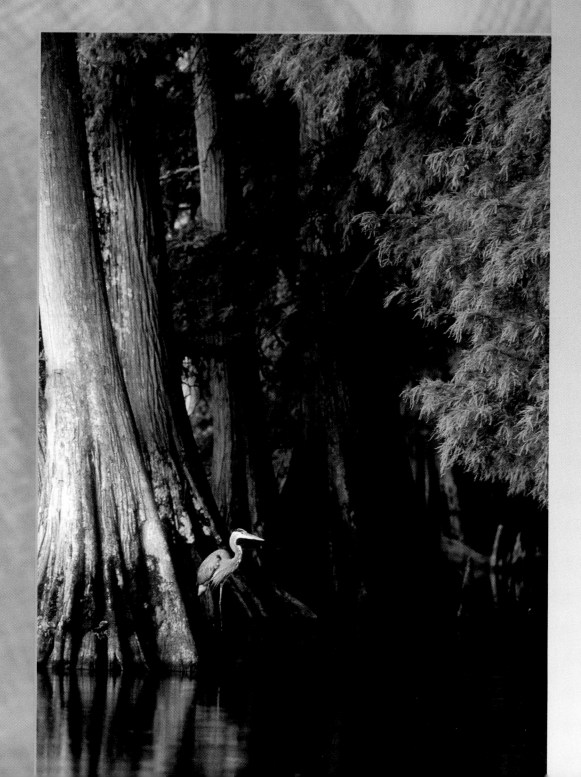

The term **environment** refers to all external physical factors that affect us. In order to survive, all animals, including human beings, require a certain amount of high quality air, water, food, and shelter. If people are deprived of any essential environmental factors, or if the environment is polluted with toxic substances, health is adversely affected. Anyone who has experienced difficulty breathing smoggy, dusty, or smoke-filled air realizes the unhealthy effects of polluted air. Anyone who has become sick from consuming contaminated food or water knows the importance of uncontaminated food and water in maintaining health.

> *I do not think that the measure of a civilization is how tall its buildings of concrete are, but rather how well its people have learned to relate to their environment and fellow man.*
>
> SUN BEAR, CHIPPEWA TRIBE

To achieve optimal health, we must live in a high quality environment. Unfortunately, the quality of many aspects of the environment is deteriorating from pollution, degradation, and depletion of natural resources. The effects of environmental pollution are long lasting and often irreversible. People and nations are just beginning to appreciate the serious consequences of ongoing air, water, and land pollution that adversely affect health. Dramatic changes in personal lifestyles and industrial technology are required to reduce existing pollution and prevent future pollution.

Environmental problems are not restricted to the United States or even to industrialized countries; environmental problems are of global concern. Worldwide problems are: (a) the threat of nuclear, biological, or chemical warfare; (b) depletion of the ozone layer from emissions of certain synthetic chemicals released into the atmosphere (since stratospheric ozone protects people from harmful ultraviolet radiation, its destruction may result in a higher incidence of skin cancer, mutations, and immune system problems); (c) global warming from increased levels of carbon dioxide in the atmosphere (global warming could damage crops, increase the frequency of violent storms and epidemics, and raise the level of the oceans, causing flooding of coastlines); (d) land degradation caused by deforestation, desertification, and soil erosion undermining the ability of many local environments to support their populations; and (e) loss of rain forests' biodiversity (the rate of species extinction is increasing as a result of overhunting, habitat destruction, and the introduction of non-native species into new environments).

Environmental health hazards stem from many different causes. Through the enactment and enforcement of environmental laws and regulations, the

Managing Stress

Honoring Mother Earth

"All things connect. Man did not weave the web of life. He is merely a strand in it. Whatever he does to the web, he does to himself."

These prophetic words were written by Chief Seattle over a century ago and still ring true today. The neglect and abuse that human beings have inflicted on the planet, primarily in the last few centuries, are beginning to take their toll. Global warming, water and air pollution, nuclear and chemical wastes, depletion of the ozone layer, deforestation, and the increased rate of extinction of plant and animal life are all signs of a sick planet.

It may seem hard to believe that the earth is a living entity. Western thought, heavily grounded in science and technology, tends to regard such an idea as foolish or more suitable to myths. But if you really pay attention to the words of Native Americans and tribal elders around the world, you begin to see the wisdom of viewing the earth as a living entity. But human beings have grown distant and separate from nature and these attitudes have caused major harm to the planet that nourishes all of us.

Whether we realize it or not, we are all connected to the earth like threads of a web. Despite all the advances of technology, we still depend on Mother Earth for the air, water, and food that keeps us alive. Wellness means living in an environment that is healthy, not one that is sick. We can begin to interact with the environment in less harmful ways; even small actions are important, as the slogan "Think globally, act locally" points out.

Here are some questions you can reflect on to become more environmentally aware and proactive.

1. How would you best describe your relationship with the earth?

2. Do you see the earth as a rock spinning in space or as a living entity that provides sustenance in one form or another to all her species of flora and fauna?

3. Getting back to nature can take many forms, from gardening to exotic vacations. What do you do to get back to nature when the urge strikes?

4. Any good relationship takes work. What steps do you feel you can take to enhance your relationship with the earth?

United States has been making progress in reducing environmental pollution and trying to stop the negative health consequences therefrom. The United Nations and the World Health Organization carry out research and sponsor programs, the aims of which are to stop environmental degradation and its health consequences. Governments and other organizations alone cannot solve environmental problems. Each individual must strive to reduce or eliminate contributions to pollution and to take steps to create a healthy environment. As the comic strip character Pogo declared years ago, *"We have met the enemy and he is us."* People's activities are at the root of almost *all* environmental pollution.

Outdoor Air Pollution

Pure air is a requirement for life. Each of us breathes about 35 pounds of air per day—more than six tons over the course of a year. Fresh, clean air consists of about 21% oxygen, 78% nitrogen, and trace amounts of seven other gases. It is the oxygen in air that is essential for human life. If the oxygen content of the air drops below 16%, body and brain functions are impaired. If breathing stops for even a few minutes, a person becomes unconscious and will die unless breathing is restored.

Terms

environment: all external physical factors that affect us

smog: air polluted by chemicals, smoke, particles, and dust

photochemical smog: air pollution from the action of sunlight on emissions from motor vehicles and industrial sources

Since the beginning of the Industrial Revolution in the 19th century, the burning of fossil fuels (coal, oil, and natural gas) to power transportation and industry has progressively polluted the air with carbon dioxide, oxides of nitrogen and sulfur, soot, and small particles, some of which cause health problems. A variety of chemical substances used in modern societies pollute the air as well (e.g., chloroflurocarbons, dioxin). Thus, technological advances over the past 200 years have created, as a by-product, pollution of the air we breathe and of Earth's atmosphere.

Smog

Everybody has heard of **smog,** a term first used in England to describe a hazardous combination of sulfurous chemicals emitted into the air from the burning of coal and water vapor in fog. Smog causes breathing problems, coughs, bronchitis, asthma, and can even result in death among people with lung diseases. In most U.S. cities, smog is not associated with fog but results from the action of sunlight on various chemicals and particles in the air that come from automobiles, oil refineries, electricity generating plants, and other industrial sources.

This is why it is called **photochemical smog.** Photochemical smog consists of ground level ozone, carbon monoxide, sulfur dioxide, nitrogen oxides, particulates, and volatile organic compounds (see Table 24.1).

Ground-Level Ozone   Ozone (O_3), consists of three atoms of oxygen as compared to the oxygen we breathe, which consists of two atoms of oxygen (O_2). Whereas ozone in the upper atmosphere benefits life on earth by shielding it from harmful ultraviolet radiation from the sun, high amounts of ozone at ground level are a major health hazard. Ground-level ozone is not emitted directly into the air from polluting

TABLE 24.1   Major Air Pollutants and Their Health Effects
These pollutants affect breathing, damage lungs, and cause a wide range of health problems. The primary sources of these air pollutants are industrial emissions, automobiles and trucks, and coal and oil burning in industry and homes.

Pollutant	Health effects and symptoms
Carbon monoxide gas	Low levels cause dizziness, headache, and fatigue. High levels lead to coma and death. Especially dangerous for persons with asthma and heart disease.
Nitrogen oxide gas	Causes a smelly brown haze that irritates the eyes, nose, and lungs.
Sulfur oxide gas	Sulfur dioxide gas is poisonous. Irritates the eyes, nose, throat, and lungs. Kills plants and rusts metals.
Particulate matter (Particles from dust and smoke that are less than 10 microns in diameter)	Causes throat irritation and permanent lung damage. Some industrial soot particulates may cause cancer.
Ozone (O_3)	In the stratosphere ozone protects us from UV light. Can be formed at ground level from nitrous oxides and organic compounds. Causes eye irritation, cough, and breathlessness.
Volatile organic compounds	Smog-forming chemicals, such as benzene, toluene, methylene chloride, and methyl chloroform. All VOCs can cause serious health problems.

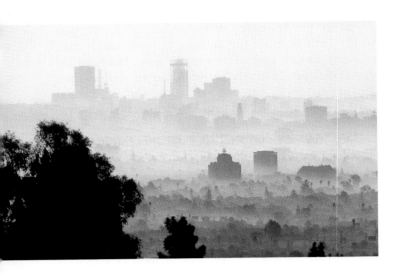

Polluted, "smoggy" air over many large cities contributes to respiratory problems and other diseases.

vehicles or industries. Instead, it is formed when sunlight acts on two other pollutants, volatile organic compounds (VOCs) and oxides of nitrogen (nitrogen oxide and nitrogen dioxide).

Ozone can damage lung tissue, reduce lung function, and sensitize the lungs to other irritants. Exposure to even relatively low amounts of ozone for several hours can reduce lung function and induce respiratory inflammation in healthy people during exercise. This decrease in lung function generally is accompanied by chest pain, coughing, sneezing, and pulmonary congestion. Ozone's effects on people with impaired respiratory systems, such as asthmatics, is usually more severe.

Carbon Monoxide　Carbon monoxide (CO) is a colorless, odorless, poisonous gas produced by incomplete burning of carbon-containing fuels. Three fourths of CO emissions in the United States are from transportation sources, mostly motor vehicle exhaust. Other major CO sources are wood-burning stoves, incinerators, and industries.

When CO enters the bloodstream, it reduces the amount of oxygen that can be delivered to the body's organs and tissues. Exposure to high levels of CO can cause impairment of visual perception, manual dexterity, learning ability, and performance of complex tasks. If the air contains 80 parts per million (ppm) of CO, the oxygen supplied to the body is reduced by 15%. In heavy freeway traffic, the levels of carbon monoxide may reach 400 ppm. It is no surprise that many commuters in large cities who get stuck in traffic jams arrive home with headaches. Car mechanics and parking garage attendants, who are exposed to high levels of carbon monoxide for long periods, may develop health problems. Health threats from CO are most serious for those with heart disease.

Sulfur Dioxide　Sulfur dioxide (SO_2) is produced when gasoline, diesel fuel, and coal or oil, all of which contain sulfur, are burned in cars, trucks, power plants, and industrial and home heating systems. Sulfur dioxide also is produced by active volcanoes. Sulfur dioxide can mix with water vapor to form sulfuric acid, a highly corrosive substance that can erode stone, pit metal, and damage living tissue. Exposure to SO_2 makes breathing difficult and aggravates existing respiratory and cardiovascular diseases. Sulfur dioxide in the air can combine with water to form acid rain (see p. 492), which damages aquatic ecosystems and forests in many parts of the world.

Nitrogen Oxides　The major sources of nitrogen oxides are from transportation, electric power plants, and industrial boilers. Nitrogen oxides consist principally of nitrogen oxide (NO) and nitrogen dioxide (NO_2). In photochemical smog, nitrogen oxide is converted to NO_2, which is a brownish, highly reactive gas that can irritate the lungs, opening the way for bronchitis, pneumonia, and other respiratory infections. Nitrogen oxides also contribute to ground-level ozone and acid rain, and they may alter both terrestrial and aquatic ecosystems.

Particulates　Particulates are microscopic particles that arise principally from the burning of diesel fuel and coal. These particles are released into the air, causing the haze associated with photochemical smog and damaging soil and structures in the process. When inhaled, microscopic particulate matter (less than 10 micrometers in diameter, called PM_{10}) damages the respiratory system and impairs breathing, aggravates existing respiratory and cardiovascular disease, alters the body's immune system, and predisposes a person to cancer. Individuals with chronic obstructive pulmonary disease (COPD), cardiovascular disease, influenza, asthma, the elderly, and children are the most sensitive to the effects of particulate matter. In smoggy, urban regions, death rates from all causes and especially respiratory and heart disease increase as the level of particulate matter increases (Samet et al., 2000).

Volatile Organic Compounds　Volatile organic compounds (VOCs) are chemical substances that exist in the air as gases. About 50% of VOCs come from industrial and commercial processes such as oil refining, printing, painting, and dry cleaning. Another 40% of VOCs come from motor vehicle exhaust. Five percent come from power generation, and the rest from miscellaneous sources. In the presence of sunlight, some VOCs (called "ozone precursors") easily combine with other air pollutants to form ground-level ozone. Besides contributing to photochemical smog, some VOCs are harmful to human health and are known as hazardous air pollutants or air toxics.

Children and Smog Children who live in smoggy cities such as Los Angeles and Mexico City suffer a 10% to 15% decrease in lung function as compared to children who grow up where the air is less polluted. Early exposure to polluted air can damage the respiratory tract and can increase the risk of respiratory disease in adult life. Children are much more likely than adults to develop smog-related lung damage because they inhale several times more air than adults, and they breathe faster, particularly during strenuous physical activity. In addition, they spend more time outdoors than any other segment of the population. To accommodate the 1996 Summer Olympics in Atlanta, citywide automobile use was reduced and, consequently, air pollution decreased by about 30%. Also during this time, the number of children seeking care for episodes of asthma declined by about 40% (Friedman et al., 2001). Cleaning the air of pollution can make a big difference in children's health.

The world's automobile "population" is exploding along with its human population. In 1950, there were about 50 million cars worldwide; by 1990, the number had increased to 400 million. As nations such as India and China, which together comprise 38% of the world's population, continue to progress economically, the car population in these and other less developed countries also will increase. Car manufacturers will rejoice, but the effects on air and land pollution will be devastating.

A modern U.S. car with a catalytic converter to reduce emissions still produces about 20 pounds of carbon dioxide for every gallon of gas that is burned; this is a significant factor in global warming. Over an average 10-year life, each American car spews 50 tons of carbon dioxide into the atmosphere. If mileage standards were increased and cars were made still more fuel efficient, CO_2 emissions could be reduced significantly.

One major victory in the battle against air pollution was the elimination of lead in gasoline in the United States. There is evidence that the phaseout of leaded gasoline, which began in 1984, has markedly reduced the blood levels of lead in the U.S. population (Figure 24.1). This battle to eliminate lead in gasoline took over 10 years to accomplish, which shows the amount of time and effort that goes into changing just one factor in air pollution. Efforts are ongoing to develop less polluting fuels.

The battle over clean air pits the Environmental Protection Agency (EPA), which is responsible for air quality and pollution standards, against much of U.S. industry, which finds flaws in the scientific research on the causes and effects of air pollution. Most industries balk at making changes that will cut into profits

and make them less competitive with foreign companies that do not have to be concerned about pollution.

The evidence that particulate matter is a health hazard is quite strong, but industries argue that other air pollutants underlie the health problems and that particulates are not responsible. It required more than 10 years of heated debate and legal wrangling to prove that lead from gasoline was damaging the brains of young children. Many years of effort and research were devoted to showing that chlorofluorocarbons (CFCs) were destroying the ozone layer that protects the earth's surface from harmful UV irradiation. Eventually, both lead in gasoline and CFCs were banned. These two examples show that improving air quality is a long and tedious process.

For several days a month the air quality over Mexico City is already so dangerous that officials limit the use of automobiles on those days. However, recent research indicates that a significant amount of Mexico City's air pollution results from leakage of gases from tanks of liquified petroleum gas that millions of people use to cook with. Solving this problem is much more difficult than banning the use of automobiles on certain days.

In the fall of 1997, the air over Southeast Asia (i.e., Indonesia, Malaysia, Thailand) was made virtually unbreathable for several months, which was caused by fires that were raging in Indonesia as a result of

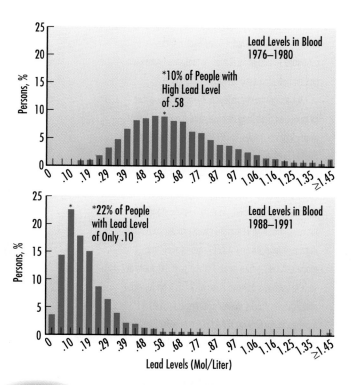

FIGURE 24.1   **Reduction in Blood Lead Levels in the U.S. Population as a Result of the Elimination of Leaded Gasoline**
Source: Data from the National Health and Nutrition Examination Survey, 1990.

agricultural burning. People had to stay indoors or move about with masks over their nose and mouth. Air quality continues to deteriorate around the world and eventually affects everyone.

Acid Rain

Acid rain is rainwater containing large amounts of sulfur dioxide and nitrogen oxides that have been released into the atmosphere. When these gases combine with water, they produce sulfuric acid and nitric acid, which are dispersed in the rain. Acid rain harms forests, and raises the acidity of lakes and rivers to levels that kill fish and vegetation. Acid rain is a global problem.

Canada and the U.S. began to monitor the extent of acid rain damage to lakes and streams in the 1970s, and both countries have since tried to reduce their emissions of sulfur dioxide gas. Since 1980, the U.S. has cut sulfur dioxide emissions by 30%, but the problem of acid rain in eastern Canada does not seem to be improving significantly. Canada has cut its sulfur dioxide emissions by much more than the U.S., but it now appears that both countries will have to make deeper cuts in sulfur dioxide emissions if lakes, streams, and forests are to be saved from further destruction.

Solutions to the acid rain problem involve difficult economic and political decisions. Acid rain can fall hundreds of miles from the source of the sulfur

Dollars and Health Sense

The United States Is the World's Biggest Energy User and Greatest Polluter

The United States is the third most populous country in the world after China and India, but Americans still have less than 5% of the world's population. However, Americans consume about 25% of the world's energy, largely in the form of gasoline. In 1997, approximately 501 million automobiles were registered in the world. About 125 million or one fourth of the total were registered in the United States. Americans' passion for bigger, more powerful passenger vehicles continues to add to increased automobile emissions and air pollution (see figure).

If cars got better mileage, there would be less air pollution, less lung disease, and a reduced threat from global warming. In 1976, the U.S. Congress tried to deal with the problem of excessive energy use by automobiles when it passed the Energy Policy and Conservation Act, a law that requires car and truck manufacturers to meet certain standards for fuel efficiency. These standards, called *corporate average fuel economy* (CAFE), are applied to a manufacturer's entire fleet. For the past 10 years or so, CAFE standards have been at 27.5 mph for cars and 20.5 for trucks. Manufacturers, however, manage to circumvent the CAFE standards. Small trucks, minivans, and SUVs are classified as trucks and thereby qualify for the lower mileage standard. Of course, as everyone knows, these vehicles are

purchased almost exclusively for use as passenger vehicles—not for use as working trucks.

Any effort by Congress to increase fleet fuel efficiency by increasing CAFE is vigorously (and successfully) lobbied against by automobile manufacturers. In 2001, increased public pressure did force a small change in the CAFE standards, but not large enough to make much difference in fuel

conservation or air pollution. Attempts to reclassify SUVs and minivans as passenger cars also have been thwarted. Manufacturers claim they are giving the American people what they want—large, heavy passenger vehicles—regardless of fuel use. As long as this philosophy prevails, America will continue to be the world's greatest user of energy and major contributor to air pollution.

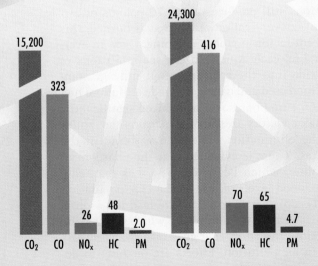

Standard Automobile   **Light truck/SUV**

Pounds of Pollutants Emitted Annually by a Standard Automobile as Compared to a Light Truck or SUV. (Emissions by light trucks and SUVs are virtually identical.)

Abbreviations: CO_2—carbon dioxide; CO—carbon monoxide; NOx—nitrogen oxides; HC—hydrocarbons; PM—particulate matter

Source: Green Guide to Cars and Trucks, 1999

dioxide emission, making it difficult to determine the exact source and responsibility. Acid rain does not observe national boundaries, so countries must cooperate if the problem is to be solved. Like other atmospheric pollution problems, acid rain is likely to fall far into the future.

Carbon Dioxide and Global Warming

Along with the gases oxygen (O_2) and nitrogen (N_2), carbon dioxide (CO_2) is a natural component of Earth's atmosphere. Plants use carbon dioxide to manufacture more plant material, and in the process, they give off oxygen that animals breathe. Carbon dioxide in air also is absorbed into oceans, where it forms carbonate-containing rocks.

Before humans began burning coal, oil, and natural gas in vast quantities to fuel the industrial revolution, the level of carbon dioxide in the atmosphere was fairly constant at about 290 parts per million (ppm) (see Figure 24.2). By 1920, the level of atmospheric CO_2 rose to about 300 ppm, and by 1950 it rose further to about 315 ppm. In the last half of the 20th century, the level of atmospheric CO_2 jumped to around 375 ppm and is still climbing.

In 1861, an English scientist pointed out that carbon dioxide is a good absorber of infrared radiation. When sunlight lands on the earth's surface, some of the energy in the light is radiated back toward space as infrared radiation or heat. Carbon dioxide absorbs the infrared radiation and thereby traps heat in the atmosphere. Because this process is analogous to how a garden greenhouse works, this phenomenon is called the **greenhouse effect** (see Figure 24.3).

In the last half of the 20th century, scientists debated whether or not the increase of atmospheric CO_2 (and other "greenhouse gases" such as methane, nitrogen oxides, etc.) would, in fact, heat up the atmosphere like the inside of a greenhouse and lead to global warming. Some argued that the earth can absorb additional CO_2 in the oceans and in additional plant material without increasing average global temperature. It became apparent in the 1990s, however, that the earth's temperature *is* increasing (see Figure 24.4) and it *is not* due to natural fluctuations in the global climate; nearly all scientists now believe that the rise

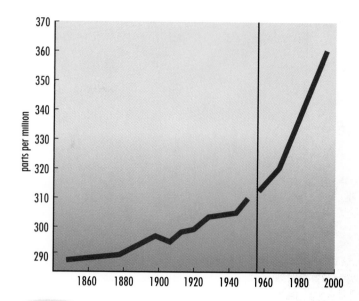

FIGURE 24.2   **Carbon Dioxide (CO_2) Levels in the Atmosphere**   Data prior to 1953 are from CO_2 measured in ice cores. Data after 1953 are direct measurements in the atmosphere. *Source:* National Oceanic and Atmospheric Administration

in global temperature is due to human activity (*Science,* 2001). If humans continue to pump greenhouse gases into the atmosphere, it is predicted that by 2100 the temperature of Earth will increase 5–10 degrees Fahrenheit. Five to ten degrees may not seem like much, but in climatic terms it is a tremendous

Terms

acid rain: rain, snow, fog, mist, etc., with a pH lower than 5.6

greenhouse effect: the ability of atmospheric carbon dioxide to reflect heat radiated from the earth back to the earth and to thereby raise the earth's temperature globally

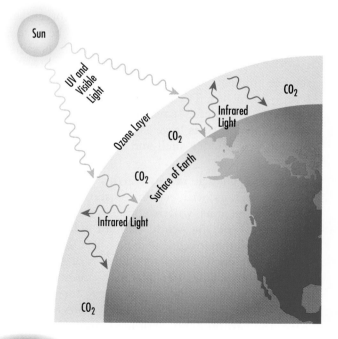

FIGURE 24.3   **Greenhouse Effect**   Carbon dioxide (CO_2) in the earth's atmosphere acts like the glass roof in a greenhouse. Carbon dioxide is transparent to the radiation from the sun and lets it pass to the ground, which warms up.

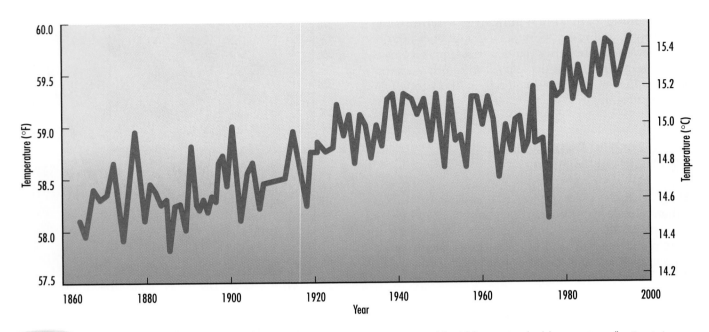

FIGURE 24.4   **Global Temperature Changes (1880–2000)**   *Almost all atmospheric scientists are convinced that global warming is real and that temperatures will continue to rise un-less CO$_2$ emissions are reduced.*   *Source:* U.S. National Climatic Data Center

change. Some of the predicted effects of such global warming include:

- **A rise in sea level from the melting of ice masses in the Arctic, Antarctic, and on mountaintops suffi-cient to flood coastal and low-lying regions all over the world.** A three-degree increase in global tem-perature will raise sea level one to three feet. People would be forced to relocate, possibly resulting in massive refugee problems. During the past century, sea level rose 4–10 inches. The Arctic Ocean and tundra no longer are completely covered with ice during win-ter. Chunks of ice as large as Delaware have broken off the Antarctic ice shelf and melted in the south-ern oceans.

> *It ain't what we don't know that gives us trouble, it's what we know that ain't so that gives us trouble.*
>
> WILL ROGERS

- **A massive change in the earth's climate.** Some tropical regions will become deserts while some temperate regions will become more tropical. In some parts of the world rainfall will increase, whereas in others it will decrease. Winters may be-come a bit more temperate with less snow, and summers may be hotter and more humid. Global climate change certainly will affect food produc-tion throughout the world in a variety of ways. Also, the natural habitats of land- and water-living plants and animals will change.

- Many diseases, particularly insect-borne diseases, will spread to new regions. Dengue fever, previously

unknown in South America, is now prevalent and has spread as far north as Texas. Malaria will spread widely to warmer areas (Patz et al., 1996).

- The number and intensity of violent storms—hurri-canes, cyclones, drought, blizzards, and wildfires—will increase globally. Since 1992, record-setting storms have struck countries around the world and produced weather changes, including record rainfall, drought, hurricanes, and tornados in regions of the United States.

At an international conference on global warming in Kyoto, Japan, in December 1997, a historic treaty was signed that will dramatically reduce the global emissions of CO$_2$ by all of the industrialized nations. The U.S., which produces about 25% of the world's CO$_2$ emissions, agreed to reduce levels to 7% below the 1990 levels by the year 2012. However in early 2001, President Bush repudiated the Kyoto agreement, arguing that the commitment to drastically curtail CO$_2$ emissions will require a complete revamping of the coal, petroleum, automotive, electricity-generat-ing, and other major industries in the United States and thus, harm the country's economy.

The opposition to such sweeping changes in the U.S. economy, which comes from these industries, la-bor unions, and a population that has become depen-dent on energy and its consequent CO$_2$ emissions, will present unprecedented political obstacles to rati-fication of the global warming treaty by the U.S. Sen-ate. Ultimately, the choice of what happens to our en-vironment will be up to the American people; if they want to protect the world for their children and grandchildren, making changes in lifestyles now is critical to reducing CO_2 emissions in the coming years.

The Ozone Layer

The **ozone layer** consists of ozone molecules (i.e., 3 atoms of oxygen bonded together: O_3) that form a layer in the outermost region of the earth's atmosphere. The ozone layer absorbs much of the dangerous ultraviolet (UV) light that is radiated from the sun, and protects us from excessive exposure to UV radiation that can increase the risk of skin cancer and cataracts in the lens of the eye. The ozone in the ozone layer is the same chemical produced in photochemical smog. However, in the upper reaches of the atmosphere ozone protects life, whereas at ground-level it is a toxic irritant.

A class of chemicals called **chlorofluorocarbons (CFCs)** have been widely used as refrigerant gases and as propellant gases in cans during the past 30 years. These CFCs escape into the atmosphere and rise to the ozone layer where they destroy ozone molecules. In the 1970s it was discovered that the ozone layer was thinning; over the Antarctic an **ozone hole** appears during the Antarctic spring (September to October) and ozone disappears completely in that region. The ozone hole has now spread over populated areas of Asia and northern Europe (Figure 24.5). The intensity of UV radiation in these areas is increasing, exposing people to a higher risk of skin cancer and cataracts.

When the seriousness of the thinning of the ozone layer was realized, 31 industrialized countries agreed in 1987 to phase out the use of CFCs. Even though CFC use has now dropped significantly, the large

TABLE 24.2   **Major Sources of Emission of a Pollutant versus Major Sources of Exposure to It***

Pollutant	Major emission sources	Major exposure sources
Benzene	Industry; automobiles	Smoking
Tetrachloroethylene	Dry-cleaning shops	Dry-cleaned clothes
Chloroform	Sewage treatment plants	Showers
p-Dichlorobenzene	Chemical manufacturing	Air deodorizers
Particulates	Industry; automobiles; home heating	Smoker at home
Carbon monoxide	Automobiles	Driving; gas stoves
Nitrogen dioxide	Industry; automobiles	Gas stoves

*For many hazardous airborne pollutants, the health risk is not related significantly to the major source of emission (as shown in Figure 24.5).

amounts of these chemicals already in the atmosphere will cause the ozone layer to continue to thin for the rest of this century and will cause health problems for millions of people.

Evaluating the Risks of Air Pollution

In evaluating the health hazards of toxic air pollutants, two important factors must be evaluated separately. **Emission** refers to the amount of a substance that is released into the atmosphere from an automobile or other source of air pollution. **Exposure** refers to the amount of the substance to which people are exposed. Frequently, emission can be high, while exposure is low. Alternatively, emission can be low, while exposure is high.

For many air pollutants, such as carbon monoxide, benzene, and chloroform, the major sources of emissions are automobiles, industry, and sewage treatment plants, respectively. However, the major health risks from these substances are *not* from the sources of highest emission, but from gas stoves, cigarettes, and chloroform in shower water, respectively (Table 24.2).

To regulate all of the possible pollutants of the air is impossible, so it is important to identify both the

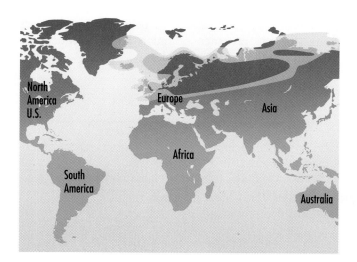

FIGURE 24.5   **The "Ozone Hole"**   Since its discovery in 1985, the ozone hole has spread dramatically. Lighter color shows the area of most damage to the ozone layer; the darker color shows somewhat less damage.

Source: NASA.

Terms

ozone layer: a layer of ozone molecules located in the stratosphere in a diffuse band extending from 10 to 30 miles above the earth's surface

chlorofluorocarbons (CFCs): chemicals formerly used as coolants that are released into the atmosphere and are responsible for destroying stratospheric ozone

ozone hole: an ozone-deficient portion of the atmosphere above Antarctica that has been steadily growing since the problem was first reported in 1985

emission: amount of substance that is released into the atmosphere

exposure: actual amount of the substance people are exposed to

sources of greatest emission and the sources of greatest exposure. For example, benzene is an important chemical used in many industrial processes; it also can cause leukemia in people who are exposed to it. Of all the benzene released into the air, 50% comes from automobiles. However, although cigarettes emit only a tiny amount of benzene compared with automobiles, at least half of the total population's exposure to benzene comes from smoking cigarettes (Figure 24.6). Even nonsmokers get most of their exposure to benzene from second-hand cigarette smoke as opposed to benzene from automobile exhausts. The most serious indoor air pollutant is cigarette smoke.

Indoor Pollution

Cigarette smoke is not only harmful to the person who smokes, but the "second-hand smoke" that is produced is harmful to others who breathe it (see chapter 17). The carbon monoxide levels in smoke-filled rooms can rise to hazardous levels. For example, in bars and conference rooms where many people are smoking, the air may contain levels of carbon monoxide as high as 50 ppm. This level is sufficient to produce headache, nausea, impaired judgment, and other symptoms (Table 24.3).

Radon

Another form of indoor air pollution is **radon**, a radioactive gas that is invisible and odorless. Radon is naturally produced in the ground in areas that contain uranium ore. In New Jersey, for example, some homes built on top of rocks that contain uranium ore have over one hundred times the safe level of radon in air inside the house. Homes also may be constructed from bricks or building materials that contain radioactive minerals, one of the decay products of which is

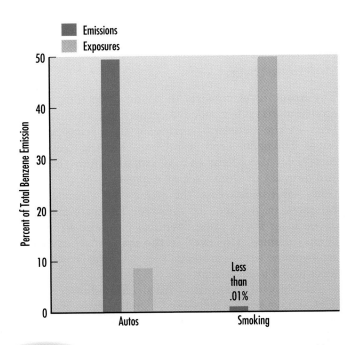

FIGURE 24.6   **Benzene Emissions**   Automobiles emit the greatest amount of benzene into the air—about 50% of the total. However, in terms of the amount of benzene that people inhale, most exposure comes from cigarette smoking.

radon gas. The radon is slowly released into the house over many years.

Long-term exposure to radon increases the risk of lung cancer. Uranium miners exposed to radon for years have a much higher risk of lung cancer than average people not occupationally exposed to the gas. Cigarette smoking seems to act synergistically with radon; smokers who also are exposed to radon get lung cancer at rates much higher than individuals whose exposure is limited solely to cigarette smoke or solely to radon. The EPA estimates that radon exposure in homes is responsible for as many as 30,000 deaths from lung cancer a year. It is possible to test one's home for the presence of radon and to reduce the amount of radon if it is found.

TABLE 24.3   **Symptoms of Carbon Monoxide (CO) Poisoning**

CO blood level (%)	Symptoms
0–2	No symptoms.
2–5	No symptoms in most people, but sensitive tests reveal slight impairment of arithmetic and other cognitive abilities. Levels of 2–5% are found in light or moderate smokers.
5–10	Slight breathlessness on severe exertion. Levels of 5–10% are found in smokers who inhale one or more packs of cigarettes per day.
10–20	Mild headache, breathlessness on moderate exertion. These levels are sometimes seen in smokers who are exposed to additional CO from other sources.
20–30	Throbbing headache, irritability, impaired judgment, defective memory, rapid fatigue.
30–40	Severe headache, weakness, nausea, dimness of vision, confusion.
40–50	Confusion, hallucinations, ataxia, hyperventilation, and collapse.
50–60	Deep coma with possible convulsions.
Above 60	Usually results in death.

TABLE 24.4   Effects of Lead in People

Lead blood level (μg/dl)	Observable effects
10	Enzyme inhibition, learning disabilities
15–40	Red blood cells affected
40–50	Anemia, infertility (men)
50–60	Central nervous system effects, cognitive disabilities
60–100	Permanent brain damage, death

Lead Pollution

Lead is a heavy metal that is a serious threat to the health of millions of Americans, especially children. Lead contaminates air, land, water, and houses that still contain lead-based paints. Early symptoms of **plumbism** (lead poisoning) are loss of appetite, weakness, and anemia (Table 24.4). Lead poisoning also causes brain damage and is responsible for an enormous number of learning problems among children. For every 10 μg/dL increase in blood lead levels, IQ test scores are reduced by two to three points.

Poor children account for 60% of 1 to 5 year olds with blood lead levels greater than 10 μg/dL; they account for 83% of children with levels greater than 20 μg/dL (Centers for Disease Control, 2000). These children live in old, decrepit inner-city housing that may contain lead-based paints that flake off. Small children may eat the paint flakes and also ingest lead in the house dust. Health policy to prevent damage from lead poisoning in children focuses on screening all children for lead and using chemicals to detoxify the lead in the body. Unfortunately, neurological damage from lead poisoning cannot be reversed by detoxification (Rosen and Mushak, 2001). The best way to prevent learning disabilities in children caused by lead pollution is to clean up the environment.

Another study has documented that attention-deficit disorders, aggression, and delinquency are associated with low levels of lead toxicity and that the higher the blood lead levels are, the greater the symptoms of aberrant behaviors among affected children (Needleman et al., 1996). Despite the progress society has made in reducing lead contamination of the environment, the neurological development of millions of children is still at risk from lead toxicity.

Terms

radon: a radioactive gas found in some homes that can increase the risk of cancer

plumbism: disease caused by lead poisoning

Lead is important to many industries, particularly the battery industry, so it is still an uphill battle to reduce the amount of lead released into the environment and to clean up all sources of lead poisoning. Most of the children who suffer from lead poisoning come from poor families with little political power, so the government has not conducted an all-out effort to further reduce the lead in the environment.

Water Pollution

After air, water is probably the body's most essential requirement. We can survive without air for only a few minutes and without water perhaps for several days. The human body is composed of about 60% water, which is essential to every function carried out by organs in the body.

Agriculture, cities, and industry in this country are enormous consumers of water. For example, producing a gallon of gasoline requires five gallons of water; brewing a barrel of beer consumes a thousand gallons; a ton of newspaper takes about 50,000 gallons; a ton of steel requires 25,000 gallons; and irrigating an acre of orange trees requires almost a million gallons of water a year. A family of four uses about 600 gallons of water daily.

Water is continuously recycled in the environment by evaporation and rain. However, as more and more water becomes polluted from pesticides, chemicals, oil spills, and sewage, less and less water is suitable for human consumption and agricultural use. Of special concern is the chemical contamination of rivers, lakes, and underground water supplies, which provide most of our water needs. Around the world, safe, sufficient water supplies are stretched to the limit (Gleick, 2000).

Waterborne diseases, such as cholera, typhoid fever, and dysentery, have been virtually eliminated in North America through sanitation and water treatment methods. In many communities, the water supplied to homes is purified by sedimentation, filtration, or chlorination. The addition of chlorine to water kills dangerous bacteria; however, it may create other health hazards. Interaction of chlorine with other chemicals in the water produces toxic substances, such as chloroform and chloramines, which are cancer-causing agents. The widespread use of detergents, herbicides, pesticides, fertilizers, and other chemicals also has contributed to increased water pollution. In 1993, more than 400,000 persons in the city of Milwaukee were made sick (and more than 50 people died) because the municipal drinking water had become contaminated by the protozoan *Cryptosporidium* which can bypass standard water treatment processes.

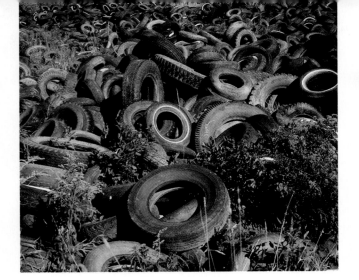

Do you ever think about what happens to your old tires? It's not a pretty picture, but it's a problem we have to solve.

In the early 1970s, the Environmental Protection Agency found that the water supplies of many towns and cities were dangerously contaminated with pathogenic organisms and toxic chemicals. As a result of these findings, Congress passed the Safe Drinking Water Act of 1974, which covers 58,000 community water supply systems and another 160,000 private systems. The Act requires that these systems meet federal drinking water safety standards; but it is one thing to pass such a law and another thing to enforce it.

In 1996, Congress renewed the Safe Drinking Water Act of 1974. Under the new act, consumers must be notified whenever contaminants are found in drinking water and not merely when the water does not meet federal standards for contamination and safety. Community water systems in the United States must be tested for 80 contaminants. Each year, about 7% of community water systems report exceeding federal safety levels for at least one contaminant.

Because millions of Americans still are supplied with water that does not meet federal standards for health and safety, people are purchasing bottled water and water purifying equipment in ever-increasing amounts.

Until relatively recently, little attention was paid to the disposal of garbage and solid wastes in landfills around the country. Now, however, we are beginning to run out of space to dump the stuff we want to get rid of. Each year in the U.S., we junk about 8 million cars and trucks; 100 billion cans, bottles, and jars; and more than 200 million tons of garbage. The average American generates more than twice as much garbage as citizens of other industrialized countries. The United States produces 1,584 pounds of trash per person annually; Japan, 902 pounds; and the European Union, 660 pounds.

Many old, abandoned solid waste disposal sites are dangerous to health because they contain hazardous materials that may be corrosive, flammable, or contain toxic chemicals (Table 24.5). In 1980, Congress passed the Superfund Act, which provides for the clean-up of the most dangerous waste sites. By 2000, only 757 of the 1,509 hazardous sites on the Superfund list had been cleaned up. The average cost to clean up a site has been $27 million. These high costs prompt many people to believe we should be looking for more environmentally safe ways of manufacturing what we need and of recycling what we discard.

For example, discarded automobile tires are a major problem for landfills. Americans throw away about 250 million tires a year. Experts have suggested that the government should investigate environmentally safe ways to use the scrapped tires to generate electricity. Each automobile tire is the equivalent of about 2.5 gallons of oil. Stacked up in landfills around the country are tires that add up to about 178 million barrels of oil. But political and economic pressures force the U.S. to import foreign oil, rather than explore new ways to clean up the environment and produce energy.

 ## Pesticides

Soil, water, and some foods have become increasingly contaminated with chemicals used to control weeds,

TABLE 24.5 Hazardous Wastes That Escape into the Environment Cause Many Health Problems
Millions of tons of these substances are discarded every year in the U.S.

Substance	Source	Health effects
Mercury	Sludge from chloralkali plants; electrical equipment, fluorescent lights	Tremors, mental retardation, loss of teeth, kidney damage, neurological damage
Arsenic	Arsenic trioxide from coal combustion and from metal smelters	Diarrhea, vomiting, paralysis, skin cancers
Cadmium	Waste from electroplating industry; paint containers, nickel-cadmium batteries	Lung diseases
Cyanide	Electroplating industry waste	Poisoning, interferes with cellular energy metabolism
Pesticides	Solid wastes and wastes in solutions	Multiple effects including rashes, respiratory and gastrointestinal symptoms, neurological disorders, hemorrhages

Wellness Guide

Precautions for Pesticide Use

- Before you buy a pesticide product, read the instructions for use and any health and safety warnings. When mixing, do not increase the concentration of the pesticide above the label-recommended amount. Do not purchase the product if you can't use the pesticide properly (you may not have the right equipment). If you don't understand or feel completely comfortable with the health and safety information provided, get more information before you buy the product. Also, consider whether you have adequate storage space for the pesticide. A bigger bottle may be cheaper, but can you store it safely?

- Use the least toxic pesticide available for your pest control problem. Try to strike a balance between effective pest control and the safety of people, pets, and other nontarget organisms. Minimize skin and respiratory contact with pesticides. Wear rubber gloves. When you select gloves, consider both the solvent used in the pesticide formulation and the possibility that the pesticide itself can penetrate skin. You may want to use a respirator to guard against inhaling pesticide spray or dust.

- Use pesticides only for the uses for which they are intended. For instance, some wood preservatives are meant for outside use only, so don't use them inside the house!

- Don't leave seemingly empty pesticide containers where children can get them. Children have been poisoned by drinking from "empty" containers that actually contained leftover pesticide.

- Never smoke, eat, or drink while using pesticides.

---

insects, and plant diseases in the environment. Any chemical capable of killing is called a **pesticide.** Specific kinds of chemicals that destroy certain kinds of organisms are **insecticides** (kills insects), **fungicides** (kills molds and fungi), **herbicides** (kills weeds), and **rodenticides** (kills rats and mice). Pesticides are important to the agriculture industry, which has claimed over the years that the abundance and quality of food grown in the United States depend on the use of chemicals to destroy crop pests. While pesticides may contribute to agricultural productivity (although this is contested by people who practice organic farming), widespread dissemination of pesticides in the environment has created health and pollution problems for people and animals.

The evidence over the safety of pesticide use is both confusing and controversial. Pesticide manufacturers claim that their products are perfectly safe when used as directed. Monitoring of pesticide residues on food shows that the levels are not dangerous. However, consumer groups and many scientists argue that pesticides cause much more harm than good both to people and to the environment and are responsible for many serious health problems.

Many pesticides have been found to be so dangerous that their use has been banned by the EPA, the federal agency that regulates pesticide use. One of the most widely used pesticides, DDT, was found to be carcinogenic and was banned by the EPA more than 20 years ago.

The use of other pesticides such as heptachlor, kepone, dieldrin, mirex, and toxophene has been banned and these chemicals have been off the market in the United States for a number of years. The quandary faced by the EPA is balancing the necessary use of

Terms

pesticide: a chemical that kills unwanted organisms
insecticide: a pesticide that kills insects
fungicide: a chemical that kills fungi
herbicide: a chemical that kills weeds
rodenticide: a chemical that kills mice and rats

Many people would like to see the use of pesticides on our food supply reduced.

chemicals by agriculture and other industries while safeguarding the public's health. Also many of the banned pesticides are still in use in other countries around the world.

Millions of homes in the United States have been treated for termite control. Until recently, the two most commonly used chemicals for killing termites were chlordane and heptachlor, both related in chemical structure to DDT. These chemicals do not break down; they persist in houses and the environment for at least 25 years. Exposure to these pesticides is claimed by some to cause headaches, breathing problems, fatigue, nervous system disorders, liver and kidney damage, and possibly cancer. Some people have had to abandon their homes because of health problems resulting from the pesticides used to kill termites.

Generally, the health effects of pesticides on people and other animals are subtle. For the most part, pesticides do not cause sudden, severe sickness or death unless the amount of exposure is extremely high. The amount of pesticide capable of causing death varies widely depending on the specific chemical as well as on individual susceptibility to these poisons. For some insecticides and rodenticides, a very small amount can kill a full-grown person. However, there is growing concern over pesticide residues in the environment that mimic hormones and may be responsible for the increase in breast and uterine cancer (Davis et al., 1993).

Year after year, thousands of tons of various pesticides are released into the environment. Most of these chemicals do not degrade easily, and they accumulate in soil, lakes, and rivers. Plants and animals in the environment absorb chemicals, which become more and more concentrated as they move up the food chain.

Many large animals, birds, and fish now have high levels of pesticides in their tissues. For example, in a lake in Florida, 80% to 95% of alligator eggs have failed to hatch in recent years, a mortality rate of 10 times normal. The alligator eggs contain abnormal levels of estrogen and testosterone, which are essential reproductive hormones in all animals. The few male and female alligators that do survive are reproductively abnormal, and males have abnormally small penises. A pesticide called **dicofol,** similar to DDT in structure, is present in the lake as a result of dumping by a chemical company that used to operate on its shore. Dicofol mimics the action of estrogen and causes abnormalities in reproduction and in sexual development (Raloff, 1995).

As a society, we are not ready to abandon the use of pesticides. However, as individuals we should restrict our use of pesticides as much as possible to protect ourselves and the environment. To achieve this goal, many people now grow their own vegetables without the use of pesticides. Others shop at stores that sell fruits and vegetables grown without the use of pesticides and herbicides.

Polychlorinated Biphenyls (PCBs)

Polychlorinated biphenyls (PCBs) belong to a family of more than 200 structurally related chemicals that were widely used from 1930 until the late 1970s as industrial coolants, especially in power transformers. PCBs were found to cause cancer in laboratory animals and have been banned for more than 20 years in the United States. However, they persist in the environment and may have contributed to the death of seals and other animals in water contaminated with PCBs. Even though use of PCBs has been banned for years, they persist in the environment and in the bodies of people who were exposed. In this century, more than 120 different kinds of PCBs have been manufactured, and the World Wildlife Fund estimates that at least a billion pounds have been dispersed into the environment worldwide.

Studies of children born in the 1980s in Michigan indicate that prenatal exposure to PCBs caused developmental delays, learning impairment, and lower IQ scores. While most of these middle-class children are still within the normal range of IQ, they are at the lower end of normal (Jacobson & Jacobson, 1996).

Endocrine Disruptors

Endocrine disruptors are chemical substances in the environment that can get into the body and interfere with the action of one or more hormones. Some endocrine disruptors mimic the effects of a hormone, causing overstimulation of a normally regulated biological process. Other endocrine disruptors block the actions of normal hormones, thereby lessening or completely inhibiting a biological process. Because hormones are present in the body in very small amounts, it does not take much for an endocrine disruptor to affect hormone signaling.

Terms

dicofol: a pesticide that mimics the action of estrogen and causes reproductive abnormalities

polychlorinated biphenyls (PCBs): a family of banned synthetic, organic chemicals that affect the human thyroid gland and reproductive systems of animals

endocrine disruptors: chemical substances in the environment that interfere with the actions of one or more of the body's hormones

electromagnetic fields (EMFs): a form of radiation produced by electrical power lines and appliances that may increase the risk of cancer

Some endocrine disruptors are well-known pollutants such as DDT, PCBs, and chlordane. These substances have been banned because of their toxicity and negative effects on the environment. However, because they were used in such large amounts, they still persist in water and soil and continue to act as endocrine disruptors. Other endocrine disruptors include dioxin, produced by incineration in industrial processes, and phthalates, chemicals used in the manufacture of plastic wrap, food containers, garden hoses, children's toys, babies' pacifiers, fingernail polish, and perfumes.

The effect of endocrine disruptors on human health is still being investigated. One study found that adolescents exposed to dioxin and PCBs from nearby waste incinerators matured sexually at an older age (and boys had smaller testicles) than children not exposed to these chemicals (Staessen et al., 2001). In another study, 75% of girls with premature breast development were found to have high levels of phthalates in their blood (Colon et al., 2000). In adults, male workers exposed to phthalates used in the manufacture of plastics had an increased risk of testicular cancer (Ohlson and Hardell, 2001).

Electromagnetic Fields (EMFs)

Electric power lines, appliances, motors, TV sets, microwave ovens, and power tools all emit very low frequency **electromagnetic fields (EMFs).** Except for the earth's electromagnetic field, all EMFs come from electricity that is generated by electrical devices of all kinds (Table 24.6). Only in the past few generations have people been exposed to the magnetic fields. Until recently, these EMFs were thought to be too weak

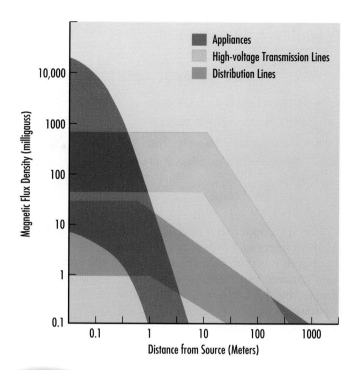

FIGURE 24.7   **Strength of Magnetic Fields from Sources of Electromagnetic Fields (EMFs)**   Small appliances produce strong fields, but the strength disappears within a few feet. High-voltage lines produce less dense magnetic fields but they cover a large area.
Source: Adapted from Keith Florig.

to affect living organisms, so their impact on health was ignored.

Some epidemiological studies have found an association between the incidence of childhood leukemia and brain tumors and exposure to EMFs. Families that live close to high voltage power lines or electrical distribution boxes tend to experience more sickness and more cancers. However, a very careful study of the risks of childhood leukemia and exposure to EMFs showed that the risk of cancer was not increased (UK Childhood Cancer Study, 1999). On the other hand, studies suggest that exposure to EMFs among adult railway workers are associated with a higher risk for leukemia (Savitz, 2001). And although there has been concern about an association of cell phone use and a higher risk of brain cancer, epidemiological studies have failed to confirm such a risk (Johansen et al., 2001).

All of us are exposed to EMFs every day. An electric shaver or hair dryer puts out a strong EMF, although users are exposed for only a few minutes a day (Figure 24.7). If a person lives near a high-voltage transmission line, exposure to EMFs may be considerable depending on the distance between the house and the wires. And the exposure goes on day and night. Calculating EMF exposure, at best, yields crude approximations, one reason why the evidence regarding EMFs and harmful health effects is conflicting.

TABLE 24.6   **Strength of Electromagnetic Fields from Household Sources**
Many electrical appliances, especially ones with motors, produce very strong magnetic fields, but the strength of the field falls rapidly with increasing distance from the appliance.

Source	Intensity (milligauss) at distance from source	
	At 4 cm	At 20 cm
100-watt bulb	2.5	—
Refrigerator (back)	11	5
200-watt stereo	27	5
80-watt fluorescent bulb	34	18
Coffeemaker	90	7
Electric drill	600	6
Hair dryer	1,000	0.1

Wellness Guide

- Don't use an electric blanket or water bed heater unless it is a newer model with reduced EMFs.
- Use battery-operated shavers and hair dryers. Battery-operated appliances and toys do not put out EMFs.

- Don't sit too close to computers, TVs, fans, or light fixtures.
- If your work requires long exposure to EMFs, look for ways to reduce it. Do not sit too close to computer screens for long periods.

- If you rent or buy a house, choose one that is not near a high-voltage line or distribution transformer.

Despite extensive research on the biological and health effects of EMFs, the only conclusions that can be drawn are that EMFs *may* increase the risk of certain cancers and *may* contribute to ill health, for example, by diminishing the functions of the immune system.

Based on current research, the risk to health from exposure to EMFs must be regarded as small compared with the risks of chemical pollutants in air, soil, water, and food. Moreover, our lives are so dependent on electricity and the gadgets that make life more comfortable that major changes in electrical use are not anticipated.

Noise Pollution

Have you ever been kept awake at night by a dripping faucet or a neighbor's party? Does the sound of sirens and horns put you on edge? Have you ever found yourself thinking, "If that noise doesn't stop, I'm going to scream"? Everyone is sensitive to noise, and excessive noise produces stress and can cause health problems. Noise interferes with sleep and over periods of time can cause fatigue, irritability, tension, and anxiety.

Sound activates the nervous system, thereby affecting functions of the endocrine, cardiovascular, and reproductive systems. Noise is a "stressor" and can increase blood pressure, alter hormone levels, constrict blood vessels, and cause intense pain at high levels.

Sound levels are measured in **decibels** (dB). The danger zone for hearing loss begins at about 85 dB, a level present on schoolbuses crowded with kids or driving in freeway traffic with the window open (Table 24.7). Many daily activities expose us to sound levels

that can permanently damage hearing. An estimated 20 million men, women, and children in the United States are exposed to dangerous levels of sound every day that can cause hearing loss (Flodin, 1992).

Rock musicians and people who listen to loud rock music are particularly at risk for hearing loss. Members of many famous rock bands suffer from **tinnitus,** a persistent ringing in the ears, or have lost a significant amount of their hearing. Children are especially prone to turning up the volume and to listening to music with earphones at dangerously high sound levels.

Many people live and work amidst the din of urban life, and have forgotten the rest and peacefulness that come with silence. If you have the good fortune to spend time at isolated spots in the woods or at the ocean, you become aware of the beneficial effects of quiet. The human need for stillness was expressed elo-

TABLE 24.7 **Noise Levels Produced by Daily Activities and Machines**
A noise level above 85 dB can damage hearing and cause hearing loss over time.

Source of noise	Sound level (dB)
Firearms	140 to 170
Jet engines	140
Rock concerts	90 to 130
Amplified car stereos	140 (at full volume)
Portable stereos (e.g., Sony Walkman)	115 (at full volume)
Power mowers	105
Jackhammers	100
Subway trains	100
Video arcades	100
Freeway driving in a convertible	95
Power saws	95
Electric razors	85
Crowded school buses	85
School recesses or assemblies	85

Terms

decibel: a measure of noise level

tinnitus: persistent ringing in the ears often caused by repeated or sudden exposure to loud noises

quently in 1854 by Chief Seattle, after whom the modern city in Washington is named:

> There is no quiet place in the white man's cities. No place to hear the unfurling of leaves in spring or the rustle of insects' wings. But perhaps it is because I am a savage and do not understand. The clatter only seems to insult the ears. And what is there to life if a man cannot hear the lonely cry of the whippoorwill or the arguments of the frogs around a pond at night?

How Human Population Growth Affects Us

According to the United Nations, on October 12, 1999, the world's human population reached 6 billion. Forty years before, in 1960, the world's human population was 3 billion. At the current fertility rate of 2.7 children per woman, it is expected to reach 9 billion by 2050 (see Figure 24.8).

What do these numbers mean with respect to environmental degradation and human health? One unresolved question of a rapidly growing population is whether the world can produce enough food to feed its people. In addition, crowding and poverty lead to disease epidemics and increased crime, conditions that are already appearing in some areas of this country and around the world.

All of the world's environmental problems stem, in one way or another, from human activities and human overpopulation (Vitousek, 1997). Deforestation; loss of native species of plants and animals; depletion of natural resources; and air, water, and land pollution are all related to too many people needing too many scarce resources. The demand for modern lifestyles and products adds to the destruction and pollution of

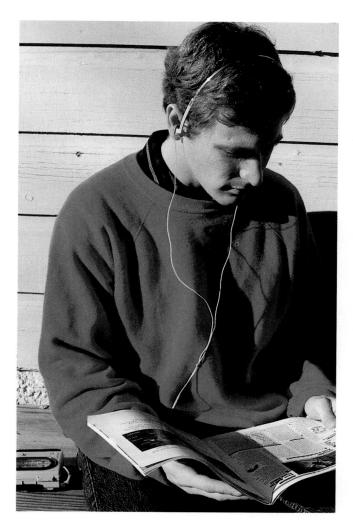

Keep the volume low to avoid hearing loss.

the environment. Indeed, as one close observer of nature has observed, we already may be witnessing the "end of nature," a process that progressed for billions of years before the emergence of human beings a few million years ago (McKibben, 1989).

The actions, needs, and goals of people are at the root of all environmental problems and the ongoing destruction of nature. As the economies of nations become stronger and aspirations of people around the globe increase, so does the rate of environmental destruction. Political and economic solutions to the population problem are discussed, but many

> *When you come to a fork in the road, take it.*
> YOGI BERRA

nations are unable or unwilling to undertake the measures that might curb population growth. Some countries have family planning programs, but the success of these programs depends on educating people and in raising their standard of living so that they understand that large families are not in their interest. Most of the world's population is opposed to any form

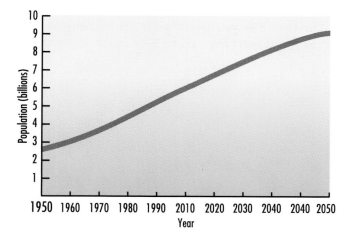

FIGURE 24.8   World Population from 1950–2050 (estimate)
Source: U.S. Bureau of the Census

of birth control, so the world's population is expected to continue to increase for at least the next 50 years.

The United States has made progress in reducing environmental pollution and in slowing population growth (the goal of most industrialized nations is zero population growth). Thanks to legislation, environmental lawsuits, and improved technology, air quality has improved, many waterways are cleaner than they were 20 years ago, and disposal of hazardous wastes has declined dramatically. While all this is good news, we have a long way to go in solving environmental and population problems. Most observers of the world's population growth are pessimistic about the future. As one physician observed: "*Homo sapiens* is destined to become *Homo extinctus* if the population increase continues without constraint and the resources of the planet are exhausted" (Wall, 1995).

> What we call the beginning is the end
> And to make an end is to make a beginning.
> The end is where we start from.
>
> —*T.S. Eliot*
> *Four Quartets*

Critical Thinking About Health

1. Check around your house or apartment, and make a list of all pesticides or herbicides that are stored anywhere. Decide which ones you really need to keep and which ones can be discarded. (Check with your local waste management authorities for proper disposal of pesticides and herbicides.) Make a list of how and when you use pesticides and what precautions you take when you use them. After doing this, write a report on how you can reduce your use and exposure to pesticides and herbicides.

2. The United States has made a commitment to lower carbon dioxide (CO_2) emissions dramatically in the next few years. To accomplish this, society must make major readjustments in the use of energy and transportation and in industrial output. Everyone will have to contribute to this effort. Begin by making a list of how you can:
   a. Reduce your electricity use by 30%. What appliances use the most electrical energy and what changes can you make to reduce their use?
   b. Reduce the use of your automobile by 30% or more. What changes in your lifestyle can you make that will reduce your dependence on car transportation?
   c. Find out what industries release the most CO_2 in manufacturing their products. Are these products essential to your life, or would you be able to live without some of them?

3. The major global threats to the environment are (a) nuclear, chemical, and biological warfare; (b) depletion of the ozone layer; (c) global warming; (d) land and ocean degradation; and (e) extinction of species of plants and animals. Indicate which of these global environmental problems is of the most concern to you personally. What can you personally do about the problem? What do you think governments should do about the problem? Discuss any effects that you think this problem will have on your life now and in the future.

4. If you had the option of living anywhere in the world, where would you choose to live? Is your choice largely determined by job opportunities, environmental concerns, access to a favorite sport (e.g., swimming), or by some other variable? Discuss your choice in detail, and explain the things that are most important to you in making your selection. Do you think your choice will be the same 10 years from now? Why might it change?

Health in Review

- To maintain good health, people require adequate unpolluted air, water, food, and shelter.
- The air we breathe is often polluted with ozone, carbon monoxide, hydrocarbons, nitrogen and sulfur oxides, lead, cigarette smoke, and other contaminants.
- Global warming is expected to cause serious environmental disruptions in the next century.
- The greenhouse effect and the ozone hole are examples of global environmental problems caused by human activities.
- Pollution of air, land, and water from heavy metals, such as lead, is particularly hazardous to health. Children with even small amounts of lead or PCBs in their bodies may suffer from learning deficits.

- Drinking water may be contaminated with particulates or microorganisms that can cause disease. Pesticides in land, water, and food that have hormone-like properties may be damaging human endocrine and reproductive systems.
- Noise pollution can cause a wide range of health problems, including stress, tinnitus, and hearing loss.
- Pesticides, some of which are endocrine disruptors, can harm health in various ways.
- World population is expected to double in the next 50 years, severely taxing an already depleted environment and creating more health and environmental problems.

Health and Wellness Online

The World Wide Web contains a wealth of information about health and wellness. By accessing the Internet using Web browser software, such as Netscape Navigator or Microsoft's Internet Explorer, you can gain a new perspective on many topics presented in *Health and Wellness, Seventh Edition*. Access the Jones and Bartlett Publishers Web site at http://www.jbpub.com/hwonline

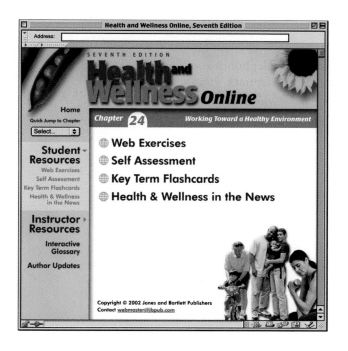

References

Centers for Disease Control (2000, December 8). Recommendations for blood lead screening of young children. *Morbidity Mortality Weekly Report, 49*.

Centers for Disease Control and Prevention. (1997). Children with elevated blood lead levels attributed to home renovation and remodeling activities—New York, 1993–1994. *Journal of the American Medical Association, 277*, 1030–1031.

Colon, I., et al. (2000). Identification of phthalate esters in the serum of young Puerto Rican girls with premature breast development. *Environmental Health Perspectives, 108*, 895–900.

Davis, D. L., et al. (1993). Medical hypothesis: Xenoestrogens as preventable causes of breast cancer. *Environmental Health Perspectives, 101*(5), 372–377.

Flodin, K. C. (1992, January/February). Now hear this. *American Health*, 59–62.

Friedman M. S., et al. (2001). Impact of changes in transportation and commuting behaviors during the 1996 summer games in Atlanta on air quality and childhood asthma. *Journal of the American Medical Association, 285*, 897–905.

Gleick, P. H. (2001, February). Making every drop count. *Scientific American*, 41–45.

Jacobson, J. L., and Jacobson, S. W. (1996). Intellectual impairment in children exposed to polychlorinated biphenyls *in utero*. *New England Journal of Medicine, 335*, 783–789.

Johansen, C., et al. (2001). Cellular telephones and cancer—a nationwide cohort study in Denmark. *Journal of the National Cancer Institute, 93*, 203–207.

McKibben, B. (1989). *The end of nature*. New York: Random House.

Needleman, H. L. (1996). Bone lead levels and delinquent behavior. *Journal of the American Medical Association, 275*, 363–369.

Ohlson, C. G., and Hardell, L. (2001). Testicular cancer and occupational exposures with a focus on xenoestrogens in polyvinyl chloride plastics. *Journal of the National Cancer Institute, 93*, 203–207.

Raloff, J. (1995). Beyond estrogens. *Science News, 148*, 44–46.

Rosen, J. F., and Mushak, P. (2001). Primary prevention of childhood lead poisoning—the only solution. *New England Journal of Medicine, 344*, 1470.

Savitz, D. A. (2001). Electromagnetic fields and cancer in railway workers. *American Journal of Epidemiology, 153*, 836–838.

Science (2001, May 18). The science of climate change. 1261.

Staessen, J. A., et al. (2001). Renal function, cytogenetic measurements, and sexual development in adolescents in relation to environmental pollutants. *Lancet, 357*, 1660–1669.

UK Childhood Cancer Study Investigators (1999). Exposure to power-frequency magnetic fields and the risk of childhood cancer. *Lancet, 354*, 1925–31

Vitousek, P. M., et al. (1997). Human domination of Earth's ecosystems. *Science, 277*, 494–499.

Suggested Readings

Epstein, P. R. (2000, August). Is global warming harmful to health? *Scientific American, 283,* 50–57. A thorough discussion of the health effects expected from an increase in global warming.

50 simple things you can do to save the earth. (1989). Berkeley, CA: The Earthworks Group. Simple, practical things each person can do to help heal the environment.

Gleick, P. H. (2001, February). Making every drop count. *Scientific American,* 41–45. Discusses the urgent need for safe, sanitary water supplies around the world.

Needleman, H. L., and Landrigan, P. J. (1994). *Raising children: Toxic free.* New York: Farrar, Straus, and Giroux. Two physicians concerned with environmental hazards to health explain how to protect children from the most dangerous ones.

Ott, W. R., and Roberts, J. W. (1998, February). Everyday exposure to toxic pollutants. *Scientific American,* 86–91. Describes the toxic substances we are exposed to in our daily routines. An excellent article if you want to learn how to avoid pollutants in the environment.

Potts, M. (2000, January). The unmet need for family planning. *Scientific American,* 88–93. Discusses the need worldwide for family planning to slow human population growth.

Web sites

Balbus, J. M. and Wilson, M. L. (2000). Human health and global climate change: a review of potential impacts in the United States. Pew Center on Global Climate Change (http://www.pewclimate.org/projects/human_health.cfm)

Intergovernment Panel on Climate Change. Expert analysis from the World Meteorological Organiza-tion (WMO) and the United Nations Environment Programme (UNEP) on the scientific, technical and socioeconomic information relevant for the understanding of the risk of human-induced climate change. (http://www.ipcc.ch)

U.S. Environmental Protection Agency (http://www.epa.gov)

Appendix A   Stress Management Techniques

This appendix contains several relaxation exercises and stress management techniques that you may find useful. As noted throughout this book, the association between stress and adverse health consequences is well documented. By incorporating relaxation and stress reduction exercises into our daily lives, we help maintain our physical, mental, and spiritual health.

You may want to try one or more of the physical and mental relaxation exercises described in this appendix. The techniques include mental imagery (Experiencing the Peacefulness of a Mountain Lake), muscular stress reduction (Progressive Muscular Relaxation), and mind-body harmony exercises (Yoga and T'ai Chi). You may want to record the instructions on an audiotape so that you can listen to the instructions while focusing on the exercise. A selection of relaxation exercises on audio CD is available from Jones and Bartlett Publishers (800-832-0034).

Exercise 1
Experiencing the Peacefulness of a Mountain Lake

Imagine yourself walking alone in the early morning along a path leading to some nearby mountains. All around you are trees rustling in the breeze; the path is covered with soft leaves and pine needles. The air is cool but not cold; your body feels relaxed as you walk slowly through the woods. You become aware of the quietness of the surroundings, how different from the constant noise of city life. As you stroll along you hear the calls of different songbirds announcing your arrival. You breathe in the cool air tinged with the fragrance of pine and eucalyptus. You walk through patches of sunlight and see the shadows of the mountain peaks in the distance.

As you gradually move higher, you notice the faint sound of water cascading over rocks and the sound mixes with the wind moving through the branches of the tall trees. Up ahead, a chipmunk is perched on an old stump of a tree, frozen in time in the moment before it decides which way to jump. Suddenly it is gone and you notice the colored insects that are buzzing around the flowers on the bushes. As the path begins to level off, your pace quickens and the air turns slightly cooler. Now the path is more rocky and, as you come around a bend a deep blue mountain lake abruptly comes into view. You climb up onto a boulder to get a better vantage point from which to view the entire lake. You sit down on the boulder weathered smooth by water, wind, and time.

Near the shore of the lake are tall green grasses and spreading back from the shore are clusters of spruce, pine, aspen, and birch. On top of one tree off in the distance a large bird is perched, possibly an eagle. As you watch, the bird spreads its wings and swoops down over the lake, soars up again, and is gone. The peaks of the mountains surrounding the lake are a mixture of grays and white, snow left over from the winter's snowfall. As your eyes move from the lake to the peaks and back to the lake again, you become aware of the harmony of nature, how each part seems to be in balance with the other parts of the scene.

The sky is cloudless except for small puffs of white clouds that circle the peaks and vanish into the endless blue. The rock you are sitting on radiates back the heat it absorbed from the sun, and you feel your body relaxing, melting into the comfortable saddle of the rock. Your eyes return to the surface of the lake and now you notice the evenly spaced ripples moving across its surface.

As your attention becomes more aware of the wind-induced ripples on the otherwise still surface of the lake, you make the symbolic association between the ripples on the lake and the tensions that move through your body. You would like your body to become as quiet and relaxed as the stillest part of the lake. As the cessation of the breeze causes the ripples to cease, so the cessation of thoughts in your mind causes the tension to disappear. As you watch the surface of the lake, all of your attention is focused on the ripples as they form, move toward the shore, and disappear.

Breathe slowly and deeply from your diaphragm and continue to focus on the stillness of the beautiful, clear mountain lake that you have created in your mind. Notice that you can make the surface of the lake as smooth as a mirror; as you do this all of your tensions, thoughts, and worries also disappear and your mind and body become fully relaxed. Hold onto this feeling of calm and relaxation for as long as your mind desires. Remind yourself that this is a place you can come back to in your mind time and time again whenever you feel tense, stressed, or angry. It's your personal safe haven that will always induce a feeling of calmness and relaxation.

Note: You can record this image-visualization exercise yourself or have a friend read it into a tape recorder so that you can simply listen to the instructions whenever you feel the need for some mental and physical relaxation. Also, the details of the image can be changed to suit your own experiences or imagination.

Exercise 2
Open Heart and Compassion Meditation

The heart is vital to life, and heart disease is still the number one cause of death in most industrialized countries. The heart is a pump; it circulates blood through the body. But symbolically, we think of the heart as the center of feeling; love flows from the heart. However, we also think of a *hardened heart,* one that may express mean, hateful, destructive, indifferent, and inconsiderate sentiments. What we feel in our heart symbolically can be manifested as stress and in physiological changes that may eventually produce illness. Feelings of anger, hate, or fear directed toward others may contribute to heart disease as well as other ailments. A healthy goal is to rid the heart of acrimonious, destructive feelings and to develop feelings of love and compassion for others, even those that hurt us either deliberately or unwittingly. The following suggestions are designed to help you open your heart to feeling love and compassion for others.

- Sit quietly for a few minutes in a comfortable position on a chair or on the floor, and pay attention to your breathing. Feel the air come in through your nose and flow down into your lungs as the lungs expand and your diaphragm moves outward. Breathe in slowly and exhale slowly to a count of ten. Repeat this a number of times while noticing your body becoming more relaxed with each breath. It may help to repeat silently in your mind, "My body is calm and relaxed."
- After your breathing has become slow and even, focus your attention on the left side of your chest where your heart is located. Picture in your mind a symbol of your heart, such as a flower or some other object you associate with love. If you visualize a

flower, imagine it starting out as a bud and opening up into a full blossom just as a rosebud opens up.
- As you breathe in and out, see the flower or other object symbolic of your heart radiating love outward through your chest.
- Bring into your mind the image of some person to whom you want to send your love or deep feeling of compassion. Use your imagination to surround that person with the rays of your love and caring.
- Make the feeling of love or compassion as profound as your mind can imagine it to be. Feel the warmth of it in your chest.
- Realize that this love can be sent both to people whom you truly love as well as to people with whom you feel angry or frustrated. Use your imagination to beam your love and caring feelings to the person whose image you have in your mind. You may want to visualize the person at work or at home and see how the person responds to the feelings you are sending.
- Feeling and sharing love and compassion with others helps to keep you emotionally and spiritually well.

Exercise 3
Progressive Muscular Relaxation

The following is a slight variation of a stress reduction technique developed by a physician, Edmund Jacobson, in 1929 in Chicago. Our technique involves deliberately tensing various muscles in the body to varying degrees. For each area of the body listed below, tense the muscles for about 5 seconds (1) as hard as you can, (2) about half as hard as the first time, and (3) just the slightest tension. In so doing, you train your mind to recognize varying degrees of tension in different parts of the body and, more importantly, how to relax the tension. After performing these exercises for a while, your mind automatically recognizes tension building up in different parts of your body and that awareness leads to relaxation of the tension.

Below we describe how to tense and relax various parts of the body that most commonly accumulate tension. After you have practiced progressive muscle relaxation exercises for a while, you can apply the same principles to any area of your body that needs to learn how to relax.

Jaws

Take a moment to feel the muscles of your jaws. Notice any tension, even the slightest amount. The jaw muscles can harbor a lot of undetected muscle tension. Now consciously tense the muscles of your jaws really tight, as tight as you can and hold it, even tighter, hold it. Now relax these muscles, exhale, and sense the tension disappear completely. You may even feel your mouth begin to open a little. Feel the difference between how these muscles feel now, compared with what you just experienced at 100 percent contraction. Feel the absence of tension. Now, contract these same muscles, but at half the full intensity, a 50 percent contraction. Hold the tension, keep holding, and now relax again. Feel how relaxed these muscles are. Compare this feeling of relaxation with what you felt before. By comparing the difference in tension levels, a greater sense of relaxation will surface. Once again, contract these same muscles, but with only a 5 percent contraction. A 5 percent contraction is a very slight twinge, with no motion whatsoever, just the acknowledgment that these muscles can contract. Now hold it, keep holding, and relax. Release any remaining tension so that these muscles are completely loose and relaxed. And sense just how relaxed these muscles are. To enhance this feeling of relaxation, take a comfortably slow, deep breath and sense how relaxed your jaw muscles have become.

Shoulders

Concentrate on the muscles of your shoulders and isolate these from the surrounding neck and upper arm muscles. Take a moment to sense these muscles. The shoulder muscles can also harbor a lot of undetected muscle tension resulting in stiffness. Symbolically, your shoulders carry the weight of all your thoughts, the weight of your worries and concerns. Now, consciously tense the muscles of your shoulder really tight, as tight as you can and hold it, even tighter, hold it. Now relax these muscles and sense the tension disappear completely. Sense the difference between how these muscles feel now compared with what you just experienced at 100 percent contraction. Once again, contract these same muscles, but this time only half as tight, a 50 percent contraction. Hold the tension, keep holding, and now completely relax these muscles. Sense how relaxed your shoulder muscles are. Compare this feeling of relaxation with what you felt before. By comparing the difference in tension levels, a greater sense of relaxation will surface. Finally, contract these same muscles at only 5 percent. A 5 percent contraction is a very slight twinge, with no motion whatsoever—just the acknowledgment that these muscles can contract, just a sense of the clothing touching the shoulder muscles. Now hold it, keep holding, and relax. Release any remaining tension so that these muscles are completely loose and relaxed. To enhance this feeling of relaxation, take a slow, deep breath and sense how relaxed your shoulder muscles have become.

Hands and Forearms

Concentrate on the muscles of your hands and forearms. Take a moment to feel these muscles including your fingers, palms, wrists, and forearms. Notice the slightest bit of tension. Now consciously tense the muscles of each hand and forearm really tight by making a fist, as tight as you can and hold it, as if you're going to punch something. Now release the fist and relax these muscles. Sense the tension disappear completely. Open the palm of each hand slowly, extend your fingers, and let them recoil just a bit. Sense the difference between how relaxed these muscles feel now compared with what you just experienced at 100 percent contraction. They should feel very relaxed. Now contract these same muscles at half the intensity, a 50 percent contraction. Hold the tension, keep holding, and now relax again. Sense how relaxed these muscles are. Compare this feeling of relaxation with what you felt before. By comparing the difference between tension and relaxation, a more profound sense of relaxation will surface. Now, barely contract these same muscles. A slight contraction is like holding an empty, delicate eggshell in the palm of your hand. Try to imagine that. Now hold it, keep holding, and relax. Release any remaining tension so that hand and arm muscles are completely relaxed. To enhance this feeling of relaxation, take a slow, deep breath and sense how relaxed your forearm and hand muscles have become.

Abdominals

Really focus your attention on your abdominal muscles. Take a moment to sense any residual tension in either the muscles or organs of the abdomen. Now consciously tense your abdominal muscles really tight as if someone is about to punch you in the stomach and you want to block that punch. Contract as tight as you can and hold it, even tighter, hold it. Now relax these muscles and sense the tension disappear completely. Feel the complete absence of tension. Compare the difference between how these muscles feel now with what you just experienced at 100 percent contraction. Once again contract these same muscles, this time at half the full intensity. A 50 percent contraction is like preparing for a false stomach punch. You know they won't make contact, but just in case you want to be ready. Hold the tension, keep holding, and now relax again. Feel how relaxed these muscles are. Compare this feeling of relaxation with what you felt before. When you compare the difference between tension levels and this current state of relaxation, a greater sense of relaxation will follow. Finally, contract these same muscles so slightly you barely feel the clothing over your stomach area. Now hold it, keep holding, and relax. Release any remaining tension so that these muscles are completely relaxed. Sense just how relaxed these muscles have become. To enhance this feeling of relaxation, take a slow, deep breath and feel how relaxed your abdominal region has become.

Feet

Focus your attention on the muscles of your feet. Typically the muscles of the feet are not tense, but standing can produce a lot of tension. In addition, in the confinement of shoes, feet muscles become tense. Now consciously contract the muscles of your feet by scrunching your toes really tight, as tight as you can. Hold it, even tighter, hold it. Now relax these muscles and sense the tension disappear completely. You may even feel your feet become warm as they relax. Feel the difference between how these muscles feel now as compared with when they were tense. Once again contract these same muscles at half the tension. Hold the tension, keep holding, and now relax again. Compare this feeling of relaxation with the tension you felt at full tension. By comparing the difference in tension levels, a greater sense of relaxation will surface. Now, contract these same muscles only slightly. Now hold it, keep holding, and relax. Release any remaining tension so that these muscles are completely relaxed. Sense just how completely relaxed these muscles are. To enhance this feeling of relaxation, take a slow, deep breath and feel how relaxed your feet and whole body are now. Your whole body feels completely relaxed and calm.

Now lie still, and enjoy the complete feeling of relaxation.

Exercise 4
Hatha Yoga Postures (Asanas)

Yoga has been used for centuries as a way to relax the mind and body and to promote health and spiritual well-being. The following hatha yoga postures (or *asanas*) were chosen and arranged to reflect a typical yoga class. Each position should be done slowly and without pain. Go only as far into the posture as you can while maintaining full complete breaths. It is very important to breathe through each posture. Hold each posture for at least thirty seconds. If you feel any pain (especially in your knees or lower back) ease out of the pose until the pain subsides. Do not judge yourself. Yoga is not about reaching an ideal or being competitive; it is about moving your body, listening to your body, and increasing your flexibility over time.

If you find these postures enjoyable and helpful in reducing tension, you may want to enroll in a yoga class, as it is very helpful to have an instructor. Also, videotapes are available that allow you to follow a course of instruction in your own home at your own convenience. To view a video of these yoga positions visit www.jbpub.com/hwonline.

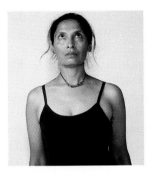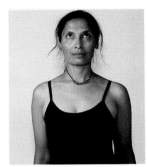

Eye exercises Sitting comfortably on a chair or on the floor, lengthen the spine and relax the facial muscles. Be sure to breathe normally throughout the exercises. Without moving the head, move the eyes slowly and smoothly: (1) look up and keep looking up without blinking for a couple breaths and then look down and hold for a couple breaths; return to a neutral gaze; (2) look to the right and hold, and then to the left and hold; return to a neutral gaze; (3) slowly circle the eyes clockwise and then counterclockwise. Finish by rubbing the palms together quickly and vigorously to create heat and lightly cup the palms over closed eyes to soothe and relax them.

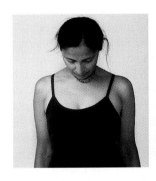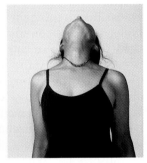
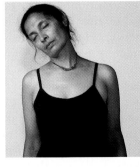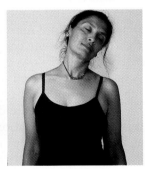

Neck exercises (1) Keeping the torso upright, gently and slowly move the head forward, easing the back neck muscles long. Use the weight of the head to lengthen the muscles as you breathe easily in and out. Roll the head back up and tilt it on the top of the spine (which is at the level of the ears) as you gently ease the chin up toward the ceiling, allowing the head to tilt back only as far as is comfortable. Be careful not to crunch the neck; keep those muscles long. Roll back up and repeat forward and backward several times. (2) Tilt the head to the right, easing the right ear toward the right shoulder. Keep the shoulders level while you breathe through the stretch. Repeat to the left side.

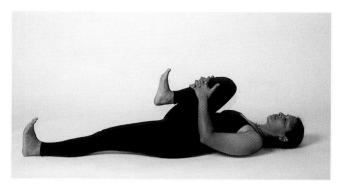

Wind relieving pose *(Pavanmuktasana)* Lie on your back, spreading your back along the floor. Bring the right knee toward the head and the right thigh toward the chest. Grasp the knee or behind the knee to pull the leg in closer, as you lengthen the left leg along the floor. Breathe easily in and out while you stay in this position. Bring the left knee up and in as you lengthen the right leg along the floor. Breathe easily in and out while you stay in this position.

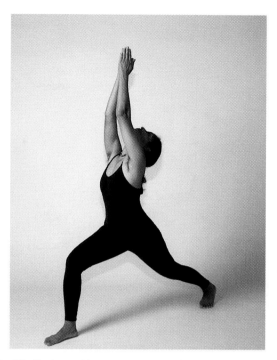

Warrior *(Virabhadrasana)* Come into Mountain pose and inhale an easy breath. Exhale on a "ha" sound as you step forward with your right leg into a lunge position. Check that your right knee is directly over your right foot (front to back and side to side). Straighten your left leg behind you as you ease the left heel toward the ground. Breathe easily a few times. If you feel comfortable, you can bring a slight arch in your back and look up at the ceiling. Lean forward over your right leg with your arms and trunk as you step your left foot forward to join your right and return to Mountain pose. Notice the sensations in your body as you allow the arms to float back down to your sides. Repeat with the left leg forward and the right leg behind.

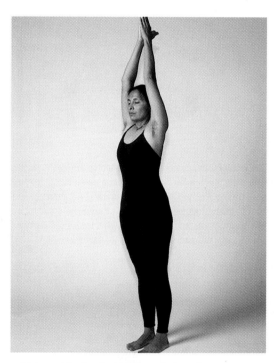

Mountain *(Tadasana)* Stand comfortably with your feet hip-width apart as you lengthen your head up off the top of the spine. Feel the weight of your arms dropping down and out to the sides of your body. Allow the arms to lengthen out wide to the sides as you float them up overhead, palms facing each other. (Be sure not to arch your back. If your back is arched, bring your hands out in front of you. Also, don't lock your knees.) Take a few easy sufficient breaths and gradually release the arms out and down to the sides.

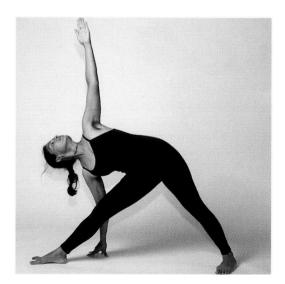

Triangle *(Trikonasana)* Come into Mountain pose. Step lightly to the right so your feet are about three feet apart and bring your arms out to the side at shoulder height, palms facing down. Rotate the right leg out from the hip joint to turn the knee and foot to the right. Inhale, and as you exhale, ease your hips to the left as you reach out with your right fingertips as far as you can. Find ease as you inhale. Exhale as you rotate the arms, the left up toward the ceiling and the right down toward your leg, palms facing forward. Turn the head to look up at your left hand. Continue to breathe. If you cannot breathe easily, bring your torso up a little. Return slowly to the upright position and repeat on the left side.

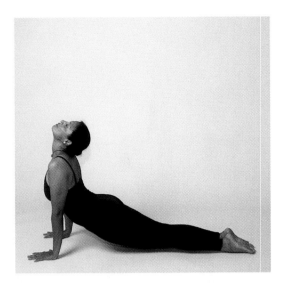

Cobra (*Bhujangasana*) Lie comfortably on the floor on your stomach, with your legs together. Soften your body into the ground as you breathe. Bring the palms to the floor under your shoulders, keeping wide between the shoulder blades. Lengthen your head forward and roll up, gently pressing the palms into the floor. Keep the elbows close to the body and ease the shoulders down, away from the ears. (Don't crunch the lower back. If you have any pain, be sure to come back down.) Breathe in and out a few times and ease down keeping the spine long.

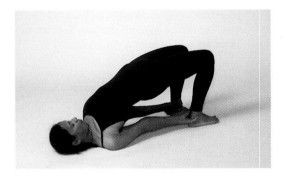

Bridge (*Setu bandhasana*) Lie on your back with your knees bent. Spread your shoulder blades wide and ease your lower back onto the floor. Slide your heels toward your buttocks, hip-width apart. Begin to lift your buttocks off the ground, sending your knees forward over your feet and gradually roll the back up off the ground toward the neck and shoulders. Clasp the hands underneath as you begin to straighten the elbows and ease the shoulder blades together behind you. Allow the breath to flow in and out with ease as you maintain this position. To come out of the pose, separate the hands, widen the shoulders and back, and slowly roll the back down onto the ground.

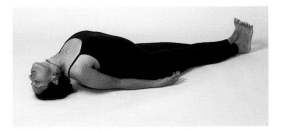

Fish (*Matsyasana*) Lie on your wide, long back with your legs together in front of you. Place your hands close together under your buttocks, palms down, arms straight, and elbows as close together as possible. Allowing the head to roll back, press your elbows into the ground as you expand your chest and torso forward and up, gently resting the crown of the head on the ground, and lengthening the front of your neck. Keep lengthening and expanding the torso as you breathe. Ease the heels of the feet forward and when you are ready, tuck the chin forward and slowly ease your back onto the ground. Release the arms out to the sides and rest, making note of the movement of your breath.

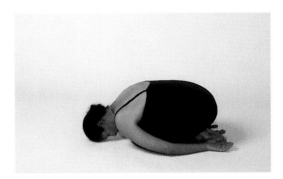

Child (*Gharbasana*) Come onto your knees and gently sit on your heels as you lengthen the spine. Lean forward as you allow your chest to come toward your knees. Rest your forehead on the ground or on a pillow. Allow your arms to lengthen in front of you, then let them rest on the ground. Soften the facial muscles, feel the massage of your organs against your thighs as you breathe. Spread your back wide and long. Stay for a couple of minutes, and when you are ready, gently and slowly support the torso with your hands as you return to kneeling.

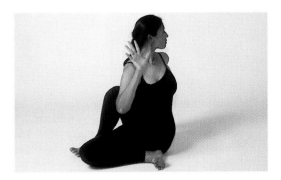

Spinal Twist (*Matsyendrasana*) Find comfort in sitting, with legs extended straight out in front of you. (If you can't sit comfortably, with your back straight, you may want to sit on the edge of a cushion or rolled up towel or blanket.) Bend the left leg and put it to the right of your right knee. Bring the left knee as close to you as you can while keeping the foot on the floor. Grab the left knee in the crook of your right arm and pull on the arm to help bring your torso forward and up. Keep the right leg extended in front of you, opening the knee toward the floor, with the foot flexed. Inhale and bring the left arm out to the side at shoulder height and with palm down. As you exhale, take your arm, eyes, and head to the left, rotating slowly through the entire spine. Place the left arm down on the floor, close to your body, and support yourself into a more upright position. Follow the movement of your body as you breathe. Ease back out by unwinding the spinal rotation. Repeat on the other side, left leg down, right knee up, and twisting to the right.

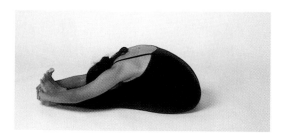

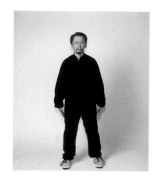

Starting Position Stand erect with feet shoulder width apart, arms by your side, palms in toward the legs, chin up, and eyes looking directly ahead.

Stretch of the West *(Paschimottanasana)* Find comfort in sitting, with legs together and extended straight out in front of you. (If you can't sit comfortably, with your back straight, you may want to sit on the edge of a cushion or rolled up towel or blanket.) Put your fists on the floor next to your hips and press them into the ground as you lengthen your torso up. Keep the spine long and, without curving the back, ease your way forward by bending in your hip joints. Go only as far as you can with a straight back and be careful not to roll the shoulders forward. Open the backs of the knees into the floor, bring the toes toward you, and find ease in the body as you breathe. Notice where you feel sensation and slowly float the head and torso back up.

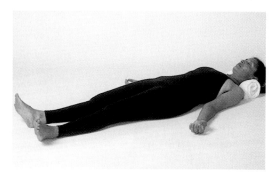

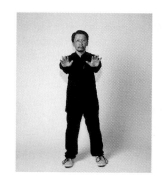

Beginning Position Leading with the wrists, raise your arms directly in front of the body to about shoulder level. Elbows should be slightly bent and shoulders relaxed. Leading with the elbows, slowly allow your arms and hands to return to starting position below waist level.

Corpse *(Savasana)* Slowly lower yourself onto your back. Resting on the floor, lengthen the neck muscles as you ease the head away from your feet. Wrap your arms around yourself and grasp your shoulder blades, easing them out to the sides. Lower the arms to the floor about 30 degrees out from the sides of the body, palms facing up. Gently press the lower back into the floor, then release it, allowing the natural curve of the spine to return. Lengthen the heels away from your torso, and let the heels roll out from the hips, feet opening out. Scan the body to find any areas of tension and let it go: in the face muscles, neck, shoulders, arms, torso, buttocks, abdomen and pelvis, legs and feet. Rest here for at least 10 minutes as you follow the flow of your breath.

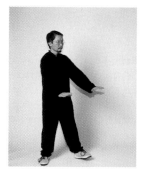

 ## T'ai Chi Movements

T'ai Chi Chuan comes from China and is based on a system of martial arts. In practicing T'ai Chi, the individual concentrates on moving the joints of the body freely and developing internal energy. The practice of T'ai Chi can be an ideal way of improving your health and staying in shape. There are several major styles of T'ai Chi (named after the families that founded them) and great variation within each style. All T'ai Chi forms are low impact, improve balance and coordination, increase mobility and reduce stress. T'ai Chi forms are sets of movements varying in length from 5 minutes to nearly one hour. The example illustrated here is an excerpt from a Yang style form. The orientation of the body is described in terms of north, south, east, and west directions. When starting, you should be facing north. Keep in mind that although the exercise is described as a series of steps the movement is continuous. To view a short video of the complete exercise visit the Jones and Bartlett Web site at www.jbpub.com/hwonline.

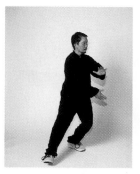

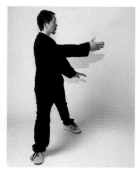

Right Hand Ward-off With your weight on your right foot pivot your body left about 90 degrees. Keep your arms in front of you, palms down and at waist level. Once you've rotated your body, shift your weight to your left foot, bending at the knee. Bring your left hand up to mid-chest level, keeping the palm turned down. Keep your right hand at waist level but turn your palm up, keeping space between your hands. Step north with the right foot. Shifting your weight back to the right leg, extend your right arm and raise your right hand to shoulder level. Lower your left hand to waist level, keeping your palm down and your arm extended.

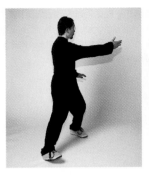 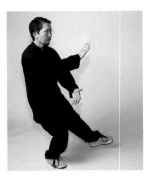   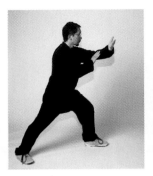 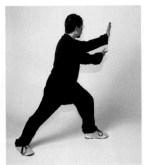

Left Hand Ward-off Shift your weight back to your left foot, bending at the knee. Pivoting on your right heel, bring your right foot in slightly toward your body. Move your right arm, bringing your arm and hand up to chin level and keeping your arm outstretched. Shift your weight to your right leg, bending at the knee. Set the left foot on its heel, pointing west. Turn the palm of your right hand outward and start pulling your arm in toward your chest, bending at the elbow. Pull your left arm across your body so that it is underneath your right arm, and turn the palm inward.

Grasp the Bird's Tail Shift your weight forward to your left foot. While doing this movement, bring your left arm, still curved, across your body with the palm facing inward at chin level. Keep your right hand in front of you, palm facing outward. Turn the left hand out to face forward while pushing outward with both arms.

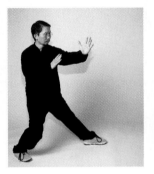 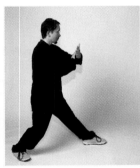 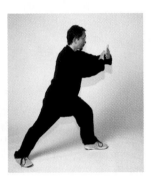

Rollback and Press Shift your weight backward onto your right leg, bending at the knee, and rotate your body to the right. Pull your right arm back toward your chest, bending at the elbow and keeping your palm facing the same direction as your body and at shoulder height. Rotate your body to the left, keeping your right arm close to your chest. Pull your left arm across your body and bring your palm toward your right hand as if the two were touching. As you shift your weight forward onto your left leg, push through the movement by pushing both arms forward in front of your body as if the right arm were pushing the left arm out at the wrist.

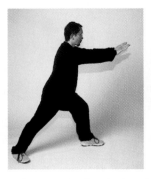 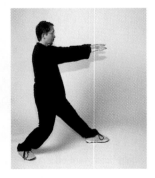 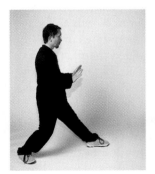 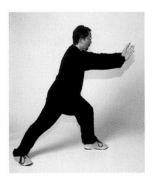

Push Continue to lean forward and extend your arms, turning both palms down with fingers pointing slightly upward. Release the wrists so the palms face down and pull back, shifting your weight to your right leg. Leading with your elbows, pull both arms down and toward your stomach. With your elbows bent, your forearms should be parallel to the floor with your palms facing forward. Shift your weight forward onto your left leg and extend your arms outward in front of you with palms continuing to face outward, as if you were pushing against a wall.

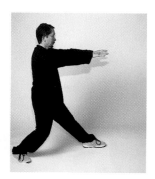
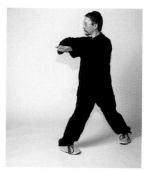
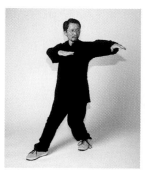
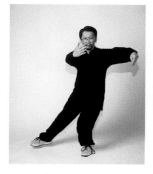
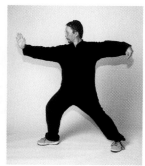

Holding a Single Whip With your arms still outstretched, release your wrists so your palms face the floor. Shift your weight back onto your right leg, bending at the knee. Keeping the right leg bent, pivot on your left heel, turning the foot in 90 degrees. Bend your right arm at the elbow and bring your right hand toward your chest, your palm continuing to face down. Keep your left arm extended out. Shift your weight to your left foot, bending at the knee, and pick up the right foot and step 45 degrees to the right. Keep your arms in the same position and rotate them around with your body. Your left hand points down toward the floor as you continue to shift your weight to your left foot, bringing the right foot off the floor and turning the leg outward (right foot points east). Turn the palm of your right hand to face toward you at chin level. Let the left wrist bend and the four fingers of the hand gather around the thumb to form a beak-hand. Shift your weight to the right onto your right leg and swing your right arm open so the palm faces outward. (The body and palm should now be facing east.) Keep your left arm out behind you.

If you are interested in studying T'ai Chi, it is important that you find a teacher because it is difficult to learn from a book or video. Find a teacher who practices the martial aspects of T'ai Chi, which can include selfdefense applications of movements from the T'ai Chi form, push-hands and boxing, and weapons forms. Though you need not become a great fighter to benefit from practicing T'ai Chi, you can gain a greater understanding of the form and the health-giving aspects of T'ai Chi by studying the martial aspects.

A second guideline to follow in finding a teacher is to go to a class and participate—don't just watch. If you feel that you have learned something from your participation and feel the teacher and other students are sincere in their efforts to learn, then you have probably found a good class and teacher. Like any activity that you enjoy and engage in fully, practicing T'ai Chi can offer immediate benefits, but it takes many years to become highly skilled. Beware of teachers who say that they have secrets or shortcuts, for there is no such thing. It is your own diligent practice that will bring you the full benefits of T'ai Chi. The teacher is there to show you the way.

January

National Volunteer Blood Donor Month
American Association of Blood Banks
8101 Glenbrook Road
Bethesda, MD 20814
301-907-6977
www.aabb.org
Contact: Public Relations

February

American Heart Month
American Heart Association
7272 Greenville Avenue
Dallas, TX 75231
800-AHA-USA1
www.americanheart.org
Contact: Local chapters

National Children's Dental Health Month
American Dental Association
211 E. Chicago Avenue
Chicago, IL 60611
312-440-2593
www.ada.org
Contact: Public Information

National Child Passenger Safety Awareness Week
US Dept. of Transportation
National Highway Traffic Safety Administration
400 Seventh Street, SW
Washington, DC 20590
202-366-9550
www.nhtsa.dot.gov

March

Hemophilia Month
National Hemophilia Foundation
116 West 32nd St
11th Floor
New York, NY 10001
800-42-HANDI
www.hemophilia.org

National Kidney Month
National Kidney Foundation
30 E. 33rd Street
New York, NY 10016
800-622-9010
www.kidney.org
Contact: Local chapters

National Chronic Fatigue Syndrome Awareness Month
National Chronic Fatigue Syndrome Association
3521 Broadway
Suite 222
Kansas City, MO 64111
816-931-4777

National Nutrition Month
American Dietetic Association
216 W. Jackson Blvd
Suite 800
Chicago, IL 60606-6995
312-899-0040
www.eatright.org/

Red Cross Month
American Red Cross
National Headquarters
430 17th Street NW
Washington, DC 20006-5307
Contact: Public Inquiries
www.redcross.org

National Poison Prevention Week
Poison Prevention Week Council
P.O. Box 1543
Washington, DC 20013
301-504-0580
Third full week in March

April

National Alcohol Awareness Month
National Council on Alcoholism and Drug Dependence
20 Exchange Place, Suite 2902
New York, NY 10005
212-269-7797
www.ncadd.org

National Cancer Control Month
American Cancer Society
1599 Clifton Road, NE
Atlanta, GA 30329-4251
800-ACS-2345
Contact: Local chapters
www.cancer.org

National Child Abuse Prevention Month
National Committee to Prevent Child Abuse
2950 Tennyson Street
Denver, CO 80212
303-433-2541
www.childabuse.org

Alcohol-Free Weekend
Rhode Island Council on Alcoholism and Drug Dependence
500 Prospect Street
Pawtucket, RI 02860
401-725-0410

World Health Day
American Association for World Health
1825 K Street, NW
Suite 1208
Washington, DC 20006
202-466-5883
www.aawhworldhealth.org

Minority Cancer Awareness Week
National Cancer Institute
Building 31 Room 10A31
31 Center Drive
Bethesda, MD 20892-2580
800-4-CANCER (Cancer Information Service)
http://nci.nih.gov

May

Clean Air Month
American Lung Association
1740 Broadway
New York, New York 10019
212-315-8700
www.lungusa.org

Mental Health Month
National Mental Health Association
1021 Prince Street
Alexandria, VA 22314-7971
703-684-7722
www.nmha.org

National High Blood Pressure Month
National Heart, Lung, and Blood Institute
P.O. Box 30105
Bethesda, MD 20824-0105
301-251-1222
www.nhlbi.nih.gov

National Physical Fitness and Sport Month
President's Council on Physical Fitness and Sport
200 Independence Avenue SW
Humphrey Building Room 738H
Washington, DC 20201
202-690-9000

Older Americans Month
Administration on Aging
330 Independence Ave, SW
Room 309F
Washington, DC 20201
202-401-7501
www.aoa.dhhs.gov

National Employee Health and Fitness Day
National Association of Governors' Councils on Physical Fitness and Sports
201 South Capitol Avenue
Suite 560
Indianapolis, IN 46225-1072
317-237-5630
www.fitnesslink.com/Govcouncil/
Third Wednesday in May

World No Tobacco Day
American Association for World Health
1825 K Street, NW
Suite 1208
Washington, DC 20006
202-466-5883
www.aawhworldhealth.org

June

Dairy Month
American Dairy Association
O'Hare International Center
10255 W. Higgins
Suite 900
Rosemont, IL 60018-5615
847-803-2000
www.dairyinfo.com

National Safety Week
American Society of Safety Engineers
1800 E. Oakton Street
Des Plaines, IL 60018-2187
847-692-4121
www.asse.org

July

National Therapeutic Recreation Week
National Therapeutic Recreation Society
22377 Belmont Ridge Road
Ashburn, VA 20148
703-858-0784
www.nrpa.org/branches/ntrs.htm

August

National Water Quality Month
Culligan International
One Culligan Parkway
Northbrook, IL 60062
847-205-6000
www.culligan.com/

September

National Cholesterol Education Month
National Cholesterol Education Program
Program Information Center
P.O. Box 30105
Bethesda, MD 20824-0105
301-251-1222
www.nhlbi.nih.gov/calendar/nhcol.htm
Contact: Information Center

National Sickle Cell Month
Sickle Cell Disease Association of America
200 Corporate Pointe
Suite 495
Culver City, CA 90230-7633
800-421-8453

Treatment Works Month
National Clearinghouse for Alcoholism and Drug Information
P.O. Box 2345
Rockville, MD 20852
800-729-6686
www.health.org

October

Family Health Month
American Academy of Family Physicians
11400 Tomahawk Creek Parkway
Leawood, KS 66211-2676
913-906-6000
www.aafp.org

National Breast Cancer Awareness Month
Susan G. Komen Breast Cancer Foundation
5005 LBJ Freeway
Suite 250
Dallas, TX 75244
972-855-1600
www.komen.org/

National Collegiate Alcohol Awareness Week
Interassociation Task Force on Campus Alcohol and Other Substance Abuse Issues
P.O. Box 100430
Denver, CO 80250
Starts the third Sunday in October

World Food Day
National Committee for World Food Day
2175 K Street, NW
Washington, DC 20437
202-653-2404

American Heart Association's Heartfest
American Heart Association
7272 Greenville Avenue
Dallas, TX 75231
800-AHA-USA1
www.americanheart.org
Contact: Local chapters

National Adult Immunization Awareness Week
National Coalition for Adult Immunization and National Foundation for Infectious Diseases
4733 Bethesda Avenue
Suite 750
Bethesda, MD 20814-5228
301-656-0003
www.nfid.org
www.medscape.com/Affiliates/NCAI/index.html
Last full week in October

November

National Alzheimer's Awareness Month
Alzheimer's Association
919 N. Michigan Avenue
Suite 1000
Chicago, IL 60611-1676
800-272-3900
www.alz.org

Great American Smokeout
American Cancer Society
1599 Clifton Road, NE
Atlanta, GA 30329-4251
800-ACS-2345
www.cancer.org
Contact: Local chapters

December

National Drunk and Drugged Driving Prevention
Month
National Coalition Against Drunk Driving
1900 L Street, NW Suite 705
Washington, DC 20036
202-223-7012
www.3dmonth.org/

World AIDS Day
American Association for World Health
1825 K Street, NW
Suite 1208
Washington, DC 20006
202-466-5883
www.aawhworldhealth.org

Glossary

abortion: the expulsion or extraction of the products of conception from the uterus before the embryo or fetus is capable of independent life; abortions may be spontaneous or induced

accident: sequence of events that produces unintended injury, death, or property damage; refers to the event, *not* the result of the event

accident mitigation: methods to reduce damage caused by unplanned events

accident prevention: ways to eliminate the occurrence of unintended injuries

acetaldehyde: a toxic substance produced when the liver breaks alcohol down

acid rain: rain, snow, fog, mist, etc., with a pH lower than 5.6

acquaintance rape: (also known as "date rape") sexual assault occurring when the victim and the rapist are known to each other and may have previously interacted in some socially appropriate manner

activators: potential stressors; occurrences, situations, or events perceived as stressful

actual effectiveness: how well a birth control method performs in actual use in a population

acupuncture: an ancient Chinese alternative medicine that uses thin needles inserted into specific points on the body to produce healing energy

addiction: physical and psychological dependence on a drug, substance, or behavior

aerobic training: exercise that increases the body's capacity to use oxygen

afterbirth: placenta and fetal membranes

ageism: prejudice against older people

aging: normal changes in body functions that begin after sexual maturity and continue until death

AIDS (acquired immune deficiency syndrome): a syndrome of more than two dozen diseases caused by HIV

AIDS antibody test: detects antibodies in blood that are produced in response to infection by HIV

alcohol abuse: frequent, continued use of alcohol; binge drinking

alcoholic: a person dependent on alcohol

alcoholism: loss of control over drinking alcohol

allergens: foreign substances that trigger an allergic response by the immune system

alpha-1-antitrypsin (AAT): a protein that inhibits destructive enzymes implicated in causing emphysema

alternative medicine: any form of therapy or healing performed by someone other than a physician

alveoli: tiny air sacs in the lungs that exchange oxygen and carbon dioxide

Alzheimer's disease: a common cause of senile dementia and other symptoms, eventually leading to death

amino acids: compounds containing nitrogen, which are the building blocks of protein

amniocentesis: a procedure that involves aspiration of amniotic fluid from the uterus to detect certain abnormalities in the fetus

amnion: the inner membrane that forms a fluid-filled sac surrounding and protecting the embryo and fetus

amniotic fluid: fluid of the amnion

amphetamines: synthetic drugs that stimulate the central nervous system and sometimes produce hallucinogenic states

amyloid protein: an abnormal protein in the brain of patients with Alzheimer's disease

anabolic steroids: synthetic male hormones used to increase muscle size and strength

analgesics: drugs that relieve pain

anaphylactic shock: a severe allergic reaction involving the whole body that can cause death

anemia: a deficiency of red blood cells; often caused by insufficient iron

aneurysm: a ballooning out of a vein or artery

angina pectoris: medical term for chest pain caused by coronary heart disease; a condition in which the heart muscle doesn't receive enough blood, resulting in chest pain

angiocardiography: an x-ray examination of the coronary arteries and heart; produces a picture called an angiogram

anorexia athletica: athletes who restrict their food intake to stay slim or lean

anorexia nervosa: emotional disorder occurring most commonly in adolescent females, characterized by abnormal body image, fear of obesity, and prolonged refusal to eat, sometimes resulting in death

antibodies: proteins that recognize and inactivate viruses, bacteria, and other organisms and toxic substances that enter the body

antigens: foreign proteins on infectious organisms that stimulate an antibody response

antioxidants: substances that in small amounts inhibit the oxidation of other compounds

anxiety: the fear of an imaginary threat

aorta: the large artery that transports blood from the heart to the body

appestat: region of the hypothalamus that controls appetite and eating behavior

appetite suppressants: drugs that diminish the sense of hunger

arteries: any one of a series of blood vessels that carry blood from the heart to all parts of the body

arteriography (cardiac catheterization): visualization of blocked coronary arteries by injecting a dye and monitoring blood flow

arteriosclerosis: hardening of the arteries

artificial fat: chemicals added to packaged foods to provide the taste and texture of fat but few or no calories

artificial insemination: introduction of semen into the uterus or oviduct by other than natural means

atherosclerosis: a disease process in which fatty deposits build up in the arteries and block the flow of blood

athletic amenorrhea: irregular or cessation of menstruation due to excessive participation in athletics

autoimmune diseases: mistakes in the functioning of the immune system that cause it to attack tissues in the body

autonomic nervous system: the special group of nerves that control some of the body's organs and their functions

average life span: the age at which half the members of a population have died

Ayurvedic medicine: a form of medicine that has its roots in the Hindu religion and is practiced widely in India

B-cells: cells of the immune system that produce antibodies

basal body temperature (BBT) method: uses daily body temperature readings taken immediately after waking to identify the time of ovulation; approximately 24 hours after ovulation, the BBT increases

basal cell carcinoma: a form of skin cancer which usually can be removed surgically

basal metabolic rate (BMR): the amount of energy needed per day to keep the body functioning while at rest

basal metabolism: the minimum amount of energy needed to keep the body alive

bender: several days of binge drinking

benign tumor: a tumor whose cells do not spread to other parts of the body

benzocaine: an anesthetic sometimes used in over-the-counter weight-control products to numb the sense of taste

binge drinking: ingesting five or more drinks on one occasion

binge eating disorder: an uncontrolled consumption of large quantities of food in a short period of time, even if the person does not feel hungry

biofeedback training: adjustment of a physiological process by using a monitor that feeds back information, allowing the mind to move the response in the desired direction

biopsy: removal of cells from a tumor for examination under a microscope

bipolar disorder: major episodes of depression accompanied by periods of excitement

bisexual: someone who is attracted to members of both genders

blackout: failure to recall normal or abnormal behavior or events that occurred while drinking

blood alcohol content (BAC): the amount of alcohol in the blood

body image: a person's mental image of his or her body

body mass index: a measure of body fatness, calculated by dividing body weight (in kilograms) by the square of height (in meters)

Braxton-Hicks contractions: normal uterine contractions that occur periodically throughout pregnancy

breasts: secondary sex characteristics; a network of milk glands and ducts in fatty tissue

bronchitis: inflammation of the bronchi of the lungs as a result of irritation; often accompanied by a chronic cough

bulimia: serious disorder, especially common in adolescents and young women, marked by excessive eating, often followed by self-induced vomiting, purging, or fasting

bulk-producing agents: agents used to promote a sense of fullness in the gastrointestinal tract, thus suppressing appetite

caffeine: a natural stimulant found in a variety of plants; commonly found in tea, coffee, chocolate, and soft drinks

calendar rhythm: estimation of fertile, or unsafe, days to have intercourse

calorie: the amount of energy required to raise 1 g of water from 14.5 °C to 15.5 °C

cancer-susceptibility gene: gene responsible for familial breast cancer and genes that cause susceptibility to colon cancer; increases the risk of a person developing cancer in his or her lifetime

cancer: unregulated growth of cells in the body

cannula: a hollow tube for insertion into the body cavity

capillaries: extremely small blood vessels that carry oxygenated blood to tissues

carbohydrates: the most economical and efficient source of energy; biological molecules consisting of one or more sugar molecules

carcinogens: any substances that can cause cancer in people and other animals

cardiologist: a physician who specializes in diseases of the heart

cardiovascular disease: any disease that causes damage to the heart or to arteries that carry blood to and from the heart

carotid endarterectomy: removal of fatty deposits in arteries in the neck to prevent a stroke

celibacy: sexual abstinence

cell-mediated immunity: the response of T-cells to infections

cellulose: a carbohydrate forming the skeleton of most plant structures and plant cells; the most abundant polysaccharide in nature and the source of dietary fiber

cervical cap: small latex cap that covers the cervix, used with spermicidal jelly or cream inside the cap

cervix: the lower, narrow end of the uterus

cesarean section: delivery of the fetus through a surgical opening in the abdomen and uterus

challenge situations: positive events that may involve major life transitions and may cause stress

chancre: the primary lesion of syphilis, which appears as a hard, painless sore or ulcer often on the penis or vaginal tissue

chemical carcinogen: a chemical that damages cells and causes cancer

chemotherapy: use of toxic chemicals to kill cancer cells and treat some forms of cancer

chewing tobacco: a form of shredded smokeless tobacco; chewed or placed in mouth between lower lip and gum

chi: a Chinese term referring to the balance of energy in the body

child abuse: physical or mental injury, sexual abuse or exploitation, maltreatment, or neglect of a child by a person who is responsible for the child's welfare; circumstances in which a child's health or welfare is harmed or threatened

chiropractic: an alternative medicine that uses manipulation of the spine and joints for healing

chlamydia: a sexually transmitted disease caused by the bacterium *Chlamydia trachomatis*

chlorofluorocarbons (CFCs): chemicals formerly used as coolants that are released into the atmosphere and are responsible for destroying stratospheric ozone

cholesterol: a fatlike compound occurring in bile, blood, brain, nerve tissue, liver, and other parts of the body

chorionic villus analysis: a prenatal procedure used to determine if genetic or anatomical defects exist in a fetus; an alternative to amniocentesis

chorionic villus sampling (CVS): a method to detect biochemical disorders and chromosomal abnormalities in the fetus

chronic obstructive pulmonary diseases (COPD): diseases that restrict the ability of the body to obtain oxygen through the respiratory structures (bronchi and lungs); including asthma, bronchitis, and emphysema

cilia: microscopic hairs in the lining of the bronchial tubes

circumcision: a surgical procedure to remove the foreskin from the penis

clitoris: small, sensitive organ located above the vaginal opening; center of sexual pleasuring

cocaine: a stimulant drug, obtained from the leaves of the coca shrub, that causes feelings of exhilaration, euphoria, and physical vigor

codependency: a relationship pattern in which the non-addicted family members identify with the alcoholic

cognition: the act or process of knowing in the broadest sense

coitus interruptus: removing the penis from the vagina just prior to ejaculation; also called withdrawal or pulling out

colostrum: yellowish liquid secreted from the breasts; contains antibodies and protein

communicable disease: an infectious disease that is usually transmitted from person to person

complex carbohydrates: a class of carbohydrates called polysaccharides; foods composed of starch and cellulose

complex diseases and **complex traits:** diseases or traits determined by many genes as well as environmental factors

computed tomographic scan: use of multiple x-ray images to construct a three-dimensional image of a diseased organ or body part

condom: a latex or polyurethane sheath worn over the penis (male condom) or inside the vagina (female condom); can be both a barrier method and act as a prophylactic against sexually transmitted diseases

congeners: flavorings, colorings, and other chemicals present in alcoholic beverages

congenital defect: any physical or biological abnormality observed in a newborn

conscious: knowing or perceiving something within oneself

consequences: the effects of one's action; the effects of stress response

contact dermatitis: an allergic reaction of the skin to something that is touched

contraindication: any medical reason for not taking a particular drug

cool-down: light or mild exercise immediately following competition or a training session; the primary purpose is to speed the removal of lactic acid from the muscles and allow the body to gradually return to a resting state

coping strategies: ways people devise to prevent, avoid, or control the emotional distress of unfulfilled needs

coping: attempts to manage a stressful situation

copulation: sexual intercourse

coronary arteries: two arteries arising from the aorta that supply blood to the heart muscle

coronary bypass surgery: surgery to improve blood supply to the heart muscle; most often performed when narrowed coronary arteries reduce the flow of oxygenated blood to the heart

cortisol: a steroid hormone secreted by the cortex (outer layer) of the adrenal gland

Cowper's glands: small glands secreting drops of alkalinizing fluid into the urethra

creatine: a natural substance in skeletal muscle tissue, which also can be taken in dietary supplement to enhance muscle performance

culpotomy: a female sterilization procedure

cumulative trauma disorders: disorders caused by repeated stress to a body part; carpal tunnel syndrome is considered a cumulative trauma disorder

cystitis: inflammation of the bladder

cytokines: small molecules that coordinate the activities of B-cells and T-cells

decibel: a measure of noise level

defense mechanisms: mental strategies for controlling anxiety

delirium tremens (DTs): hallucinations and uncontrollable shaking sometimes caused by withdrawal of alcohol in alcohol-dependent individuals

denial: refusal to admit you (or someone else) have a drinking problem

deoxyribonucleic acid (DNA): a nucleic acid of complex molecular structure occurring in cell nuclei; carrier of the genes; present in all body cells of every species

Depo-Provera: injectable form of medroxyprogesterone acetate

depression: a mental disorder characterized by sadness, feelings of inadequacy, and low self-esteem

diagnosis: the cause of a disease or illness as determined by a physician

diaphragm: a soft, rubber, dome-shaped contraceptive device worn over the cervix and used with spermicidal jelly or cream

diastole: the pressure in the arteries when the heart relaxes (the lower number)

dicofol: a pesticide that mimics the action of estrogen and causes reproductive abnormalities

dietary supplements: products that provide one or more of the 40 essential nutrients or nonessential vitamins, minerals, enzymes, amino acids, herbs, hormones, and nucleic acids

dilation and curettage (D and C): dilation of the cervix with use of a wand or laminaria and scraping the uterine lining; this procedure is often used during abortion

dilation and evacuation (D and E): dilation of the cervix and evacuation of the uterine contents using vacuum techniques

direct-to-consumer advertising: the marketing of prescription drugs to consumers in order to stimulate demand for a drug

disabling injury: an injury causing death, permanent disability, or any degree of temporary total disability beyond the day of the injury

distress: stress resulting from unpleasant stressors

diuretics: drugs that increase urine production

DNA (deoxyribonucleic acid): a chemical substance in chromosomes that carries genetic information

dose: amount of drug that is administered

double-blind: when neither the person receiving the drug nor the person administering the drug know whether it is a placebo or the real drug

douching: rinsing the vaginal canal with a liquid; not an effective means of birth control or STD prevention

drug: a single chemical substance in a medicine that alters one or more of the body's biological functions

drug abuse: persistent or excessive use of a drug without medical or health reasons

drug hypersensitivity: an allergic reaction to a drug

dysthymia: a long-lasting, mild form of depression

eclampsia: A late stage of toxemia characterized by blurred vision, headaches, convulsions, coma, and possibly death

ectopic pregnancy: a pregnancy occurring outside the uterus, usually in the fallopian tubes

elder abuse: physical, sexual, or emotional maltreatment or financial exploitation of an adult age 60 or older

electromagnetic fields (EMFs): a form of radiation produced by electrical power lines and appliances that may increase the risk of cancer

embryo: the developing infant during the first two months of conception

emission: amount of substance that is released into the atmosphere

emotional wellness: understanding emotions and knowing how to cope with problems that arise in everyday life, and how to endure stress

emphysema: a progressive degeneration of the lung alveoli, causing breathing and oxygen assimilation to become more and more difficult

enabling: denial of, or excuses for, the excessive drinking by an alcoholic to whom one is close

endocrine disruptors: chemical substances in the environment that interfere with the action of one or more of the body's hormones

endometrium: the inner lining of the uterus

endorphins and **enkephalins:** morphine-like substances that are secreted by the brain that mitigate pain; produced during strenuous exercise and childbirth

endurance: the ability to work out over a period of time without fatigue

energy balance: when energy consumed as food equals the energy expended in living

environment: all external physical factors that affect us

environmental model: modern analyses of ecosystems and environmental risks to health, such as socioeconomic status, education, and various environmental factors that affect health

enzymes: proteins in cells that carry out and speed up chemical reactions

epidemiology: a branch of science that studies the causes and frequencies of diseases in human populations

epididymitis: inflammation of the epididymis (a structure that connects the vas deferens and the testes)

epinephrine: hormone secreted principally by the adrenal medulla with a wide variety of functions, such as stimulating the heart, making carbohydrates available in the liver and muscles, and releasing fat from fat cells

episiotomy: an incision in the perineum to facilitate passage of the baby's head during childbirth, while minimizing injury to the woman

essential amino acids: amino acids that cannot be synthesized by the body and must be provided by food

essential fat: necessary and required fat in the diet; required for normal physiological functioning

essential hypertension: high blood pressure that is not caused by any observable disease

essential nutrients: chemical substances obtained from food and needed by the body for growth, maintenance, or repair of tissues; not made by the body; must be obtained from food

ethyl alcohol (ethanol): the consumable type of alcohol that is the psychoactive ingredient in alcoholic beverages; often called grain alcohol

etiology: specific cause of disease

eugenics: the science of improving human beings by selective breeding of people with desirable traits

eustress: stress resulting from pleasant stressors

euthanasia: helping someone who is on the verge of death or in a coma to die without suffering

exposure: actual amount of the substance people are exposed to

failure rate: likelihood of becoming pregnant if using a birth control method for one year

fallopian tubes: the usual site of fertilization; a pair of tube-like structures that transport ova from the ovaries to the uterus

familial hyperlipidemia (FH): an inherited disease causing extremely high levels of cholesterol in the blood

fat-soluble vitamins: soluble in fat; there are four fat-soluble vitamins

fatness set point: the physiologically regulated amount of fat on the body

fatty acids: naturally occurring in fats, either saturated or unsaturated (monounsaturated or polyunsaturated)

feedback: response of the receiver of a message to let the sender know he or she received the message and what the message was

fertility awareness methods: methods of birth control in which a couple charts the cyclic signs of the woman's fertility and ovulation, using basal body temperature, mucus changes, and other signs to determine fertile periods

fertilization: the fusion of a sperm cell and an ovum

fetal alcohol syndrome: birth defects and mental retardation caused by ingestion of alcohol during pregnancy

fiber: a group of compounds that make up the framework of plants; fiber cannot be digested

fibrillation: rapid, erratic contraction of the heart

fight-or-flight response: a defensive reaction that prepares the organism for conflict or escape by triggering hormonal, cardiovascular, metabolic, and other changes

first-stage labor: the beginning of labor during which there are regular contractions of the uterus

fitness: the extent to which the body can respond to the demands of physical effort

fixation: the restricted movement of one or more vertebrae

flavonoids: substances that may reduce the risk of heart disease

flexibility: the ability of a joint to move through its range of motion

follicle-stimulating hormone: stimulates ovaries to develop mature follicles (with eggs); the follicle produces estrogen

food allergies: allergic responses to something that is eaten

forcible rape: sexual assault using force or threat of force and involving sexual penetration of the victim's vagina, mouth, or rectum

foreskin: a fold of skin over the end of the penis

free radicals: oxidizing substances in the body that can damage blood vessels and tissues

fructose: a simple sugar found in fruits and honey

functional food: a food to which additional vitamins, minerals, herbs or other substances are added to allow the manufacturer to make health claims

fungicide: a chemical that kills fungi

galactose: a monosaccharide derived from lactose

gametes: sex cells, either sperm or ova, that fuse at fertilization; gametes carry a complete set of genetic information from each parent that is passed on to the child

gamma irradiation: nonchemical method of food preservation

gangrene: decay of tissue when the blood supply is restricted

gender identity: awareness of being male or female

gender role: behaviors specific to a gender

gene therapy: a technique for replacing defective genes with normal ones in certain tissues of a person affected with a hereditary disease

generalized anxiety disorder: persistent and often nonspecific worry and anxiety

genetic counseling: information to help prospective parents evaluate the risks of having or delivering a genetically handicapped child

genetically modified food (GMF): any edible plant or animal that carries one or more genes derived from a different organism (foreign genes)

gerontology: science that studies the causes and mechanisms of aging

glucose: the principal source of energy in all cells; also called dextrose

glycogen: the form in which carbohydrate is stored in humans and animals

goiter: an enlargement of the thyroid gland resulting from lack of iodine, causing a swelling in the front part of the neck

gonadotropin-releasing hormone: hormone that directs the release of pituitary sex hormones

gonorrhea: sexually transmitted disease caused by gonococcal bacteria *(Neisseria gonorrhea)*

greenhouse effect: the ability of atmospheric carbon dioxide to reflect heat radiated from the earth back to the earth and to thereby raise the earth's temperature globally

growth needs: a human need that includes social belonging, self-esteem, and spiritual growth

habituation: psychological dependence arising from repeated use of a drug

hallucinogens: psychoactive substances that alter sensory processing in the brain; produce visual or auditory sensations that are not real (i.e., that are hallucinatory)

hangover: unpleasant physical sensations resulting from excessive alcohol consumption

harm-and-loss situations: stressful events that include death, loss of property, injury, and illness

hashish: the sticky resin of the *Cannabis* plant

health maintenance organization (HMO): an organization (either nonprofit or for-profit) of physicians, hospitals, and support staff that provides medical services to members

health: state of sound physical, mental, and social well-being

heart attack: death of, or damage to, part of the heart muscle caused by an insufficient blood supply

heavy drinkers: people who drink more than 14 alcoholic drinks a week

hemicellulose: substances found in plant cell walls that are composed of various sugars chemically linked together

hemophilia: a hereditary disease (primarily in men) caused by lack of an essential blood clotting factor; results in excessive bleeding in response to any scratch or injury

herbal medicines: materials derived from plants and other organisms that are made into teas, powders, and salves to treat diseases and injuries

herbicide: a chemical that kills weeds

hereditary (genetic) disease: any disease resulting from the inheritance of defective genes or chromosomes from one or both parents

herpes: sexually transmitted disease caused by *Herpes simplex virus*, HSV

heterosexual: someone who is attracted to people of the opposite gender

hierarchy of needs: a progression of human requirements, including physiological needs, safety, love, self-esteem, and self-actualization

high-density lipoprotein (HDL): the carrier of cholesterol from tissues to the liver for removal from the circulation; carrier of "good" cholesterol

histamine: a chemical released by cells in an allergic response; causes inflammation

histocompatibility: the degree to which the antigens on cells of different persons are similar

HIV (human immunodeficiency virus): the virus defined as the cause of AIDS

HLA (human leukocyte antigens): antigens that are measured to determine the suitability of an organ for transplantation from donor to recipient

holistic model: encompasses the physiological, mental, emotional, social, spiritual, and environmental aspects of health

homeopathy: an alternative medicine that administers very dilute solutions of substances that mimic the patient's symptoms

homeostasis: the tendency for body systems to interact in ways that maintain a constant physiological state

homocysteine: a substance derived from the amino acid methionine; high blood levels increase the risk of heart disease; blood levels are reduced with adequate intake of folic acid

homosexual: someone who is attracted to people of the same gender

hormone replacement therapy (HRT): administration of estrogen to menopausal and postmenopausal women to help prevent symptoms of menopause, osteoporosis, and heart disease

hormones: complex chemicals, produced and secreted by endocrine glands, that travel through the bloodstream and regulate body functions

hospice: a place for terminally ill patients to spend the time before death in an environment that attends to their physical, emotional, and spiritual needs but no further treatments are administered; hospice care also can be given in a patient's home

human chorionic gonadotropin (HCG): a hormone produced during the first stages of pregnancy; it is used as a basis for pregnancy tests

human immunodeficiency virus (HIV): the virus that causes AIDS; it causes a defect in the body's immune system by invading and then multiplying within the white blood cells

human papillomavirus (HPV): a genus of viruses including those causing papillomas (small nipple-like protrusions of the skin or mucous membrane) and warts

humoral immunity: the response of B-cells to infections

hypertension: high blood pressure

hypnotherapy: the use of hypnosis to treat sickness

hypnotics: CNS depressants used to induce drowsiness and encourage sleep

hypothalamus: a part of the brain that activates, controls, and integrates the autonomic nervous system, the endocrine system, and other bodily functions

hysterectomy: surgical removal of the uterus

I-statements: statements beginning with "I"; positive communication skill

image visualization: use of mental images to promote healing and change behaviors

immune system: an interacting system of organs and cells that protect the body from infectious organisms and harmful substances

immunizations: vaccinations to prevent a variety of serious diseases caused by both bacteria and viruses

immunosuppressive drugs: drugs to suppress the functions of the immune system (e.g., after organ transplants)

incidence: frequency of occurrence of a particular disease

infarction: death of heart cells resulting from a blocked blood supply

infertile: unable to become pregnant or to impregnate

ingredient label: label on a manufactured food that lists the ingredients in descending order by weight

inhalants: vaporous substances that, when inhaled, produce alcohol-like intoxication

injury epidemiology: the study of the occurrence, causes, and prevention of injury

insecticide: a pesticide that kills insects

insemination: introduction of semen into the uterus or oviduct

insoluble fiber: cannot be dissolved in water

insomnia: prolonged inability to obtain adequate sleep

integrative medicine: conventional medicine practiced in conjunction with alternative medicine (herbal remedies, acupuncture, massage) to treat sickness

intellectual wellness: having a mind open to new ideas and concepts

intrauterine device (IUD): a flexible, usually plastic, device inserted into the uterus to prevent pregnancy

***in vitro* fertilization (IVF):** a procedure in which an egg is removed from a ripe follicle and fertilized by a sperm cell outside the human body; the fertilized egg is allowed to divide in a protected environment for about 2 days and then is inserted back into the uterus

ionizing radiation: radiation, such as x-rays, that can damage cells and cause cancer; also used to treat cancer

ischemia: an insufficient supply of blood to the heart

isometric training: another term for strength training

isoprenoids: fat-soluble substances that may reduce the risk of some cancers

isopropyl alcohol: rubbing alcohol, sometimes used as an anesthetic

karyotype: visual display of all of a person's chromosomes that can detect chromosomal abnormalities characteristic of inherited diseases

kilocalorie: unit of energy; the amount of heat needed to raise one kilogram of water 1 °C, equivalent to 1000 calories

labia majora: a pair of fleshy folds that cover the labia minora

labia minora: a pair of fleshy folds that cover the vagina

labor: the process of childbirth

lactase: enzyme secreted by glands in the small intestine that converts lactose (milk sugar) into simple sugars

lacto-ovo-vegetarian: one who excludes meats, poultry, and fish, but includes eggs and dairy products

lacto-vegetarian: one who excludes meat, poultry, fish, and eggs, but includes dairy products

lactose: a molecule of glucose and galactose chemically bonded together; found primarily in milk

laminaria: a plug of sterile dried kelp (seaweed), which expands when in contact with water and can thus be placed in the cervical canal to dilate the cervix

laparoscopy: a surgical incision into the abdomen used to visualize internal organs

laryngospasm: spasm of the larynx

Leading Health Indicators: ten categories of health goals that represent the major public health concerns in the United States

lecithin: an essential component of cell membranes

leptin: a hormone that controls appetite

leukocytes: white blood cells that fight infections

life expectancy: average number of years a person can expect to live

lightening: the positioning of the fetus for birth by descent in the uterus

linoleic acid: an essential fat that must be obtained from food

lipids: fats such as cholesterol and triglycerides

liposuction: surgery used to remove fat under the skin in order to reshape parts of the body

literal message: a message that is conveyed by symbols

living will: a legal document that expresses your wishes regarding treatment if you become unable to make your own medical decisions

low-density lipoprotein (LDL): the carrier of "bad" cholesterol in blood

lowest observed failure rate: likelihood of becoming pregnant if using a birth control method consistently and as intended

LSD: a powerful hallucinogenic chemical; ingestion alters brain chemistry and produces a variety of hallucinogenic and behavioral effects

lupus erythematosus: an autoimmune disease that mostly affects women

luteinizing hormone: anterior pituitary hormone that causes a follicle to release a ripened ovum and become a corpus luteum; in the male, it stimulates testosterone production and the production of sperm cells

Lyme disease: a serious, difficult-to-diagnose infectious disease caused by bacteria deposited by ticks when they bite

lymph nodes: nodules spaced along the lymphatic vessels that trap infectious organisms or foreign particles

lymphatic system: a system of vessels in the body that trap foreign organisms and particles; the immune system is part of the lymphatic system

macrophages: specialized cells that destroy and eliminate foreign particles and microorganisms from the body

magnetic resonance imaging: use of a strong magnetic field to produce images of internal parts of the body; especially useful for soft tissues

maintenance needs: human needs that include physical safety and survival requirements, such as food and water

malaria: a disease of red blood cells that produces fever, anemia, and death

malignant tumor: a tumor whose cells spread throughout the body

mammogram: x-ray picture used to detect tumors in the breast

managed care: systems of health care in which the primary goal is to reduce costs

mandala: an artistic, religious design used as an object of meditation

mantra: a sound or phrase that is repeated in the mind to help produce a meditative state

marijuana: a psychoactive substance present in the dried leaves, stems, flowers, and seeds of plants of the genus *Cannabis*

masturbation: self-induced sexual stimulation

maximum life span: the theoretical maximum number of years that individuals of a species can live

medical model: interprets health in terms of the absence of disease and illness

medicine: drugs used to prevent, treat, or cure illness; aid healing; or supress symptoms

meditation: relaxed state of mind produced by focusing the mind on internal images, sounds, or passing thoughts

melanoma: a particularly dangerous form of skin cancer

menarche: the beginning of menstruation

menopause: the cessation of menstruation in mid-life

menstruation: the regular sloughing of the uterine lining via the vagina

meridians: the channels along the body where energy flows and where acupuncture points are located

mesothelioma: a form of lung cancer caused by asbestos

meta-analysis: statistical methods used to evaluate many studies (sometimes hundreds) of a particular treatment, drug effectiveness, or alternative medicine; meta-analysis attempts to resolve conflicting studies and to arrive at a statistical summary of effectiveness

metabolism: the process of obtaining energy and matter from the chemical breakdown of molecules obtained from food or from the body

metamessage: how the message is interpreted between sender and receiver

metastasis: the process by which cancer cells spread throughout the body

methyl alcohol: wood alcohol or methanol

minerals: inorganic elements found in the body both in combination with organic compounds and alone

minilaparotomy: female sterilization procedure in which the fallopian tubes are ligated or cauterized through a small abdominal incision

moist snuff: a form of snuff made from air- and fire-cured tobacco leaves; most hazardous form of smokeless tobacco

mononucleosis: an infectious disease caused by the Epstein-Barr virus, common among college-age adults

monounsaturated fatty acid: carries one less than all the hydrogen atoms it possibly could

morbidity: ratio of persons who are diseased to those who are well in a given community

mortality: death rate: number of deaths per unit of population (e.g., per 100; 10,000; or 1,000,000) in a specific region, age range, or other group

multiple sclerosis (MS): an autoimmune disease that affects the central nervous system

mutation: a permanent change in the genetic information in a cell; only mutations in sperm and eggs are inherited

mutual empathy: both partners care and understand about each other

myelin: a substance that sheaths and insulates nerve fibers in the brain and spinal cord

myocardium: muscular wall of the heart that contracts and relaxes

myotonia: muscle tension

narcolepsy: extreme tendency to fall asleep during the day

naturopathy: an alternative medicine that uses nutrition, herbs, massage, and other techniques to promote healing

neuropeptides: small molecules that circulate throughout the body and bind to cells in the emotional center of the brain and to many organs, especially cells of the gut and immune system; these molecules are used in mind-body communications

neutraceutical: a dietary supplement intended to prevent or treat an illness or disease

nicotine: an addicting chemical in tobacco that produces rapid pulse, increased alertness, and a variety of other physiological effects

nicotine replacement therapy: using nicotine-containing gum, skin patch, nasal spray, or inhaler to temper the symptoms of nicotine withdrawal when quitting smoking

nitrates: preservatives containing any salt or ester of nitric acid. Some individuals are sensitive to nitrates and may suffer from headache, diarrhea, or urticaria after ingesting them

nitrites: preservatives containing any salt or ester of nitrous acid

nonessential amino acids: eleven amino acids required for protein synthesis that are synthesized by humans and are not specifically required in the diet

norepinephrine: hormone that has many of the same effects as epinephrine

Norplant: hormone-containing capsule inserted under the skin

nosocomial diseases: an infectious disease contracted while in the hospital for an unrelated disease or problem

nutrition facts label: label on a manufactured food that lists the quantity of certain nutrients in the food and the percent daily value for those nutrients

nutritional calorie: unit of energy; often used interchangeably with the term kilocalorie

obesity: the condition of having a BMI of more than 30 or weighing more than 20% (men) or 30% (women) of the recommended weight-for-height

obsessive-compulsive disorder: persistent, unwelcome thoughts or images and the urgent need to engage in certain rituals that cannot be controlled

occupational wellness: enjoyment of what you are doing to earn a living and contribute to society

open-heart surgery: surgery performed on the opened heart while the blood supply is diverted through a heart-lung machine

opiates: CNS depressants derived from the opium poppy

opportunistic infections: any infectious disease in a patient with a weakened immune system; often occurs in AIDS patients

orgasm: the climax of sexual responses and the release of physiological and sexual tensions

osteopathy: an alternative medicine that uses manipulation and medicines for healing; osteopaths receive training comparable to that of physicians and can prescribe drugs

osteoporosis: a condition in older people, particularly women, in which bones lose density and become porous and brittle

ova: a term for female eggs (singular, *ovum*)

ovaries: a pair of almond-shaped organs in the female abdomen that produce egg cells (ova) and female sex hormones

over-the-counter (OTC) drugs: drugs that do not require a prescription

overuse syndromes: injuries to muscles, tendons, ligaments, and joints resulting from too much exercise

ovulation: release of an egg (ovum) from the ovary

oxytocin: hormone that promotes release of milk; also can cause muscles in the uterine wall to contract

ozone hole: an ozone-deficient portion of the atmosphere above Antarctica that has been steadily growing since the problem was first reported in 1985

ozone layer: a layer of ozone molecules located in the stratosphere in a diffuse band extending from 10 to 30 miles above the earth's surface

pacemaker: an electrical device implanted in the chest to control the heartbeat

panic disorder: severe anxiety accompanied by physical symptoms

parasomnias: activities that interrupt restful sleep

parasympathetic nervous system: a division of the autonomic nervous system that tones down the excitatory effects of the sympathetic nervous system; slows metabolism and restores energy reserves

Parkinson's disease: a neurodegenerative disease in which brain functions that control movements of the body gradually are lost

pathogen: a disease-causing organism

pathologist: a physician who specializes in the causes of diseases

pelvic inflammatory disease (PID): inflammation of the pelvic structures, especially the uterus and fallopian tubes; often caused by a sexually transmitted disease

penicillin: an antibiotic produced by mold and capable of curing many bacterial infections

penis: the male's organ of copulation and urination

percent daily value: percentage of the recommended daily amount of a particular nutrient found in a food

percutaneous transluminal coronary angioplasty (PTCA): a procedure to open blocked arteries

pesticide: a chemical that kills unwanted organisms

phencyclidine (PCP): drug that, depending on the route of administration and dose, can be a stimulant, depressant, or hallucinogen; originally developed as an animal anesthetic

phenylpropanolamine (PPA): active ingredient in over-the-counter weight-control products

phobia: a powerful and irrational fear of something

photochemical smog: air pollution from the action of sunlight on emissions from motor vehicles and industrial sources

physical dependence: a physiological state that depends on the continuous presence of a drug; absence of the drug may cause discomfort, nervousness, headaches, and sweating (withdrawal symptoms) and sometimes death

physical wellness: maintenance of your body in good condition by eating right, exercising regularly, avoiding harmful habits, and making informed responsible decisions about your health

physician-assisted suicide: a form of active euthanasia in which a physician helps a patient who no longer desires to live because of pain or an incurable illness to commit suicide

phytochemicals: chemicals produced by plants

phytosterols: sterols of plant origin

placebo effect: healing that results from a person's belief in a treatment that has no medicinal value

placenta: the flat circular vascular structure within the pregnant uterus that provides nourishment to and eliminates wastes from the developing embryo and fetus and is passed as afterbirth after the baby is born

plaque: deposit of fatty substances in the inner lining of arteries

platelets: cells in the blood that are essential for clotting

plumbism: disease caused by lead poisoning

poison: any chemical substance that causes illness, injury, or death

polychlorinated biphenyls (PCBs): a family of banned synthetic, organic chemicals that affect the human thyroid gland and reproductive systems of animals

polyunsaturated fatty acid: carries at least two fewer hydrogen atoms than it would if saturated

post-traumatic stress disorder (PTSD): physical and mental illnesses resulting from severe trauma

prana: the life force in the body that is derived from cosmic consciousness

preeclampsia: an early stage of toxemia characterized by protein in the urine, high blood pressure, and edema

preferred provider organization (PPO): physicians who belong to the organization provide medical care at reduced costs that are negotiated by the organization

prevalence: predominance of a particular disease

prions: proteinaceous infectious particles that contain no genetic information, yet can cause some rare infectious diseases

progestin-only contraceptives: work by inhibiting ovulation and thickening of the cervical mucus; completely reversible

progressive muscle relaxation: a specific technique that produces relaxation by tensing and relaxing muscles

prolactin: a hormone produced by the anterior lobe of the pituitary gland that promotes milk production

proof: a number assigned to an alcoholic product that is twice the percentage of alcohol in that product

prostate gland: gland at the base of the bladder providing seminal fluid

prostate-specific antigen: a blood test that detects a protein associated with abnormal growth of the prostate gland

proteins: the foundation of every body cell; biological molecules composed of chains of amino acids

psychoactive: any substance that primarily alters mood, perception, and other brain functions

psychological dependence: dependence that results because a drug produces pleasant mental effects

psychosomatic illnesses: physical illnesses brought on by negative mental states such as stress or emotional upset

pubic lice: small insects that live primarily in hair in the genital and rectal regions

puerperium: the 6 weeks after childbirth, also called postpartum period

radiation therapy: use of high-energy radiation, such as x-rays, to kill cancer cells and treat some forms of cancer

radon: a radioactive gas found in some homes that can increase the risk of cancer

rapid eye movement (REM) sleep: stage of sleep in which dreams occur

reactions: interpretations of activators as taxing or overwhelming

reactive hypoglycemia: occurring after the ingestion of carbohydrate, with consequent release of insulin

receptor: protein on the surface or inside a cell to which a drug or natural substance can bind and thereby affect cell function

recommended [daily] dietary allowances (RDA): levels of nutrients recommended by the Food and Nutrition Board of the National Academy of Sciences for daily consumption by healthy individuals, scaled according to gender and age

relaxation response: the physiological changes in the body that result from mental relaxation techniques

rodenticide: a chemical that kills mice and rats

safety: an ever-changing condition in which one attempts to minimize the risk of injury, illness, or property damage from the hazards to which one may be exposed

saturated fat: generally solid at room temperature; comes from animal sources

scabies: infestation of the skin by microscopic mites (insects)

schizophrenia: a mental disorder that involves a disturbance in thinking, in perceiving reality, and in functioning

scrotum: the sac of skin that contains the testes

secondary hypertension: high blood pressure caused by a recognizable disease

secondary sex characteristics: anatomical features appearing at puberty that distinguish males from females

secondhand binge effects: negative experiences caused by another's binge drinking

second-stage labor: the stage during which the baby moves out through the vagina and is delivered

sedatives: CNS depressants used to relieve anxiety, fear, and apprehension

self-actualization: a state in which a person has achieved the highest level of growth in Maslow's hierarchy of needs

self-disclosure: sharing personal experiences and feelings with someone

self-efficacy: your belief that you are capable of handling the situation; self-esteem

semen: a whitish, creamy fluid containing sperm

seminal vesicles: sac-like structures that secrete a fluid that activates the sperm

seminiferous tubules: convoluted tubules in the testicles that produce sperm

senile dementia: loss of cognitive functions in elderly people

sepsis syndrome: bacterial infection of the blood; may be fatal

sex: has several definitions: (a) an individual's classification as male or female based on anatomical characteristics; (b) a set of behaviors; (c) the experience of erotic pleasure

sexual: characterized by or having the qualities of sex; the opposite is asexual

sexual assault: violent actions that include rape, incest, attempted rape, and unwanted sexual touching

sexual orientation: attraction toward and interest in members of one or both genders

sexual response cycle: the physiological response in both men and women as described in four phases

sexuality: a person's sense of self that is used to create sexual experiences

sexually transmitted diseases (STDs): infections passed from person to person by sexual contact

sexually transmitted warts: hard growths caused by an infection with human papillomavirus (HPV) that appears on the skin of the genitals or anus

sick building syndrome: collection of symptoms reported by workers in some modern buildings

side effects: unintended and often harmful actions of a drug

sidestream smoke (passive smoking): smoke released into the environment directly from lighted tip of cigarettes

simple sugars: a class of carbohydrates called monosaccharides; all carbohydrates must be reduced to simple sugars to be digested

sinoatrial node: the region of the heart that produces an electrical signal that causes the heart to contract

sleep apnea: state of troubled or interrupted breathing while sleeping

smegma: a white, cheesy substance that accumulates under the foreskin of the penis

smog: air polluted by chemicals, smoke, particles, and dust

snuff: a form of smokeless tobacco; made from powdered or finely cut leaves

social phobia: fear of being observed and evaluated by others in social situations

social wellness: ability to perform the expectations of social roles effectively, comfortably, and without harming others

soluble fiber: can be dissolved in water

somatization: occurrence of physical symptoms without any bodily disease or injury being present

somatization disorder: prolonged pain and other symptoms that are not due to disease or injury

somnambulism: sleepwalking

specific metabolic rate: the amount of energy per gram of body weight consumed per day

spectatoring: observing one's own sexual experience rather than fully taking part in it

spermicide: a chemical that kills sperm; particularly foams, creams, gels, and suppositories used for contraception

spiritual wellness: state of balance and harmony with yourself and others

squamous cell carcinoma: cancer of the bottom layer of skin; most are curable if removed early

starch: complex chain of glucose molecules

sterility: not being able to be impregnated or impregnate

stimulants: drugs that produce nervous system excitement; including cocaine, caffeine, and amphetamines

storage fat: also called depot fat; energy stored as fat in various parts of the body

strength training: the use of resistance to increase one's ability to exert or resist force for the purpose of improving performance

stress: the sum of physical and emotional reactions to any stimulus that disturbs the organism's homeostasis

stressor: any physical or psychological event or condition that produces stress

stroke: an insufficient supply of blood to the brain, resulting in loss of muscle function, loss of speech, or other symptoms

subluxation: partial displacement of a vertebra from its correct position

sucrose: common refined "table" sugar; a molecule of glucose and a molecule of fructose chemically bonded together

sulfites: used as preservatives for salad, fresh fruits and vegetables, wine, beer, and dried fruit; in susceptible individuals, especially those with asthma, they can cause a severe reaction

suppositories: a medicine placed in a body orifice to dissolve and sometimes to be absorbed; birth control suppositories contain spermicidal chemicals

sympathetic nervous system: a division of the autonomic nervous system that reacts to danger or challenges by almost instantly putting body processes into high gear

sympto-thermal method: using both the BBT and the mucus methods at the same time

syphilis: a sexually transmitted disease caused by spirochete bacteria *(Treponema pallidum)*

systole: the pressure in the arteries when the heart contracts (the higher number)

T-cells: cells of the immune system that attack foreign organisms that infect the body

tar: the yellowish brown residue of tobacco smoke

tartrazine: a yellow food dye, referred to by the FDA as "FD&C yellow No. 5"

teratogen: any environmental agent that causes abnormal development of a fetus

testes: a pair of male reproductive organs that produce sperm cells and male sex hormones

theoretical effectiveness: how well a birth control method performs if it is used as intended and consistently

third-stage labor: the stage during which the afterbirth is expelled

threat situations: events that cause stress because of a perception that harm or loss may occur

thyroxin: a hormone produced by the thyroid gland

tinnitus: persistent ringing in the ears often caused by repeated or sudden exposure to loud noises

tocotrienols: have some biological vitamin E activity

tolerance: a condition in which increased amounts of a drug or increased exposure to an addictive behavior are required to produce desired effects

toxemia: an infrequent complication of pregnancy characterized by high blood pressure and fluid retention

trachea: upper part of respiratory tract

training effect: beneficial physiological changes as a result of exercise

tranquilizers: central nervous system depressants that relax the body and calm anxiety

trans-fatty acid: an artificial fatty acid manufactured by chemically modifying monounsaturated and polyunsaturated fatty acids

triglyceride: a storage form of fat

tubal ligation: a surgical procedure in women in which the fallopian tubes are cut, tied, or cauterized to prevent pregnancy; a form of sterilization

tumor viruses: viruses that infect cells, change their growth properties, and cause cancer

tumor: a mass of abnormal cells

type A behavior: behaviors characterized by traits, such as anger or hostility, that contribute to the risk of heart disease

typical failure rate: likelihood of becoming pregnant considering all the potential problems associated with a birth control method

ulcers: open sores that occur in the stomach or small intestine for reasons largely unknown

ultrasound scanning: use of sound waves to visualize the fetus in the womb

unconscious: whatever is in the mind but out of conscious awareness

undernutrition: restricting the daily caloric intake of an animal or person without causing malnutrition

unintentional injury: preferred term for accidental injury; result of an accident

universal donor: a person whose blood is accepted by everyone during transfusion

universal recipient: a person whose blood type is compatible with anyone else's blood

urethra: a tube that carries urine from the bladder to the outside

urethritis: an irritation or infection of the urethra caused by bacteria

uterus: the female organ in which a fetus develops

vaccines: inactivated bacteria or viruses that are injected or taken orally; the body responds by producing antibodies and cells that provide lasting immunity

vacuum (suction) curettage: removal of fetal tissue by suctioning off contents of the uterus

vagina: a woman's organ of copulation and the exit pathway for the fetus at birth

vaginitis: an infection of the vagina

varicose veins: swelling of veins (usually in the legs) resulting from defective valves

vasectomy: a surgical procedure in men in which segments of the vas deferens are removed and the ends tied to prevent the passage of sperm

vasocongestion: the engorgement of blood vessels in particular body parts in response to sexual arousal

vector: the carrier of infectious organisms from animals to people or from person to person

vegan: one who excludes all animal products from the diet, including milk, cheese, eggs, and other dairy products

vegetarian: one who consumes no meat, poultry, or fish

veins: blood vessels that return blood from tissues to the heart

violence: a physical or verbal behavior, in which the aim is to harm, injure, or destroy someone or something

vital statistics: numerical data relating to birth, death, disease, marriage, and health

vitamins: essential organic substances needed daily in small amounts to perform specific functions in the body

vulva: the female external genital structures

warm-up: low-intensity exercise done before full-effort physical activity to improve muscle and joint performance, prevent injury, reinforce motor skills, and maximize blood flow to the muscles and heart

water-soluble vitamins: soluble in water; there are nine water-soluble vitamins

weaned: to discontinue breast-feeding, using other means to provide nutrients

wellness: emphasizes individual responsibility for well-being through the practice of health-promoting lifestyle behaviors

Western blot test: a test to determine the presence of specific HIV proteins; very accurate

withdrawal symptoms: uncomfortable and sometimes dangerous reactions that occur after a person stops taking a physically addicting drug

xenoestrogens: environmental chemicals that mimic the effects of natural estrogen

yoga: a combination of physical movements and mental exercises that relax the mind and the body

you-statements: statements beginning with "You"; negative communication skill

zygote: the first cell of a new person, formed at fertilization

Chapter ①

Review the learning objectives and key terms for this chapter to test your knowledge of the material.
The key terms are available in a flash card format on our Web site.   www.jbpub.com/hwonline

Learning Objectives

1. Describe what it means to be healthy.

2. Describe the medical, environmental, and holistic, or wellness, models of health.

3. Explain the wellness continuum and its impact on personal health.

4. Identify and describe the six dimensions of wellness.

5. Describe the personal qualities that are associated with the six dimensions of wellness.

6. Explain the philosophy of holistic health.

7. List the three most common actual causes of death and explain how lifestyles and behaviors contribute to disease.

8. Explain how modern lifestyles contribute to nearsightedness (myopia).

9. Understand how spirituality enhances health.

10. Explain the importance of the national health objectives for the year 2010.

Key Terms (page)

Emotional wellness (7)

Environmental model (5)

Health (4)

Holistic model (6)

Incidence (5)

Intellectual wellness (7)

Leading health indicators (14)

Medical model (4)

Morbidity (5)

Mortality (5)

Occupational wellness (7)

Physical wellness (7)

Prevalence (5)

Social wellness (7)

Spiritual wellness (7)

Vital statistics (5)

Wellness (4)

Study Guide and Self Assessment

Exploring Your Health

How Well Are You?

Complete the following health and wellness inventory to gauge your present degree of wellness. For each of the questions, circle the number

5 if the statement is ALWAYS true

4 if the statement is FREQUENTLY true

3 if the statement is OCCASIONALLY true

2 if the statement is SELDOM true

1 if the statement is NEVER true

1. I am able to identify the situations and factors that overstress me.   5 4 3 2 1

2. I eat only when I am hungry.   5 4 3 2 1

3. I don't take tranquilizers or other drugs to relax.   5 4 3 2 1

4. I support efforts in my community to reduce environmental pollution.   5 4 3 2 1

5. I avoid buying foods with artificial colorings.   5 4 3 2 1

6. I rarely have problems concentrating on what I'm doing because of worrying about other things.   5 4 3 2 1

7. My employer (school) takes measures to ensure that my work (study) place is safe.   5 4 3 2 1

8. I try not to use medications when I feel unwell.   5 4 3 2 1

9. I am able to identify certain bodily responses and illnesses as my reactions to stress.   5 4 3 2 1

10. I question the use of diagnostic X-rays.   5 4 3 2 1

11. I try to change personal habits that are risk factors for heart disease, cancer, and other lifestyle diseases.   5 4 3 2 1

12. I avoid taking sleeping pills to help me sleep.   5 4 3 2 1

13. I try not to eat foods with refined sugar or corn sugar as ingredients.   5 4 3 2 1

14. I accomplish goals I set for myself.   5 4 3 2 1

15. I stretch or bend for several minutes each day to keep my body flexible.   5 4 3 2 1

16. I support immunization of all children for common childhood diseases.   5 4 3 2 1

17. I try to prevent friends from driving after they drink alcohol.   5 4 3 2 1

18. I minimize my salt intake.   5 4 3 2 1

19. I don't mind when other people and situations make me wait or lose time.   5 4 3 2 1

20. I climb four or fewer flights of stairs rather than take the elevator.   5 4 3 2 1

21. I eat fresh fruits and vegetables.   5 4 3 2 1

22. I use dental floss at least once a day.   5 4 3 2 1

23. I read product labels on foods to determine their ingredients.   5 4 3 2 1

24. I try to maintain a normal body weight.   5 4 3 2 1

25. I record my feelings and thoughts in a journal or diary.   5 4 3 2 1

26. I have no difficulty falling asleep.   5 4 3 2 1

27. I engage in some form of vigorous physical activity at least three times a week.   5 4 3 2 1

28. I take time each day to quiet my mind and relax.   5 4 3 2 1

29. I want to make and sustain close friendships and intimate relationships.   5 4 3 2 1

30. I obtain an adequate daily supply of vitamins from my food or vitamin supplements.   5 4 3 2 1

31. I rarely have tension or migraine headaches or pain in the neck or shoulders.   5 4 3 2 1

32. I wear a safety belt when driving.   5 4 3 2 1

33. I am aware of the emotional and situational factors that lead me to overeat.   5 4 3 2 1

34. I avoid driving my car after drinking any alcohol.   5 4 3 2 1

35. I am aware of the side effects of the medicines I take.   5 4 3 2 1

36. I am able to accept feelings of sadness, depression, and anxiety, realizing that they are almost always transient.   5 4 3 2 1

37. I would seek several additional professional opinions if my doctor recommended surgery for me.   5 4 3 2 1

38. I agree that nonsmokers should not have to breathe the smoke from cigarettes in public places.   5 4 3 2 1

39. I agree that pregnant women who smoke harm their babies.   5 4 3 2 1

40. I feel I get enough sleep.   5 4 3 2 1

41. I ask my doctor why a certain medication is being prescribed and inquire about alternatives.   5 4 3 2 1

42. I am aware of the calories expended in my activities.   5 4 3 2 1

43. I am willing to give priority to my own needs for time and psychological space by saying "no" to others' requests of me.   5 4 3 2 1

44. I walk instead of drive whenever feasible.   5 4 3 2 1

45. I eat a breakfast that contains about one-third of my daily need for calories, proteins, and vitamins.   5 4 3 2 1

46. I prohibit smoking in my home.   5 4 3 2 1

47. I remember and think about my dreams.   5 4 3 2 1

48. I seek medical attention only when I have symptoms or feel that some (potential) condition needs checking, rather than have routine yearly checkups.   5 4 3 2 1

49. I endeavor to make my home accident-free.   5 4 3 2 1

50. I ask my doctor to explain the diagnosis of my problem until I understand all that I care to.   5 4 3 2 1

51. I try to include fiber or roughage (whole grains, fresh fruits, vegetables, or bran) in my daily diet.   5 4 3 2 1

52. I can deal with my emotional problems without alcohol or other mood-altering drugs.   5 4 3 2 1

53. I am satisfied with my school or job.   5 4 3 2 1

54. I require children riding in my car to be in infant seats or in shoulder harnesses.   5 4 3 2 1

55. I try to associate with people who have a positive attitude about life.   5 4 3 2 1

56. I try not to eat snacks of candy, pastries, and other "junk" foods.   5 4 3 2 1

57. I avoid people who are "down" all the time and who bring down those around them.   5 4 3 2 1

58. I am aware of the calorie content of the foods I eat.   5 4 3 2 1

59. I brush my teeth after meals.   5 4 3 2 1

60. *(for women only)* I routinely examine my breasts.   5 4 3 2 1

    (for men only) I am aware of the signs of testicular cancer.   5 4 3 2 1

How to Score

Enter the numbers you've circled above next to the question number in the columns below and total your score for each category. Then use the wellness status key to determine your degree of wellness for each category.

Emotional health	Fitness and body care	Environmental health	Stress	Nutrition	Medical self-responsibility
6 ____	15 ____	4 ____	1 ____	2 ____	8 ____
12 ____	20 ____	7 ____	3 ____	5 ____	10 ____
25 ____	22 ____	17 ____	9 ____	13 ____	11 ____
26 ____	24 ____	32 ____	14 ____	18 ____	16 ____
36 ____	27 ____	34 ____	19 ____	21 ____	35 ____
40 ____	33 ____	38 ____	28 ____	23 ____	37 ____
47 ____	42 ____	39 ____	29 ____	30 ____	41 ____
52 ____	44 ____	46 ____	31 ____	45 ____	48 ____
55 ____	58 ____	49 ____	43 ____	51 ____	50 ____
57 ____	59 ____	54 ____	53 ____	56 ____	60 ____
Total ____	Total ____	Total ____	Total ____	Total ____	Total ____

Wellness Status

To assess your status in each of the six categories, compare your total score in each column to the following key: **0–34,** need improvement; **35–44,** good; **45–50,** excellent.

Contracting with Yourself

Based on your wellness status results, make appropriate changes in categories you would like to improve. List the changes you wish to make, set a time to begin making them, and decide when you want the change to be fully integrated into your life.

For example:

Change Desired

• quit smoking

• take up meditation

• record dreams

Begin Change

• in 1 week

• immediately

• after quitting smoking

Time Allotted

• 1 month

• 2 weeks

• 1 week

Do not try to make all the changes on your list at the same time. Begin with either the one or two most important or the one or two you know you can accomplish. Then make one or two changes at a time after that.

Study Guide and Self Assessment

Chapter 2

Review the learning objectives and key terms for this chapter to test your knowledge of the material.
The key terms are available in a flash card format on our Web site. www.jbpub.com/hwonline

Learning Objectives

1. Describe how the mind and body communicate (chemically and electrically) to enhance physical and mental well-being.

   _____

   _____

2. Explain homeostasis and the role it plays in maintaining health.

   _____

   _____

3. Describe the function(s) of the autonomic nervous system.

   _____

   _____

4. Explain the Chinese ideas of yin and yang and chi energy.

   _____

   _____

5. Describe the relationship between hormones and certain body functions.

   _____

   _____

6. Explain what is meant by somatization disorder.

   _____

   _____

7. Describe ways to relieve test anxiety.

   _____

   _____

8. Discuss how prayer and hypnosis are used in healing.

   _____

   _____

9. Describe how image visualization can promote behavioral changes.

   _____

   _____

Key Terms (page)

Autonomic nervous system (24)

_____

Biofeedback training (24)

_____

Chi (23)

_____

Homeostasis (23)

_____

Hormones (25)

_____

Hypnotherapy (32)

_____

Image visualization (35)

_____

Mandala (34)

_____

Mantra (34)

_____

Meditation (33)

_____

Neuropeptides (24)

_____

Placebo effect (28)

_____

Progressive muscle relaxation (34)

_____

Psychosomatic illnesses (26)

_____

Relaxation response (33)

_____

Somatization (27)

_____

Somatization disorder (27)

_____

Yoga (33)

_____

Study Guide and Self Assessment

Exploring Your Health

Visualization Eliminates the Pain

Everyone can learn to reduce or eliminate the pain of minor surgery and dental procedures. One way to reduce pain is to imagine it as a *discomfort;* most people can handle discomfort even if they have difficulty coping with pain. Self-induced deep mental relaxation, or self-hypnosis, can effectively control most pain, even that of terminal cancer. One woman describes her use of visualization to control the pain of dental surgery.

> Just two days ago, before going for extraction of a molar, I relaxed and imagined painless, bloodless surgery. It came to pass just as I had programmed it.

No bleeding and no pain, in spite of having the bone scraped and the gum stitched. The prescription given me for codeine was not necessary. Prior to my recent understanding, my threshold for pain was practically nonexistent. For years I bled excessively at the dentist's office or while having minor surgery. Now I am no longer a "bleeder" but a believer.

- Describe two other instances in which image visualization could prevent pain.
- Describe an incident in which you used visualization to decrease pain (e.g., sports, injury, doctor's office visit).

Review the learning objectives and key terms for this chapter to test your knowledge of the material. The key terms are available in a flash card format on our Web site.   www.jbpub.com/hwonline

Learning Objectives

1. Define the terms stress, stressor, eustress, distress, and stress-related illness.

   _____

   _____

2. Describe the changes in behavior, autonomic nervous system, and immune system that are caused by stress.

   _____

   _____

3. Name several stress-related illnesses.

   _____

   _____

4. Identify and explain the three components of stress.

   _____

   _____

5. Explain how frustration, inner conflict, and social pressures cause stress.

   _____

   _____

6. Discuss three common reactions to stress.

   _____

   _____

7. Discuss several factors that influence the degree of stress a person experiences.

   _____

   _____

8. Explain the fight-or-flight response.

   _____

   _____

9. Describe the three phases of the general adaptation syndrome.

   _____

   _____

10. Describe how stress affects the immune system.

    _____

    _____

11. Explain how stress can be managed.

    _____

    _____

Key Terms (page)

Activators (43)

_____

Challenge situations (48)

_____

Consequences (43)

_____

Coping (48)

_____

Cortisol (49)

_____

Distress (48)

_____

Epinephrine (49)

_____

Eustress (48)

_____

Fight-or-flight response (49)

_____

Harm-and-loss situations (47)

_____

Hypothalamus (49)

_____

Parasympathetic nervous system (49)

_____

Posttraumatic stress disorder (PTSD) (51)

_____

Reactions (43)

_____

Self-efficacy (54)

_____

Stress (42)

_____

Stressor (42)

_____

Sympathetic nervous system (49)

_____

Threat situations (48)

_____

Study Guide and Self Assessment

Study Guide and Self Assessment

Exploring Your Health

What Are Your Stress Reactions?

Many people experience particular physical reactions to excessive stress. Here's a list of some common stress reactions. Which ones do you frequently experience? Can you add some reactions that are not on the list?

Reaction	Once a day	Once every 2–3 days	Once a week	Once a month	Not in the last 2 months
Headaches	____	____	____	____	____
Nervous tics and twitches	____	____	____	____	____
Blurred vision	____	____	____	____	____
Dizziness	____	____	____	____	____
Fatigue	____	____	____	____	____
Coughing	____	____	____	____	____
Wheezing	____	____	____	____	____
Backache	____	____	____	____	____
Muscle spasms	____	____	____	____	____
Itching	____	____	____	____	____
Excessive sweating	____	____	____	____	____
Palpitations	____	____	____	____	____
Constipation	____	____	____	____	____
Jaw tightening	____	____	____	____	____
Rapid heart rate	____	____	____	____	____
Impotence	____	____	____	____	____
Pelvic pain	____	____	____	____	____
Stomachache	____	____	____	____	____
Diarrhea	____	____	____	____	____
Frequent urination	____	____	____	____	____
Dermatitis (rash)	____	____	____	____	____
Hyperventilation	____	____	____	____	____
Irregular heart rhythm	____	____	____	____	____
High blood pressure	____	____	____	____	____
Delayed menstruation	____	____	____	____	____
Vaginal discharge	____	____	____	____	____
Nail biting	____	____	____	____	____
Heartburn	____	____	____	____	____

How Susceptible Are You to Stress?

Some persons are more susceptible to the harmful effects of stress than others. The following inventory can give you an indication of your susceptibility. Score each item from 1 (almost always) to 5 (never) as it applies to you. A total score lower than 50 indicates you are not particularly vulnerable to stress. A score of 50 to 80 indicates moderate vulnerability, and a score of more than 80, high vulnerability—time to make some changes.

_____ 1. I eat at least one hot, nutritious meal a day.
_____ 2. I get 7 to 8 hours sleep at least 4 nights a week.
_____ 3. I am affectionate with others regularly.

_____ 4. I have at least one relative within 50 miles on whom I can rely.
_____ 5. I exercise to the point of sweating at least twice a week.
_____ 6. I smoke fewer than 10 cigarettes a day.
_____ 7. I drink fewer than five alcoholic drinks a week.
_____ 8. I am about the proper weight for my height and age.
_____ 9. I have enough money to meet basic expenses and needs.
_____ 10. I feel strengthened by my religious beliefs.
_____ 11. I attend club or social activities on a regular basis.
_____ 12. I have several close friends and acquaintances.
_____ 13. I have one or more friends to confide in about personal matters.

_____ 14. I am basically in good health.

_____ 15. I am able to speak openly about my feelings when angry or worried.

_____ 16. I discuss problems about chores, money, and daily living issues with the people I live with.

_____ 17. I do something just for fun at least once a week.

_____ 18. I am able to organize my time and do not feel pressured.

_____ 19. I drink fewer than three cups of coffee (or tea or cola drinks) a day.

_____ 20. I allow myself quiet time at least once during each day.

TOTAL

SCORE _____

Source: Adapted from a test developed by L. H. Miller and A. D. Smith.

Do You Have "Hurry Sickness"?

Behavior	Almost always	Only sometimes	Almost never
1. Do you interrupt other people before they have finished speaking?	_____	_____	_____
2. Are you irritated when you have to wait in line?	_____	_____	_____
3. Do you eat fast?	_____	_____	_____
4. Do you try to do more than one thing at a time?	_____	_____	_____
5. Are you annoyed if you lose at sports or games?	_____	_____	_____
6. How often do you forget what you were going to say?	_____	_____	_____
7. Do you tap your fingers or bounce your feet while sitting?	_____	_____	_____
8. Do you speed up and drive through yellow caution lights at intersections?	_____	_____	_____
9. Do you race the car engine while waiting for the signal to change?	_____	_____	_____
10. Do you fall behind in the things you need to accomplish?	_____	_____	_____

Here's how to determine your score: If you checked *Almost always,* give yourself 3 points; if you checked *Only sometimes,* 2 points; and if *Almost never,* 1 point. Add up all the points. If you scored 25 to 30, you probably have hurry sickness (don't worry, it's not fatal) and need to work on slowing down or relaxing more. If you scored 16 to 24, you have a potential for hurry syndrome. If you scored less than 16, you are probably pretty laid back.

Study Guide and Self Assessment

Chapter 4

Review the learning objectives and key terms for this chapter to test your knowledge of the material. The key terms are available in a flash card format on our Web site.   www.jbpub.com/hwonline

Learning Objectives

1. Explain Maslow's hierarchy of needs and the role it plays in emotional wellness.

   _____

   _____

2. Identify several strategies for coping with emotional distress.

   _____

   _____

3. Identify several defense mechanisms.

   _____

   _____

4. Identify and explain fear and phobia.

   _____

   _____

5. Explain the characteristics of depression.

   _____

   _____

6. Discuss the prevalence and several signs of suicide.

   _____

   _____

7. Discuss the importance of sleep for mental well-being.

   _____

   _____

8. Identify characteristics of schizophrenia.

   _____

   _____

Key Terms (page)

Anxiety (64)

_____

Bipolar disorder (68)

_____

Cognition (60)

_____

Conscious (60)

_____

Coping strategies (62)

_____

Defense mechanisms (63)

_____

Depression (67)

_____

Dysthymia (68)

_____

Growth needs (60)

_____

Hierarchy of needs (60)

_____

Insomnia (72)

_____

Maintenance needs (60)

_____

Narcolepsy (72)

_____

Obsessive-compulsive disorder (66)

_____

Panic disorder (65)

_____

Parasomnias (72)

_____

Phobia (64)

_____

Rapid eye movement (REM) (73)

_____

Schizophrenia (74)

_____

Self-actualization (60)

_____

Sleep apnea (72)

_____

Social phobia (64)

_____

Somnambulism (72)

_____

Unconscious (61)

_____

Study Guide and Self Assessment

Identify Your Fears or Phobias

Frightening situations or objects	No fear	Mild fear	Strong fear
Airplanes	____	____	____
Birds	____	____	____
Bats	____	____	____
Blood	____	____	____
Cemeteries	____	____	____
Dead animals	____	____	____
Insects	____	____	____
Crowds of people	____	____	____
Dark places	____	____	____
Dentists or doctors	____	____	____
Hospitals	____	____	____
Dirt or germs	____	____	____
Lakes or oceans	____	____	____
Dogs or cats	____	____	____
Other animals	____	____	____
Guns	____	____	____
Closets or elevators	____	____	____
Heights	____	____	____
Public presentations	____	____	____
Loud noises	____	____	____
Driving in a car	____	____	____
Being shouted at	____	____	____
Being rejected	____	____	____
Walking alone at night	____	____	____
Other fears	____	____	____

Keep a Sleep and Dream Record

Each morning for 1 week, assess your sleep behavior with the aid of a chart like the one below; also record the details of your dreams in your journal or notebook. Hints for dream recording:

1. Keep a pen or a pencil and a pad of paper near your bed.
2. Remind yourself before going to sleep that you want to remember your dreams.
3. Write down your dreams immediately upon awakening.

Sleep Assessment Chart

	Sun	Mon	Tues	Wed	Thurs	Fri	Sat
Time to bed							
Time fell asleep (estimate on waking)							
Feelings before falling asleep							
Trouble falling asleep? (yes or no)							
Take sleeping aid? (e.g., milk or pills)							
Number of times awake in the night							
Time woke up							
Time arose							
Feelings on awakening							
Dreams? (yes or no)							
Total sleep time							

Saying No

Many people have a hard time saying *no* to the requests and demands made by others and an equally hard time saying *yes* to themselves for something they want. To be generous with time and energy is thought to be a virtue; to accommodate your own wishes, selfish. There are times, however, when saying *no* to others and *yes* to yourself is highly appropriate. Your emotions tell you those times. The time to say *no* is when saying *yes* makes you feel angry and resentful. The time to say *yes* to yourself is when it increases your inner feelings of love and peace.

Think about some recent times when you said *yes* to others when you really wanted to say *no*. Write them down like this: I would have liked to have said *no* when _____ asked me to_____ .

Prepare yourself to say *no* to the same or other requests the next time they occur. Imagine yourself saying *no* to another and firmly and politely dealing with the other person's response.

Learning to say *no* may take practice, so don't get discouraged if at first you find it difficult.

Chapter 5

Review the learning objectives and key terms for this chapter to test your knowledge of the material.
The key terms are available in a flash card format on our Web site.   www   www.jbpub.com/hwonline

Learning Objectives

1. Discuss the various factors that influence dietary choices.

2. Describe the dietary guidelines proposed by health organizations.

3. Describe the three kinds of vegetarian diets and several reasons for vegetarianism.

4. Describe which foods are at the bottom of the food guide pyramid and which are at the top and give the reasons for that placement.

5. Describe the ingredients and nutrition facts labels on manufactured foods.

6. Describe the three functions of food.

7. Define calorie.

8. List the seven components of food, and identify common foods that contain each component.

9. Describe the difference between simple and complex carbohydrates.

10. Define and identify sources of antioxidants.

Key Terms (page)

Amino acids (90)

Anemia (86)

Antioxidants (97)

Artificial fat (96)

Basal metabolic rate (BMR) (89)

Basal metabolism (89)

Calorie (88)

Carbohydrates (93)

Cellulose (95)

Cholesterol (96)

Complex carbohydrates (94)

Deoxyribonucleic acid (DNA) (93)

Essential amino acids (90)

Essential nutrients (85)

Fat-soluble vitamins (97)

Fatty acids (96)

Fiber (94)

Flavonoids (99)

Fructose (94)

Study Guide and Self Assessment

Galactose (94)

_____

Gamma irradiation (104)

_____

Glucose (94)

_____

Glycogen (95)

_____

Goiter (86)

_____

Hemicellulose (95)

_____

Homocysteine (97)

_____

Ingredients label (84)

_____

Insoluble fiber (95)

_____

Kilocalorie (89)

_____

Lactase (94)

_____

Lacto-ovo-vegetarian (107)

_____

Lactose (94)

_____

Lacto-vegetarian (107)

_____

Lecithin (96)

_____

Linoleic acid (96)

_____

Lipids (96)

_____

Metabolism (89)

_____

Minerals (97)

_____

Monounsaturated fatty acid (96)

_____

Nitrates (92)

_____

Nitrites (92)

_____

Nonessential amino acids (90)

_____

Neutraceutical (100)

_____

Nutrition facts label (84)

_____

Nutritional calorie (89)

_____

Percent daily value (84)

_____

Phytochemicals (98)

_____

Polyunsaturated fatty acid (96)

_____

Proteins (90)

_____

Reactive hypoglycemia (107)

_____

Recommended [daily] dietary allowances (RDA) (86)

_____

Saturated fat (96)

_____

Simple sugars (94)

_____

Soluble fiber (95)

_____

Starch (94)

_____

Sucrose (94)

_____

Sulfites (102)

_____

Tartrazine (103)

_____

Trans-fatty acid (96)

_____

Veganism (107)

_____

Vegetarian (107)

_____

Vitamins (97)

_____

Water-soluble vitamins (97)

_____

Exploring Your Health

Food Diary

Data Collection

For 2 days, keep a list of *everything* you eat. You should choose days that are representative of your usual food consumption patterns. You should also record the quantity of each food item, the time of day it was consumed, whether consumption was part of meal or a snack, whether you ate because of hunger or for other reasons, your feelings at the time you ate, and the social circumstances surrounding eating (e.g., alone, with friends, family).

Food	Quantity	Time of day	Meal or snack	Hungry? Other?	Feelings?	Social?
cereal	bowlful	6:30 AM	meal	hungry	sleepy	alone
banana	one	"	"	"	"	"
milk, skim	cup	"	"	"	"	"

Data Analysis

Analyze the nutrient content of a representative meal from your food diary.

1. Choose a representative meal.
2. Log on to the Nutritional Analysis Calculator at the University of Illinois and submit your meal for a nutrition analysis. You can find the link to the calculator on the *Health and Wellness* Web site.
3. Print out the analysis.
4. Write a one-page paper in which you compare your food intake (the number of servings in each category) with the guidelines offered by the "Food Guide Pyramid" (see page 84).

My Eating Habits: Some Clues to Calories

Calories come from food—all kinds of food. Do you get enough? Or more than you need? Think about your eating patterns—and why you eat what you eat. Check all the answers that describe your eating patterns.

What Do I Usually Eat?

_____ A varied and balanced diet.
_____ A diet with only moderate amounts of fats and sugars.
_____ Deep-fat-fried and breaded foods.
_____ "Extras," such as salad dressings, potato toppings, spreads, sauces, and gravies.
_____ Sweets and rich desserts, such as candies, cakes, and pies.
_____ Snack foods high in fat and sodium, such as chips and other "munchies."
_____ Soft drinks.

When Do I Usually Eat?

_____ At mealtime.
_____ While studying.
_____ While preparing meals or clearing the table.
_____ When spending time with friends.
_____ While watching TV or participating in other activities.
_____ Anytime.

Where Do I Usually Eat?

_____ At home at the kitchen or dining room table.
_____ In the school cafeteria.
_____ In fast-food places.
_____ In front of the TV or while studying.
_____ Wherever I happen to be when I'm hungry.

Why Do I Usually Eat?

_____ It's time to eat.
_____ I'm hungry.
_____ Foods look tempting.
_____ Everyone else is eating.
_____ Food will get thrown away if I don't eat it.
_____ I'm bored or frustrated.

Changes I Want to Make

1. _____
2. _____
3. _____

Source: U.S. Department of Agriculture, *Dietary Guidelines and Your Health: Health Educator's Guide to Nutrition and Fitness* (Washington, D.C.: U.S. Government Printing Office, 1992).

Eat for Good Nutrition

Are you "in action"? Are you ready to stay in shape—for a lifetime? From these statements, check seven sense guidelines for smart eating that can help you stay healthy.

_____ Use salt and sodium only in moderation.
_____ Choose a diet low in fat, saturated fat, and cholesterol.
_____ Avoid snacking.
_____ Eat an apple a day for good health.
_____ Use sugars only in moderation.
_____ Avoid desserts.
_____ Maintain a healthy weight.
_____ Avoid alcoholic beverages.
_____ Eat green vegetables every day.
_____ Avoid candy, chips, and soft drinks.
_____ Choose a diet with plenty of vegetables, fruits, and grain products.
_____ Eat a variety of foods.
_____ Avoid fast foods.

Study Guide and Self Assessment

I want to follow the dietary guidelines so I stay healthy. Here's how I'll eat smart:

_____

_____

_____

_____

SIGNED _____

DATE _____

Source: U.S. Department of Agriculture, *Dietary Guidelines and Your Health: Health Educator's Guide to Nutrition and Fitness* (Washington, D.C.: U.S. Government Printing Office, 1992).

How Does Your Diet Rate for Variety?

A varied diet is a healthful diet. How would you describe the variety in your food choices?

	Seldom or never	1 or 2 times a week	3 to 4 times a week	Almost daily
How often do you eat:				
1. At least six servings of breads, cereals, rice, crackers, pasta, or other foods made from grains (a serving is one slice of bread or a half cup of cereal or rice) per day?	☐	☐	☐	☐
2. Foods made from whole grains?	☐	☐	☐	☐
3. Three different kinds of vegetables per day?	☐	☐	☐	☐
4. Cooked dry beans or peas?	☐	☐	☐	☐
5. A dark-green vegetable, such as spinach or broccoli?	☐	☐	☐	☐
6. Two kinds of fruit or fruit juice per day?	☐	☐	☐	☐
7. Three servings of milk, yogurt, or cheese per day?	☐	☐	☐	☐
8. Two servings of lean meat, poultry, or fish, or eggs, dry beans, or nuts per day?	☐	☐	☐	☐
Count the number of check marks in each column. TOTAL	_____	_____	_____	_____

To eat a varied diet, I will _____

_____

Chapter 6

Review the learning objectives and key terms for this chapter to test your knowledge of the material.
The key terms are available in a flash card format on our Web site.   www.jbpub.com/hwonline

Learning Objectives

1. Describe the extent and causes of overweight in American society.

   _____

   _____

2. Describe the significance of body mass index (BMI) to health.

   _____

   _____

3. Explain the concept of fatness set point.

   _____

   _____

4. Explain why calorie-restricting weight-loss programs fail.

   _____

   _____

5. Discuss why exercise (and *not* calorie restriction) is the key to healthy weight maintenance.

   _____

   _____

6. List the psychological factors that contribute to weight problems.

   _____

   _____

7. Discuss the advantages and disadvantages of the medical treatments for overweight.

   _____

   _____

8. Describe the signs of anorexia nervosa and bulimia.

   _____

   _____

Key Terms (page)

Anorexia athletica (127)

_____

Anorexia nervosa (128)

_____

Appestat (118)

_____

Appetite suppressants (124)

_____

Benzocaine (125)

_____

Binge eating disorder (129)

_____

Bulk-producing agents (126)

_____

Body image (127)

_____

Body mass index (115)

_____

Bulimia (128)

_____

Energy balance (118)

_____

Essential fat (115)

_____

Fatness set point (117)

_____

Glycogen (117)

_____

Hormones (126)

_____

Leptin (119)

_____

Liposuction (124)

_____

Storage fat (115)

_____

Triglyceride (117)

_____

Study Guide and Self Assessment

Exploring Your Health

What Are Your Weight Statistics?

Fill in the blanks below.

Your height in inches
(without shoes) _____ inches (multiply by .0254 = _____ meters)

Your weight (with
clothes) _____ pounds (divide by 2.2 = _____ kilograms)

Highest adult weight _____ pounds, when age_____

Lowest adult weight _____ pounds, when age_____

Recommended weight for height (see page 116) _____

Body mass index (see page 117) _____ Divide your weight (in kilograms)
by your height (in meters, squared)

Watching Your Weight

Refer to your food diary to complete the following assessment:

1. List all the feelings other than hunger that are associated with your eating be-havior. Does one feeling predominate?

2. Make a list of activities that you can do instead of eating when you are not hungry.

Body Image

How do you feel about the appearance of these regions of your body?

	Quite satisfied	Somewhat satisfied	Somewhat dissatisfied	Very dissatisfied
Hair	☐	☐	☐	☐
Arms	☐	☐	☐	☐
Hands	☐	☐	☐	☐
Feet	☐	☐	☐	☐
Waist	☐	☐	☐	☐
Buttocks	☐	☐	☐	☐
Hips	☐	☐	☐	☐
Legs and ankles	☐	☐	☐	☐
Thighs	☐	☐	☐	☐
Chest or breasts	☐	☐	☐	☐
Posture	☐	☐	☐	☐
General attractiveness	☐	☐	☐	☐

1. Which of your thoughts and actions enhance your body image?

_____

_____

2. Which of your thoughts and actions are detrimental to your body image?

_____

_____

3. What societal forces (expectations of friends and parents, advertising,

celebrities and professional athletes, etc.) influence your body image most strongly?

_____

_____

4. What could you do to become more satisfied with your body image?

_____

_____

Chapter

Review the learning objectives and key terms for this chapter to test your knowledge of the material. The key terms are available in a flash card format on our Web site.   **www.jbpub.com/hwonline**

Learning Objectives

1. Define physical activity.

   _____

   _____

2. Describe the health benefits of physical activity.

   _____

   _____

3. Describe the psychological benefits of physical activity.

   _____

   _____

4. Define aerobic training and strength training.

   _____

   _____

5. Make a plan for incorporating physical activity into your life.

   _____

   _____

6. Describe common overuse syndromes.

   _____

   _____

Key Terms (page)

Aerobic training (140)

_____

Anabolic steroids (142)

_____

Athletic amenorrhea (147)

_____

Cool-down (145)

_____

Creatine (143)

_____

Endorphins and enkephalins (140)

_____

Endurance (144)

_____

Epinephrine (140)

_____

Fitness (140)

_____

Flexibility (144)

_____

Isometric training (142)

_____

Norepinephrine (140)

_____

Overuse syndromes (147)

_____

Strength training (141)

_____

Training effect (141)

_____

Warm-up (145)

_____

Study Guide and Self Assessment

Study Guide and Self Assessment

Exploring Your Health

Determine Your Fitness Index

The Harvard Step Test is a standardized measure of cardiorespiratory fitness. To carry out the Harvard Step Test, you need to be comfortably dressed (athletic clothes are best); and you need a chair, stool, or bench 12 to 18 inches high, a stopwatch or clock with a second hand, a pencil and paper, and a metronome or some other method to produce a rhythmic 100 to 120 beats per minute, such as a recording of a march or some disco music. Once all this is assembled, you can begin.

1. Make a 15-second recording of your resting pulse and multiply by 4 to obtain your heartbeat rate per minute.

2. Start the metronome or music at 120 beats per minute.

3. Step completely up on the bench with the left leg first, followed by your right leg, then step back down with the left leg first, followed by the right. The stepping should be done on a four-count: up-up-down-down; up-up-down-down . . .

4. Continue the exercise for 3 minutes unless you are over 30 years old and have been rather inactive for more than 6 months. In that case, do the test for only a minute or two, whichever you think you can do. If you are sure you cannot do the test for even a few seconds, don't.

5. When the 3 minutes of exercise are through, immediately take your pulse. Record the number of heartbeats between 15 and 30 seconds after exercising. Make additional heart rate measurements between 60 and 75 seconds, 120 and 135 seconds, 180 and 195 seconds, 240 and 255 seconds, and a final measurement between 300 and 315 seconds.

6. Multiply each of the 15-second heart rates by 4 to give the beats per minute. Record your data on a graph below.

7. Compute your fitness index: Add the per-minute heart rates for the first 3 minutes after exercise. Then divide that number into 30,000.

Fitness index	Rating
Above 90	Excellent
80–89	Good
65–79	Average
55–64	Low Average
Below 55	Poor

Harvard Step Test data record

Time	Heartbeats per 15 seconds		Heartbeats per minute
At rest	_____	× 4 =	_____
15–30 sec	_____	× 4 =	_____
60–75 sec	_____	× 4 =	_____
120–135 sec	_____	× 4 =	_____
180–195 sec	_____	× 4 =	_____
240–255 sec	_____	× 4 =	_____
300–315 sec	_____	× 4 =	_____

Determine Your Flexibility Index

Body flexibility is a fundamental aspect of feeling good and keeping your body young. Use this simple YMCA test to determine your degree of body flexibility, and continue to use it to determine your progress in becoming more limber. You can consult exercise and yoga books to find exercises that will help you improve your flexibility.

1. Warm up with some stretching before the test.

2. Sit on the floor with your legs extended and feet a few inches apart.

3. With a piece of adhesive tape, mark the place where your heels touch the floor. Your heels should touch the near edge of the tape.

4. Place a yardstick on the floor between your legs and parallel to them. The beginning of the yardstick should be closest to you and the 15-inch mark should align with the near edge of the tape.

5. Slowly reach with both hands as far forward as possible. Touch your fingers to the yardstick to determine the distance reached. Do not jerk to increase your distance—this may cause damage to your leg muscles.

6. Repeat the exercise two or three times and record your best score.

Inches reached		Rating
Men	Women	
22–23	24–27	Excellent
20–21	21–23	Good
14–19	16–20	Average
12–13	13–16	Fair
0–11	0–12	Poor

<u>Chapter</u>   **8**

Review the learning objectives and key terms for this chapter to test your knowledge of the material.
The key terms are available in a flash card format on our Web site.   www.jbpub.com/hwonline

Learning Objectives

1. Define the terms sex, sexuality, sexual, menopause, masturbation, gender role, gender identity, sexual orientation, heterosexual, homosexual, bisexual.

   _____

   _____

2. Compare and contrast traditional gender roles for males and females.

   _____

   _____

3. Describe the male reproductive system.

   _____

   _____

4. Describe the female reproductive system.

   _____

   _____

5. Explain the menstrual cycle.

   _____

   _____

6. Explain the sexual response cycle.

   _____

   _____

7. Identify and discuss several different sexual difficulties.

   _____

   _____

8. Describe an intimate relationship.

   _____

   _____

9. Identify and describe the essential components of good communication.

   _____

   _____

   _____

Key Terms (page)

Bisexual (158)

_____

Breasts (162)

_____

Celibacy (167)

_____

Cervix (160)

_____

Circumcision (165)

_____

Clitoris (161)

_____

Copulation (164)

_____

Cowper's glands (165)

_____

Cystitis (162)

_____

Endometrium (163)

_____

Fallopian tubes (160)

_____

Feedback (174)

_____

Fertilization (156)

_____

Follicle-stimulating hormone (163)

_____

Foreskin (165)

_____

Gametes (156)

_____

Gender identity (157)

_____

Gender role (157)

_____

Heterosexual (158)

_____

Homosexual (158)

_____

I-statements (174)

_____

Labia majora (161)

_____

Labia minora (161)

_____

Study Guide and Self Assessment

Literal message (173)

Luteinizing hormone (163)

Masturbation (167)

Menarche (163)

Menopause (163)

Menstruation (163)

Metamessage (173)

Mutual empathy (174)

Myotonia (166)

Orgasm (167)

Ova (159)

Ovaries (160)

Ovulation (160)

Penis (164)

Prostate gland (165)

Scrotum (164)

Secondary sex characteristics (159)

Self-disclosure (171)

Semen (165)

Seminal vesicles (165)

Sex (156)

Sexual (156)

Sexual orientation (158)

Sexual response cycle (166)

Sexuality (156)

Smegma (165)

Spectatoring (167)

Testes (164)

Urethra (161)

Urethritis (162)

Uterus (160)

Vagina (160)

Vaginitis (161)

Vasocongestion (166)

Vulva (161)

You-statements (174)

Exploring Your Health

How Realistic Are Your Attitudes About Love?

By now you probably understand that *love* does not mean the same thing to everyone, even professionals in the field of human sexuality. As individuals, we carry concepts of love that range from romantic to realistic to cynical, depending largely on our life experiences.

For each of the following statements, circle the number that most closely approximates your response.

	Strongly agree	Somewhat agree	Strongly disagree
1. I don't believe that research should be done on love, because love should remain mysterious.	3	2	1
2. Love is the most important thing in my life.	3	2	1
3. My life is very unhappy when I am not in love.	3	2	1
4. I am able to function very well without someone to love.	1	2	3
5. Love is a fantasy that is popular with 13-year-old girls.	1	2	3
6. Each of us has our "one and only" somewhere out there, if only we can find that person.	3	2	1
7. Once you find your "one and only," you will never feel attracted to anyone else.	3	2	1
8. If you love too much, you will only get hurt.	1	2	3
9. I am able to function very well without someone loving me.	1	2	3
10. The smartest people don't get hung up on someone.	1	2	3
11. You can tell when you first see someone if you are going to love that person.	3	2	1
12. The best relationships have some basis more important than love.	1	2	3
13. If you love someone enough, any kind of problem in the relationship can be overcome.	3	2	1
14. If I had to choose between living in poverty or living without love, I would choose to love in poverty.	3	2	1
15. As soon as someone thinks you love them, they will start to take advantage of you.	1	2	3
16. You're a sucker if you fall in love with someone who has no money.	1	2	3

TOTAL POINTS: _____

Interpretation:

40 to 48 points: You have very romantic ideas about love. You might put too much emphasis on love as a basis for a partnership, while ignoring other important considerations.

24 to 39 points: You have more realistic ideas about love. Love is important to you, but you also are aware of the many other bases of a smoothly functioning partnership.

16 to 23 points: You appear to be pretty cynical about love. Maybe you previously have been hurt or come from a family where romance was not emphasized. Your attitudes might insulate you from getting hurt again but could also be preventing you from enjoying the benefits of a loving relationship.

Source: Byer, C. O., Shainberg, L. W., & Galliano, G. (1999). *Dimensions of Human Sexuality.* Boston, MA: McGraw-Hill College, p. 86.

Study Guide and Self Assessment

An Assessment of Sexual Communication

Communication skills contribute to rewarding relationships in many ways. Many of the problems couples experience could be avoided or easily resolved with more effective communication skills. How are your communication skills? For each statement, circle the appropriate number of points.

	Usually	Sometimes	Seldom
1. I find it easy to express my nonsexual needs and feelings to others.	2	1	0
2. I find it easy to express my sexual needs and feelings to others.	2	1	0
3. I am sensitive to the needs and feelings expressed by others, and especially their nonverbal expressions.	2	1	0
4. My relationships with other people are pleasant and rewarding.	2	1	0
5. When a conflict arises in one of my relationships, it is resolved with ease.	2	1	0
6. I find it easy to communicate with people of both genders.	2	1	0
7. I can communicate effectively with people of various ethnic groups.	2	1	0
8. I can find the right words to express the ideas I want to convey.	2	1	0
9. I am good at interpreting nonverbal messages from other people.	2	1	0
10. I try very hard not to interrupt someone who is speaking to me.	2	1	0
11. I try very hard to be nonjudgmental in my responses when people share their ideas and feelings with me.	2	1	0
12. When a discussion is causing me to feel uncomfortable, I try hard not to withdraw from the discussion or change the subject.	2	1	0
13. I try to help people open up by asking open-ended, rather than yes-or-no questions.	2	1	0
14. When I want to express my feelings, I try to phrase them as "I" statements, rather than "you" statements.	2	1	0
15. I feel that I am adequately assertive.	2	1	0
16. I let someone know when they are not respecting my rights or feelings.	2	1	0
17. I find it easy to say no to pressure for unwanted sexual activity.	2	1	0
18. I find it easy to talk to a potential sexual partner about prevention of sexually transmitted diseases.	2	1	0
19. When conflicts arise in my relationships, I am, if necessary, willing and able to make a compromise to resolve the conflict.	2	1	0
20. When conflicts arise in my relationships, I try to find a resolution that satisfies the needs of both persons involved.	2	1	0

TOTAL POINTS: _____

Interpretation:

36 to 40 points: You have developed highly effective patterns of communication and assertiveness.

32 to 35 points: You have above-average communication and assertiveness skills.

28 to 31 points: You have about average communication and assertiveness skills. Sharpening these skills will improve your relationships and need fulfillment.

27 points or less: It would be very rewarding for you to improve your communication skills. Your relationships would function much better, and you would experience much greater need fulfillment.

Source: Byer, C. O., Shainberg, L. W. & Galliano, G. (1999). *Dimensions of Human Sexuality*. Boston, MA: McGraw-Hill College, p. 68.

Gender Roles and Society

Purpose: This inventory will aid you in becoming aware of your attitudes toward stereotypical masculine and feminine roles in society. The views of many people in regard to these traditional roles are changing but not necessarily in the same way. Therefore, it is important that you understand your own values as well as the values of those with whom you interact.

Directions: Read each statement carefully and respond by using the scale given below. Use the first column of blanks for your own responses. Then use a sheet of paper to cover your responses and have your partner or friend use the second column of blanks to respond to the statements.

You	Friend	Strongly agree 1	Agree 2	Disagree 3	Strongly disagree 4

_____ _____ 1. Men should feel comfortable receiving flowers from a woman.

_____ _____ 2. Women should take the steps necessary to prevent pregnancy, as contraception is the woman's responsibility.

_____ _____ 3. The woman's role is to stay home, take care of the children, and support her husband in his work; the man's role is to support the family financially.

_____ _____ 4. A man should be open to relocating because of his wife's job, regardless of whose salary is higher.

_____ _____ 5. Men should be expected to stand when a woman enters the room and to open doors for women.

_____ _____ 6. Men and women should share equally in the role of decision maker in the home.

_____ _____ 7. Women should pay their half of the expenses on dates.

_____ _____ 8. Women should be able to ask men for dates.

_____ _____ 9. A woman who pursues a career cannot be a good mother.

_____ _____ 10. Men should be free to express their emotions as openly as women do.

_____ _____ 11. Women should be free to initiate the sex act.

_____ _____ 12. Education is equally important for husband and wife.

_____ _____ 13. Only men should be drafted into the army.

_____ _____ 14. Society discriminates against women in certain occupations.

_____ _____ 15. Society discriminates against men in certain occupations.

_____ _____ 16. Parents should allow their sons to play with dolls.

_____ _____ 17. A woman should be free to pursue whatever interest or career she would like, as long as it does not inconvenience her husband.

_____ _____ 18. Girls should be raised feeling proud to say that their vocation is wife and mother.

_____ _____ 19. The movement toward desexualization in clothes, jobs, recreation, and education is dangerous.

_____ _____ 20. Maternal and nurturing feelings are instinctive only to women.

_____ _____ 21. Men are sexual, women are productive.

_____ _____ 22. Boys play at love when what they desire is sex, and girls play at sex when they desire love.

_____ _____ 23. Married women should feel comfortable keeping their maiden names.

_____ _____ 24. Men stand to gain just as much from the women's movement as women do.

_____ _____ 25. The ideal couple should go everywhere together.

_____ _____ 26. Women should be allowed to serve in combat in the armed forces.

Reactions: Use the space provided to respond to the following questions.

1. For which statements were your responses different from those of your partner?

2. After discussing the differences in your responses, decide if these are potential problem areas. Explain why or why not.

3. Discuss whether you feel your beliefs regarding these statements are the same as those of most people your age.

Source: Valois, R.F. & Kammerman, S. (1992). *Your Sexuality* (2nd ed.). New York, NY: McGraw-Hill, 4–6.

Study Guide and Self Assessment

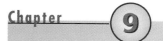

Chapter   9

Review the learning objectives and key terms for this chapter to test your knowledge of the material.
The key terms are available in a flash card format on our Web site.   www.   **www.jbpub.com/hwonline**

Learning Objectives

1. Discuss reasons for and against becoming pregnant.

   _____

   _____

2. Explain what takes place during pregnancy, beginning with fertilization.

   _____

   _____

3. Identify and briefly describe four important health habits during pregnancy.

   _____

   _____

4. Discuss childbirth preparation.

   _____

   _____

5. Identify three risks to fetal development.

   _____

   _____

6. Discuss two ways to detect birth defects.

   _____

   _____

7. Identify and briefly explain four potential problems during pregnancy.

   _____

   _____

8. Describe the birthing process.

   _____

   _____

9. Discuss several methods of medical intervention in childbirth.

   _____

   _____

10. Identify the pros and cons of breast-feeding.

    _____

    _____

11. Identify several reasons for infertility and options for infertile couples.

    _____

    _____

12. Discuss types of adoption.

    _____

    _____

Key Terms (page)

Afterbirth (192)

_____

Amniocentesis (189)

_____

Amnion (184)

_____

Amniotic fluid (184)

_____

Artificial insemination (196)

_____

Braxton-Hicks contractions (191)

_____

Cesarean section (194)

_____

Chorionic villus sampling (CVS) (189)

_____

Colostrum (194)

_____

Eclampsia (187)

_____

Ectopic pregnancy (184)

_____

Embryo (183)

_____

Episiotomy (193)

_____

Fertilization (182)

_____

First-stage labor (191)

_____

Human chorionic gonadotropin (HCG) (183)

_____

In vitro fertilization (IVF) (196)

_____

Infertile (195)

_____

Insemination (196)

_____

Study Guide and Self Assessment

Labor (191)

Lightening (191)

Placenta (184)

Preeclampsia (187)

Prolactin (194)

Puerperium (194)

Second-stage labor (192)

Seminiferous tubules (183)

Third-stage labor (192)

Toxemia (187)

Weaned (195)

Zygote (182)

Exploring Your Health

To Be or Not to Be Parents

Purpose: Since two people are needed to conceive a child, two people should decide whether and when to conceive. With the advent of more reliable birth control methods, couples may spend years deciding whether or not to become parents. If or when you consider having a child, this exercise provides a chance to examine your and your partner's expectations of parenthood. *Even if you feel parenthood is far in your future,* this will help you determine your current expectations.

Directions: On another sheet of paper, you and your partner should independently write a sentence or two in answer to each question. Then *go through what you have written* and indicate, by a check in the proper column, whether each *prediction* would make you pleased, unhappy, or neither if it came true. Pick out which of the areas covered in the questions are most important to you in your decision.

	Pleased	Unhappy	Neither
1. How will having a child affect my partner's and my career and education?	____	____	____
2. How will a child affect our financial situation now and later?	____	____	____
3. How will the child affect our relationship with each other?	____	____	____
4. How will the child affect our relationship with family and friends?	____	____	____
5. How will the child affect our freedom, privacy, and spontaneity?	____	____	____
6. How will my partner and I deal with the pregnancy and birth?	____	____	____
7. How will each of us deal with supervising, training, and being with a young child (birth to age 8)?	____	____	____
8. How will we each deal with supervising, training, and being with an older child or teenagers?	____	____	____
9. How will we deal with possible problems of health and personality our child could have?	____	____	____
10. How do we feel about bringing up a child in today's world (i.e., what kinds of problems and solutions are there for the child's future world)?	____	____	____

Scoring: Compare answers with your partner. Discussing realistic predictions of parenthood can quell some fears (or bring others to mind) and be a starting point for making a decision.

Reactions: Use the space provided to respond to the following questions.

1. Which of the areas covered in the questions are most important to your decision?

2. At this time, do you foresee children in your future? Explain.

Source: Valois, R. F. & Kammerman, S. (1992). *Your Sexuality* (2nd ed.). New York, NY: McGraw-Hill, pp. 239–240.

Study Guide and Self Assessment

Chapter 10

Review the learning objectives and key terms for this chapter to test your knowledge of the material.
The key terms are available in a flash card format on our Web site.   www.jbpub.com/hwonline

Learning Objectives

1. Identify the advantages and disadvantages of the following fertility control methods: male condom, female condom, spermicides, diaphragm, cervical cap, hormonal contraceptives, Norplant, Depo-Provera, intrauterine device, abstinence, sterilization, withdrawal, and postcoital methods.

_____

2. Identify several different types of fertility awareness methods.

_____

3. Identify the most effective and least effective fertility control method.

_____

4. Determine the best fertility control method for your sexual lifestyle.

_____

5. Discuss the importance of communication when determining the right fertility control method to use with your partner.

_____

6. Explain why some sexually active people do not use fertility control.

_____

7. Define abortion and describe the different types of abortion procedures.

_____

_____

Key Terms (page)

Abortion (220)

_____

Basal body temperature (BBT) method (213)

_____

Calendar rhythm (213)

_____

Cannula (220)

_____

Cervical cap (209)

_____

Coitus interruptus (203)

_____

Condom (210)

_____

Culpotomy (215)

_____

Depo-Provera (206)

_____

Diaphragm (207)

_____

Dilation and curettage (D and C) (221)

_____

Dilation and evacuation (D and E) (221)

_____

Douching (203)

_____

Ectopic pregnancy (207)

_____

Failure rate (202)

_____

Fertility awareness method (212)

_____

Hysterectomy (215)

_____

Intrauterine device (IUD) (206)

_____

Laminaria (220)

_____

Laparoscopy (215)

_____

Lowest observed failure rate (202)

_____

Luteinizing hormone (214)

_____

Minilaparotomy (215)

_____

Norplant (206)

_____

Pelvic inflammatory disease (PID) (207)

_____

Progestin-only contraceptives (206)

_____

Spermicide (209)

_____

Sterility (214)

_____

Suppositories (209)

_____

Sympto-thermal method (214)

_____

Tubal ligation (215)

_____

Typical failure rate (202)

_____

Vacuum (suction) curettage (220)

_____

Vasectomy (214)

_____

Exploring Your Health

Contraceptive Comfort and Confidence Scale

In assessing your answers to these questions, you will be helping yourself decide whether the method of control you are using or considering is a realistic choice. (Members of a couple should answer these questions separately.)

Method of birth control you are considering using: _____

Length of time you used this method in the past: _____

Check **Yes** or **No** for each of the following questions:	Yes	No
1. Have I had problems using this method before?	____	____
2. Have I or my partner ever become pregnant while using this method?	____	____
3. Am I afraid of using this method?	____	____
4. Would I really rather not use this method?	____	____
5. Will I or my partner have trouble remembering to use this method?	____	____
6. Will I or my partner have trouble using this method correctly?	____	____
7. Do I still have unanswered questions about this method?	____	____
8. Does this method make menstrual periods longer or more painful?	____	____
9. Does this method cost more than I can afford?	____	____
10. Could this method cause me or my partner to have serious complications?	____	____
11. Am I opposed to this method because of my religious or moral beliefs?	____	____
12. Is my partner opposed to this method?	____	____
13. Am I using this method without my partner's knowledge?	____	____
14. Will using this method embarrass my partner?	____	____
15. Will using this method embarrass me?	____	____
16. Will I or my partner enjoy intercourse less because of this method?	____	____
17. If this method interrupts lovemaking, will I avoid it?	____	____
18. Has a nurse or physician ever told me or my partner NOT to use this method?	____	____
19. Is there anything about my or my partner's personality that could lead me or my partner to use this method incorrectly?	____	____
20. Am I or is my partner at risk of being exposed to HIV or another STD if I use or my partner uses this method?	____	____

Most persons will have a few "yes" answers. "Yes" answers mean that problems might arise. If you have more than a few "yes" responses, you may want to talk with a physician, counselor, partner, or friend to help you decide whether to use this method or how to use it so that it will really be effective for you. In general, the more "yes" answers you have, the less likely you are to use this method consistently and correctly at every act of intercourse.

Source: Byer, C. O., Shainberg, L. W., & Galliano, G. (1999). _Dimensions of Human Sexuality._ Boston, MA: McGraw-Hill College, p. 455.

Chapter   11

Review the learning objectives and key terms for this chapter to test your knowledge of the material.
The key terms are available in a flash card format on our Web site.   www.jbpub.com/hwonline

Learning Objectives

1. Describe the impact of sexually transmitted diseases (STDs) on society.

   _____

   _____

2. List the risk factors for contracting an STD.

   _____

   _____

3. Identify the causative agent, symptoms, and treatment for the following diseases: trichomonas vaginitis and gardnerella vaginitis, chlamydia, gonorrhea, syphilis, genital herpes, genital warts, pubic lice, scabies, and AIDS.

   _____

   _____

4. Explain the importance of testing for HIV infection and the proper testing procedures.

   _____

   _____

5. Identify several "safer sex" practices.

   _____

   _____

6. Describe the importance of effective communication in reducing the risk of STDs and AIDS.

   _____

   _____

Key Terms (page)

Chancre (229)

_____

Chlamydia (228)

_____

Epididymitis (229)

_____

Genital warts (231)

_____

Gonorrhea (229)

_____

Hemophilia (236)

_____

Herpes (230)

_____

Human immunodeficiency virus (HIV) (233)

_____

Human papillomavirus (HPV) (231)

_____

Pubic lice (232)

_____

Scabies (233)

_____

Sexually transmitted diseases (STDs) (226)

_____

Syphilis (229)

_____

Exploring Your Health

Home Test for HIV

A home test kit for HIV is distributed by Home Access Health Corporation and can be purchased at pharmacies or obtained by calling 1-800-HIV-TEST. A blood sample is taken at home and mailed to a laboratory along with an anonymous identification number. The results can be obtained by phone in 3 to 7 days. A phone counseling service is available 24 hours a day and anyone with a positive result is automatically connected with a counselor. Anyone can speak with a counselor and receive information before or after the test.

Study Guide and Self Assessment

Chapter **12**

Review the learning objectives and key terms for this chapter to test your knowledge of the material.
The key terms are available in a flash card format on our Web site.   www.jbpub.com/hwonline

Learning Objectives

1. Define pathogen, communicable disease, vector, immunizations, opportunistic infections, nosocomial disease, immune system, antibodies, antigens, and autoimmune diseases.

2. Identify and explain how infectious diseases are prevented and treated.

3. Discuss the importance of antibiotics with regard to bacterial infections and the implications of antibiotic-resistant strains of bacteria.

4. Discuss how immunizations prevent infections.

5. Discuss the etiology, symptoms, and treatments for cold and flu, Lyme disease, mononucleosis, and ulcers.

6. Explain how antibodies battle infectious diseases.

7. Describe how unwanted activities of the immune system cause allergies.

8. Discuss organ transplants, blood transfusions, and the Rh factor.

9. Describe how HIV causes AIDS.

Key Terms (page)

AIDS (acquired immune deficiency syndrome) (269)

AIDS antibody test (271)

Allergens (262)

Anaphylactic shock (263)

Antibodies (258)

Antigens (260)

Autoimmune diseases (265)

B-cells (260)

Cell-mediated immunity (260)

Cilia (251)

Communicable disease (247)

Contact dermatitis (262)

Cytokines (261)

DNA (deoxyribonucleic acid) (247)

Etiology (264)

Food allergies (264)

Hepatitis (255)

Histamine (262)

Histocompatibility (267)

Study Guide and Self Assessment

HIV (human immunodeficiency virus) (269)

_____

HLA (human leukocyte antigens) (267)

_____

Humoral immunity (260)

_____

Immune system (258)

_____

Immunizations (261)

_____

Immunosuppressive drugs (268)

_____

Leukocytes (251)

_____

Lupus erythematosus (265)

_____

Lyme disease (253)

_____

Lymph nodes (259)

_____

Lymphatic system (259)

_____

Macrophages (251)

_____

Malaria (247)

_____

Mononucleosis (253)

_____

Multiple sclerosis (MS) (266)

_____

Myelin (266)

_____

Nosocomial diseases (258)

_____

Opportunistic infections (270)

_____

Pathogen (246)

_____

Penicillin (248)

_____

Prions (256)

_____

T-cells (260)

_____

Ulcers (254)

_____

Universal donor (268)

_____

Universal recipient (268)

_____

Vaccines (261)

_____

Vector (247)

_____

Western blot test (271)

_____

Exploring Your Health

Are You Current on All Your Vaccines?

Adult Vaccination Schedules

Vaccine	Indication	Precautions and contraindications
Bacille Calmette-Guérin	Debatable benefits for adults at high risk of multiple drug-resistant tuberculosis	Immunocompromised
Hæmophilus influanzae type B	Patients with splenic dysfunction, other at-risk conditions	Safety in pregnancy unknown
Hepatitis A	Adults at increased risk, e.g., travelers to endemic areas, gay men, injecting drug users, day care workers	Pregnancy risk not fully evaluated
Hepatitis B	Healthcare workers in contact with blood, persons residing for ≥ 6 months in areas of high endemicity, others at high risk	Safety to fetus unknown, pregnancy not a contraindication in high-risk persons
Influenza	Adults with high-risk conditions, healthy persons ≥ 65 years, health care personnel	Anaphylaxis in response to eggs, first trimester of pregnancy (relative contraindication)
Measles	Adults born after 1956 without measles (diagnosed by a physician or immunologic test) or live-virus immunization, for revaccination of persons given killed measles vaccine (1963–1967)	Pregnancy, immunocompromised, history of anaphylaxis to eggs or neomycin
Meningococcal polysaccharide	Travel to areas with epidemic meningococcal disease	Safety in pregnancy unknown
Mumps	Susceptible adults	Pregnancy, immunocompromised, history of anaphylaxis in response to eggs or neomycin
Pneumococcal polysaccharide	Persons at increased risk of pneumococcal disease and its complications, healthy adults ≥ 65 years	Safety in pregnancy unknown
Polio (inactivated)	Preferred for ≥ 18-year-olds for primary immunization; one-time booster dose for travelers	Safety to fetus unknown, anaphylactic reactions to streptomycin or neomycin
Polio (oral)	One-time booster for previously immunized persons, completion of the series in partially immunized adults, alternative to inactivated polio vaccine when there is < 1 month before travel, not used for primary immunization in persons ≥ 18 years	Immunocompromised host or contact
Rubella	Susceptible adults, particularly women of childbearing age	Pregnancy, immunocompromised, history of anaphylactic reaction to neomycin
Tetanus-diphtheria	Adults	First trimester of pregnancy, hypersensitivity or neurologic reaction to previous doses, severe local reaction
Varicella	Susceptible adolescents and adults, especially health care workers and others likely to be exposed	Pregnancy, immunocompromised

Source: Adapted in part from data of the Centers for Disease Control and Prevention.

Study Guide and Self Assessment

Chapter **13**

Review the learning objectives and key terms for this chapter to test your knowledge of the material.
The key terms are available in a flash card format on our Web site.   www   www.jbpub.com/hwonline

Learning Objectives

1. Identify and describe the most important ways to prevent cancer.
   _____
   _____

2. Briefly discuss the incidence of cancer today and why mortality has not fallen.
   _____
   _____

3. Define the following terms: cancer, tumor, benign tumor, malignant tumor, metastasis, and xenoestrogen.
   _____
   _____

4. Explain the difference between inherited diseases and genetic diseases.
   _____
   _____

5. Describe the kinds of environmental agents that cause cancer.
   _____
   _____

6. Explain ways to prevent skin cancer.
   _____
   _____

7. Discuss some risk factors associated with breast cancer.
   _____
   _____

8. Describe how to do a breast self-exam (BSE).
   _____
   _____

9. Discuss how cigarette smoke contributes to cancer.
   _____
   _____

10. Discuss the association between diet and cancer.
    _____
    _____

11. Briefly describe the three medical treatments for cancer.
    _____
    _____

12. Describe several coping mechanisms for someone with cancer.
    _____
    _____

13. Explain the risks and benefits of being tested for a cancer susceptibility gene.
    _____
    _____

Key Terms (page)

Basal cell carcinoma (290)
_____

Benign tumor (278)
_____

Biopsy (280)
_____

Cancer (278)
_____

Cancer-susceptibility gene (282)
_____

Chemical carcinogen (285)
_____

Chemotherapy (292)
_____

Epidemiology (283)
_____

Ionizing radiation (283)
_____

Malignant tumor (279)
_____

Mammogram (288)
_____

Melanoma (290)
_____

Mesothelioma (285)
_____

Metastasis (279)
_____

Mutation (283)
_____

Pathologist (279)
_____

Prostate-specific antigen (289)
_____

Study Guide and Self Assessment

Radiation therapy (292)

_____

Squamous cell carcinoma (290)

_____

Tumor (278)

_____

Tumor viruses (284)

_____

Xenoestrogens (286)

_____

Exploring Your Health

Reduce Environmental Cancer Risks
Make a list of environmental agents and substances that are known to be carcinogenic that you think you have been exposed to within the past 6 months.

1. _____

2. _____

3. _____

4. _____

5. _____

6. _____

7. _____

8. _____

9. _____

10. _____

Hint: some common examples are x-rays, cigarette smoke, asbestos dust, and household pesticides.

In what ways can you reduce your exposure to these and other carcinogenic substances?

Study Guide and Self Assessment

Chapter **14**

Review the learning objectives and key terms for this chapter to test your knowledge of the material.
The key terms are available in a flash card format on our Web site.   www   www.jbpub.com/hwonline

Learning Objectives

1. Describe how the heart functions.

   _____

   _____

2. Define cardiovascular disease, infarction, coronary heart disease, stroke, and heart attack.

   _____

   _____

3. Explain the role atherosclerosis plays in heart disease.

   _____

   _____

4. Identify and explain types of heart surgeries used to repair blocked arteries.

   _____

   _____

5. Identify the major risk factors of heart disease that cannot be changed, major risk factors that can be changed, and other contributing factors.

   _____

   _____

6. Explain the role of homocysteine in heart disease.

   _____

   _____

7. Discuss various ways to reduce cholesterol levels.

   _____

   _____

8. Explain how stress contributes to hypertension.

   _____

   _____

9. List dietary supplements and foods that help maintain a healthy cardiovascular system.

   _____

   _____

Key Terms (page)

Aneurysm (310)

_____

Angina pectoris (305)

_____

Angiocardiography (307)

_____

Aorta (303)

_____

Arteries (303)

_____

Arteriography (cardiac catheterization) (307)

_____

Arteriosclerosis (305)

_____

Atherosclerosis (305)

_____

Capillaries (305)

_____

Cardiologist (303)

_____

Cardiovascular disease (302)

_____

Carotid endarterectomy (310)

_____

Coronary arteries (302)

_____

Coronary bypass surgery (308)

_____

Diastole (314)

_____

Essential hypertension (313)

_____

Familial hyperlipidemia (FH) (312)

_____

Fibrillation (303)

_____

Free radicals (318)

_____

Study Guide and Self Assessment

Study Guide and Self Assessment

Exploring Your Health

Testing for Risk of Heart Disease

Total the Points for All Your Risk Factors from the Tables Below

Age	
HDL Cholesterol	+
Total Cholesterol	+
Syst. Blood Press.	+
Cigarette Smoker	+
Diabetes	+
LVH	+
POINT TOTAL	+

Note: Add plus points and subtract minus points

Age Risk

Find the Points That Correspond to Your Age			
Men		**Women**	
Age	**Points**	**Age**	**Points**
30	−2	≤30	−12
31	−1	31	−11
32–33	0	32	−9
34	1	33	−8
35–36	2	34	−6
37–38	3	35	−5
39	4	36	−4
40–41	5	37	−3
42–43	6	38	−2
44–45	7	39	−1
46–47	8	40	0
48–49	9	41	1
50–51	10	42–43	2
52–54	11	44	3
55–56	12	45–46	4
57–59	13	47–48	5
60–61	14	49–50	6
62–64	15	51–52	7
65–67	16	53–55	8
68–70	17	56–60	9
71–73	18	61–67	10
74	19	68–74	11

Blood Lipid Risks

HDL Cholesterol		Total Cholesterol	
HDL	Points	Total	Points
25–26	7	139–151	−3
27–29	6	152–166	−2
30–32	5	167–182	−1
33–35	4	183–199	0
36–38	3	200–219	1
39–42	2	220–239	2
43–46	1	240–262	3
47–50	0	263–288	4
51–55	−1	289–315	5
56–60	−2	316–330	6
61–66	−3		
67–73	−4		
74–80	−5		
81–87	−6		
88–96	−7		

Blood Pressure Risks

Systolic Blood Pressure	
SBP	Points
98–104	−2
105–112	−1
113–120	0
121–129	1
130–139	2
140–149	3
150–160	4
161–172	5
173–185	8

Other Risks

Factor	Points
Cigarette smoker	4
Diabetic male	3
Diabetic female	6
Left ventricular hypertrophy (LVH)	9

Measure the Risk Corresponding to Your Point Total

	Probability of developing heart disease	
Points	5-Yr. Risk	10-Yr. Risk
1 or less	Less than 1%	Less than 2%
2	1%	2%
3	1%	2%
4	1%	2%
5	1%	3%
6	1%	3%
7	1%	4%
8	2%	4%
9	2%	5%
10	2%	6%
11	3%	6%
12	3%	7%
13	3%	8%
14	4%	9%
15	5%	10%
16	5%	12%
17	6%	13%
18	7%	14%
19	8%	16%
20	8%	18%
21	9%	19%
22	11%	21%
23	12%	23%
24	13%	25%
25	14%	27%
26	16%	29%
27	17%	31%
28	19%	33%
29	20%	36%
30	22%	38%
31	24%	40%
32	25%	42%

Compare Your Risk to 10-Year Average Risks for U.S. Population

	Average 10-year risks	
Age	Women	Men
30–34	less than 1%	3%
35–39	less than 1%	5%
40–44	2%	6%
45–49	5%	10%
50–54	8%	14%
55–59	12%	16%
60–64	13%	21%
65–69	9%	30%
70–74	12%	24%

Study Guide and Self Assessment

Review the learning objectives and key terms for this chapter to test your knowledge of the material. The key terms are available in a flash card format on our Web site.   www.jbpub.com/hwonline

Learning Objectives

1. Identify and describe several congenital birth defects.

   _____

   _____

2. Identify and describe several chemical substances that cause birth defects.

   _____

   _____

3. Explain what a hereditary disease is.

   _____

   _____

4. Discuss the importance of genes in health and disease.

   _____

   _____

5. Explain prenatal testing for genetic diseases and discuss the importance of genetic counseling.

   _____

   _____

6. Describe how some hereditary diseases can be treated.

   _____

   _____

7. Describe several kinds of genetic discrimination.

   _____

   _____

8. Explain genetic testing and gene therapy.

   _____

   _____

Key Terms (page)

Amniocentesis (332)

_____

Chorionic villus analysis (332)

_____

Congenital defect (326)

_____

DNA (deoxyribonucleic acid) (330)

_____

Enzymes (331)

_____

Eugenics (325)

_____

Gene therapy (334)

_____

Genetic counseling (331)

_____

Genetically modified food (GMF) (335)

_____

Hereditary (genetic) disease (329)

_____

Karyotype (330)

_____

Teratogen (327)

_____

Ultrasound scanning (332)

_____

Study Guide and Self Assessment

Chapter ⑯

Review the learning objectives and key terms for this chapter to test your knowledge of the material. The key terms are available in a flash card format on our Web site.   www.jbpub.com/hwonline

Learning Objectives

1. Explain the difference between a drug and a medicine.

   _____

   _____

2. Explain the concept of a drug receptor and its relation to drug side effects.

   _____

   _____

3. Describe the logic of a double-blind drug effectiveness study.

   _____

   _____

4. Give examples of the overuse of legal drugs in American society and the influences of drug advertising on drug use.

   _____

   _____

5. Define the terms addiction, physical dependence, habituation, tolerance, and withdrawal.

   _____

   _____

6. Describe the different effects of the major classes of psychoactive drugs: stimulants, depressants, marijuana, hallucinogens, PCP, and inhalants.

   _____

   _____

7. Describe the health hazards of using anabolic steroids.

   _____

   _____

Key Terms (page)

Addiction (351)

_____

Amphetamines (355)

_____

Analgesics (345)

_____

Caffeine (357)

_____

Cocaine (354)

_____

Contraindication (345)

_____

Direct-to-consumer advertising (350)

_____

Diuretics (345)

_____

Dose (346)

_____

Double-blind (346)

_____

Drug (344)

_____

Drug abuse (351)

_____

Drug hypersensitivity (345)

_____

Ephedrine (357)

_____

Habituation (354)

_____

Hallucinogens (360)

_____

Hashish (359)

_____

Hypnotics (358)

_____

Inhalants (361)

_____

LSD (361)

_____

Marijuana (359)

_____

Medicine (345)

_____

Opiates (359)

_____

Over-the-counter (OTC) drugs (348)

_____

Phencyclidine (PCP) (361)

_____

Physical dependence (352)

_____

Study Guide and Self Assessment

Psychoactive (348)

_____

Psychological dependence (354)

_____

Receptor (345)

_____

Sedatives (358)

_____

Side effects (345)

_____

Stimulants (354)

_____

Teratogen (345)

_____

Tolerance (353)

_____

Tranquilizers (358)

_____

Withdrawal symptoms (353)

_____

Exploring Your Health

The Drugs You Take

Keep a list of all the nonessential drugs that you ingest for a week. Be sure to include coffee, tea, and cola drinks (which contain caffeine); alcohol; nicotine; and pain relievers. After the first week, look at your list. Are you surprised by how many of these nonessential drugs you use? Now, keep the list for another week, but eliminate just one of the nonessential drugs that you ingest and make notes about how you feel.

Week 1	Sun	Mon	Tues	Wed	Thurs	Fri	Sat
Caffeine (How many cups of coffee or 12-oz. servings of cola drinks per day?)							
Alcohol (How many 12-oz. beers, glasses of wine, or mixed drinks per day?)							
Nicotine (How many cigarettes, cigars, pipes, or dips of snuff or chewing tobacco per day?)							
Pain relievers (How many tablets per day?)							
Other:							
Other:							

Week 2	Sun	Mon	Tues	Wed	Thurs	Fri	Sat
Caffeine (How many cups of coffee or 12-oz. servings of cola drinks per day?)							
Alcohol (How many 12-oz. beers, glasses of wine, or mixed drinks per day?)							
Nicotine (How many cigarettes, cigars, pipes, or dips of snuff or chewing tobacco per day?)							
Pain relievers (How many tablets per day?)							
Other:							
Other:							

Be a Knowledgeable Consumer

If you are taking a prescribed drug, consult the library or your pharmacist or physician to find out any side effects and contraindications of the drug.

Drug	Side Effects	Contraindications

1. Evaluate the risks of taking the drug in relationship to its therapeutic benefits.

2. Discuss with your physician ways to deal with your medical needs without the use of drugs.

Study Guide and Self Assessment

Chapter

Review the learning objectives and key terms for this chapter to test your knowledge of the material.
The key terms are available in a flash card format on our Web site.   www.jbpub.com/hwonline

Learning Objectives

1. Describe the hazards of cigarette smoking.

   _____

   _____

2. Describe the hazards of smokeless tobacco use.

   _____

   _____

3. Identify and explain the physiological effects of tobacco.

   _____

   _____

4. Differentiate the different types of smokeless tobacco.

   _____

   _____

5. Discuss the short-term and long-term health-related and social consequences of tobacco use.

   _____

   _____

6. Discuss the effects of smoke on nonsmokers, and the implications for both smokers and nonsmokers.

   _____

   _____

7. Explain why some people smoke.

   _____

   _____

8. Identify advertising themes targeted at young men and women.

   _____

   _____

9. Identify ways to quit smoking.

   _____

   _____

10. Briefly discuss tobacco legislation and its effect on the society as a whole.

    _____

    _____

11. Discuss the role of the U.S. government in tobacco production and laws regulating tobacco use.

    _____

    _____

Key Terms (page)

Alpha-1-antitrypsin (AAT) (373)

_____

Alveoli (373)

_____

Bronchitis (372)

_____

Carcinogens (372)

_____

Chewing tobacco (370)

_____

Chronic obstructive pulmonary disease (COPD) (372)

_____

Emphysema (372)

_____

Moist snuff (370)

_____

Nicotine (369)

_____

Nicotine replacement therapy (375)

_____

Snuff (370)

_____

Tar (370)

_____

Trachea (373)

_____

Study Guide and Self Assessment

Exploring Your Health

Commit to Quit

Check off each item as you go to complete your *Commit to Quit* plan and begin your smoke-free life (http://www.cancer.org).

1. Deciding to quit.
- ☐ Decide what your reasons are for quitting.
- ☐ Choose the date. Mark it on a calendar.
- ☐ Say it as if you mean it. Repeat your reasons for quitting 10 times each night before going to bed.

2. Preparing to quit.
- ☐ Choose a smoking cessation method. Discuss your options with your pharmacist or doctor.
- ☐ Sign on the dotted line. Put your intention to quit in writing—and sign it.

- ☐ Don't go it alone. Reach out to family members, and try to recruit other smokers you know to join you in quitting.
- ☐ Remove triggers. Get rid of cigarettes, smoking paraphernalia and that stale, smoky smell from your home, car, office, and clothes.
- ☐ Plan alternative activities. Avoid places where smokers congregate in favor of places where smoking isn't allowed. Find a hobby that keeps your mind occupied and your hands busy.

3. Following through.
- ☐ Enroll in a counseling support program either through your local American Cancer Society office or as part of an over-the-counter nicotine replacement therapy.
- ☐ Fight cravings by practicing the 4Ds (deep breathe; drink lots of water; do something; delay reaching for a cigarette).
- ☐ Reward yourself for not smoking.

Chapter 18

Review the learning objectives and key terms for this chapter to test your knowledge of the material. The key terms are available in a flash card format on our Web site.   www.jbpub.com/hwonline

Learning Objectives

1. Discuss the prevalence of drinking, types of drinking, reasons for drinking, and attitudes toward drinking among college students.

2. Explain the effects of alcohol on the body.

3. Describe how alcohol is absorbed into the body and how this absorption relates to blood alcohol concentration.

4. Discuss the effects of alcohol on behavior, including sexual behavior.

5. Describe the long-term effects of alcohol overconsumption.

6. Define alcohol abuse, alcohol addiction, and alcoholism.

7. Explain the phases of alcoholism.

8. Describe how alcohol affects one's significant others and the help that is available for both the family and the alcoholic.

Key Terms (page)

Acetaldehyde (388)

Alcohol abuse (392)

Alcoholic (392)

Alcoholism (392)

Bender (393)

Binge drinking (386)

Blackout (393)

Blood alcohol content (BAC) (387)

Codependency (394)

Congeners (388)

Delirium tremens (DTs) (392)

Denial (394)

Enabling (394)

Ethyl alcohol (ethanol) (387)

Fetal alcohol syndrome (391)

Hangover (388)

Isopropyl alcohol (387)

Methyl alcohol (387)

Proof (387)

Secondhand binge effects (386)

Study Guide and Self Assessment

Exploring Your Health

How to Cut Down on Your Drinking

If you are drinking too much, you can improve your life and health by cutting down. How do you know if you drink too much? Read these questions and answer *yes* or *no*:

- Do you drink alone when you feel angry or sad?
- Does your drinking ever make you late for work?
- Does your drinking worry your family?
- Do you ever drink after telling yourself you won't?
- Do you ever forget what you did while you were drinking?
- Do you get headaches or have a hangover after you have been drinking?

If you answered *yes* to any of these questions, you may have a drinking problem. Check with your doctor to be sure. Your doctor will be able to tell you whether you should cut down or abstain. If you are alcoholic or have other medical problems, you should not just cut down on your drinking—you should stop drinking completely. Your doctor will advise you about what is right for you.

If your doctor tells you to cut down on your drinking, these steps can help you:

1. **Write your reasons for cutting down or stopping.**
2. **Set a drinking goal.**
Choose a limit for how much you will drink. You may choose to cut down or not to drink at all. If you are cutting down, keep below these limits:

- Women: No more than one drink a day
- Men: No more than two drinks a day

Now write your drinking goal on a piece of paper. Put it where you can see it, such as on your refrigerator or bathroom mirror. Your paper might look like this:

My drinking goal

I will start on this day_____ .

I will not drink more than _____ drinks in 1 day.

I will not drink more than _____ drinks in 1 week.

or

I will stop drinking alcohol.

3. **Keep a "diary" of your drinking. Write down every time you have a drink for 3 to 4 weeks.**

Week:

	No. of drinks	Type of drinks	Place consumed
Mon			
Tues			
Wed			
Thurs			
Fri			
Sat			
Sun			

Now you know why you want to drink less and you have a goal. There are many ways you can help yourself to cut down. Try the tips.

4. **Watch it at home.**
Keep a small amount or no alcohol at home. Don't keep temptations around.

5. **Drink slowly.**
When you drink, sip your drink slowly. Take a break of 1 hour between drinks. Drink soda, water, or juice after a drink with alcohol. Do not drink on an empty stomach! Eat food when you are drinking.

6. **Take a break from alcohol.**
Pick a day or two each week when you will not drink at all. Then, try to stop drinking for 1 week. Think about how you feel physically and emotionally on these days. When you succeed and feel better, you may find it easier to cut down for good.

7. **Learn how to say *NO*.**
You do not have to drink when other people drink. You do not have to take a drink that is given to you. Practice ways to say *no* politely. For example, you can tell people you feel better when you drink less. Stay away from people who give you a hard time about not drinking.

8. **Stay active.**

9. **Get support.**
Cutting down on your drinking may be difficult at times. Ask your family and friends for support to help you reach your goal. Talk to your doctor if you are having trouble cutting down. Get the help you need to reach your goal.

10. **Watch out for temptations.**
Watch out for people, places, or times that make you drink when you do not want to. Stay away from people who drink a lot or bars where you used to go. Plan ahead of time what you will do to avoid drinking when you are tempted.

Do not drink when you are angry or upset or have a bad day. These are habits you need to break if you want to drink less.

11. **DO NOT GIVE UP!**
Most people do not cut down or give up drinking all at once. Just like a diet, it is not easy to change. That is okay. If you do not reach your goal the first time, try again. Remember, get support from people who care about you and want to help.

Source: National Institute on Alcohol Abuse and Alcoholism, National Institutes of Health, March 1996, NIH Publication No. 96-3770.

<u>Chapter</u> **19**

Review the learning objectives and key terms for this chapter to test your knowledge of the material.
The key terms are available in a flash card format on our Web site.   www.jbpub.com/hwonline

Learning Objectives

1. Describe what you need to know to be an intelligent health care consumer.

   _____

   _____

2. Distinguish between different types of health care professionals.

   _____

   _____

3. Compare and contrast private health insurance, preferred provider organizations, and health maintenance organizations.

   _____

   _____

4. Explain why health care costs have escalated.

   _____

   _____

5. Discuss health care reform and its effect on personal health care.

   _____

   _____

6. Discuss what you believe should be the essential elements of health care for all Americans.

   _____

   _____

Key Terms (page)

Diagnosis (404)

_____

Health maintenance organization (HMO) (406)

_____

Magnetic resonance imaging (409)

_____

Managed care (406)

_____

Preferred provider organization (PPO) (407)

_____

Study Guide and Self Assessment

Exploring Your Health

Intelligent Health Consumer Profile

This exercise can help determine the extent to which consumers act intelligently when exposed to misleading and inaccurate information, health fraud, and health quackery. Place an X in the column to the right that best represents your answer:

	VM	M	S	L	N
Are you sufficiently informed to be able to make sound decisions?					
Where do you go for information when needed?					
Professional health organizations or individuals					
Health books, magazines, newsletters					
Government health agencies					
Advertisements					
Newspapers or magazines					
Radio or television					
People you know					
To what extent do you accept statements appearing in news reports or advertisements at face value?					
To what extent can you identify quacks, quackery, fraudulent schemes, and hucksters?					
When selecting health practitioners to what extent do you:					
Talk with or visit before first appointment					
Check or inquire regarding qualifications or credentials					
Ask friend or neighbor about reputation					
Inquire about fees and payment procedures					
When you have been exposed to a fraudulent practice, quack, quackery, or a poor product or service, to what extent do you report your experience?					

Key: *VM* = very much; *M* = much; *S* = some; *L* = little; *N* = none.

Source: H. J. Cornacchia and S. Barrett, *Consumer Health: A Guide to Intelligent Decisions,* 5th ed. (St. Louis, MO: Mosby, 1993), p. 11.

Chapter (20)

Learning Objectives

1. Describe the main differences between modern medical care and alternative medicines.

   _____

   _____

2. Define the four categories of alternative medicines.

   _____

   _____

3. Discuss the philosophy and method of treatment in acupuncture, chiropractic, herbal medicine, and homeopathy.

   _____

   _____

4. Discuss the reasons why some people choose an alternative medicine in addition to, or instead of, modern medicine.

   _____

   _____

5. List some diseases that can be treated successfully by alternative medicines.

   _____

   _____

6. Describe an alternative medicine that you regard as fraudulent and explain your reasons.

   _____

   _____

7. Explain how you can protect yourself from being victimized by health fraud.

   _____

   _____

Key Terms (page)

Acupuncture (421)

_____

Alternative medicine (416)

_____

Aromatherapy (426)

_____

Ayurvedic medicine (417)

_____

Chiropractic (420)

_____

Herbal medicine (423)

_____

Homeopathy (419)

_____

Integrative medicine (416)

_____

Meridians (421)

_____

Naturopathy (424)

_____

Osteopathy (421)

_____

Subluxation (426)

_____

Therapeutic massage (425)

_____

Study Guide and Self Assessment

Exploring Your Health

Alternative Therapies Checklist

The decision to use alternative treatments is an important one. The following topics should be considered before selecting an alternative therapy—the safety and effectiveness of the therapy or treatment, the expertise and qualifications of the health care practitioner, and the quality of the service delivery. Consider these when selecting any practitioner or therapy.

Assess the Safety and Effectiveness of the Therapy

Generally, *safety* means that the benefits outweigh the risks of a treatment or therapy. A safe product or practice is one that does no harm when used under defined conditions and as intended.

Effectiveness is the likelihood of benefit from a practice, treatment, or technology applied under typical conditions by the average practitioner for the average patient.

Examine the Practitioner's Expertise

Health consumers may want to take a close look into the background, qualifications, and competence of any potential health care practitioner, whether a physician or a practitioner of alternative health care.

This can be accomplished by contacting a state or local regulatory agency with authority over practitioners who practice the therapy or treatment you want. However, the practice of alternative medicine is usually not as regulated as the practice of conventional medicine. So, it may be helpful to talk both with other health practitioners and with patients who have had experience with the practitioner you are considering. Find out whether there have ever been any complaints from patients. Finally, talk to the practitioner in person. Find out how open the practitioner is to communicating with patients about technical aspects of methods, possible side effects, and potential problems.

Consider the Service Delivery

The quality of the service delivery, or how the treatment or therapy is given and under what conditions, is an important issue. However, quality of service is not necessarily related to the effectiveness or safety of a treatment or practice.

Visit the practitioner's office, clinic, or hospital. Ask the practitioner how many patients are typically seen in a day or week and how much time is spent with each patient. Look at the conditions in the office or clinic. Consider whether the service delivery adheres to regulated standards for medical safety and care.

Consider the Costs

Costs are an important factor to consider, because many alternative treatments are not currently reimbursed by health insurance. Many patients pay directly for these services. Ask your practitioner and your health insurer which treatments or therapies are reimbursable. Also, find out what several practitioners charge for the same treatment to assess the appropriateness of costs.

Consult Your Health Care Provider

Most importantly, discuss all issues concerning treatments and therapies with your health care provider, whether a physician or practitioner of alternative medicine. A complete picture of your treatment plan requires knowledge of both conventional and alternative therapies you are undergoing.

Review the learning objectives and key terms for this chapter to test your knowledge of the material. The key terms are available in a flash card format on our Web site.   www.jbpub.com/hwonline

Learning Objectives

1. Define safety, accidents, and unintentional injuries.

   _____

   _____

2. Describe various strategies to prevent unintentional injuries.

   _____

   _____

3. Use the epidemiological triad to identify unintentional injury risk factors.

   _____

   _____

4. Describe the Haddon matrix and explain why it was developed.

   _____

   _____

5. Discuss various ways to prevent motor vehicle crashes, motorcycle accidents, bicycle accidents, and pedestrian accidents.

   _____

   _____

6. Describe various strategies to improve home and work safety.

   _____

   _____

Key Terms (page)

Accident (433)

_____

Accident mitigation (433)

_____

Accident prevention (433)

_____

Cumulative motion disorders (443)

_____

Injury epidemiology (434)

_____

Laryngospasm (440)

_____

Poison (440)

_____

Safety (432)

_____

Sick building syndrome (443)

_____

Unintentional injury (433)

_____

Exploring Your Health

Prevention of Unintentional Injury

Answer *yes* or *no* to the following questions.

1. I abuse alcohol or other drugs.	Y	N
2. I wear seat belts when driving or riding in a car.	Y	N
3. I have a car with front air bags.	Y	N
4. I drive defensively rather than competitively.	Y	N
5. I drive appropriately for weather conditions.	Y	N
6. I maintain my car's tires, wipers, brakes, and lights.	Y	N
7. I wear a helmet when riding on a bicycle, motorcycle, or roller blades.	Y	N
8. I follow safety rules when riding a bicycle.	Y	N
9. I keep gasoline, paint, oily rags, newspapers, plastics, and other flammable materials away from sources of heat.	Y	N
10. I avoid overloading electrical circuits.	Y	N
11. I use only safe sources of heat in my living quarters.	Y	N
12. I avoid smoking in bed.	Y	N
13. I have a smoke detector on each floor of my house.	Y	N
14. I have a fire extinguisher in my house.	Y	N
15. I keep a first-aid kit at home and in my car.	Y	N
16. I post local emergency numbers and the poison control center number.	Y	N
17. I follow safety procedures when involved in recreational activities.	Y	N

Based on your responses to the questions above, are there behaviors or situations in your life that need to be addressed?

_____

_____

_____

What concerns do you have, both as an individual and a member of the community, related to unintentional injury and death?

_____

_____

_____

Study Guide and Self Assessment

Exploring Your Health

Prevention of Intentional Injury

Answer yes or no to the following questions.

1. I have guns in my home.   Y   N
   If yes, are they stored safely?   Y   N
   When used, are they always used safely?   Y   N
2. I am involved in an abusive relationship.   Y   N
3. I live in a heavy-crime area.   Y   N
4. I abuse alcohol or other drugs.   Y   N
5. I work in a high-risk job.   Y   N
6. I clearly communicate my intentions and boundaries in a dating
   situation.   Y   N
7. I know, and have immediate access to, emergency phone
   numbers.   Y   N
8. I have sources of personal support.   Y   N
9. I know the warning signs of suicide.   Y   N
10. I know resources for mental health counseling in my community. Y   N

Based on your responses to the questions above, are there behaviors or situations in your life that need to be addressed? If so, what are they?

_____

_____

_____

_____

_____

What concerns do you have, both as an individual and a member of your community, related to intentional injury and death?

_____

_____

_____

_____

_____

Source: Birch and Creary, *Managing Your Health: Assessment and Action,* © 1996 by Jones and Bartlett Publishers, Inc.

Chapter ___ (22)

Learning Objectives

1. Describe some of the biological changes that occur with aging.

   _____

   _____

2. Define aging, maximum life span, average life span, life expectancy, ageism, and gerontology.

   _____

   _____

3. Discuss some of the health related and social implications of the average increase in age of the U.S. population.

   _____

   _____

4. Briefly explain two theories of aging.

   _____

   _____

5. Explain how undernutrition affects the aging process.

   _____

   _____

6. Discuss Alzheimer's disease and senile dementia.

   _____

   _____

7. Describe several ways to prevent osteoporosis.

   _____

   _____

8. Identify the stages of dying as defined by Elizabeth Kubler-Ross.

   _____

   _____

9. Explain differences between euthanasia and physician-assisted suicide.

   _____

   _____

10. Compare palliative care with physician-assisted suicide.

    _____

    _____

11. Describe factors involved in healthy aging.

    _____

    _____

Key Terms (page)

Aging (451)

_____

Alzheimer's disease (455)

_____

Amyloid protein (455)

_____

Average life span (451)

_____

Euthanasia (460)

_____

Gerontology (452)

_____

Hormone replacement therapy (458)

_____

Hospice (462)

_____

Life expectancy (451)

_____

Living will (460)

_____

Maximum life span (451)

_____

Osteoporosis (457)

_____

Parkinson's disease (PD) (456)

_____

Physician-assisted suicide (460)

_____

Senile dementia (455)

_____

Specific metabolic rate (453)

_____

Undernutrition (454)

_____

Study Guide and Self Assessment

Exploring Your Health

A Simple Test for Loss of Cognitive Function

Forgetting a person's name or an appointment is not a sign that you are "losing your mind." Loss of cognitive function as a result of disease or injury can prevent a person from answering even simple questions. Following is a simple test to determine loss of some cognitive functions. Score 1 point for each correct answer. Most older persons score at least 17 points out of a possible 19 points.

- Name the season, year, date, month, and day.   (5 answers)
- Name three objects that you see.   (3 answers)
- Name the last five letters of the alphabet backwards.   (5 answers)
- Repeat the sentence: "No ifs, ands, or buts."   (3 answers)
- Repeat the three objects that you mentioned before.   (3 answers)

Chapter **23**

Review the learning objectives and key terms for this chapter to test your knowledge of the material. The key terms are available in a flash card format on our Web site.   www.jbpub.com/hwonline

Learning Objectives

1. Describe the different kinds of interpersonal violence.

   _____

   _____

2. Explain ways that violence affects health.

   _____

   _____

3. Discuss the symptoms and long-term effects of post-traumatic stress disorder.

   _____

   _____

4. Describe the different forms of child abuse and why the incidence is different in different cultures.

   _____

   _____

5. Define sexual assault, forcible rape, and acquaintance rape.

   _____

   _____

6. Discuss the reasons that underlie forcible rape and acquaintance rape.

   _____

   _____

7. Define elder abuse and the factors that contribute to it.

   _____

   _____

8. Discuss the ways in which firearm abuse affects the health of individuals and disrupts society.

   _____

   _____

Key Terms (page)

Acquaintance rape (476)

_____

Child abuse (473)

_____

Elder abuse (478)

_____

Forcible rape (475)

_____

Post-traumatic stress disorder (PTSD) (470)

_____

Sexual assault (475)

_____

Violence (470)

_____

Exploring Your Health

Crime Prevention Tips

Be streetwise and safe:

- Stand tall and walk confidently. Watch where you're going and what's happening around you.
- Stick to well-lit and busy streets. Walk with friends. Avoid shortcuts through a dark alley or deserted street.
- If harassed from a car, walk quickly or run in the opposite direction to safety. If you are really scared, scream.
- Never hitchhike. Accept rides only from people you know and trust.
- Don't flash your cash. Always have *emergency* change for a telephone call.
- Know your neighborhood. What hours are stores and restaurants open? Where are the police and fire stations, libraries, and schools? You might need them in an emergency.
- If you go out for a late night snack or a midnight movie, take a friend. Don't go alone. Most assaults happen to a lone victim.
- Let someone know where you are going and when you will come back. Call if you're going to be late.
- If you are driving, park your car in well-lit places and lock it when you leave. Check for uninvited passengers in the back seat or on the floor before you get in.
- Have your keys in hand when approaching your car. Don't wait until you get to the car to look for your keys.
- Alter your routine. Change daily patterns and, if possible, take different routes to work or to school. Park in different locations.

When jogging or bicycling:

- Go with a friend and take familiar and well-traveled routes.
- Don't jog or bike at night.
- Try it without your stereo headphones. It's safer to remain alert to what's around and behind you.

If you are the victim of a crime:

- If someone attacks you, try not to panic. Look at the attacker carefully so you can give a good description to the police. Try to remember key things like age, race, complexion, body build, clothing, height and weight, hair, eyes, or unusual features.

Study Guide and Self Assessment

- Report all crimes to your local police. For life-threatening emergencies, call 911.
- If the attacker has a weapon and only wants your money or possessions, don't fight. Your life and safety are more important.

- If you're harassed by a gang, go to an open store, gas station, firehouse, or anywhere there are people present.

Source: Courtesy of the Columbus, Ohio, Police Department, 1998.

Study Guide and Self Assessment

Chapter (24)

Review the learning objectives and key terms for this chapter to test your knowledge of the material.
The key terms are available in a flash card format on our Web site.   www.jbpub.com/hwonline

Learning Objectives

1. Discuss the relationship between environment and health.
   _____
   _____

2. Describe the health effects of air pollution, including smog and the hole in the ozone layer.
   _____
   _____

3. Explain the greenhouse effect and the predicted consequences of global warming.
   _____
   _____

4. Describe the effects of lead on children's health and intelligence.
   _____
   _____

5. Describe substances that pollute water in the United States.
   _____
   _____

6. Discuss the impact of land pollution on food production and health.
   _____
   _____

7. Describe sources of pesticide contamination and their effects on health.
   _____
   _____

8. Identify the potential health problems associated with noise pollution and EMFs.
   _____
   _____

9. Discuss how human population growth will affect global health and environmental issues.
   _____
   _____
   _____

Key Terms (page)

Acid rain (492)
_____

Chlorofluorocarbons (CFCs) (495)
_____

Decibel (502)
_____

Dicofol (500)
_____

Electromagnetic fields (EMFs) (501)
_____

Emission (495)
_____

Endocrine disruptors (500)
_____

Environment (488)
_____

Exposure (495)
_____

Fungicide (499)
_____

Greenhouse effect (493)
_____

Herbicide (499)
_____

Insecticide (499)
_____

Ozone hole (495)
_____

Ozone layer (495)
_____

Pesticide (499)
_____

Photochemical smog (489)
_____

Plumbism (497)
_____

Polychlorinated biphenyls (PCBs) (500)
_____

Radon (496)
_____

Rodenticide (499)
_____

Smog (489)
_____

Tinnitus (502)
_____

Study Guide and Self Assessment

Exploring Your Health

How Do You Score on Environmental Awareness?

Circle the number that is your most appropriate response to each question.

Do you use pesticides in the house to kill insects, such as ants, roaches, or flies?

1. Frequently
2. Occasionally
3. Almost never

Do you use pesticides or herbicides around the garden and yard to kill insects and weeds?

1. Frequently
2. Occasionally
3. Almost never

Do you recycle newspapers or other kinds of paper?

1. Almost never
2. Sometimes
3. Regularly

Do you recycle bottles, cans, or plastics?

1. Hardly ever recycle these items
2. Some of these items sometimes
3. Most of the items regularly

When you go on a picnic or hike do you pack out and dispose of all trash in proper trash receptacles?

1. Very infrequently
2. Sometimes
3. All the time

If you need to run an errand that is less than a half mile away, do you walk or bike instead of drive?

1. Almost never
2. Occasionally
3. Most of the time

Do you conserve electricity by turning off unneeded lights and by not running appliances when you don't really need to (like the air conditioner)?

1. Hardly ever
2. Some of the time
3. Almost always

Do you make an effort to conserve water when showering, flushing, washing the car, etc.?

1. Almost never
2. Sometimes
3. Almost always

Do you pour dangerous chemicals like gasoline or paint solvents down the drain or into sewer systems instead of arranging for proper disposal?

1. Often
2. Sometimes
3. Almost never

Have you thrown an empty can or bottle into the environment?

1. Within the past week
2. Within the past month
3. Not within the past year that you can remember

If you smoke, do you throw your butts into the environment when smoking outside?

1. Usually
2. Occasionally
3. Never

What kind of mileage does your automobile average?

1. Less than 20 miles per gallon
2. 20 to 30 miles per gallon
3. More than 30 miles per gallon

If you play a radio outdoors, how loud do you play it?

1. About as loud as it will go
2. Just loud enough for me to hear
3. Never play a radio outdoors where it might disturb others

When shopping for needed products, do you look for environmentally safe ones?

1. Never, just look for the cheapest and best product
2. Sometimes, depends on what is needed
3. Almost always, if I can find one

How many motor vehicles do you own, including cars, motorcycles, motorboats, jet skis, and others?

1. More than four
2. Two to four
3. Only one

A perfect score on these specific environmental questions is 45, but remember that no one is perfect. Perhaps by reviewing your answers you can find ways to improve your environmental awareness—and also contribute to your own health.

Index

Photo Credits

p. 3, Bill Bachman/Photo Network/PNI; p. 6, Frank Priegue/International Stock; p. 7, Mark N. Boulton/Photo Researchers; p. 9, Art Stein/Science Source/Photo Researchers; p. 11, (left) NovaStock/Photo Researchers; (center) Hazel Hankin/Stock Boston/PNI; (right) Michael Newman/PhotoEdit/PNI; p. 14, © Skip Nall/PhotoDisc; p. 15, © Karl Weatherly/PhotoDisc; p. 21, A. Ramey/Stock Boston; p. 29, Stephen Collins/Photo Researchers; p. 33, Rafael Macia/Photo Researchers; p. 34, Courtesy of Gordon Edlin; p. 41, Russell D. Curtis/Photo Researchers; p. 44, Sheila Terry/Science Source/Photo Researchers; p. 49, © William Bacon III/AllStock/PNI ; p. 50, © Owen Franken/Stock, Boston/PNI; p. 53, Gunther/Explorer/Photo Researchers; p. 59, Stewart Cohen/Tony Stone Images; p. 64, Richard T. Nowitz/Science Source/Photo Researchers; p. 67, Ex-Rouchon 03/Explorer/Photo Researchers; p. 71, Richard Hutchings/Photo Researchers; p. 74, Richard Hutchings/Photo Researchers; p. 81, Charles Gupton/Stock Boston/PNI; p. 88, Anthony Blake/Tony Stone Worldwide; p. 113, © Kevin Morris/AllStock/PNI; p. 115, Robert W. Ginn/PhotoEdit; p. 118, Rhoda Sidney/Stock Boston; p. 119, (left) SPL/Custom Medical Stock Photo; (right) SPL/Custom Medical Stock Photo; p. 120, © Stock South/PNI ; p. 123, Chuck Pefley/Stock Boston; p. 126, Jen Morin; p. 135, Norm Thomas/Photo Researchers; p. 137, © Michael Philip Manheim/Photo Network/PNI; p. 141, David Weintraub/Stock Boston; p. 146, (left) © Seth Resnick/Stock Boston/PNI; (right) © Charles Gupton/Stock Boston/PNI; p. 155, B. Seitz/Photo Researchers; p. 157, Lawrence Migdale/Photo Researchers; p. 158, Phyllis Picardi/The Picture Cube; p. 170, Frank Siteman/Tony Stone Images; p. 172, Lori Adamski Peek/Tony Stone Images; p. 174, P.P. A/Explorer/Photo Researchers; p. 181, James Davis/International Stock; p. 188, © Annie Griffiths Belt/Aurora/PNI ; p. 191, Roger Tully/Tony Stone Images; p. 195, © Jeffry W. Myers/Stock Boston/PNI; p. 201, Frank Siteman/Stock Boston/PNI ; p. 210, © Cindy Karp/Black Star/PNI; p. 216, Kevin Horan/Stock Boston/PNI; p. 221, © Meryl Levin, 1994; p. 225, Vanessa Vick/Photo Researchers; p. 229, Roswell Angier/Stock Boston/PNI; p. 230, lft Biophoto Associates/Photo Researchers; p. 230, CDC/Science Source/Photo Researchers; p. 231, Dr. P. Marazzi/Science Photo Library/Photo Researchers; p. 238, © W. L. McCoy/Stock South/PNI; p. 245, Russell D. Curtis/Science Source/Photo Researchers; p. 247, (left) NIBSC Science Photo Library/Photo Researchers, Inc.; (right) A.B. Dowsett/Science Photo Library/Photo Researchers, Inc.; p. 251, David M. Phillips/Photo Researchers, Inc.; p. 256, Phil Schofield/Tony Stone Images; p. 269, CDC/Science Source/Photo Researchers, Inc.; p. 277, AP Photo/Khue Bui; p. 278, SIU/Photo Researchers, Inc.; p. 280, NCI/Science Source/Photo Researchers; p. 289, Spencer Grant/Stock Boston; p. 290, William Gage/Custom Medical Stock Photo; p. 301, Berta A. Daniels; p. 310, M. Bernsau/The Image Works, Inc.; p. 317, Blair Seitz/Photo Researchers; p. 325, © Charles Gupton/Stock Boston/PNI; p. 326, © 1998 PhotoDisc, Inc; p. 333, Med. Illus. SBHS/Tony Stone Images; p. 343, © Pete Winkel/Stock South/PNI; p. 348, David R. Frazier/Science Source/Photo Researchers; p. 357, Robert V. Eckard, Jr./Stock Boston; p. 358, © Michael Hardy/Woodfin Camp & Associates/PNI; p. 361, Custom Medical Stock Photo; p. 367, Corbis Digital Stock; p. 372, courtesy the Bridgeman Art Library and Kunsthistorisches Museum, Vienna, Australia; p. 374, Jeffrey Dunn/The Picture Cube; p. 375, Richard T. Nowitz/Science Source/Photo Researchers; p. 379, AP Photo; p. 383, David Harry Stewart/Tony Stone Images; p. 387, PhotoDisc, Inc.; p. 387, PhotoDisc, Inc; p. 387, PhotoDisc, Inc; p. 390, Christopher Brown/Stock Boston; p. 392, Don Smetzer/Tony Stone Images; p. 401, Blair Seitz/Science Source/Photo Researchers; p. 405, Bill Horsman/Stock Boston; p. 410, Owen Franken/Stock Boston; p. 415, Chave/Jennings/Tony Stone Images; p. 420, Ouellette/Science Source/Photo Researchers; p. 423, Paul Biddle/Science Source/Photo Researchers; p. 431, David J. Sams/Stock Boston/PNI; p. 436, Oli Tennent/Tony Stone Images; p. 439, Bob Daemmrich/Stock Boston; p. 441, Judy Gelles/Stock Boston; p. 442, Robert Rathe/Stock Boston; p. 443, AP Photo/Mark Duncan; p. 449, Bachman/Photo Researchers; p. 452, Bruce Ayres/Tony Stone Images; p. 454, Laurence B. Aiuppy/Tony Stone Images; p. 457, Sean O'Brien/Custom Medical Stock Photo; p. 462, Mimi Cotter/International Stock; p. 469, Rick Reinhard/Impact Visuals/PNI; p. 473, Sean O'Brien/Custom Medical Stock Photo; p. 475, © Bob Daemmrich/Stock Boston/PNI; p. 476, Rhoda Sidney/Stock Boston/PNI; p. 479, © Copyright Ted Curtin/Stock Boston; p. 487, Byron Jorjorian/Tony Stone Images; p. 490, Tom McHugh/Photo Researchers; p. 498, Laurence Pringle/Photo Researchers; p. 499, Andy Sacks/Tony Stone Images; p. 503, Margot Granitsas/Photo Researchers.